PAIN MEDICINE AND MANAGEMENT
Just the Facts

Mark S. Wallace, MD

Program Director
Center for Pain and Palliative Medicine
University of California, San Diego
La Jolla, California

Peter S. Staats, MD, MBA

Associate Professor, Division of Pain Medicine
Department of Anesthesiology and Critical Care Medicine
and Department of Oncology
Johns Hopkins University
Baltimore, Maryland

McGraw-Hill

Medical Publishing Division

New York   Chicago   San Francisco   Lisbon   London   Madrid   Mexico City
Milan   New Delhi   San Juan   Seoul   Singapore   Sydney   Toronto

Pain Medicine and Management
Just the Facts

1 2 3 4 5 6 7 8 9 0   QPDQPD   0 9 8 7 6 5 4

ISBN: 0-07-141182-8

This book was set in Times New Roman by Macmillan India Limited.
The editors were James Shanahan and Michelle Watt.
The production supervisor was Rick Ruzycka.
Project management was provided by Roundhouse Editorial Services.
The cover designer was Aimee Nordin.
The indexer was Andover Publishing Services.
Quebecor Printing Dubuque was printer and binder.

This book is printed on acid-free paper.

Library of Congress Cataloging-in-Publication Data

Pain medicine and management : just the facts / edited by Mark Wallace and Peter Staats.
   p. ; cm.
  Includes bibliographical references and index.
  ISBN 0-07-141182-8
    1. Pain medicine—Handbooks, manuals, etc. I. Wallace, Mark S. II. Staats, Peter.
    [DNLM: 1. Pain—drug therapy—Handbooks. 2. Analgesics—Handbooks.
    WL 39 P1444 2004]
RB127.P33249 2004
616'.0472—dc22
                                               2003059313

To my loving wife, Anne, and my two sons, Zachary and Dominick
—MSW

To my wife, Nancy, my parents, and my children, Alyssa, Dylan, and Rachel
—PSS

CONTENTS

Contributors   xi
Foreword   xvii
Preface   xix

Section I
TEST PREPARATION AND PLANNING   1

1   Test Preparation and Planning   *Stephen E. Abram, MD*   1

Section II
BASIC PHYSIOLOGY   7

2   Nociceptive Pain   *Linda S. Sorkin, PhD*   7
3   Neuropathic Pain   *Tony L. Yaksh, PhD*   9

Section III
EVALUATION OF THE PAIN PATIENT   15

4   History and Physical Examination
        Brian J. Krabak, MD, Scott J. Jarmain, MD   15
5   Electromyography/Nerve Conduction Studies
        Nathan J. Rudin, MD, MA   20
6   Quantitative Sensory Testing   *Mark S. Wallace, MD*   26
7   Radiologic Evaluation
        Marcus W. Parker, MD, Kieran J. Murphy, MD   28
8   Psychological Evaluation   *Robert R. Edwards, PhD,*
        Michael T. Smith, PhD, Jennifer A. Haythornthwaite, PhD 30

Section IV
ANALGESIC PHARMACOLOGY   37

9   Topical Agents   *Bradley S. Galer, MD,*
        Arnold R. Gammaitoni, PharmD   37

10 Acetaminophen and Nonsteroidal Anti-Inflammatory
Drugs *Michael W. Loes, MD*   46

11 Antidepressants *Michael R. Clark, MD, MPH*   52

12 Anticonvulsant Drugs *Misha-Miroslav Backonja, MD* 56

13 Sodium and Calcium Channel Antagonists
Mark S. Wallace, MD   59

14 Tramadol *Michelle Stern, MD,
Kevin Sperber, MD, Marco Pappagallo, MD*   63

15 Opioids *Tony L. Yaksh, PhD*   67

16 Miscellaneous Drugs *Mark S. Wallace, MD*   74

Section V
ACUTE PAIN MANAGEMENT   77

17 Intravenous and Subcutaneous Patient-Controlled
Analgesia *Anne M. Savarese, MD*   77

18 Epidural Analgesia *Jeffrey M. Gilfor, MD,
Eugene R. Viscusi, MD*   82

19 Intrathecal Therapy for Cancer Pain
Peter S. Staats, MD, Frederick W. Luthardt, MA   90

20 Interpleural Analgesia *Michael D. McBeth, MD*   99

21 Peripheral Nerve Blocks and Continuous Catheters
Eric Rey Amador, MD, Sean Mackey, MD, PhD   102

Section VI
REGIONAL PAIN   107

22 Abdominal Pain *Alan Millman, MD,
Elliot S. Krames, MD*   107

23 Upper Extremity Pain *Matthew Meunier, MD*   125

24 Lower Extremity Pain *William Tontz, Jr., MD,
Robert Scott Meyer, MD*   128

25 Headaches *Joel R. Saper, MD, FACP, FAAN*   131

26 Low Back Pain *Michael J. Dorsi, MD,
Allan J. Belzberg, MD, FRCSC*   141

27 Neck and Shoulder Pain *Donlin Long, MD*   147

28 Orofacial Pain *Bradley A. Eli, DMD, MS*   151

29 Pelvic Pain *Ricardo Plancarte, MD,
Francisco Mayer, MD, Jorge Guajardo Rosas, MD,
Alfred Homsy, MD, Gloria Llamosa, MD*   154

30 Thoracic Pain *P. Prithvi Raj, MD*   167

Section VII
CHRONIC PAIN MANAGEMENT   175

31 AIDS-Related Pain Syndromes
Benjamin W. Johnson, Jr., MD, MBA, DAPBM   175

32 Arthritis *Zuhre Tutuncu, MD, Arthur Kavanaugh, MD* 179

33 Cancer Pain *Bradley W. Wargo, DO,*
    Allen W. Burton, MD   183

34 Central Pain *Michael G. Byas-Smith, MD*   189

35 Complex Regional Pain Syndrome
    Paul J. Christo, MD, Srinivasa N. Raja, MD   195

36 Geriatric Pain *F. Michael Gloth III, MD, FACP, AGSF*   200

37 Myofascial Pain and Fibromyalgia
    Robert D. Gerwin, MD   204

38 Pediatric Pain *Robert S. Greenberg, MD*   210

39 Peripheral Neuropathy *Mitchell J. M. Cohen, MD*   218

40 Postsurgical Pain Syndromes *Amar B. Setty, MD,*
    Christopher L. Wu, MD   220

41 Pregnancy and Chronic Pain *James P. Rathmell, MD,*
    Christopher M. Viscomi, MD, Ira M. Bernstein, MD   225

42 Sickle Cell Anemia *Richard Payne, MD*   234

43 Spasticity *R. Samuel Mayer, MD*   237

44 Substance Abuse *Steven D. Passik, PhD,*
    Kenneth L. Kirsh, PhD   240

45 Biopsychosocial Factors in Pain Medicine
    Rollin M. Gallagher, MD, MPH, Sunil Verma, MBBS   244

Section VIII
SPECIAL TECHNIQUES IN PAIN MANAGEMENT   255

46 General Principles of Interventional Pain Therapies
    Richard L. Rauck, MD, Christopher Nelson, MD   255

47 Acupuncture *Albert Y. Leung, MD*   260

48 Botulinum Toxin Injections *Charles E. Argoff, MD*   266

49 Neurolysis *Richard B. Patt, MD*   272

50 Complementary and Alternative Medicine
    Maneesh Sharma, MD   277

51 Cryoneurolysis *Lloyd Saberski, MD*   282

52 Spinal Cord Stimulation *Richard B. North, MD*   285

53 Epidural Steroid Injections *John C. Rowlingson, MD*   289

54 Facet Joint Blocks *Somayaji Ramamurthy, MD*   295

55 Intravenous Drug Infusions *Theodore Grabow, MD*   296

56 Neurosurgical Techniques *Kenneth A. Follett, MD, PhD* 301

57 Radiofrequency Ablation *Sunil J. Panchal, MD,*
    Anu Perni, MD   309

58 Peripheral Nerve Stimulation *Lew C. Schon, MD,*
    Paul W. Davies, MD   315

59 Prolotherapy *Felix Linetsky, MD,*
    Michael Stanton-Hicks, MB, BS, Conor O'Neill, MD   318

60 Rehabilitation Evaluation and Treatment in Patients
    with Low Back Pain *Michael Kaplan, MD*   325

61 Piriformis Syndrome *Wesley Foreman, MD,*
    Gagan Mahajan, MD, Scott M. Fishman, MD   331

62 Sacroiliac Joint Dysfunction   *Norman Pang, MD,*
        Gagan Mahajan, MD, Scott M. Fishman, MD   336
63 Spinal Drug Delivery   *Stuart Du Pen, MD*   341
64 Sympathetic Blockade
        Mazin Elias, MD, FRCA, DABA   344
65 Transcutaneous Electrical Nerve Stimulation
        Gordon Irving, MD   349
66 Discography/Intradiscal Electrothermal Annuloplasty
        Richard Derby, MD, Sang-Heon Lee, MD, PhD   350
67 Nucleoplasty   *Philip S. Kim, MD*   354
68 Lysis of Adhesions   *Carlos O. Viesca, MD,*
        Gabor B. Racz, MD, Miles R. Day, MD   360

Section IX
DISABILITY EVALUATION   365

69 Disability/Impairment   *Gerald M. Aronoff, MD*   365
70 Medical/Legal Evaluations   *Richard L. Stieg, MD, MHS* 368

Index   373

CONTRIBUTORS

Stephen E. Abram, MD, Professor, Department of Anesthesiology, University of New Mexico School of Medicine, Albuquerque, New Mexico

Eric Rey Amador, MD, Clinical Instructor, Department of Anesthesia, Lucile Packard Children's Hospital at Stanford, Stanford, California

Charles E. Argoff, MD, Director, Cohn Pain Management Center, North Shore University Hospital; Assistant Professor of Neurology, New York University School of Medicine, Bethpage, New York

Gerald M. Aronoff, MD, Chairman, Department of Pain Medicine, Presbyterian Orthopedic Hospital, Charlotte, North Carolina

Misha-Miroslav Backonja, MD, Associate Professor, Department of Neurology, University of Wisconsin, Madison, Wisconsin

Allan J. Belzberg, MD, FRCSC, Associate Professor of Neurosurgery, School of Medicine, Johns Hopkins University, Baltimore, Maryland

Ira M. Bernstein, MD, Department of Obstetrics/Gynecology, University of Vermont College of Medicine, Burlington, Vermont

Allen W. Burton, MD, Associate Professor of Anesthesiology, Section Chief, Cancer Pain Management Section, University of Texas MD Anderson Cancer Center, Houston, Texas

Michael G. Byas-Smith, MD, Assistant Professor of Anesthesiology, Emory University School of Medicine Hospital, Atlanta, Georgia

Paul J. Christo, MD, Department of Anesthesiology and Critical Care Medicine, Johns Hopkins University School of Medicine, Baltimore, Maryland

Michael R. Clark, MD, MPH, Associate Professor and Director, Chronic Pain Treatment Programs, Department of Psychiatry and Behavioral Sciences, The Johns Hopkins Medical Institutions, Baltimore, Maryland

Mitchell J. M. Cohen, MD, Department of Psychiatry and Human Behavior, Jefferson Medical College, Philadelphia, Pennsylvania

Paul W. Davies, MD, Department of Orthopedic Surgery, The Union Memorial Hospital, Baltimore, Maryland

Miles R. Day, MD, Texas Tech University Health Service Center, Lubbock, Texas

Richard Derby, MD, Medical Director, Spinal Diagnostics and Treatment Center, Daly City, California

Michael J. Dorsi, MD, Department of Neurosurgery, Johns Hopkins University School of Medicine, Baltimore, Maryland

Stuart Du Pen, MD, Associate Director of Research, Pain Management Service, Swedish Medical Center, Seattle, Washington

Robert R. Edwards, PhD, Research Fellow, Department of Psychiatry and Behavioral Sciences, Johns Hopkins University School of Medicine, Baltimore, Maryland

Bradley A. Eli, DMD, MS, Scripps Hospital Pain Center, La Jolla, California

Mazin Elias, MD, FRCA, DABA, Director, Pain Management Clinic, Green Bay, Wisconsin

Scott M. Fishman, MD, Chief, Division of Pain Medicine, Associate Professor of Anesthesiology, Department of Anesthesiology and Pain Medicine, University of California, Davis, California

Kenneth A. Follett, MD, PhD, Professor, Department of Neurosurgery, University of Iowa Hospitals and Clinics, Iowa City, Iowa

Wesley Foreman, MD, Pain Medicine Fellow, Department of Anesthesiology and Pain Medicine, University of California, Davis, California

Bradley S. Galer, MD, Endo Pharmaceuticals, Inc., Chadds Ford, Pennsylvania; Adjunct Assistant Professor of Neurology, University of Pennsylvania School of Medicine, Philadelphia, Pennsylvania

Rollin M. Gallagher, MD, MPH, Pain Medicine and Rehabilitation Center, Medical College of Pennsylvania Hospital, Philadelphia, Pennsylvania

Arnold R. Gammaitoni, PharmD, Endo Pharmaceuticals, Inc., Chadds Ford, Pennsylvania

Robert D. Gerwin, MD, Department of Neurology, Johns Hopkins University School of Medicine, Baltimore, Maryland

Jeffrey M. Gilfor, MD, Department of Anesthesiology, Thomas Jefferson University Hospital, Philadelphia, Pennsylvania

F. Michael Gloth III, MD, FACP, AGSF, Associate Professor of Medicine, Johns Hopkins University School of Medicine, Baltimore, Maryland

Theodore Grabow, MD, Assistant Professor, Department of Anesthesiology and Critical Care Medicine, Johns Hopkins University School of Medicine, Baltimore, Maryland

Robert S. Greenberg, MD, Assistant Professor of Anesthesiology and Critical Care Medicine, Johns Hopkins University School of Medicine, Baltimore, Maryland

Jennifer A. Haythornthwaite, PhD, Associate Professor, Department of Psychiatry and Behavioral Sciences, Johns Hopkins University School of Medicine, Baltimore, Maryland

Alfred Homsy, MD, Assistant Professor of Anesthesia, Université de Montréal, Montréal, Quebec, Canada

Gordon Irving, MD, Medical Director, Pain Center, Swedish Medical Center, Seattle, Washington

Scott J. Jarmain, MD, Sports/Musculoskeletal Fellow, Johns Hopkins Physical Medicine & Rehabilitation, Johns Hopkins University School of Medicine, Baltimore, Maryland

Benjamin W. Johnson, Jr., MD, MBA, DAPBM, Department of Anesthesiology, Vanderbilt University School of Medicine, Nashville, Tennessee

Michael Kaplan, MD, Rehabilitation Team, Catonsville, Maryland

Arthur Kavanaugh, MD, The Center for Innovative Therapy, Division of Rheumatology, School of Medicine, University of California, San Diego, La Jolla, California

Philip S. Kim, MD, Director, Center for Pain Medicine, Bryn Mawr, Pennsylvania

Kenneth L. Kirsh, PhD, Director, Symptom Management and Palliative Care Program, Markey Cancer Center, University of Kentucky, Lexington, Kentucky

Brian J. Krabak, MD, Assistant Professor of Physical Medicine & Rehabilitation, Assistant Professor of Orthopedic Surgery, Associate Residency Program Director, Physical Medicine & Rehabilitation, Johns Hopkins University School of Medicine, Baltimore, Maryland

Elliot S. Krames, MD, Pacific Pain Treatment Center, San Francisco, California

Sang-Heon Lee, MD, PhD, Spinal Diagnostic and Treatment Center, Daly City, California

Albert Y. Leung, MD, Assistant Clinical Professor, Center for Pain and Palliative Medicine, Department of Anesthesiology, University of California, San Diego, La Jolla, California

Felix Linetsky, MD, Private Practice, Palm Harbor, Florida

Gloria Llamosa, MD, Neurologist, Hospital Central, Norte Petróleos Mexicanos, Mexico

Michael W. Loes, MD, Director, Arizona Pain Institute, Phoenix, Arizona

Donlin Long, MD, Department of Neurosurgery, Johns Hopkins University School of Medicine, Baltimore, Maryland

Frederick W. Luthardt, MA, Clinical Research Associate, Department of Anesthesiology and Critical Care Medicine, Johns Hopkins University School of Medicine, Baltimore, Maryland

Sean Mackey, MD, PhD, Assistant Professor, Department of Anesthesiology, Division of Pain Medicine, Stanford University School of Medicine, Stanford, California

Gagan Mahajan, MD, Director, Pain Medicine Fellowship Program, Assistant Professor of Anesthesiology, Department of Anesthesiology and Pain Medicine, University of California, Davis, California

Francisco Mayer, MD, Assistant Professor Algology, Universidad Nacional Autónoma de México, Medical Coordinator, Palliative Care, Instituto Nacional de Cancerología, Mexico

R. Samuel Mayer, MD, Department of Physical Medicine and Rehabilitation, Johns Hopkins University School of Medicine, Baltimore, Maryland

Michael D. McBeth, MD, Director, Pain Management Group, Kaiser Permanente, San Diego, California; Clinical Instructor (Voluntary), Department of Anesthesiology, Center for Pain and Palliative Medicine, School of Medicine, University of California, San Diego, La Jolla, California

Matthew Meunier, MD, University of California, San Diego, La Jolla, California

Robert Scott Meyer, MD, Department of Orthopedics, University of California, San Diego, La Jolla, California

Alan Millman, MD, San Francisco, California

Kieran J. Murphy, MD, Department of Radiology, Johns Hopkins University School of Medicine, Baltimore, Maryland

Christopher Nelson, MD, Fellow, Pain Control Center, Wake Forest University Medical Center, Winston Salem, North Carolina

Richard B. North, MD, Professor of Neurosurgery, Anesthesiology, and Critical Care Medicine, Johns Hopkins University School of Medicine, Baltimore, Maryland

Conor O'Neill, MD, Spinal Diagnostic Center, Daly City, California

Sunil J. Panchal, MD, Director, Division of Pain Medicine, Weill Medical College of Cornell University, New York City, New York

Norman Pang, MD, Pain Medicine Fellow, Department of Anesthesiology and Pain Medicine, University of California, Davis, California

Marco Pappagallo, MD, Director, Comprehensive Pain Treatment Center, Associate Professor of Neurology, New York University School of Medicine, Hospital for Joint Diseases, New York City, New York

Marcus W. Parker, MD, Johns Hopkins University School of Medicine, Baltimore, Maryland

Steven D. Passik, PhD, Symptom Management and Palliative Care Program, Markey Cancer Center, University of Kentucky, Lexington, Kentucky

Richard B. Patt, MD, President and Chief Medical Officer, The Patt Center for Cancer Pain and Wellness, Houston, Texas

Richard Payne, MD, Chief, Pain & Palliative Care Service, Memorial Sloan-Kettering Cancer Center; Professor of Neurology and Pharmacology, Weill Medical College at Cornell University, New York City, New York

Anu Perni, MD

Ricardo Plancarte, MD, Professor Algology, Universidad Nacional Autónoma de México; Medical Director, Pain Clinic and Palliative Care, Instituto Nacional de Cancerología, Mexico

Gabor B. Racz, MD, Grover Murray Professor and Chair Emeritus, Director, Pain Services, Texas Tech University Health Sciences Center, Lubbock, Texas

P. Prithvi Raj, MD, Department of Anesthesiology, Texas Tech University Health Sciences Center, Lubbock, Texas

Srinivasa N. Raja, MD, Department of Anesthesiology and Critical Care Medicine, Johns Hopkins University School of Medicine, Baltimore, Maryland

Somayaji Ramamurthy, MD, Professor, Department of Anesthesiology, University of Texas Health Science Center at San Antonio, San Antonio, Texas

James P. Rathmell, MD, Department of Anesthesiology, University of Vermont College of Medicine, Burlington, Vermont

Richard L. Rauck, MD, Co-Director, Wake Forest University Pain Control Center, Piedmont Anesthesia and Pain Consultants, Director, Center for Clinical Research, Clinical Associate Professor, Wake Forest University Medical Center, Winston Salem, North Carolina

Jorge Guajardo Rosas, MD, Resident on Trainee Pain Clinic, Universidad Nacional Autónoma de México; Pain Clinic and Palliative Care, Instituto Nacional de Cancerología, Mexico

John C. Rowlingson, MD, Professor of Anesthesiology, Director, Pain Medicine Services, Department of Anesthesiology, University of Virginia Health System, Charlottesville, Virginia

Nathan J. Rudin, MD, MA, Assistant Professor, Rehabilitation Medicine, Department of Orthopedics and Rehabilitation, University of Wisconsin Medical School; Medical Director, Pain Treatment and Research Center, University of Wisconsin Hospitals and Clinics, Madison, Wisconsin

Lloyd Saberski, MD, Advanced Diagnostic Pain Treatment Center, New Haven, Connecticut

Joel R. Saper, MD, FACP, FAAN, Director, Michigan Head Pain and Neurological Clinic, Ann Arbor, Michigan

Anne M. Savarese, MD, Assistant Professor of Anesthesiology & Pediatrics, Division Head, Pediatric Anesthesiology, Clinical Director, Acute Pain Management & PCA Services, University of Maryland Medical Center, Baltimore, Maryland

Lew C. Schon, MD, Department of Orthopedic Surgery, The Union Memorial Hospital, Baltimore, Maryland

Amar B. Setty, MD, Senior Resident, Anesthesiology, Johns Hopkins Hospital, Baltimore, Maryland

Maneesh Sharma, MD, Fellow, Pain Medicine, Johns Hopkins University Hospital, Baltimore, Maryland

Michael T. Smith, PhD, Assistant Professor, Department of Psychiatry and Behavioral Sciences, Johns Hopkins University School of Medicine, Baltimore, Maryland

Linda S. Sorkin, PhD, Department of Anesthesiology, University of California, San Diego, La Jolla, California

Kevin Sperber, MD, Clinical Instructor, New York University School of Medicine; Director of Inpatient Services, Comprehensive Pain Treatment Center, Hospital for Joint Diseases, New York City, New York

Peter S. Staats, MD, MBA, Associate Professor, Division of Pain Medicine, Department of Anesthesiology and Critical Care Medicine and Department of Oncology, Johns Hopkins University, Baltimore, Maryland

Michael Stanton-Hicks, MB, BS, Division of Pain Medicine, Department of Anesthesia, Cleveland Clinic Foundation, Cleveland, Ohio

Michelle Stern, MD, Assistant Clinical Professor of Physical Medicine and Rehabilitation, Columbia University College of Physicians and Surgeons, New York Presbyterian Hospital, New York City, New York

Richard L. Stieg, MD, MHS, Associate Clinical Professor of Neurology, University of Colorado Health Sciences Center, Denver, Colorado

William Tontz, Jr., MD, Department of Orthopedics, School of Medicine, University of California, San Diego, La Jolla, California

Zuhre Tutuncu, MD, The Center for Innovative Therapy, Division of Rheumatology, School of Medicine, University of California, San Diego, La Jolla, California

Sunil Verma, MBBS, Pain Medicine and Rehabilitation Center, Medical College of Pennsylvania Hospital, Philadelphia, Pennsylvania

Carlos O. Viesca, MD, Texas Tech University Health Service Center, Lubbock, Texas

Christopher M. Viscomi, MD, Department of Anesthesiology, University of Vermont College of Medicine, Burlington, Vermont

Eugene R. Viscusi, MD, Thomas Jefferson University Hospital, Department of Anesthesiology, Philadelphia, Pennsylvania

Mark S. Wallace, MD, Program Director, Center for Pain and Palliative Medicine, University of California, San Diego, La Jolla, California

Bradley W. Wargo, DO, Pain Management Fellow, Cancer Pain Management Section, University of Texas MD Anderson Cancer Center, Houston, Texas

Christopher L. Wu, MD, Associate Professor of Anesthesiology, Director, Regional Anesthesia, Johns Hopkins University Hospital, Baltimore, Maryland

Tony L. Yaksh, PhD, Department of Anesthesiology, School of Medicine, University of California, San Diego, La Jolla, California

This concise volume, edited by two of today's leading pain clinician-scientists, represents the culmination of several forces.

First and foremost is the recognition that the knowledge and skills supporting current medical management of pain have grown sufficiently large that this field has become a discipline in its own right. Accordingly, candidates who meet the requirements of the American Board of Anesthesiology may now become board-certified in Pain Management and achieve diplomate status just as their colleagues in other areas have done for years. The American Academy of Pain Medicine has been recognized to provide equivalent rigor in its certification process and many physicians (including this writer!) hold diplomate status through both mechanisms, and are active both in AAPM and its anesthesia-centered counterpart, the American Society of Regional Anesthesia and Pain Management.

Drs. Wallace and Staats have wisely drawn on the expertise and scholarship of a galaxy of "stars" from these two overlapping groups to achieve an amazing harmony between conciseness of each chapter and a comprehensive scope of chapters. In aggregate, the 70 chapters in this volume suffice to prepare candidates to sit successfully for either board examination, and in the future for the conjoined board, if both accreditation mechanisms were to coalesce.

The second trend, evident throughout medical education and clinical care, is to take stock of the evidence for the concepts and interventions covered so as to practice "evidence-based" pain medicine. This trend is clearly subscribed to by the editors, with many of their contributors frankly and objectively spelling out which of their recommendations is supported by consensus alone and which have experimental support in the form of randomized controlled trials, quasi-experimental studies, and case series. In an era of pervasive managed care, and its frequent need to justify—or at least provide a basis for—all medical, behavioral, and procedural interventions, this information is indispensable.

Third is the rise of "knowledge distilleries" in the form of published materials and Internet sites, whose genesis lies in clinicians' pleas for help in sorting out high-quality evidence from low-quality evidence and simply in wading through the flood of information from all sources. The literature on pain control has recently doubled in size about every five years, preventing any one person from absorbing, or even skimming, this vast amount of information. Pain-related knowledge distilleries include the Cochrane Collaboration, which emphasizes formal systematic reviews and, whenever possible, quantitative syntheses (meta-analyses) of randomized controlled trials. Relevant Cochrane Collaborative Review Groups include that on Pain, Palliative, and Supportive Care (PaPaS) as well as others such as Anesthesia, Spine, and Musculoskeletal Disorders.

A less structured approach to literature synthesis has been followed by governmental agencies such as the Agency for Healthcare Research and Quality in the United States. Interested clinicians may go to www.ahrq.gov to review evidence reports on pain relief in patients with cancer or after spinal cord injury. Professional organizations such as the American Society of Anesthesiologists, the American Society of Regional Anesthesia and Pain Medicine, and the American Pain Society have expended great human and financial resources to prepare rigorous, evidence-based practice guidelines. Others, such as the AAPM, have fashioned consensus statements collaboratively with other professional groups as evidence-based as the literature permits. And finally, there are a multitude of Internet sites prepared and maintained by for-profit and nonprofit groups, ranging from patient organizations (www.theacpa.org) to academic centers such as Oxford University (www.jr2.ox.ac.uk/bandolier/). By drawing on the knowledge, judgment, and wisdom of earnest and current clinical authorities and by asking them to "bullet" their messages, the editors have squeezed an immense amount of material into a very small space!

Both Drs. Wallace and Staats are known for their work in translating preclinical advances into improved therapies, in large part through conducting rigorous clinical studies that have had great impact on their peers and medicine in general. This perspective is evident in their having assembled for this text an extremely talented and diverse group of contributors whose accomplishments span preclinical research to clinical medicine to health policy and economics. It would be dangerous to single out any single contributor by name, because nearly all are of international status and those that are not yet, will certainly become so. The authors and editors alike should be proud of this volume, which will prove useful not only in passing examinations but also in rendering high-quality, up-to-date clinical care.

Daniel B. Carr, MD
Diplomate, American Board of Internal Medicine, with subspecialty
qualification in Endocrinology & Metabolism
Diplomate, American Board of Anesthesiology, with added
qualification in Pain Management
Diplomate, American Board of Pain Medicine
Honorary Fellow, Faculty of Pain Medicine, Australia and New Zealand
College of Anaesthetists

PREFACE

The latter part of the 20th century produced great achievements in our understanding of pain mechanisms and treatment. Prior times were difficult for the patient suffering from pain. Now, with the increased awareness and better understanding of pain, the pain practitioner has a full armamentarium for the management of pain and suffering. There are numerous textbooks focusing on various aspects of pain management including pharmacologic, psychologic, interventional, and rehabilitative aspects; however, with the vastness of knowledge, much detail must be sifted through to get to the facts.

This book, *Pain Medicine and Management: Just the Facts,* is intended to be a study guide for the pain physician who is studying for the board certification or recertification exam. Thus, Dr. Abram provides the initial chapter on "Test Preparation and Planning." Each chapter contains key points that are presented in bulleted form making it easier to use as a study aid. The unique format of the book also allows it to be used as an effective clinical aid when time is tight and authoritative information is needed quickly.

We have invited experts from all over the country to contribute to this important book. Each chapter contains information that in the author's opinion were the most important points for the chosen topic. We are confident that the resulting book will be an important contribution to your pain library.

We would like to thank all of the authors for their commitment and dedication to this book. We are also grateful to numerous individuals who assisted us with this project, especially Linda Sutherland at the UCSD School of Medicine. We would also like to thank our families who are always there for us and whose understanding made this project possible. MSW would like to thank his wife, Anne, and his two sons, Zachary and Dominick. PSS would like to thank his wife, Nancy, his parents, and his children, Alyssa, Dylan, and Rachel, for their unyielding support and for taking the pain out of his life.

1 TEST PREPARATION AND PLANNING

Stephen E. Abram, MD

SUBSPECIALTY CERTIFICATION EXAMINATION IN PAIN MEDICINE

The American Board of Anesthesiology offers a written examination in pain medicine designed to test for the presence of knowledge that is essential for a physician to function as a pain medicine practitioner. Certification awarded by the ABA on successful completion of the examination is time limited, and expires in 10 years. For that reason, the ABA offers a pain medicine recertification examination as well.

The examination required for the Certificate of Added Qualifications in Pain Management was initially offered in 1993 by the ABA, 1 year after the Accreditation Council for Graduate Medical Education approved the first accredited pain fellowship programs. Entrance into the examination up until 1998 was dependent on either completion of a 1-year fellowship in pain management or the equivalent of at least 2 years of full-time pain management practice. Subsequent to the 1998 exam, ABA diplomates were required to complete an ACGME-approved pain fellowship. The name of the certification process has recently been changed to Subspecialty Certification in Pain Medicine.

Beginning with the year 2000 examination, the ABA Pain Medicine Examination was made available to diplomates of the American Board of Psychiatry and Neurology and the American Board of Physical Medicine and Rehabilitation. For a period of 5 years, physicians from these specialties may be admitted to the examination system on the basis of temporary criteria similar to the process in place for ABA diplomates during the first 5 years of the examination system. Eventually, successful completion of an ACGME-approved fellowship in pain medicine will be required. Candidates from ABPN and ABPMR are awarded subspecialty certification by their respective boards, not by the ABA, on successful completion of the examination.

With the expansion of the examination system to diplomates of the other two boards, there was a broadening of the scope of the examination. Question writers and editors from Neurology, Psychiatry, and PM&R were added to the examination preparation process. Although previous examinations included material from all aspects of pain management practice, the infusion of new expertise produced a more diverse question bank. The examination should, and does, contain information from all of the disciplines involved in the multidisciplinary treatment of pain. The areas of knowledge that are tested can be found in the ABA Pain Medicine Certification Examination Content Outline. This document is revised periodically and can be found on the ABA web site, *http://www.abanes.org*. An approximation of the distribution of questions from each section of the Content Outline, also found on the ABA web site, is shown in Table 1–1.

The Pain Medicine Certification Examination is a 200-question exam, administered by computer. The examination uses two question formats. The A-type question is a "choose the best answer" format with four or five possible answers. The K-type question contains four answers with five possible combinations of correct answers:

A. 1, 2, and 3 are correct
B. 1 and 3 are correct
C. 2 and 4 are correct
D. 4 is correct
E. All are correct

The ABA certificates in pain medicine are limited to a period of 10 years, after which diplomates are required

TABLE 1–1   Pain Medicine Examination Specifications*

CONTENT OUTLINE	TOPIC	PERCENTAGE OF EXAM
I–IX	Anatomy	10%
X	Neuroanatomy and function	10%
XI–XXV	Pain states	20%
XXVI	Diagnosis and therapy	20%
XXVII	Pharmacology	10%
XXVIII	Pregnancy and nursing	5%
XXVIX	Pediatrics	5%
XXX	Geriatrics	5%
XXXI	Critical care	5%
XXXII	Ethics	5%
XXXIII	Record keeping, controlled drugs, quality assurance	5%
		100%

*Revised June 22, 1999. Copyright, American Board of Anesthesiology. Reprinted with permission.

to pass a recertification examination. The recertification process uses the 200-question certification exam. The success rates for the pain medicine examination through 2001 are as follows:

	1993	1994	1996	1998	2000	2001
Certification	94%	94%	89%	81%	71%	72%
Recertification	—	—	—	—	63%	75%

PREPARING FOR THE EXAM

A reasonable first step in the study process is to identify areas of weakness. A good place to start is with the ABA Content Outline. The first nine sections cover various body regions. One might begin with a review of the topographical anatomy and imaging techniques, followed by a review of the more common regional block techniques used for pain management. Keep in mind that the exam covers acute pain management as well as chronic and cancer pain, and anesthetic techniques begun in the operating room and continued into the postoperative period are part of the required knowledge base. Next is Section X, which lists a number of aspects of neuroanatomy and neurophysiology, pain mechanisms, and the pathophysiology of painful conditions.

Sections XI through XXV form a comprehensive list of pain states. For each of the painful conditions listed, you should review the diagnostic features and techniques and therapy, including medications, physical therapy, nerve blocks, surgical interventions, and psychotherapy. Section XXVI provides a list of diagnostic and therapeutic techniques that may be used throughout the entire range of painful conditions.

Review of the pharmacology of the drugs listed in Section XXVII is essential. The examination contains questions regarding the indications, pharmacokinetics,

pharmacodynamics, drug interactions, and adverse effects of the entire range of medications used in pain medicine. Substance abuse and dependence are covered as well.

Then follow special problems (Sections XVII–XXXI) concerning treatment of pain in specific populations, for example, pregnant patients, children, and the elderly, and in critically ill or severely injured patients in a critical care setting. Finally there are sections on ethics and record keeping.

Selection of study materials is always a dilemma. A useful source is the *Core Curriculum for Professional Education in Pain*, published by the International Association for the Study of Pain. It is organized somewhat differently than the ABA Core Curriculum, and has a less extensive list of topics. It is very useful, however, in that it emphasizes the important aspects of each area of study, and provides concise information about each target area as well as extensive bibliographies for each section. The latest version is the second edition, published in 1995.[1] Watch for a third edition, which was in preparation at the time this chapter was prepared.

There are a growing number of textbooks on pain medicine, each with its own strengths and weaknesses. It is reasonable to use comprehensive textbooks as a study source, keeping in mind that, by definition, information is somewhat outdated by the time a large textbook is printed. While the examination tends not to use extremely new findings, there is an effort to keep information current, particularly if there are strong data from multiple sources. It may be helpful, therefore, to supplement the use of textbooks with recent review articles, particularly for topics in fields that are changing rapidly, such as the basic sciences related to pain. These are available through medical literature search instruments, such as Medline, which can be limited to English language, review articles, and, where appropriate, discussions of human subjects or patients.

Some students retain information best from written material, others from spoken lectures. Often a combination of both sources results in the most effective retention. Participation in pain medicine review courses provides both visual and auditory inputs. Such courses are offered by the American Pain Society, the International Association for the Study of Pain, the American Society of Regional Anesthesia and Pain Medicine, and the American Academy of Pain Medicine. Many of the specialty societies offer topics in acute, chronic, and cancer pain management at their annual meetings as well. High-quality courses are also offered by both academic and private practice groups. Many review courses offer audio tapes of lectures. A major advantage of this medium is the ability to use commuting time to review pertinent topics. Hearing material that has previously been read tends to solidify one's learning.

Perhaps the best learning method is to review the available information regarding a patient one is currently managing. Application of this knowledge in the clinical setting is clearly the best way to learn and to retain knowledge. Therefore, you should review the available literature on a given condition in anticipation of a particular patient coming into the clinic or hospital with that condition or shortly after seeing a patient with the condition. Problem-based learning sessions, which are becoming more prevalent in clinical meetings and symposia, are also effective in focusing on a clinical condition and linking that clinical situation to a knowledge base.

Question-and-answer textbooks may be helpful in identifying gaps in knowledge and, if self-testing is done periodically, may be a measure of study progress. Practice examinations increase one's confidence in the test-taking process and increase familiarity with the format.

GENERAL STUDY TECHNIQUE

PLANNING MATERIAL TO COVER

The material to be studied will depend to a great extent on the range and depth of material covered in residency and fellowship training. Study of material covered in depth during training need only be reviewed briefly, while material covered only superficially needs to be studied in depth. Much of this decision is dictated by the candidate's specialty. An anesthesiologist probably needs to spend considerable time on headache management or rehabilitation of the spinal cord-injured patient, while a neurologist needs to study indications of and techniques for nerve blocks. As noted above, a grid, such as the ABA Core Curriculum, can be used to select topics for review versus in-depth study.

PLANNING STUDY TIME

Once you begin the study process, it is helpful to evaluate the amount of time available for study and to schedule your available time. Very short study sessions tend to be ineffective, whereas 1- to 2-hour sessions are probably optimal. Daily sessions of an hour or two are more productive than weekly sessions of 5 or 6 hours. According to Sherman and Wildman,[2] the best schedule is an hour or two daily for many days, ending in a concentrated review session shortly before the examination.

Early in the study process, considerable time should be devoted to surveying the material to be learned, whereas later in the process reading and reviewing

material should be used more frequently. It is helpful to develop a routine for each study session. An example[2] follows:

- Briefly review previously studied material.
- Survey new material to study.
- Review study questions on the topic, or create study questions.
- Study the material.
- Review the material studied.

STUDY SKILLS

Look for the main ideas in what you read. When reading about the management of a specific syndrome, what is the principal treatment modality? For a chronic condition, the primary goal may be regaining strength and flexibility, while many of the specific treatments merely provide the means to achieve this primary goal. Understanding the pathophysiology of a specific condition helps you remember the clinical features of and management principles of the disorder.

Assess your confidence in your knowledge and understanding of a topic. If you feel good about that material, go on to a different topic. If not, continue to read and review. Write out a brief summary of the material you have studied. Include the main ideas and the most important details. If possible, discuss the material with other trainees or with colleagues. Ask others about their understanding of a topic. If their ideas conflict with yours, reread the material. Read additional material on important topics. This will reinforce learning and may uncover areas where controversy and differences of opinion exist.

A variety of techniques have been devised to help us remember important information.[2] One helpful technique is to organize information being learned. The Content Outline can be helpful in organizing information by topic. There are a number of specific techniques for aiding memory and recall. Overlearning refers to the repetitive study of a topic that is already familiar. As stated previously, listening to an audio tape of a lecture subsequent to reading about the topic can reinforce learning. Analogies can be helpful. You can compare a topic being learned to a topic with which one is familiar. For instance, you might think of certain types of neuropathic pain caused by an ectopic focus of nociceptor activity as analogous to a seizure. Such an analogy may be particularly useful, as both conditions may benefit from the same type of drugs. Imagery can be a powerful memory technique. Creation of a visual image that describes a condition, a theory, or a treatment can be a very effective aid to learning and recall. Some students find the use of acronyms helpful. I occasionally find myself using mnemonics and acronyms I learned many years ago in medical school. The ones that are a bit risqué seem to be the easiest to remember. Recitation of material aloud multiple times is an effective way of improving retention. If the recited material rhymes or is connected to a vivid mental picture, it will be still easier to remember. If you are in an academic setting, teaching the material you have just learned to other trainees can be an extremely powerful technique, as it requires organization as well as understanding of the material.[3] Restating information, such as rewriting certain key aspects of a learned topic, can be a powerful tool. Restating a concept in your own words is most effective. Quiz yourself on the material. This is particularly important for auditory learners. Note taking is particularly important for visual learners. Notes should be brief, clear, and succinct. This is much more effective than underlining, and notes can be reviewed shortly after the reading session, and may be used for self-testing. Review should be done immediately after completion of a learning session. Practice should then be repeated periodically.

Intent to learn is important. Reading and listening to new information with the active intent to learn is key to the memory process. Some of the techniques stated above should be coupled with this active intent to remember. Attention and interest are critical. As the pain medicine examination covers material that is vitally important to future practice, interest should be a given. There may, however, be material outside your proposed area of expertise or practice that stirs little interest. Consider situations in which such material might become important to your practice.

There are a number of reasons why we forget learned material. First, we may not have learned the material well. During the learning process, the material must be given interest and attention. Subsequently, questioning oneself about the material and periodically reviewing are critical. Disuse leads to loss of memory. We forget the most in the first 24 hours after learning, and it is during this period that review is most helpful. Interference is another source of forgetting. Interference may be related to anxiety, distraction, emotional disturbance, and intellectual interference. Intellectual interference, or mental overcrowding, is related to loss of memory during subsequent intellectual activity.[4] This can be minimized by reflecting on what has just been learned, and by synthesizing and organizing the material before moving on to other topics. Another strategy is to follow a learning session with sleep or nonintellectual activities, such as exercise, and recreation. A lack of attention or effort during the learning process is very detrimental. There must be concentration without distraction during the learning process, and a conscious effort to learn and remember.

STRESS AND ANXIETY

Stress that occurs during preparation for an exam is related primarily to anxiety over the possibility of failing the exam and the consequences of that failure. The best way to deal with this is through adequate preparation and the use of practice tests to demonstrate preparedness. There are a number of techniques for dealing with the remaining anxiety and stress.[4] If anxiety interferes with the study process, meditation, relaxation exercises, and massage can be helpful. Many individuals find that aerobic exercise works best. If you begin to panic during test preparation or the test itself, it is helpful to focus your attention away from the anxiety-provoking topic. Breathing exercises, with concentration on breathing alone, can be beneficial. Another technique is to concentrate on a muscle group, first contracting then relaxing those muscles. Make a tight fist, hold it for a few seconds, then open and relax your hand, watching the blood return to the palm.

Negative thoughts about the exam or about poor performance ("catastrophizing") can increase anxiety and fear, increase catecholamine levels, and interfere with performance. Mental practice or mental rehearsal, a technique often used by athletes, can replace negative thoughts, and can be adapted to the examination process.[5] Visualize yourself sitting in the exam setting calmly and confidently, focusing all your attention on the examination. You will thus create a vivid mental image of positive outcomes, such as successfully answering a question. The technique needs to be repeated on multiple occasions. It is most successful when it is preceded by relaxation exercises.[3]

TAKING THE EXAM

Reviewing of important information the day before the exam can be beneficial, but keep the sessions to an hour or two and do not let them compete with needed recreation, relaxation, and sleep. Eat regular, moderate-sized meals. Use stress-reducing techniques. If you do aerobic exercise regularly, continue it the day before the exam.

On the day of the exam, avoid last-minute cramming. It is probably best not to study at all in the last hours before the exam. You may want to avoid caffeine, even if you use it regularly, as the combination of examination anxiety and caffeine may produce overstimulation.

Arrive at the examination site early enough that you are not rushed or stressed. Assess the number of questions on the exam and calculate the amount of time you can spend per question. Read the directions carefully. Computer-based exams usually provide a brief practice exam that can be used prior to the start of the actual exam. Be sure to participate in this exercise.

Read each question or stem carefully. Note questions asking for "all are correct <u>except</u>" answers. Think of your own answer or answers to the questions before reading the examination answers and choose responses that are closest to yours. Eliminate choices that you know are incorrect. This is particularly helpful for K-type questions, but will also help narrow the field for A-type questions. Read all of the possible responses before selecting an answer. Some questions ask for the <u>best</u> answer among responses that may have more than one correct answer.

For examinees who are prone to test anxiety, it may be helpful to read through but not answer difficult questions initially, answering the easier questions first. This technique provides momentum and confidence to complete the exam initially. Later items may provide cues for answering skipped items. Answer all questions unless there is a penalty for wrong responses (this should be made clear from the test instructions). Use all of the allotted time. Rework difficult questions and look for errors on easy questions, such as selection of the wrong letter or misreading of the stem.

REFERENCES

1. **Fields HL, ed.** *Core Curriculum for Professional Education in Pain*. 2nd ed. Seattle, Wash: IASP Press; 1995.

2. **Sherman TM, Wildman TM.** *Proven Strategies for Successful Test Taking*. Columbus, Oh: Charles E. Merrill; 1982.
3. **Davies D.** *Maximizing Examination Performance. A Psychological Approach*. London: Kogan Page; 1986.
4. **Longman DC, Atkinson RH.** *College Learning and Study Skills*. 3rd ed. Minneapolis, Minn: West; 1993.
5. **Suinn RM.** *Psychology in Sports*. Minneapolis, Minn: Burgess; 1980.

ONLINE RESOURCES

University of New Mexico Center for Academic Program Support
http://www.unm.edu/~caps/strategies.html

University of South Australia Learning Connection
http://www.unisanet.unisa.edu.au/learningconnection/students.htm
http://www.unisanet.unisa.edu.au/examsuccess/

Dartmouth Academic Skills Center
http://www.dartmouth.edu/admin/acskills/

University of Minnesota Learning and Academic Skills Center
http://www.ucs.umn.edu/lasc/OnlineLearn.htmlx

Study Skills Assessment Instrument
http://www.hhpublishing.com/_assessments/LASSI/index.html

2 NOCICEPTIVE PAIN

Linda S. Sorkin, PhD

INTRODUCTION

- Information regarding pain (nociception) is transmitted from the injured tissue (skin, muscle, or viscera) to the cerebral cortex.
- The fastest path involves three neurons: the primary afferent fiber that goes from the skin to the spinal cord, the spinal cord projection neuron (usually thought to project to the contralateral thalamus), and the thalamocortical neuron.
- At each point along the pathway there are several options for longer routes and for modulation and/or integration of the information.

TISSUE INJURY

- Nociceptive pain is initiated by tissue injury; it can be secondary to an incision, inflammation, or disease.
- Action potentials are generated in nerve fibers that respond exclusively to potentially tissue-damaging stimuli—mechanical, thermal, or chemical. These receptors and associated fibers are called nociceptors. While some are specific to one modality (eg, cold or a particular chemical like histamine) the majority are polymodal and respond to multiple types of inputs.
- Active factors released as a direct consequence of the injury or peptides released from collaterals of activated nociceptive nerve terminals (eg, calcitonin gene-related peptide [CGRP] and substance P) induce increased vascular permeability and escape of plasma proteins into the tissue. This causes edema at the injury site and the flare around it. Primary afferent

peptides and/or neurotransmitters and injury products like prostaglandins, as well as infiltrating immune cells and blood products (eg, bradykinin) escaping from the vasculature, make important contributions to inflammation and to the pain resulting from the injury.
- Activation of receptors on peripheral terminals of "pain fibers" can initiate action potentials. Endogenous prostaglandins, bradykinin, and cytokines have strong peripheral actions and can sensitize as well as excite nociceptors. If thermal threshold is reduced such that body temperature initiates neural activity, this looks like spontaneous pain. Reduction of thresholds of nociceptors to temperature and pressure to the innocuous range is manifested as allodynia and is also called primary hyperalgesia.
- Peripheral terminals also have functional receptors for inhibitory agents (eg, μ opiates and γ-aminobutyric acid [GABA]). This provides the rationale for intraarticular opiates during knee surgery and for local patch application of some antihyperalgesic agents.

AFFERENT PAIN FIBERS

- Most fibers that transmit acute nociceptive pain are Aδ (small myelinated) or C (unmyelinated) fibers. Not all Aδ and C fibers transmit pain information; many code for innocuous temperature, itch, and touch.
- Some afferent fibers, "silent nociceptors," signal only after there has been overt tissue damage. Many of these are thought to play a prominent role in arthritis pain and other diseases associated with tissue damage or inflammation. The viscera contain a particularly large proportion of silent nociceptors.
- Parallel experiments comparing electrophysiological data in single C nociceptive fibers with human

psychophysical data show a very high correlation between activity in primary afferent fibers and perception of pain. This suggests that nociceptive primary afferent fiber activity mediates pain and that inhibition of this activity diminishes pain.

- Within cutaneous C nociceptive fibers, some are activated by capsaicin and contain a variety of neuropeptides, while others are capsaicin insensitive. All have monosynaptic terminations in laminae I and II of the spinal dorsal horn. Aδ nociceptors terminate in laminae I and V of the dorsal horn. C fibers have polysynaptic connections with neurons in lamina V as well as with neurons in deeper dorsal horn. Many nociceptive afferents from viscera have monosynaptic input to lamina X around the central canal as well as throughout the dorsal horn.
- Many nociceptive fibers fire in response to tissue injury products (K^+, prostaglandins), mast cell products (cytokines, histamine), and substances that migrate into the tissue when the vasculature becomes more leaky (serotonin, bradykinin).
- Activity in C fibers produces local release of substance P and CGRP from axon terminal collaterals.

SPINAL CORD SENSORY CELLS

- The afferent fibers terminate either directly or indirectly on transmission cells that convey their information up to the brainstem and midbrain. Some neurons project to various thalamic nuclei that serve as way stations for the discriminative and affective components of pain. These ascending pathway nuclei are predominantly crossed and ascend in the anterolateral quadrant of the spinal cord contralateral to the cell body and the innervated body part.
- Other neurons project to autonomic centers that regulate increases in cardiovascular function and respiration in tandem with nociceptive transmission; these pathways tend to be bilateral. In addition to ascending pathways, intrinsic pathways in the spinal cord connect to motor neurons that participate in reflex motor activity.
- The majority of projection cells in laminae I and II (superficial dorsal or posterior horn) respond exclusively to noxious stimulation (high-threshold or nociception-specific cells). Many are multimodal and respond to both intense mechanical and thermal inputs. Others respond exclusively to noxious heat or cold. There are also cells here that respond to only chemical stimulation, including histamine release in the skin, for example, itch. A small population of nociception-specific cells are located in the deep dorsal horn.

- Cells in the deeper dorsal horn (laminae IV–VI) may receive input exclusively from low-threshold mechanoreceptors or thermoreceptors or they may exhibit convergence; that is, they receive input from more than one kind of primary afferent fiber (low threshold and nociceptive). If these convergent cells fire significantly more action potentials in response to noxious stimuli, they are called wide dynamic range (WDR) cells. A small number of WDR cells are found in lamina I.
- Convergence of input from the outer body surface (skin) and from viscera onto individual spinal neurons also occurs. When activity is initiated in viscera, pain is referred to the portion of the body surface that "shares" those neurons. This is one explanation for referred pain.

SPINAL CELL PHARMACOLOGY

- Afferent nociceptive fibers release glutamate and peptides from their central terminals in the spinal cord. Some of the peptides are released along with the glutamate only when the afferent fibers fire action potentials at high frequencies (equivalent to severe injury).
- Glutamate produces a fast response (depolarization) in the spinal neurons via receptors linked to ion channels. These are called non-NMDA-type glutamate receptors. Some peptides, like substance P, prolong the initial depolarization; this change in transmembrane voltage enables another subtype of glutamate receptor, the *N*-methyl-D-aspartate (NMDA) receptor, to become activated. NMDA receptors are also linked to ion channels; however, these channels allow influx of Ca^{2+} in addition to the Na^+ and K^+ transmembrane movement that occurs through the non-NMDA receptors. Increased intracellular calcium leads to a magnification of the incoming response, such that each incoming signal results in successively more output ("windup").
- If high-frequency C-fiber activity persists, intracellular biochemical cascades that also magnify and enhance the response become triggered and a long-lasting spinal sensitization resulting in allodynia and or hyperalgesia results. If this activity is the result of tissue injury, the allodynia or secondary hyperalgesia usually extends into uninjured tissue. This increased sensitivity is only to mechanical stimuli; thermal thresholds are usually unchanged distant from the injury site.
- One such cascade includes Ca^{2+} activation of the enzyme phospholipase A$_2$ (PLA$_2$); this frees arachadonic acid from plasma membranes, thus

making it available as a substrate for the enzyme cyclooxygenase and results in the production of prostaglandins. Prostaglandins (PGs) diffuse out of the spinal neurons and back to the central terminal of the afferent nociceptive fibers (retrograde neurotransmission). There, they act on specific PG receptors to increase the amount of neurotransmitter released per action potential invading the terminal. Other enzymes, including nitric oxide synthase, are activated by Ca^{2+} in a similar manner, also resulting in a magnification of the transmitted response.

- Prostaglandins also act via specific PG receptors on astrocytes to activate them and cause them to release additional neuroactive substances including proinflammatory cytokines.
- The original thought behind preemptive analgesia was that use of local anesthetics around the incision (injury site) would block the high-frequency C-fiber discharge that occurred at the time of injury and, thus, block or reduce the resultant spinal sensitization, pain, and analgesic requirements. Clinical trials of preemptive analgesia have not proved this to be the case. Studies with maintained peripheral blockade of afferent input are under way.
- Spinal opiates inhibit C fiber-mediated nociceptive activity in two ways. They bind to μ and κ opiate receptors on the central terminal of nociceptive primary afferent fibers (presynaptic) and, by reducing Ca^{2+} entry when the action potential invades the terminal, reduce the amount of neurotransmitter released per action potential. Opiates also bind postsynaptically (on the dorsal horn neurons) to μ and δ opiate receptors. Here, opiates increase permeability to K^+, which hyperpolarizes the neurons and results in an inhibition of acute nociceptive transmission. Aβ fibers do not have presynaptic opiate receptors. Thus, if Aβ (touch) fibers mediate pain (allodynia), spinal opiates have only a postsynaptic action and exert less analgesic effect than they would on C fiber-mediated pain. This is one theory of why Aβ-mediated pain is relatively opiate resistant.
- Serotonin and norepinephrine also inhibit nociceptive transmission both pre- and postsynaptically. These monoamines are released primarily from axons whose cell bodies are located in various branstem nuclei. Analgesic actions are potentiated by monoamine reuptake (tricyclic antidepressants) inhibitors and are synergistic with morphine.

SUPRASPINAL PROJECTIONS

- There is a strong projection from both superficial and deep dorsal horn to the lateral thalamus (spinothalamic tract). This "classical" pathway projects to somatosensory (S1) cortex and is postulated to be integral in sensory discrimination of pain, that is, where is it, is it sharp, is it hot, and so on.
- Superficial dorsal horn has a unique projection to posterior thalamus (VMpo); this nucleus, in turn, projects to posterior insula cortex. This area has recently been proposed to be a unique cortical pain center as well as to be involved in homeostatic control of the internal environment, including tissue integrity. This alternative hypothesis proposes that dorsal posterior insula rather than S1 cortex is the primary focus of the sensory-discriminative aspect of pain.
- The ventrocaudal portion of the medial dorsal thalamus (MDvc) also receives an exclusive input from lamina I. This area projects to the anterior cingulate cortex. This medial pathway is likely to represent the motivational affective component of pain.
- Other pathways contribute to changes in autonomic function concomitant with pain, including the spinoreticular and spinomesencephalic tracts.

FURTHER READING

Sorkin LS, Wallace MS. Acute pain mechanisms. *Surg Clin North Am*. 1999;79:213–230.

Wallace MS, Dunn JS, Yaksh TL. Pain: Nociceptive and neuropathic mechanisms with clinical correlates. *Anesthesiol Clin North Am*. 1997;15:229–334.

Yaksh TL, Lynch C, Zapol WM, Maze M, Biebuyck JF, Saidman LJ. *Anesthesia: Biologic Foundations*. Philadelphia: Lippincott–Raven; 1998:471–718.

3   NEUROPATHIC PAIN

Tony L. Yaksh, PhD

NERVE INJURY PAIN STATES

- Following soft tissue injury and inflammation, pain is a common symptom, the disappearance of which is considered to be a consequence of the healing process.
- In contrast, over time after a variety of injuries to the peripheral nerve, animals and humans often manifest a constellation of pain events.

- Frequent components of this evolving syndrome are (1) ongoing sharpshooting sensations referred to the peripheral distribution of the injured nerve, and (2) abnormal painful sensations in response to light tactile stimulation of the peripheral body surface.[1] The latter phenomenon is called tactile allodynia.
- This composite of sensory events was first formally recognized by Silas Weir-Mitchell in the 1860s.[2]
- The psychophysics of this state clearly emphasize that the pain is evoked by the activation of low-threshold mechanoreceptors (Aβ afferents).
- This ability of light touch to evoke this anomalous pain state is *de facto* evidence that the peripheral nerve injury has led to a reorganization of central processing; that is, it is not a simple case of peripheral sensitization of otherwise high-threshold afferents.
- In addition to these behavioral changes, the neuropathic pain condition may display other contrasting anomalies, including, on occasion, an ameliorating effect of sympathectomy of the afflicted limb[3] and an attenuated responsiveness to analgesics such as opiates.[4]

MORPHOLOGICAL AND FUNCTIONAL CORRELATES

- The mechanisms underlying this spontaneous pain and the miscoding of low-threshold afferent input are not completely understood.
- As an overview, these events are believed to reflect:
  - An increase in spontaneous activity in axons in the injured afferent nerve and or the dorsal horn neurons
  - An exaggerated response of dorsal horn neurons to normally innocuous afferent input
- Following peripheral nerve ligation or section, several events occur signaling long-term changes in peripheral and central processing.
- In the periphery after an acute mechanical injury of the peripheral afferent axon:
  - There will be an initial dying back (retrograde chromatolysis) that proceeds for some interval at which time the axon begins to sprout, sending growth cones forward.
  - The growth cone frequently fails to make contact with the original target and displays significant proliferation.
  - Collections of these proliferated growth cones form structures called neuromas.[5]
- Within the spinal cord, a variety of events are observed to occur secondary to the nerve injury. These changes are considered below and include sprouting of axon terminals and altered expression of a variety of peptides, receptors, and channels.

- These phenomena are believed to reflect mechanisms that underlie the sensory experience resulting from a discrete injury to the peripheral nerve.

SPONTANEOUS PAIN STATE

- Under normal conditions, primary afferents show little if any spontaneous activity.
- Following an acute injury to the nerve, afferent axons display:
  - An initial burst of afferent firing secondary to the injury
  - Silence for an interval of hours to days
  - Followed over time by the development of a measurable level of spontaneous afferent traffic in both myelinated and unmyelinated axons[6]
- This ongoing input is believed to provide the source of the afferent activity that leads to spontaneous ongoing sensation.

SITE OF ORIGIN OF SPONTANEOUS AFFERENT TRAFFIC
- Single-unit recording from the afferent axon has indicated that the origin of the spontaneous activity in the afferent arises from the neuroma and from the dorsal root ganglia of the injured axon.
- Activity in sensory afferents originates after an interval of days to weeks from the lesioned site (neuroma) and from the dorsal root ganglion (DRG) of the injured nerve.[7]

INCREASED SODIUM CHANNEL EXPRESSION
- Voltage-sensitive sodium channels mediate the conducted potential in myelinated and unmyelinated axons.
- Cloning has emphasized that there are multiple populations of sodium channels, differing in their current activation properties and structure.
- Following peripheral injury there is an increase in the expression of sodium channels in the neuroma and the dorsal root ganglia.
- This increased ionic conductance may result in the increase in spontaneous activity that develops in a sprouting axon.
- Alternatively, a reduction in potassium channel activity would similarly lead to increased afferent excitability.[8]

CHANGES IN AFFERENT TERMINAL SENSITIVITY
- The sprouted terminals of the injured afferent axon display a characteristic growth cone that possesses transduction properties that were not possessed by the original axon.
- These include significant mechanical and chemical sensitivity.

- Thus, these spouted endings may have sensitivity to a number of humoral factors, such as prostanoids, catecholamines, and cytokines such as tumor necrosis factor α (TNFα).[9]
- This evolving sensitivity is of particular importance given that current data suggest that following local nerve injury there occurs the release of a variety of cytokines, particularly TNFα, which can thus directly activate the nerve and neuroma.
- In addition, following nerve injury, there is significant sprouting of postganglionic sympathetic efferents which can lead to the local release of catecholamines.
- This scenario is consistent with the observation that following nerve injury, the postganglionic axons can initiate excitation in the injured axon.[10]
- These events are believed to contribute to the development of spontaneous afferent traffic after peripheral nerve injury.

EVOKED HYPERPATHIA

- The observation that low-threshold tactile stimulation yields pain states has been the subject of considerable interest.
- As noted, there is considerable agreement that these effects are often mediated by low-threshold afferent stimulation.
- Several underlying mechanisms have been proposed to account for this seemingly anomalous linkage.

DORSAL ROOT GANGLION CELL CROSS-TALK
- Following nerve injury, there is evidence suggesting that "cross-talk" develops between populations of afferents in the DRG and in the neuroma.
- Depolarizing currents in one axon would generate a depolarizing voltage in an adjacent quiescent axon.
- This proximal depolarization would permit activity arising in one axon to drive activity in a second.
- In this manner, it is hypothesized that a large low-threshold afferent would drive activity in an adjacent high-threshold afferent.[11]
- Alternatively, it is appreciated that DRG cells in vitro can release a variety of transmitters and express excitatory receptors.

AFFERENT SPROUTING
- In normal circumstances, large myelinated (Aβ) afferents project into the spinal Rexed lamina III and deeper.
- Small afferents (C fibers) tend to project into spinal laminae I and II, a region consisting mostly of nocisponsive neurons.

- Following peripheral nerve injury, it has been argued that the central terminals of these myelinated afferents (A fibers) sprout into lamina II of the spinal cord.[12]
- With this synaptic reorganization, stimulation of low-threshold mechanoreceptors (Aβ fibers) could produce excitation of these neurons and be perceived as painful.
- The degree to which this sprouting occurs is a point of current discussion, and although it appears to occur,[13] it may be less prominent than originally reported.

DORSAL HORN REORGANIZATION
- Following peripheral nerve injury, a variety of events occur in the dorsal horn which suggest altered processing wherein the response to low-threshold afferent traffic can be exaggerated.

Spinal Glutamate Release
- There is little doubt that the post-nerve injury pain state is dependent on an important role of spinal glutamate release.
- Recent studies have emphasized that after nerve injury there is a significant enhancement of resting spinal glutamate secretion.
- This release is in accord with (1) increased spontaneous activity in the primary afferent, and (2) a loss of intrinsic inhibition which may serve to modulate resting glutamate secretion (see below).
- The physiological significance of this release is emphasized by two convergent observations: (1) Intrathecally delivered glutamate evokes a powerful tactile allodynia and thermal hyperalgesia though the activation of spinal N-methyl-D-aspartate (NMDA) and non-NMDA receptors, and (2) the spinal delivery of NMDA antagonists has been shown to attenuate the hyperapathic states arising in animal models of nerve injury.[14]
- NMDA receptor activation mediates an important facilitation of neuronal excitability.
- In addition, the NMDA receptor is a calcium ionophore which, when activated, leads to prominent increases in intracellular calcium.[15]
- This increased calcium serves to initiate a cascade of events that includes the activation of a variety of enzymes (kinases), some of which phosphorylate membrane proteins (eg, calcium channels and the NMDA receptors), and others, such as the mitogen-activated protein kinases (MAP kinases), which serve to mediate the intracellular signaling that leads to the altered expression of a variety of proteins and peptides (eg, cyclooxygenase and dynorphin).[16]
- This downstream nuclear action is believed to herald long-term and persistent changes in function.

- A variety of factors have been shown to enhance glutamate release. Two examples are discussed further, below.

Nonneuronal Cells and Nerve Injury

- Following nerve injury (section or compression), there is a significant increase in activation of spinal microglia and astrocytes in spinal segments receiving input from the injured nerves.
- Of particular interest is that in the face of pathology such as bone cancer, such upregulation has been clearly shown.[17]
- Astrocytes are activated by a variety of neurotransmitters and growth factors.[18]
- While the origin of this activation is not clear, it leads to increased spinal expression of cyclooxygenase (COX)/nitric oxide synthetase (NOS)/glutamate transporters/proteinases.
- Such biochemical components have previously been shown to play an important role in the facilitated state.

Loss of Intrinsic GABAergic/Glycinergic Inhibitory Control

- In the spinal dorsal horn are a large number of small interneurons that contain and release GABA and glycine.[19]
- GABA/glycine-containing terminals are frequently presynaptic to the large central afferent terminal complexes and form reciprocal synapses, while GABAergic axosomatic connections on spinothalamic cells have also been identified.
- Accordingly, these amino acids normally exert important tonic or evoked inhibitory control over the activity of Aβ primary afferent terminals and second-order neurons in the spinal dorsal horn.[20]
- The relevance of this intrinsic inhibition to pain processing is provided by the observation that the simple intrathecal delivery of GABA-A receptor or glycine receptor antagonists leads to a powerful behaviorally defined tactile allodynia.[21]
- Similarly, animals genetically lacking glycine binding sites often display a high level of spinal hyperexcitability.[22]
- These observations led to the consideration that following nerve injury, there may be a loss of GABAergic neurons.[23]
- Although there are data that do support a loss of such GABAergic neurons, the loss typically appears to be minimal and transient.[24]
- Recent observations now suggest a second alternative. After nerve injury, spinal neurons may regress to a neonatal phenotype in which GABA-A activation becomes excitatory.[25] This excitatory effect is secondary to reduced activity of the membrane Cl^- transporter which changes the reversal current for the Cl^- conductance. Here increasing membrane Cl^- conductance, as occurs with GABA-A receptor activation, results in membrane depolarization.

Spinal Dynorphin

- Following peripheral nerve injury, there occur a wide variety of changes in the expression of dorsal horn factors.
- One such example is increased expression of the peptide dynorphin.
- Nerve injury leads to a prominent increase in spinal dynorphin expression.
- Intrathecal delivery of dynorphin can initiate the concurrent release of spinal glutamate and a potent tactile allodynia; the latter effect is reversed by NMDA antagonists.

SYMPATHETIC DEPENDENCY OF NERVE INJURY PAIN STATE

- After peripheral nerve injury, there is increased innervation of the peripheral neuroma by postganglionic sympathetic terminals.
- More recently, it has been shown that there is a growth of postganglionic sympathetic terminals into the dorsal root ganglia of the injured axons.[26]
- These postganglionic fibers form baskets of terminals around the ganglion cells.
- Several properties of this innervation are interesting:
  - They invest all sizes of ganglion cells, but particularly type A (large) ganglion cells.
  - The innervation occurs principally in the DRG ipsilateral to the lesion, but in addition, there is innervation of the contralateral ganglion cell.
  - Stimulation of the ventral roots of the segments, containing the preganglionic efferents, produces activity in the sensory axon either by an interaction at the peripheral terminal at the site of injury or by an interaction at the level of the DRG.
  - This excitation is blocked by intravenous phentolamine and typically α_2-preferring antagonists, emphasizing an adrenergic effect.[27]

PHARMACOLOGY OF NERVE INJURY PAIN STATE

- The ability of low-threshold stimuli to evoke pain behavior after peripheral nerve injury has been a subject of interest and led to the development of several models of nerve injury.

- Three commonly used models are those developed by:
  - Bennett and Xie (four loose ligatures around the sciatic nerve)[28]
  - Seltzer and Shir (hemiligation of the sciatic nerve)[29]
  - Kim and Chung (tight ligation of the L5 and L6 nerves just peripheral to the ganglion)[30]
- The Bennett model is widely used to study thermal hyperalgesia while the Chung model displays a well-defined tactile allodynia.
- These models are of particular importance as they have been widely employed to investigate the pharmacology of the pain states associated with the particular nerve injury.
- Spinal actions of drugs in ameliorating these pain states vary somewhat between the models.
- Of particular interest, these models show sensitivity to NMDA antagonists, α_2 agonists, and anticonvulsants such as gabapentin and low doses of intravenous lidocaine.
- In contrast, while thermal hyperalgesia in the Bennett model is sensitive to intrathecal morphine, tactile allodynia in the Chung model is not.
- This difference may reflect the fact that large low-threshold afferents are not thought to possess opiate receptors and hence terminal excitability is not altered by opiates.[31]

CONCLUSION

- The preceding text covers a number of mechanisms that have been shown to occur after nerve injury.
- It is not at present clear to what degree some or all of these mechanisms are brought into play in any given post-nerve injury state in humans.
- It is clear, for example, that not all post-nerve injury states possess a sensitivity to sympathetic blockade.
- Moreover, some neuropathic states are opiate-sensitive and some are not.
- Similarly, it seems certain that after nerve injury a degree of sensitivity to NMDA receptor blockade may occur in humans as well as animals.
- Such observations provide support for the idea that at least some human states have mechanisms that appear in the preclinical model.

REFERENCES

1. **Jensen TS, Gottrup H, Sindrup SH, Bach FW.** The clinical picture of neuropathic pain. *Eur J Pharmacol.* 2001;429:1–11.

2. **Weir-Mitchell S, Moorhouse GR, Keen WW.** *Gunshot Wounds and Other Injuries of Nerves.* Philadelphia: Lippincott; 1864:164.

3. **Furlan AD, Lui PW, Mailis A.** Chemical sympathectomy for neuropathic pain: does it work? Case report and systematic literature review. *Clin J Pain.* 2001;17:327–336.

4. **Wiesenfeld-Hallin Z, Aldskogius H, Grant G, Hao JX, Hokfelt T, Xu XJ.** Central inhibitory dysfunctions: Mechanisms and clinical implications. *Behav Brain Sci.* 1997; 20:420–425.

5. **Stoll G, Jander S, Myers RR.** Degeneration and regeneration of the peripheral nervous system: From Augustus Waller's observations to neuroinflammation. *J Peripher Nerv Syst.* 2002;7:13–27.

6. **Burchiel KJ, Ochoa JL.** Pathophysiology of injured axons. *Neurosurg Clin North Am.* 1991;2:105–116.

7. **Chul Han H, Hyun Lee D, Mo Chung J.** Characteristics of ectopic discharges in a rat neuropathic pain model. *Pain.* 2000;84:253–261.

8. **Rasband MN, Park EW, Vanderah TW, Lai J, Porreca F, Trimmer JS.** Distinct potassium channels on pain-sensing neurons. *Proc Natl Acad Sci USA.* 2001;98: 13373–13378.

9. **Liu B, Li H, Brull SJ, Zhang JM.** Increased sensitivity of sensory neurons to tumor necrosis factor alpha in rats with chronic compression of the lumbar ganglia. *J Neurophysiol.* 2002;88:1393–1399.

10. **Shinder V, Govrin-Lippmann R, Cohen S, et al.** Structural basis of sympathetic–sensory coupling in rat and human dorsal root ganglia following peripheral nerve injury. *J Neurocytol.* 1999;28:743–761.

11. **Devor M, Wall PD.** Cross-excitation in dorsal root ganglia of nerve-injured and intact rats. *J Neurophysiol.* 1990; 64:1733–1746.

12. **Woolf CJ, Shortland P, Coggeshall RE.** Peripheral nerve injury triggers central sprouting of myelinated afferents. *Nature.* 1992;355:75–78.

13. **Tong YG, Wang HF, Ju G, Grant G, Hokfelt T, Zhang X.** Increased uptake and transport of cholera toxin B-subunit in dorsal root ganglion neurons after peripheral axotomy: possible implications forsensory sprouting. *J Comp Neurol.* 1999;404:143–158.

14. **Parsons CG.** NMDA receptors as targets for drug action in neuropathic pain. *Eur J Pharmacol.* 2001;429:71–78.

15. **Stephenson FA.** Subunit characterization of NMDA receptors. *Curr Drug Targets.* 2001;2:233–239.

16. **Svensson CI, Yaksh TL.** The spinal phospholipase–cyclooxygenase–prostanoid cascade in nociceptive processing. *Annu Rev Pharmacol Toxicol.* 2002;42:553–583.

17. **Watkins LR, Maier SF.** Beyond neurons: Evidence that immune and glial cells contribute to pathological pain states [review]. *Physiol Rev.* 2002;82:981–1011.

18. **Sonnewald U, Qu H, Aschner M.** Pharmacology and toxicology of astrocyte–neuron glutamate transport and cycling. *J Pharmacol Exp Ther.* 2002;301:1–6.

19. **Todd AJ.** Anatomy of primary afferents and projection neurones in the rat spinal dorsal horn with particular emphasis on substance P and the neurokinin 1 receptor [review]. *Exp Physiol.* 2002;87:245–249.

20. **Rudomin P.** Selectivity of the central control of sensory information in the mammalian spinal cord. *Adv Exp Med Biol.* 2002;508:157–170.

21. **Zhang Z, Hefferan MP, Loomis CW.** Topical bicuculline to the rat spinal cord induces highly localized allodynia that is mediated by spinal prostaglandins. *Pain.* 2001;92:351–361.

22. **Gundlach AL.** Disorder of the inhibitory glycine receptor: Inherited myoclonus in Poll Hereford calves. *FASEB J.* 1990;4:2761–2766.

23. **Moore KA, Kohno T, Karchewski LA, Scholz J, Baba H, Woolf CJ.** Partial peripheral nerve injury promotes a selective loss of GABAergic inhibition in the superficial dorsal horn of the spinal cord. *J Neurosci.* 2002;22:6724–6731.

24. **Ibuki T, Hama AT, Wang XT, Pappas GD, Sagen J.** Loss of GABA-immunoreactivity in the spinal dorsal horn of rats with peripheral nerve injury and promotion of recovery by adrenal medullary grafts. *Neuroscience.* 1997;76: 845–858.

25. **Ben-Ari Y.** Excitatory actions of gaba during development: The nature of the nurture. *Nat Rev Neurosci.* 2002; 3:728–739.

26. **Michaelis M, Devor M, Janig W.** Sympathetic modulation of activity in rat dorsal root ganglion neurons changes over time following peripheral nerve injury. *J Neurophysiol.* 1996;76:753–763.

27. **Chen Y, Michaelis M, Janig W, Devor M.** Adrenoreceptor subtype mediating sympathetic–sensory coupling in injured sensory neurons. *J Neurophysiol.* 1996;76:3721–3730.

28. **Bennett GJ, Xie YK.** A peripheral mononeuropathy in rat that produces disorders of pain sensation like those seen in man. *Pain.* 1988;33:87–107.

29. **Shir Y, Seltzer Z.** A-fibers mediate mechanical hyperesthesia and allodynia and C-fibers mediate thermal hyperalgesia in a new model of causalgiform pain disorders in rats. *Neurosci Lett.* 1990;115:62–67.

30. **Kim SH, Chung JM.** An experimental model for peripheral neuropathy produced by segmental spinal nerve ligation in the rat. *Pain.* 1992;50:355–363.

31. **Yaksh TL.** Preclinical models of nociception. In: Yaksh TL, Lynch III C, Zapol WM, Maze M, Biebuyck JF, Saidman LJ, eds. *Anesthesia: Biologic Foundations.* Philadelphia: Lippincott–Raven; 1997:685–718.

EVALUATION OF THE PAIN PATIENT

4   HISTORY AND PHYSICAL EXAMINATION

Brian J. Krabak, MD
Scott J. Jarmain, MD

INITIAL UNDERSTANDING

- The importance of the initial evaluation in increasing successful outcomes in pain management cannot be overstated. This evaluation should be treated as an opportunity to acquaint oneself with a patient and come to an understanding of his or her condition.
- By eliciting useful information and examining the patient in an orderly and logical fashion, the diagnosis or a short differential list can usually be made, and an effective management plan can frequently be chosen with confidence.
- In Western countries, the prevalence of chronic pain in the adult population ranges from 2 to 40%.[1]
- The estimated cost of chronic back pain[2] is more than $33.6 billion for health care, $11 to $43 billion for disability compensation, $4.6 billion for lost productivity, and $5 billion in legal services.

HISTORY

CHIEF COMPLAINT

- Transcribe the chief complaint succinctly using the patient's own words.
- Include the patient's expectations and goals.

HISTORY OF PRESENT ILLNESS

- A thorough history should document and characterize the potential pain symptoms[3]:
  - Date of onset of the pain: atraumatic versus traumatic, acute versus insidious.
  - Character and severity of the pain: achy, allodynia (due to nonnoxious stimuli), burning, dull, dysesthesia (unpleasant abnormal sensation), electrical, hyperalgesia (increased response to a painful stimuli), lancinating, paresthesia (abnormal sensation), neuralgia (pain in a distribution of a nerve), sharp.
  - Location of pain in its entirety.
  - Associated factors, including any associated neurologic symptoms, such as weakness, numbness, and motor control or balance problems.
  - Aggravating and alleviating factors.
  - Chronicity.
  - Previous investigative tests and treatments provided, including results and responses.
- Investigate any litigation or secondary gain issues. The compensation system can promote pain behavior patterns in the injured worker, which is why an early and accurate diagnosis with appropriate intervention is essential.[4]
- Document functional losses resulting from the pain or injury and the use of assistive devices. Include changes in mobility, cognition, and activities of daily living; household arrangements; and community and vocational activities.[5]
- Explore the history in detail and document any inconsistencies in the patient's reported mechanism of injury or complaints.
- Rule out potential surgical emergencies, such as unstable fractures and aggressively progressing neurologic symptoms that may be associated with cauda equina syndrome.

MEDICAL AND SURGICAL HISTORY

• Sometimes the etiology of pain may be uncovered by a thorough review of prior medical illnesses and surgical interventions, including subsequent outcomes.

PSYCHOSOCIAL HISTORY

• The psychosocial history provides vital information necessary for understanding how pain is affecting the patient and his or her family. Roles may change and new stressors may alter family dynamics, which may influence the outcome of any treatment program.[6]
• A history of substance abuse (alcohol, tobacco, or illegal drugs) should raise the suspicion of drug-seeking behavior and secondary gain. Proper identification of substance abuse issues allows the proper treatment of pain symptoms and facilitates future counseling.
• Identify a primary caregiver, when appropriate, and family and friends who can and are willing to provide support and assistance.
• Identify housing or other living conditions that may exacerbate the pain for modification as appropriate.
• Restrictions in the ability to participate in previous hobbies and social activities can be stressful to a patient. Return to these activities should be a goal of a treatment and rehabilitation program. Feasible substitute hobbies should be identified in the interim.
• Psychiatric problems, such as depression, anxiety, and suicidal or homicidal ideation, can have a major negative influence on an individual's motivation and ability to cooperate with a treatment program. The stress of a new pain condition or injury can trigger a recurrence of a previous psychiatric problem. Supportive psychotherapy or psychiatric medications can prevent or treat problems that could interfere with successful pain management.
• Loss of income due to a new pain condition or injury can cause stress-related problems in the patient and his or her family. Early identification of such issues can facilitate a referral to a social worker as appropriate.

VOCATIONAL HISTORY AND BACK PAIN

• In a study by Suter, the risk of back injury was greater in those below the age of 25 years, but the greatest number of compensation claims occurred in workers between 30 and 40 years of age.[7]
• Handling materials, especially lifting associated with bending or twisting, is the most common work activity associated with back injuries.[7]

• In a study of sewage workers with low back pain, work disability was associated with age, the weekly duration of stooping and lifting in the previous 5 years, and high abnormal illness–behavior scores.[8]
• Occupations with the largest incidences of back injuries for which the workers receive compensation include machine operation, truck driving, and nursing.
• Factors in the work environment that are associated with the potential for delayed recovery include job satisfaction; monotonous, boring, or repetitive work; new employment; and recent poor job rating by a supervisor.[7]

MEDICATIONS AND ALLERGIES

• Obtain a complete list of prescribed and over-the-counter medications and "home remedies" that are being taken or were taken to manage the pain symptoms. (A recent study revealed that 14% of the US population use herbs/supplements and 26% use vitamins.[9])
• Review this list for each medication's indication, dosage, duration, effectiveness, and side effects.
• Reduction or avoidance of medications with unwanted cognitive and physical side effects is recommended.

FAMILY HISTORY

• Always review the medical history of family members and relatives so as not to miss genetic diseases, some of which include pain in their symptom complex.

REVIEW OF SYSTEMS

• A comprehensive review of systems may uncover problems not previously noted that may be related to the pain condition or can affect the patient's clinical course. Follow routine history-taking format to inquire about problems in all systems of the body and note psychiatric, cardiovascular, pulmonary, gastrointestinal, neurologic, rheumatologic, genitourinary, endocrine, and/or musculoskeletal symptoms.
• Constitutional symptoms, such as unexpected weight loss, night pain, and night sweats, require further investigation.

PAIN SCALES

• Pain diagrams (Figure 4–1) are helpful in visualizing the patient's symptoms.

Please draw the location of your pain on the diagram below. Mark painful areas as follows:

000 = pins and needles   /// = "lightning" or "shooting" pain   TTT = throbbing
xxx = sharp pain   AAA = aching pain

Feel free to use other symbols or words as necessary.

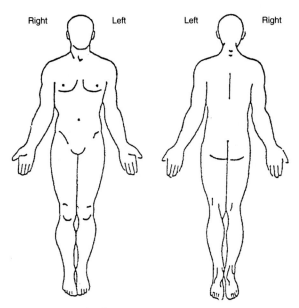

Right   Left   Left   Right

FIGURE 4–1 Pain diagram.

- Other pain and functional scales include the visual analog scale (VAS) (Figure 4–2), the Oswestry Disability Questionnaire, and the Short Form-36 Quality of Life Scale.

PHYSICAL EXAMINATION

GENERAL

- The patient should be appropriately gowned to allow proper visualization of any pertinent areas during the examination. Use a chaperone as appropriate.
- Record the patient's temperature, blood pressure, pulse, height, and weight during each evaluation.
- Examine the patient's entire body for any skin lesions, such as surgical scars, hyperpigmentation, ulcerations, and needle marks. In addition, look for bony malalignments or areas of muscle atrophy, fasciculations, discoloration, and/or edema.

MENTAL STATUS

- A thorough mental status evaluation should include a mini-mental examination to assess the patient's orien-

Please rate the intensity of your pain by making a mark on this scale

NO PAIN ————————————————— WORST PAIN IMAGINABLE

FIGURE 4–2 Visual analog scale.

tation, immediate and short- and long-term memory, comprehension, and cognition.
- Assess the patient's emotional well-being, including concurrent signs of depression, hopelessness, or anxiety.

JOINT EXAMINATION

- Always examine both sides of the patient when appropriate to detect any asymmetries.
- Record the active motion of all joints, noting any obvious limitations, dyskinesis, grimacing, or asymmetry.
- Record the passive range of pertinent joints or joints that appear abnormal during active testing, once again noting limitations, grimacing, or asymmetry.
- Palpate each joint to assess for specific areas of pain.
- Joint stability testing identifies any underlying ligamentous injuries.

MOTOR EXAMINATION

- Document manual muscle testing as outlined below, noting any give-away pain. Be sure to test all myotomal levels to help distinguish peripheral nerve, plexus, or root injuries (Tables 4–1 and 4–2).

GRADE	DEFINITION
5	Complete joint range of motion against gravity with full resistance
4	Complete joint range of motion against gravity with moderate resistance
3	Full joint range of motion against gravity
2	Full joint range of motion with gravity eliminated
1	Visible or palpable muscle contraction; no joint motion produced
0	No visible or palpable muscle contraction

SENSORY EXAMINATION

- A thorough sensory exam requires testing light touch, pin prick, vibration, and joint position, as certain fibers or columns may be preferentially affected. Be sure to test all dermatomal levels (Figure 4–3).[10]

TABLE 4–1   Upper Extremity Muscles and Innervations

MUSCLE	NERVE	ROOT	TRUNK	DIVISION	CORD
Trapezius	Spinal accessory	C2,C3,C4			
Rhomboid	Dorsal scapular	C4,C5			
Serratus anterior	Long thoracic	C5,C6,C7,C8			
Supraspinatus	Suprascapular	C4,C5,C6	Upper		
Infraspinatus	Suprascapular	C5,C6	Upper		
Pectoralis major	Medial/lateral pectoral	C5–T1	U/M/L	Anterior	Medial/lateral
Pectoralis minor	Medial pectoral	C7,C8,T1	U/M/L	Anterior	Medial/lateral
Latissmus dorsi	Thoracodorsal	C6,C7,C8	U/M/L	Posterior	Posterior
Teres major	Lower subscapular	C5,C6,C7	Upper	Posterior	Posterior
Teres minor	Axillary	C5,C6	Upper	Posterior	Posterior
Deltoid	Axillary	C5,C6	Upper	Posterior	Posterior
Biceps	Musculocutaneous	C5,C6	Upper	Anterior	Lateral
Triceps	Radial	C6,C7,C8,T1	Middle/lower	Posterior	Posterior
Anconeus	Radial	C7,C8	Middle/lower	Posterior	Posterior
Brachioradialis	Radial	C5,C6	Upper	Posterior	Posterior
Supinator	Radial (post. inter.)	C5,C6	Upper	Posterior	Posterior
ECR	Radial (post. inter.)	C5,C6,C7,C8	Upper/middle	Posterior	Posterior
EDC	Radial (post. inter.)	C6,C7,C8	Middle/lower	Posterior	Posterior
EIP	Radial (post. inter.)	C6,C7,C8	Middle/lower	Posterior	Posterior
Pronator teres	Median	C6,C7	Middle/lower	Anterior	Lateral
FCR	Median	C6,C7,C8	U/M/L	Anterior	Medial/lateral
FPL	Median (ant. inter.)	C7,C8,T1	Middle/lower	Anterior	Medial/lateral
FDS	Median	C7,C8,T1	Middle/lower	Anterior	Medial/lateral
FDP (Nos. 1,2)	Median (ant. inter.)	C7,C8,T1	Middle/lower	Anterior	Medial
Pronator quadratus	Median (ant. inter.)	C7,C8,T1	Middle/lower	Anterior	Medial/lateral
APB	Median	C6,C7,C8,T1	Lower	Anterior	Medial
Opponens pollicis	Median	C6,C7,C8,T1	Lower	Anterior	Medial
FPB (sup.)	Median	C6,C7,C8,T1	Lower	Anterior	Medial
FCU	Ulnar	C7,C8,T1	Lower	Anterior	Medial
FDP (Nos. 3,4)	Ulnar	C8,T1	Middle/lower	Anterior	Medial
AbDM	Ulnar	C8,T1	Lower	Anterior	Medial
Interossei	Ulnar	C8,T1	Lower	Anterior	Medial
FPB (deep)	Ulnar	C8,T1	Lower	Anterior	Medial

ECR, extensor carpi radialis; EDC, extensor digitorum communis; EIP, extensor indicis proprius; FCR, flexor carpi radialis; FPL, flexor policis longus; FDS, flexor digitorum superficialis; FDP, flexor digitorum profundus; APB, abductor policis brevis; FPB, flexor policis brevis; FCU, flexor carpi ulnaris; AbBM, abductor digiti minimi; sup., superior; post., posterior; ant., anterior; inter., interosseous.

OTHER NEUROLOGIC EXAMINATIONS

- Evaluate cranial nerves I through XII, especially in the setting of cervical or facial pain and headaches.
- Check muscle stretch reflexes (Table 4–3), noting asymmetry and clonus. Clonus requires more than four muscle contractions following a stimulus.
- Check for the presence of Babinski's plantar reflex and Hoffman's thumb reflex, both of which may be present in an upper motor neuron syndrome.
- Assess the patient's gait and identify cerebellar deficits by asking the patient to do dysmetric tests (finger-to-nose motion and heel-to-shin motion), rapid alternating movement of the fingers and hand (dysdiadochokinesia), and balance tests with the eyes open and closed.

SPECIAL TESTS

- Wadell et al. described five nonorganic signs that help identify patients with physical symptoms without anatomic etiology.[11] They identified a constellation of hypochondriasis, hysteria, and depression in patients with three of the five signs. These five signs help indicate when factors other than anatomic concerns should be addressed:
  - Superficial or nonanatomic distribution of tenderness
  - Nonanatomic (regional) motor or sensory impairment
  - Excessive verbalization of pain or gesturing (overreaction)
  - Production of pain complaints by tests that simulate only a specific movement (simulation)
  - Inconsistent reports of pain when the same movement is carried out in different positions (distraction)

CONCLUSION

- A thorough history and physical examination provide the foundation for the proper diagnosis of pain patients.

TABLE 4–2 Lower Extremity Muscles and Nerve Innervations

MUSCLE	NERVE	ROOT
Psoas major	Ventral primary rami	L2,L3,L4
Iliacus	Femoral	L2,L3,L4
Sartorius	Femoral	L2,L3,L4
Quadriceps femoris	Femoral	L2,L3,L4
Hip adductors	Obturator	L2,L3,L4
Adductor magnus	Sciatic (tibial) Obturator	L2,L3,L4,L5,S1
Piriformis	Nerve to piriformis	S1,S2
Gluteus minimus	Superior gluteal	L4,L5,S1
Gluteus medius	Superior gluteal	L4,L5,S1
Gluteus maximus	Inferior gluteal	L5,S1,S2
Hamstrings	Sciatic (tibial)	L4,L5,S1,S2
Biceps femoris (SH)	Sciatic (peroneal)	L5,S1,S2
Peroneii	Superficial peroneal	L4,L5,S1
Tibialis anterior	Deep peroneal	L4,L5,S1
Extensor hallucis longus	Deep peroneal	L4,L5,S1
Extensor digitorum brevis	Deep peroneal	L4,L5,S1
Tibialis posterior	Tibial	L5,S1
Soleus	Tibial	L5,S1,S2
Gastrocnemius	Tibial	S1,S2
Abductor hallucis	Tibial (medial plantar)	L4,L5,S1
Flexor digitorum brevis	Tibial (medial plantar)	L4,L5,S1
Flexor hallucis brevis	Tibial (medial plantar)	L4,L5,S1
Abductor digiti minimi	Tibial (lateral plantar)	S1,S2
Interossei	Tibial (lateral plantar)	S1,S2

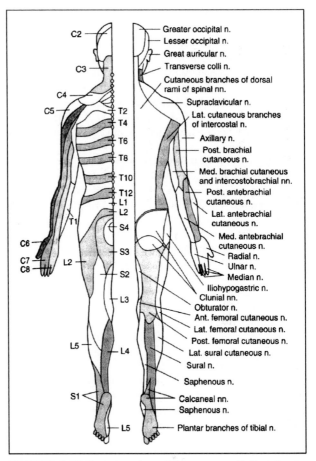

FIGURE 4–3B Posterior view of dermatomes (*left*) and cutaneous areas supplied by individual peripheral nerves (*right*). Modified with permission from Carpenter and Sutin.[10]

TABLE 4–3 Muscle Stretch Reflexes

MUSCLE STRETCH REFLEX	SPINAL SEGMENT
Biceps	C5
Brachioradialis	C6
Triceps	C7
Patella tendon	L4
Medial hamstring	L5
Achilles	S1

- Such an evaluation must include physical, mental, and emotional factors.
- When developing a treatment plan, a physician should understand the patient's goals.

REFERENCES

1. **Verhaak PFM, Kerssens JJ, Dekker J, et al.** Prevalence of chronic benign pain disorder among adults: a review of the literature. *Pain.* 1998;77:231.

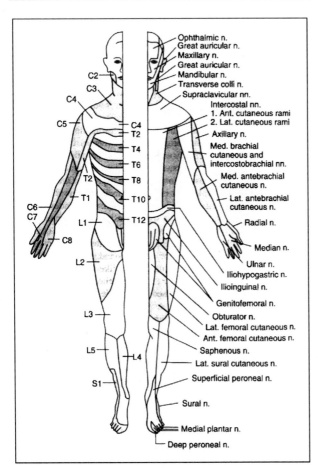

FIGURE 4–3A Anterior view of dermatomes (*left*) and cutaneous areas supplied by individual peripheral nerves (*right*). Modified with permission from Carpenter and Sutin.[10]

2. **Frymoyer J, Durett C.** The economics of spinal disorders. In: Frymoyer J, ed. *The Adult Spine*. Philadelphia: Lippincott–Raven; 1997:143.

3. Adapted from Members of the Department of Neurology, Mayo Clinic and Mayo Clinic Foundation for Medical Education and Research. *Clinical Examination in Neurology*. 6th ed. Philadelphia: Saunders; 1991.

4. **Bigos SJ, Spengler DM, Martin NA, et al.** Back injuries in industry: a retrospective study. III. Employee-related factors. *Spine*. 1986;11:252.

5. **Walker WC, Cifu DX, Gardner M, et al.** Functional assessment in patients with chronic pain: Can physicians predict performance? *Am J Phys Med Rehabil*. 2001;80:162.

6. **Linton SJ.** A review of psychological risk factors in back and neck pain. *Spine*. 2000;25:1148.

7. **Suter PB.** Employment and litigation: Improved by work, assisted by verdict. *Pain*. 2002;100:249.

8. **Friedrich M, Cermak T, Heiller I.** Spinal troubles in sewage workers: Epidemiological data and work disability due to low back pain. *Int Arch Occup Environ Health*. 2000; 73:245.

9. **Kaufman DW, Kelly, JP, Rosenberg L, et al.** Recent patterns of medication use in the ambulatory adult population of the United States: The Slone survey. *JAMA*. 2002;16;287:337.

10. **Carpenter MB, Sutin J.** In: *Human Neuroanatomy*. 8th ed. Baltimore: Williams & Wilkins; 1983.

11. **Wadell G, McCulloh JA, Kummel E, et al.** Nonorganic physical signs in low-back pain. *Spine*. 1980;5:117.

5 ELECTROMYOGRAPHY/NERVE CONDUCTION STUDIES

Nathan J. Rudin, MD, MA

OBJECTIVES

This article is intended to:
- Familiarize the reader with the basic principles of electrodiagnostic testing.
- Provide the basic knowledge necessary to interpret an electrodiagnostic report.
- Teach when and how to apply electrodiagnostic testing in patients with pain.

GLOSSARY

- *Action potential*: the electrical phenomenon generated by threshold or suprathreshold depolarization of a nerve cell or muscle cell.
- *Antidromic*: moving in the opposite direction from normal physiologic function.
- *Compound muscle action potential* (CMAP): the potential generated by a muscle when its supplying motor nerve is stimulated; formed by the summation of multiple motor unit action potentials (see below).
- *Fibrillation potential*: a type of spontaneous activity.
- *Insertional activity*: the brief burst of electrical activity following movement of a needle electrode within muscle; may be increased in irritable or damaged muscle and decreased in fibrotic muscle.
- *Motor unit*: a motor neuron and the group of muscle fibers it supplies.
- *Motor unit action potential* (MUAP): the potential generated by the firing of a single motor unit.
- *Nerve conduction velocity* (NCV): speed of nerve conduction in meters per second; can be calculated during nerve conduction studies.
- *Orthodromic*: moving in the direction typical of normal physiologic function.
- *Phase*: the portion of a (MUAP) waveform existing between departure from and return to baseline.
- *Positive sharp wave*: a type of spontaneous activity.
- *Recruitment*: characteristic firing pattern of motor units during voluntary muscle contraction; units are added in a predictable fashion as the strength of contraction increases.
- *Sensory nerve action potential* (SNAP): the potential generated in a sensory nerve when it is stimulated.
- *Spontaneous activity*: electrical potentials occurring in a skeletal muscle in the absence of voluntary effort; almost always an indicator of abnormality.

ELECTRODIAGNOSTIC TESTING

- Electrodiagnostic testing is an extension of the history interview and physical examination.
  - It can help explain the causes of acute or chronic pain.
  - It can identify focal or diffuse areas of nerve and muscle injury.
  - It can identify or rule out processes amenable to rehabilitation, injection, surgery, or drug therapy.
  - It can significantly narrow a differential diagnosis or confirm a diagnosis.
  - It supplements information gleaned from imaging studies.
  - By defining the type and extent of injury, it can provide prognostic information.
  - Serial examinations can be useful in monitoring recovery and therapeutic outcome.
- The two basic components of electrodiagnostic testing are *nerve conduction studies* and *needle electromyography*.

NERVE CONDUCTION STUDIES

Nerve conduction studies (NCSs) permit the noninvasive assessment of nerve physiology and function.
- Slowed conduction velocity or delayed response latency may reflect injury to myelin.
- Diminished response amplitude or temporally dispersed waveforms may reflect axonal injury or loss.
- The distribution of abnormalities can differentiate between focal and diffuse neuropathic processes.

INDICATIONS

- Suspected nerve entrapments or other mononeuropathies.
- Suspected polyneuropathies.
- Suspected radiculopathy or plexopathy.
- Suspected neuromuscular junction disease.

CONTRAINDICATIONS

- Pacemaker, automatic implantable cardioverter/defibrillator (AICD), spinal cord stimulator, or other electrosensitive implants. Stimulation distant from the implant may not pose a problem; check with the electromyographer.
- Marked edema or skin damage (likely to impede data acquisition).

GENERAL PRINCIPLES

- A pickup electrode is placed over the desired recording area, and a reference electrode is placed nearby. A ground electrode is also affixed to the patient.
- The nerve is electrically stimulated to generate an action potential, which is propagated down the nerve and detected at the pickup electrode.
- Potentials are visually displayed, recorded, and analyzed.
- The action potential's latency (time for stimulus-generated potential to reach the active electrode) and amplitude are measured. Nerve conduction velocity (NCV) is calculated.
- Electrical stimulation is delivered as a short-duration shock (usually 0.1–0.2 ms), usually perceived as mildly uncomfortable. Transcutaneous stimulation is most commonly used. The practitioner can also use a fine needle to stimulate deeper nerves. Stimulation is performed at a standard distance from the active electrode.

- Stimulation may be repeated at a different point along the nerve to measure conduction characteristics along a particular nerve segment. This may help to identify focal lesions.
- Each laboratory should consistently use the same techniques and compare results against the same preestablished norms, permitting meaningful data interpretation.[1]

STUDY TYPES

- Motor nerve conduction studies (MNCSs) (Figure 5–1) measure the CMAP produced by depolarization of muscle fibers in response to electrical stimulation. CMAP is recorded using electrodes positioned over the muscle of interest.
- Sensory nerve conduction studies (SNCSs) (Figure 5–2) measure the SNAP produced as depolarization propagates along nerve. SNAP is recorded using electrodes positioned directly over the nerve, at a point distal or proximal to the stimulation site.[2]

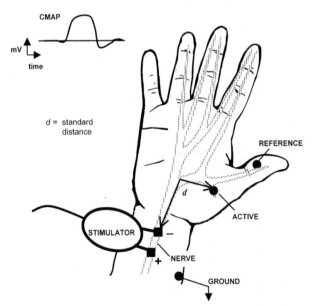

FIGURE 5–1 Median motor nerve conduction study. The active electrode is placed over the belly of the muscle to be studied. The reference electrode is placed over an electrically neutral landmark, in this case the IP joint of the thumb. Transcutaneous electrical stimulation is applied over the nerve at a standard distance (*d*) from the active electrode. CMAP is detected at the active electrode, amplified, and displayed (upper left). CMAP amplitude and latency are recorded and compared with laboratory norms. NCV cannot be calculated over this most distal segment of the nerve because it includes the time for transmission at the neuromuscular junction. One can calculate NCV over more proximal segments by stimulating proximally to the wrist, measuring interstimulus distance, and subtracting distal from proximal latency.

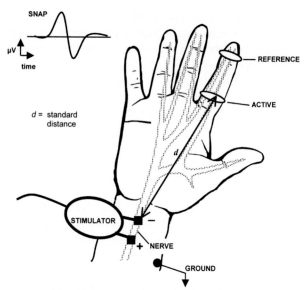

FIGURE 5–2 Median sensory nerve conduction study. Active and reference electrodes are placed along the course of the nerve to be studied. Transcutaneous electrical stimulation is applied over the nerve at a standard distance (*d*) from the active electrode. SNAP is detected at the active electrode, amplified, and displayed (upper left). SNAP amplitude and latency are recorded and compared with laboratory norms. Nerve conduction velocity (m/s) is calculated by dividing *d* (in mm) by onset latency (in ms).

LIMITATIONS

- NCSs measure only the fastest-conducting fibers; injury to the smallest (unmyelinated or lightly myelinated) fibers may go undetected.
- NCS results, particularly for SNCSs, are sensitive to temperature. If the skin and underlying nerves are too cool, conduction velocity and response latency may be slowed, but amplitude may paradoxically increase. Skin should be warmed (to at least 32°C for upper limbs, 30°C for lower limbs) prior to testing.
- SNCSs assess the function of primary afferent neurons, that is, the pathway distal to the dorsal root ganglion (DRG). In radiculopathies, where injury often occurs proximal to the DRG, the SNCS may be normal.

F WAVE

- The F wave is a special NCS that assesses motor conduction along the most proximal segment of the nerve. Antidromic stimulation of a peripheral nerve sends an action potential to the spinal cord, where it activates a small number of anterior horn cells. The resultant action potential is transmitted orthodromically and triggers a small motor response (F wave) in the same peripheral nerve territory.

- F-wave latencies are length-dependent, and normal values must be adjusted for patient height or limb length.
- F waves are frequently abnormal (delayed or absent) in polyneuropathies, entrapment neuropathies, radiculopathies, and motor neuron disease (eg, amyotrophic lateral sclerosis).[3]

H REFLEX

- The H reflex (Figure 5–3) is the electrical equivalent of a muscle stretch reflex elicited by tendon tap. It is examined using a modified MNCS technique.
- In adults, the H reflex is most often present in the soleus muscle and, at times, in the forearm flexor muscles. It may be more widespread in hyperreflexic conditions (eg, myelopathy) and in children.[3]
- H reflex latencies are length-dependent, and normal values must be adjusted for patient height or limb length.[3]
- The soleus H reflex is the most frequently studied. It may be delayed or absent in S1 radiculopathy.

REPETITIVE NERVE STIMULATION

- Repetitive nerve stimulation (RNS) is an invaluable technique for assessing neuromuscular junction physiology.
- Two main factors affect neurotransmitter release at the normal neuromuscular junction: the amount of acetylcholine (Ach) available for release and the amount of available calcium (Ca^{2+}), which affects the probability of transmitter release.[4]

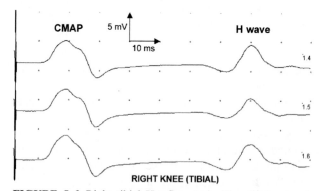

FIGURE 5–3 Right tibial H-reflex study. The tibial nerve is stimulated in the popliteal fossa with the cathode directed proximally. The electrical stimulus proceeds bidirectionally along the nerve. Distal spread produces a CMAP in the soleus muscle. Proximal spread reaches the spinal cord and triggers a spinal reflex, which sends a motor signal distally and produces an H wave. Delay or absence of the tibial H wave may reflect S1 radiculopathy or another neuropathic process.

- When MNCS is performed using rapid RNS (usually 2–3 Hz), the amplitude of the CMAP normally does not change.
- In many types of neuromuscular disease, repetitive stimulation can deplete available Ach to the point where a decrement is seen in CMAP amplitude with successive stimuli. Depending on the disease, a brief period of sustained muscle contraction, which increases the availability of Ca^{2+}, may reverse the decrement (eg, myasthenia gravis) or cause an increment in baseline amplitude (eg, Lambert–Eaton myasthenic syndrome).[4]

NEEDLE ELECTROMYOGRAPHY

- Needle electromyography (EMG) uses needle electrodes to evaluate the electrical activity of muscle fibers. It provides copious information about the integrity, function, and innervation of motor units and (using special techniques) individual muscle fibers.[5] The wealth of information is such that EMG has been called "the electrophysiologic biopsy."[6]
- The skilled electromyographer can identify processes causing muscle denervation (neuropathies), muscle destruction (myopathies), and failure of neuromuscular transmission (eg, myasthenia gravis).
- EMG can provide information about the extent of injury. Serial examinations allow monitoring of recovery or disease progression.

INDICATIONS

- Suspected mononeuropathy or polyneuropathy.
- Suspected radiculopathy or plexopathy.
- Suspected myopathy.
- Suspected neuromuscular junction disease.
- Suspected motor neuron disease.

CONTRAINDICATIONS

- Anticoagulant therapy (depends on planned test location, degree of anticoagulation).
- Coagulopathy.
- Implanted hardware at or near desired exam site.
- Muscle to be biopsied as the exam may introduce abnormalities.

GENERAL PRINCIPLES

- Surface landmarks and physical examination are used to isolate the desired muscle(s). After skin steriliza-

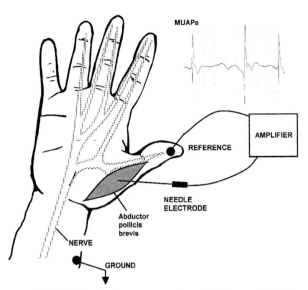

FIGURE 5–4 Needle electromyography of abductor pollicis brevis. The reference electrode is placed over an electrically neutral landmark. The needle (active electrode) is inserted into the resting muscle and moved in small increments to assess for spontaneous activity. The subject then performs graded muscle contraction to assess MUAP morphology and recruitment.

tion, a needle electrode is advanced into the muscle. Muscle potentials are monitored visually and audibly (Figure 5–4).
- The needle is moved through the muscle in small increments. This elicits spontaneous activity in abnormal muscle.
- The patient then voluntarily activates the muscle at mild and strong levels of contraction. MUAP morphology, number, and recruitment are assessed.[7]

SPONTANEOUS ACTIVITY

- A normal muscle produces short bursts of insertional activity when the needle is moved, with electrical silence between insertions.
- A denervated or damaged muscle produces spontaneous activity, which may persist after the needle is moved. Different potentials have characteristic appearances (Figure 5–5) and sounds. Spontaneous potentials may include fibrillation potentials, positive sharp waves, and complex repetitive discharges.[7]
- The amount and frequency of spontaneous activity provide information about the severity or acuity of a disease process. Spontaneous activity is graded using this scale:

0 = none
1+ = transient but reproducible discharges after moving needle

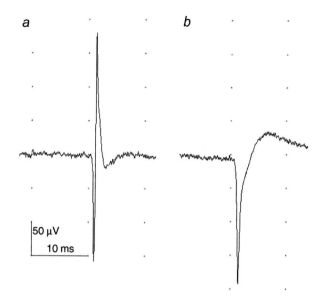

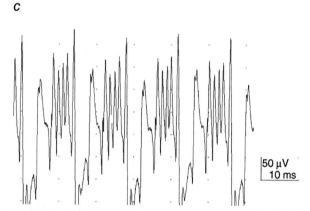

FIGURE 5–5 Examples of spontaneous activity. Fibrillation potentials (*a*) are short-duration potentials occurring in a regular pattern. Positive sharp waves (*b*) are similar to fibrillation potentials but have no negative spike component. Complex repetitive discharges (*c*) may be the result of ephaptic transmission causing repetitive, rhythmic firing of irritable muscle fibers. Their rhythmic "buzzsaw" sound is easily recognizable.

2+= occasional discharges at rest in more than two different sites

3+= spontaneous activity at rest regardless of needle position

4+= abundant, constant spontaneous activity[3]

EMG ANALYSIS

- A normal MUAP has a characteristic amplitude, duration, and number of phases. The EMG signal as a whole has a characteristic appearance and recruitment pattern. Abnormalities in any of these parameters help to diagnose the type and chronicity of disease (Table 5–1).

- The skilled electromyographer tailors the choice of muscles to the patient's situation. By carefully selecting muscles and observing the distribution of abnormalities, the electromyographer can distinguish among radiculopathy, plexopathy, myopathy, and many other conditions.

USING ELECTRODIAGNOSIS IN PAIN MEDICINE

- Electrodiagnosis is useful when pain is thought to originate from neurologic, intrinsic muscular, or neuromuscular junction disease.
- Before ordering electrodiagnostic testing, identify the specific question you want to answer. Remember that electrodiagnostic testing is uncomfortable. As with all medical interventions, before ordering, ask yourself: Will the test be of practical value? Will an accurate diagnosis change any aspect of the treatment plan or provide other benefits?
- State the question clearly on the referral. If you wish to look for or rule out particular conditions, mention them.
- Be sure that you are comfortable with your chosen electrodiagnostic laboratory and its practices. A well-run electrodiagnostic laboratory should:
  ○ Ensure the most comfortable experience possible for the patient.
  ○ Control for skin temperature during NCS, and record temperatures in the report.
  ○ Have a consistent set of norms for NCS data, and present these norms in the report for comparison. Abnormal data should be clearly marked.
  ○ Compare abnormal results against the contralateral side wherever possible.
  ○ Present the findings clearly.
  ○ Make sure the referring provider receives the results quickly.

SELECTED CLINICAL CONDITIONS

CARPAL TUNNEL SYNDROME

- Median MNCS and SNCS confirm a clinical diagnosis of carpal tunnel syndrome (CTS) with high sensitivity (>85%) and specificity (95%).[8]
- EMG of the thenar muscles is quite painful and should be reserved for atypical or unusual presentations where additional information is needed.[9]
- When abnormalities are found on one limb, the contralateral limb should also be studied.[9]

TABLE 5–1   Clinical Significance of EMG Parameters Commonly Mentioned in Electrodiagnostic Reports*

EMG PARAMETER	DECREASED	INCREASED
Amplitude	Loss or denervation of muscle fibers, eg, myopathy, axonal neuropathy, motor neuron disease	Reinnervation after injury, with spatially larger motor units; hypertrophied muscle fibers (eg, recovery from myopathy or neuropathy)
Duration	Loss or atrophy of muscle fibers, as in myopathy	Reinnervation after injury, with spatially dispersed muscle fibers (myopathy or neuropathy)
Number of phases	Normal units have three or four phases; fewer phases are not generally seen	Increased variability of fiber diameter (myopathy); increased width of MUP endplate zone (neuropathy)
Recruitment	Usually reflects muscle denervation (loss of motor units); initial units fire very rapidly before the next unit is recruited, characteristic of neuropathic processes	Usually reflects muscle damage (fewer motor units per muscle); more units are needed to achieve a given strength of contraction, characteristic of myopathic processes
Spontaneous activity	No spontaneous activity seen in normal muscle	May be caused by myopathy, neuropathy, direct trauma (including surgery)

*This table is provided as a guide to interpretation. The list is incomplete; interested readers are referred to more comprehensive texts.

- While NCS is helpful diagnostically, the final decision to proceed with surgery versus conservative treatment should be based primarily on symptoms and functional impact.[10]

COMPLEX REGIONAL PAIN SYNDROME

- Electrodiagnosis can help distinguish between complex regional pain syndrome (CRPS, "reflex sympathetic dystrophy") subtypes I (no specific nerve injury identified) and II (causalgia, specific nerve injury identified).[11]
- Cases of this severe neuropathic pain syndrome have been linked to radiculopathy, brachial plexitis, and many other neuropathic conditions.
- Treatment of the underlying nerve injury, where possible, may provide some relief for the CRPS II patient.
- Reserve electrodiagnostic testing for patients with a suspected definable nerve injury. EMG and NCS may be extremely painful in the CRPS patient, and increased analgesic therapy may be required.

RADICULOPATHY

- It is essential to tailor the EMG exam to the patient's presentation and physical findings. No one exam method is appropriate for all patients.
- The needle EMG examination is the most useful for identifying radiculopathy, but sensitivity is limited. Screening six or more muscles optimizes identification of radiculopathies.[12]
- SNCSs are frequently normal, as spinal lesions causing radiculopathy often spare the dorsal root ganglion.
- MNCSs may be abnormal, particularly in advanced cases.
- EMG findings can help target the site for diagnostic/therapeutic image-guided spinal injection.

- When performed before and after decompressive surgery, EMG and NCS can monitor recovery and provide prognostic information.
- Neither EMG nor MRI is superior in the diagnosis of radiculopathy; they remain complementary diagnostic tools.[13,14]

GENERALIZED NEUROMUSCULAR DISEASE

- Electrodiagnostic testing remains an important tool for diagnosing muscular dystrophies, inflammatory myopathies, neuromuscular junction disease, hereditary neuropathies, and other generalized neuromuscular disorders.
- To be helpful, testing must be conducted in the context of the patient's physical exam and clinical situation.[15]

MYOFASCIAL PAIN AND FIBROMYALGIA SYNDROME

- Electrodiagnosis is normal in these musculoskeletal pain syndromes unless there are comorbid conditions, such as carpal tunnel syndrome.
- Generalized neuromuscular disorders such as myopathies, myasthenia gravis, and peripheral neuropathies may mimic fibromyalgia or myofascial pain.
- If the exam and other workup raise concern about neuromuscular disease, electrodiagnosis can provide valuable information.[15]

PAINFUL NEUROPATHY

- When neuropathy is suspected as a cause of pain, NCS and EMG can help confirm the diagnosis and identify the type and bodily distribution of neuropathy (eg, axonal, demyelinating, mixed; sensory, motor, mixed; uniform, segmental).

- Electrodiagnostic testing can help identify treatable neuropathies (eg, metabolic, toxic, vitamin deficiency; nerve transections).
- Electrodiagnostic testing provides valuable prognostic information, and serial examinations can document disease progression or recovery.
- When polyneuropathy is suspected, complete examination requires both MNCS and SNCS, preferably on multiple nerves in both upper and lower limbs.[16]
- When abnormalities are observed, the same nerve on the contralateral side should be examined to differentiate between symmetric and asymmetric processes.

REFERENCES

1. **Wang SH, Robinson LR.** Considerations in reference values for nerve conduction studies. *Phys Med Rehabil Clin North Am.* 1998;9:907.
2. **Kimura J.** Kugelberg lecture: Principles and pitfalls of nerve conduction studies. *Electroencephalogr Clin Neurophysiol.* 1998;106:470.
3. **Kimura J.** *Electrodiagnosis in Diseases of Nerve and Muscle: Principles and Practice.* 2nd ed. Philadelphia: Davis; 1989.
4. **Keesey JC.** AAEM Minimonograph #33: Electrodiagnostic approach to defects of neuromuscular transmission. *Muscle Nerve.* 1989;12:613.
5. **Kraft GH.** An approach to electrodiagnostic medicine: The power of needle electromyography. *Phys Med Rehabil Clin North Am.* 1994;5:495.
6. **Barkhaus PE, Nandedkar SD.** EMG evaluation of the motor unit: The electrophysiologic biopsy. *eMedicine.com;* 2003.
7. **Daube JR.** AAEM Minimonograph #11: Needle examination in clinical electromyography. *Muscle Nerve.* 1991;14:685.
8. **Jablecki CK, et al.** Practice parameter for electrodiagnostic studies in carpal tunnel syndrome: Summary statement. *Muscle Nerve.* 2002;25:918.
9. **Mazur A.** Role of thenar electromyography in the evaluation of carpal tunnel syndrome. *Phys Med Rehabil Clin North Am.* 1998;9:755.
10. **Stevens JC.** AAEM Minimonograph #26: The electrodiagnosis of carpal tunnel syndrome. *Muscle Nerve.* 1987; 10:99.
11. **Bruehl S, Harden RN, Galer BS, et al.** External validation of IASP diagnostic criteria for complex regional pain syndrome and proposed research diagnostic criteria. International Association for the Study of Pain. *Pain.* 1999;81:147.
12. **Dillingham TR.** Electrodiagnostic approach to patients with suspected radiculopathy. *Phys Med Rehabil Clin North Am.* 2002;13:567.
13. **McDonald CM, Carter GT, Fritz RC, et al.** Magnetic resonance imaging of denervated muscle: Comparison to electromyography. *Muscle Nerve.* 2000;23:1431.
14. **Nardin RA, Patel MR, Gudas TF, et al.** Electromyography and magnetic resonance imaging in the evaluation of radiculopathy. *Muscle Nerve.* 1999;22:151.
15. **Dillingham TR.** Electrodiagnostic approach to patients with suspected generalized neuromuscular disorders. *Phys Med Rehabil Clin North Am.* 2001;12:253.
16. **Donofrio PD, Albers JW.** AAEM Minimonograph #34: Polyneuropathy: Classification by nerve conduction studies and electromyography. *Muscle Nerve.* 1990;13:889.

6 QUANTITATIVE SENSORY TESTING

Mark S. Wallace, MD

- Quantitative sensory testing is used to evaluate the function of individual nerve fibers (large myelinated, Aβ; small myelinated, Aδ; and small unmyelinated, C). The correlation between sensation and nerve fiber activity has been extensively studied and no definite conclusions can be made as to what nerve fibers correlate with certain sensations.[1]
- Methods used for quantitative sensory testing include mechanical nonpainful sensation (vibratory, von Frey hair), mechanical painful sensation (pinch, pressure), thermal sensation, and current perception sensation (Table 6–1).

MECHANICAL NONPAINFUL SENSATION

- Mechanical nonpainful sensation is used to measure large myelinated (Aβ) fiber function.[2]

TABLE 6–1 Summary of Quantitative Sensory Testing[1–12]

Thermal thresholds	
Cool	Aδ
Warm	C
Cold pain	Interaction between Aδ and C
Heat pain (at threshold)	C
Heat pain (supramaximal)	Aδ
Mechanical painful	
Single stimuli	Aδ and C
Repetitive stimuli	C
Mechanical nonpainful	
Vibratory	Aβ
Von Frey	Aβ
Current perception monitor	
5 Hz	C
250 Hz	Aδ
2000 Hz	Aβ

- Of all the sensations, mechanical nonpainful sensation is the most vulnerable to nerve ischemia and decreases within minutes of nerve ischemia.[3,4]
- Large myelinated fiber function is often the most decreased after peripheral nerve injury.
- Vibratory thresholds are most often tested using a C tuning fork but this method is crude and unreliable. More sophisticated equipment is available but expensive.
- Von Frey hairs are a good, cheap method of measuring large myelinated fiber function. Calibrated von Frey hairs are filaments of varying size. The filaments are selected at random and three successive stimuli are applied for 2 seconds at 5-second intervals per filament applied in an ascending pattern of thickness of the hair fiber. The patient is not able to witness application of the hair fiber and is simply asked to report when a stimulus is felt. Thresholds are expressed in millinewtons and measured as positive if the patient feels one of the three successive stimuli. At the stimulus intensity evoking a report of sensation, the next hair fiber stimulus used is one unit smaller. This stimulus reversal is repeated twice, and the average reversal intensity is defined as the threshold.[5]

MECHANICAL PAINFUL SENSATION

- A single stimulus measures small myelinated (Aδ) and small unmyelinated (C) fiber function. Repetitive stimuli measure C fiber function.[6,7]
- A pinch or pressure algometer is most often used. A pinch algometer consists of a pistol-shaped handle and a shaft with two circular probes facing each other (area = 1 cm^2). A fold of skin is placed between the two probes and one is displaced slowly and evenly (rate 30 kPa/s) toward the other, pinching the skin. A transducer in one of the probes provides constant feedback of the pressure exerted. The subject is instructed to press a switch at the very instant of pain experience. The trial is then terminated. Mechanical pain threshold is defined as the mean pressure for three trials. Stimuli are given at 1-minute intervals.

THERMAL SENSATION

Thermal sensation is used to measure the function of small myelinated (Aδ) and small unmyelinated (C) fibers.[8–11]

- *Cool Sensation*: Measures Aδ fiber function. Of all the thermal sensations, cool sensation is the first to decrease after peripheral nerve injury, depends the most on spatial summation so small probes falsely decrease the sensation, and is the most vulnerable to nerve ischemia.
- *Warm Sensation*: Measures C fiber function. Warm sensation is the second thermal sensation to decrease after peripheral nerve injury. It is less dependent on spatial summation than cool sensation but more dependent than heat pain, and is less vulnerable to nerve ischemia than cool sensation but more vulnerable than heat pain.
- *Cold Pain Sensation*: Results from an interaction between Aδ and C fiber function. Of all the thermal stimuli, it is the least reproducible between subjects. Evidence suggests that Aδ fibers transmit the cool portion and C fibers transmit the pain portion of the sensation. In peripheral nerve injury, cold pain thresholds can approach cool sensation thresholds, resulting in *cold allodynia.*
- *Heat Pain Sensation*: Just painful thresholds measure C fiber function. Supramaximal painful thresholds measure Aδ fiber function. In the early stages of complex regional pain syndrome, heat pain thresholds approach warm sensation thresholds, resulting in *heat hyperalgesia.* As disease progresses, heat pain sensation normalizes (Table 6–2).

CURRENT PERCEPTION THRESHOLD

- Recent technological advances allow quantitative measurement of the functional integrity of both large- and small-diameter sensory nerve fibers using the current perception threshold (CPT) sensory testing device. CPT evaluation is a noninvasive, painless, quantitative sensory test that provides a functional assessment of the sensory nervous system. The CPT is the minimum amount of a transcutaneously applied current that an individual perceives as evoking a sensation. CPT evaluation is performed using the Neurometer CPT/C (Neurotron, Inc., Baltimore, Md) neuroselective diagnostic stimulator, which uses a microprocessor-controlled constant current sine wave stimulus to obtain CPT measures. The constant-current feature compensates for alterations in skin resistance and standardizes the stimulus between skin thickness and degree of skin moisture. This device is

TABLE 6–2 Mechanical/Thermal Thresholds in Normal and Neuropathic Patients[13,14]

	NORMAL	NEUROPATHIC
Cool thresholds (°C)	30	23
Warm thresholds (°C)	34.5	41
Cold pain (°C)	12	22
Hot pain (°C)	45	45
Von Frey (mN)	3.8	4.2

currently used as a clinical evaluation tool in assessing differential nerve fiber thresholds. CPT uses three frequencies, 5, 250, and 2000 Hz, specific to the C fiber, Aδ fiber, and Aβ fiber, respectively.[12]

REFERENCES

1. **Gruener G, Dyck PJ.** Quantitative sensory testing: Methodology, applications, and future directions. *J Clin Neurophys*. 1994;11:568–583.
2. **Torebjork HE, Vallbo AB, Ochoa JL.** Intraneural microstimulation in man: Its relation to specificity of tactile sensations. *Brain*. 1987;110:1509–1529.
3. **Yarnitsky D, Ochoa JL.** Differential effect of compression-ischemia block on warm sensation and heat-induced pain. *Brain*. 1991;114:907–913.
4. **Yarnitsky D, Ochoa JL.** Release of cold-induced burning pain by block of cold-specific afferent input. *Brain*. 1990;113:893–902.
5. **Olmos PR, Cataland S, O'Dorisio TM, Casey CA, Smead WL, Simon SR.** The Semmes–Weistein monofilament as a potential predictor of foot ulceration in patients with noninsulin-dependent diabetes. *Am J Med Sci*. 1995;309:76–82.
6. **Nordin, N.** Low-threshold mechanoreceptive and nociceptive units with unmyelinated C fibers in the human supraorbital nerve. *J Physiol*. 1990;426:229–240.
7. **Ochoa JL, Torebjork E.** Sensations evoked by intraneural microstimulation of single mechanoreceptor units innervating the human hand. *J Physiol Lond*. 1993;342:465–472.
8. **Konietzney F.** Peripheral neural correlates of temperature sensation in man. *Hum Neurobiol*. 1984;3:21–32.
9. **Ochoa JL, Torebjork E.** Sensations evoked by intraneural microstimulation of C nociceptor fibers in human skin nerves. *J Physiol*. 1989;415:583–599.
10. **Verdugo R, Ochoa JL.** Quantitative somatosensory thermotest: A key method for functional evaluation of small calibre afferent channels. *Brain*. 1992;115:893–913.
11. **Yarnitsky D, Ochoa JL.** Warm and cold specific somatosensory systems, psychophysical thresholds, reaction times and peripheral conduction velocities. *Brain*. 1991;114:1819–1826.
12. **Katims JJ.** Electrodiagnostic functional sensory evaluation of the patient with pain: A review of the neuroselective current perception threshold and pain tolerance thresholds. *Pain Digest*. 8:219–230.
13. **Wallace MS, Laitin S, Licht D, Yaksch TL.** Concentration-effect relationships for intravenous lidocaine infusions in human volunteers: Effect upon acute sensory thresholds and capsaicin-evoked hyperpathia. *Anesthesiology*. 1997;86:1262–1272.
14. **Wallace MS, Magnuson S, Ridgeway B.** Oral mexiletine in the treatment of neuropathic pain. *Reg Anesth Pain Med*. 2000;25:459–467.

7 RADIOLOGIC EVALUATION

Marcus W. Parker, MD
Kieran J. Murphy, MD

INTRODUCTION

- Low back pain has a lifetime prevalence of approximately 80%, and the resulting medical costs exceed $8 billion annually.
- Low back pain is also the most frequent reason for work disability in the United States.[1]
- Thus, this chapter focuses on the radiologic evaluation of pain resulting from degenerative diseases of the spine.

INDICATIONS FOR THE USE OF IMAGING

- Most cases of back pain do not require imaging. In patients with typical, uncomplicated back pain, imaging studies should only follow failure of a 4-week trial of conservative management as symptoms resolve in 90% of cases.[2]
- It is important to rule out nondegenerative causes, including neoplasm, infection, inflammatory disease, and vascular causes. A history consistent with these pathologic processes and/or unremitting pain should prompt a thorough laboratory and radiologic workup.
- Radiologic studies are also indicated for patients with motor, bowel, bladder, or sexual neurologic deficits; previous spinal fusion surgery; or symptoms persisting more than 4 weeks.[2]
- If a patient has nerve root compression symptoms that indicate a possible surgically treatable cause, consult with a surgeon to determine the type of study needed.
- It is critical to remember that radiologic studies cannot image pain, and asymptomatic lesions can mislead physicians. An MRI study, for example, found disc bulges in 52%, disc protrusions in 27%, and disc extrusions in 1% of asymptomatic adults.[3]
- The location and type of suspected tissue injury guide the choice of imaging study.

PLAIN RADIOGRAPHY

- Plain radiography is an inexpensive, rapid, readily available technique for initial screening of the spine for fractures, misalignment of vertebrae, spondylolisthesis and spondylolysis, and other bone pathologies.

It may also detect an underlying infection or neoplastic process.

- The low sensitivity and nonspecificity of findings, lack of detail, and poor imaging of soft tissue limit the usefulness of plain films.
- Plain films should be obtained to rule out fractures in patients presenting with back pain and recent trauma or a history suggesting osteoporosis and compression fractures. Such patients usually also require CT and MRI if spinal cord damage is suspected.
- Flexion–extension views may provide additional information in patients with spondylolisthesis or a prior spinal fusion surgery.

MAGNETIC RESONANCE IMAGING

- MRI is the most useful tool in the evaluation of the spine.
- The advantages of MRI are that it is noninvasive, can image in sagittal and axial planes, can be used in patients allergic to iodinated contrast, uses no ionizing radiation, produces no beam-hardening artifact, and provides the best soft tissue contrast and visualization of the spinal ligaments.
- Contraindications to the use of MRI include the presence of cardiac pacemakers, ferromagnetic aneurysm clips, ferromagnetic cochlear implants, and intraocular metallic foreign bodies. Claustrophobic patients may be unable to tolerate the procedure unmedicated, but administration of 5 mg diazepam before leaving for the MRI and 5 mg in the MRI suite usually controls symptoms. Open MRI may also be available for these patients, but image quality is inferior.
- Limitations of MRI are the expense, long procedure times, limited availability in some localities, inability to detect calcification, and inability to visualize cortical bone directly.
- MRI is equal to CT in evaluation of a herniated disc and spinal stenosis. The reported sensitivity and specificity are 0.6–1.0 for MRI and 0.43–0.97 for CT for a herniated disc and 0.9 for MRI and 0.72–1.0 for CT for spinal stenosis.[4]
- MRI is more sensitive and specific than other techniques in detecting osteomyelitis, disc space infection, or malignancy.[4] It is also very useful in evaluating arachnoiditis and is the best method of assessing spinal cord compression and damage.
- T1-weighted images provide good anatomic detail in the imaging of end-plate reactive changes, osteophytic narrowing, lateral disc herniation, postoperative scarring, spondylolisthesis, and infiltrative disease.
- T2-weighted images are more time-consuming to obtain but are useful in intramedullary disease,

infection, and inflammation because of the increased sensitivity to the higher water content in these conditions.
- Gadolinium-DTPA contrast should be used in postoperative patients to differentiate scarring from the intervertebral discs and also in patients with infection, inflammation, and/or cancer.
- In the cervical region, thin-section axial images (1.5 mm) should be obtained, but 3- to 5-mm sections usually suffice in the lumbar spine.

COMPUTED TOMOGRAPHY

- Compared with MRI, CT is more rapid, more available, and less expensive and provides superior bone detail.
- CT can be used in patients with ferromagnetic devices that preclude the use of MRI.
- CT can also be combined with myelography for increased sensitivity in certain situations (see below).
- Standard CT is well-suited for the evaluation of spinal trauma: CT can clearly establish the extent of fractures seen on plain film, detect subtle fractures not previously seen, and determine the degree to which bony fragments impinge on the spinal canal. The neural damage in as many as half of patients with cervical spine bone injuries, however, requires MRI for accurate evaluation.[5]
- As mentioned above, CT is equivalent to MRI in facilitating diagnosis of disc herniation and spinal stenosis. CT can also accurately depict nerve root impingement but is inferior to MRI in detecting infection and neoplasm.
- Thin CT sections from pedicle to pedicle should be obtained in the region of suspected spinal damage.

MYELOGRAPHY

- Myelography involves the intrathecal injection of a contrast agent followed by plain film or, more usually, CT imaging.
- Although relatively safe, myelography is an invasive procedure with risks and side effects. The most common side effect is a postprocedure headache, but the incidence of headache can be reduced to 10% of patients by using a 26-gauge needle and having the patient remain prone for 4–8 hours following the procedure.[6]
- Postmyelography CT has a high sensitivity in detecting cervical radiculopathy, osteophytic impingement, and disc herniation and can also identify subarachnoid tumor spread and arachnoiditis.

- This test is the definitive preoperative study, although it is usually not necessary before an operation.
- Myelography may be indicated in patients with ambiguous diagnoses from MRI and standard CT as well as in those unable to undergo MRI.
- CT without intrathecal contrast should be used for the lumbar spine because the natural contrast of fat with bone and disc is sufficient in this region.

RADIONUCLIDE SCANNING

- Injection of technetium-99*m*-labeled phosphate complexes followed by a whole-body bone scan is a very sensitive method of detecting regional changes in bone metabolism. These bone scans are useful in the detection of early osteomyelitis, compression and small stress fractures, primary malignancy, and skeletal metastasis in patients with back pain of unknown origin. Plain films are negative in 10–40% of metastases identified using bone scans, while a bone scan is falsely negative in 5% of spinal metastases identified by plain film.[7]
- The disadvantages of nuclear bone scans are poor detail and specificity. Usually a positive result necessitates further studies to confirm the cause, and MRI is more sensitive as well as the test of choice in patients with a strong suspicion of spinal metastases or infection.[8]
- Combining radionuclide imaging with single-proton emission CT improves spatial resolution.

DISCOGRAPHY

- Discography is the injection of contrast under fluoroscopic guidance into the center of the nucleus pulposus of an intervertebral disc.
- The appearance of contrast accumulation and the pain response to a given force of injection are used to determine if a particular disc is causing the patient's pain.
- This technique can be combined with CT.
- Although it is the only imaging study that seeks to establish a causal relationship between anatomic abnormalities and pain, discography is not often used in clinical practice.

ARTERIOGRAPHY

- Spinal arteriography is the intraarterial injection of iodinated contrast into spinal arteries.
- This test is generally used only to improve preoperative or preembolization visualization or to identify the cause when MRI reveals a possible vascular tumor or malformation.
- Arteriography carries the risks of spinal stroke causing neurologic deficits as well as the nonneurologic complications associated with an invasive procedure.

REFERENCES

1. **Salkever D.** *Morbidity Cost: National Estimates and Economic Determinants.* Report No. (PHS) 86-3343;1985.
2. **Bigos S, Bowyer O, Braen G, et al.** *Clinical Practice Guideline Number 14: Acute Low Back Problems in Adults.* Rockville, Md: Agency for Health Care Policy and Research, Public Health Service, US Department of Health and Human Services; 1994. AHCPR publication 95-0642.
3. **Jensen M, Brant-Zawadzki M, Obuchowski N, et al.** Magnetic resonance imaging of the lumbar spine in people without back pain. *N Engl J Med.* 1994;331:69.
4. **Jarvik J, Deyo R.** Diagnostic evaluation of low back pain with emphasis on imaging. *Ann Intern Med.* 2002;137:586.
5. **Riggins RJ, Krause JF.** The risk of neurologic damage with fractures of the vertebra. *J Trauma.* 1977;17:126.
6. **Vezina JL, Fontaine S, Laperriere J.** Outpatient myelography with fine-needle technique: An appraisal. *AJR Am J Roentgenol.* 1989;153:383.
7. **Alazraki N.** Radionuclide techniques. *Bone Joint Imaging.* 1989;16:185.
8. **Avrahami E, Tadmor R, Dally O, et al.** Early MR demonstration of spinal metastases in patients with normal radiographs and CT and radionuclide bone scans. *J Comput Assist Tomogr.* 1989;13:598.

8 PSYCHOLOGICAL EVALUATION

Robert R. Edwards, PhD
Michael T. Smith, PhD
Jennifer A. Haythornthwaite, PhD

OVERVIEW: BIOPSYCHOSOCIAL MODEL OF PAIN

- The experience of pain is not equivalent to nociception, and tissue damage is only one of the factors influencing the experience of pain.
- Biological, psychological, and social factors interact in complex and incompletely understood ways to produce the experience of pain and pain-related sequelae.

- A comprehensive assessment of the patient with chronic pain should attend to mood, pain-coping strategies, areas of disability, and the social environment. Additional consideration should be given to secondary gain and patient–provider interactions.

CRITICAL PSYCHOSOCIAL AND BEHAVIORAL FACTORS

MOOD

FEAR/ANXIETY

- Anxiety in acute pain settings is associated with longer hospital stays, greater acute pain, and increased use of pain medications.
- Fear of pain, particularly activity-related pain such as low back pain, can lead to a debilitating cycle in which the individual becomes increasingly debilitated and pain becomes chronic.[1]
- Pain-related fear may be more disabling than the pain itself.

Assessment Questions
- What activities do you avoid because of your pain?
- What are you worried will happen if you do [this activity]?
- If you do [this activity], do you become anxious or worried about the pain?

DEPRESSION

- Symptoms of depression in the context of chronic pain are associated with increased pain intensity, increased pain behavior, lower daily activity levels and function, and greater interference of pain in daily activities.[2]
- Depression is associated with greater chronicity of pain, and depression has been implicated as a risk factor for the development of chronic pain following acute injury.
- Higher levels of depressive symptoms predict poorer outcome from surgical, medical, and psychological treatment of pain.
- Chronic pain and chronic depression are both risk factors for suicide; the presence of these factors together may be especially dangerous.

Assessment
- The assessment of depression should focus on questions about interest in previously pleasurable activities (eg, sexual activity, hobbies, time with family), changes in concentration, and thoughts about dying, as well as the usual assessment of mood, sleep, appetite, and energy.

Assessment Questions
- *Interest*: Have you experienced any change in your interest or pleasure in activities you used to enjoy? (*Note*: Be careful to distinguish between interest and ability.)
- *Concentration/Memory*: Have you noticed any change in your memory or concentration? Can you follow news stories in the newspaper or on television?
- *Thoughts of Dying*: Have you had thoughts of dying? If yes, what have you thought? How frequently do you have these thoughts? (*Note*: Once or twice is not uncommon, but regular thoughts of dying are a signal to obtain a formal consultation for assessment of depression.)

COPING

- Much of the pain-coping literature distinguishes between active coping strategies (ie, doing something directly about the pain) and passive coping (eg, responding to the pain by cutting back on activities, resting, or looking to others to control the pain).
- Although frequently debated, in general, active coping strategies are associated with better outcomes and higher function, and passive coping strategies are associated with poorer outcomes and lower function in patients with chronic pain syndromes.

CATASTROPHIZING

- The most important dimension of pain coping identified during the past few decades is *catastrophizing*, an emotional, cognitive, and attitudinal response to pain that consistently is associated with greater pain and disability, more pain behavior, negative mood, and worsening depression.[1]
- Although experts debate the conceptual details, catastrophizing appears to serve as a coping strategy by activating negative emotions, which may motivate the individual to deal with the pain or, when expressed to others, may elicit social responses to pain such as emotional support.

Assessment
- Key components of catastrophizing include hypervigilance to bodily sensations, helplessness about controlling the pain, fear that the pain cannot be controlled and will get worse, and pessimism that the pain will never go away.

Assessment Questions
- How frequently do you feel that you cannot stand the pain?
- How often do you feel overwhelmed by the pain?
- How frequently do you worry that the pain will never go away?

- How often do you feel that there is nothing you can do to reduce the pain?

COPING SELF-STATEMENTS

- Coping self-statements are realistic statements individuals make to motivate themselves to deal with pain.
- Some studies have found that the use of coping self-statements is associated with lower pain, less distress, and higher function.[3]
- Training in use of these statements is an integral part of cognitive-behavioral therapy (CBT) for pain management, and these thoughts increase as a result of CBT treatment, although such changes are not consistently associated with better long-term outcomes.

Assessment

- Measuring this coping strategy focuses on the individual's ability to see pain as a challenge that can be dealt with and will improve in the future.

Assessment Questions

- Are there times when you are able to consider the pain as a challenge?
- How often do you think of the pain as something you can deal with?
- How often do you think that the pain will get better in the future?

DISABILITY

GENERAL ISSUES

- Chronic pain is associated with widespread impairment in multiple domains of functioning, ranging from disruption in basic activities of daily living to disruption in psychosocial functioning and work-related activities.[4]
- Physical disability can lead to a debilitating cycle in which the individual becomes increasingly deconditioned and pain is exacerbated.[1]
- A subset of chronic pain patients with high levels of pain, affective distress, and maladaptive coping are at greatest risk for increased disability.[3]

Assessment

- Aside from evaluating the specific domains already addressed, evaluation of pain-related disability should focus on identifying how the pain condition impacts multiple dimensions of the patient's life.

Assessment Questions

- Please describe a typical day.
- What aspects of your daily life are disrupted by your pain?

- What activities do you no longer do because of your pain?

FEAR-AVOIDANCE MODELS OF PAIN-RELATED DISABILITY

- Fear-avoidance models of pain-related disability have received substantial empirical support.[5]
- The extent to which individuals believe that engaging in physical activities will increase pain or result in harm or reinjury is independently associated with self-reported disability and physical capacity evaluations.[5]
- Pain self-efficacy beliefs, that is, an individual's confidence in his or her ability to perform a range of specific tasks despite pain, are inversely related to pain and avoidance behaviors.[6]
- Changes in fear-avoidance beliefs during pain treatment are associated with improvements in disability.[7]

Assessment

- Assessment should focus on eliciting *specific* beliefs and avoiding *specific* physical activities.
- An evaluation of the degree of conviction of fear-avoidance beliefs and the reasons patient give for holding these beliefs is essential.
- Leading with open-ended questions and following up with specific closed-ended questions can be helpful.

Assessment Questions

- Which activities do you believe are likely to cause your pain to worsen?
- Have you had some bad experiences trying to do these kinds of activities?
- How certain are you that engaging in these activities will lead to pain and reinjury?
- What are you concerned might happen if you were to engage in [this particular activity]?

SLEEP DISTURBANCE

- Sleep disturbance is a highly prevalent and often ignored correlate of chronic pain, and sleep problems are associated with increased disability, pain severity, and psychosocial impairment.[8]
- Often a consequence of pain and mood disturbance, sleep disturbance itself may reciprocally exacerbate pain and negative mood.
- Chronic insomnia is often maintained in part by cognitive-behavioral factors in addition to or independent from actual pain.
- Aggressive treatment of sleep disturbance is recommended and often includes: a sleep disorder center evaluation, use of sedating tricyclic antidepressants,

and/or referral for behavioral treatment for insomnia by a behavioral sleep medicine specialist.

Assessment
- Assessing sleep disturbance associated with chronic pain should include consideration of the many contributing factors, including: psychiatric disturbance, intrinsic sleep disorders, medications, substance use, and cognitive-behavioral factors.

Assessment Questions
- Tell me about your sleep. How long does it take you to fall asleep?
- About how long are you awake in the middle of the night or early morning?
- During the daytime, are you often so sleepy that you have to fight to stay awake or do you fall asleep at inappropriate times?
- Are you bothered by intrusive thoughts or worries at night?

WORK-RELATED ISSUES
- Chronic pain conditions often impact a person's ability to work, and work-related factors such as workers' compensation and disability payments can sometimes influence pain behavior and motivation for treatment.
- Predictors of return to work are multifactorial and involve a combination of pain-related factors, nonclinical factors (such as age and education), patients' goals and beliefs about work, and work-related factors (such as availability of modified work programs and workers' compensation status).
- Modified work programs may improve return-to-work rates for workers with work-related injuries.[9,10]

Assessment
- Determine whether the patient's pain condition is associated with a work-related injury, if the patient is receiving disability compensation, and whether legal claims or actions are pending.
- Identify intentions, goals, and barriers related to return to work, bearing in mind that such issues can often be an extreme source of stress to patients.

Assessment Questions
- Were you injured on your job?
- Are you receiving any workers' compensation or other disability payments due to your injury?
- Do you have any pending legal action related to your injury?
- Do you think you will be able to return to work?
- If so, in what capacity?
- What kinds of things do you anticipate will make it difficult for you to resume working?

SOCIAL ENVIRONMENT

FAMILY HISTORY
- Individuals undergoing chronic pain treatment have a disproportionately high likelihood of having a family history of a similar pain condition. This finding is consistent for headache, abdominal pain, and fibromyalgia.
- Chronic pain patients are more likely than controls without pain to report a family history of at least one psychiatric disorder.[11]
- A family history of pain is associated with poor health, more pain complaints, and enhanced sensitivity to pain compared with controls.[12]
- Longitudinal studies suggest that parental modeling and reinforcement of illness behavior in children are related to increased risk of chronic pain as an adult and to health care-seeking behavior.[13]

Assessment
- A standardized assessment of the patient's family history of pain may yield insight into the contribution of social learning to the patient's pain behavior.

Assessment Questions
- Have others in your family had pain conditions?
- How did they cope with the pain?

SOCIAL SUPPORT
- Individuals with chronic pain are more likely than controls to report current and past distress related to family relationships.[11]
- Perceived social support is positively related to health and inversely related to pain and disability ratings across a number of chronic pain conditions, and poor social support is associated with greater use of inpatient and outpatient medical services.
- The relationship between distress and pain is strongest in those with minimal social support[14]; a positive social environment may buffer the negative effects of pain-related distress.
- Interventions that enhance social support can reduce pain and disability.

Assessment
- An assessment should take into account the amount and the perceived quality of social relationships as well as the patient's preferences regarding the degree of social contact (eg, "I would like to have other people to talk to").

Assessment Questions
- How are the social and family relationships in your life?

- How has your pain affected those relationships?
- Are the people in your life providing the support you need?

SOCIAL INTERACTIONS

- Pain behavior is, like all behavior, at least partially under operant control. That is, it is influenced by the response of the environment to the behavior. In fact, researchers have found that chronic back pain patients are more susceptible to operant conditioning than are controls.[15]
- Solicitous behavior (attention to pain and, sometimes, encouragement of disability) on the part of a spouse or significant other is associated with higher ratings of pain among chronic pain patients, and greater marital satisfaction is associated with increased severity of pain, presumably because it is associated with solicitous behavior.[16]
- Marital conflict and negative responses by a spouse are also associated with higher reports of pain among pain patients (possibly as a result of increased distress).
- In contrast, family members who support a patient's efforts to cope with pain may promote improved adjustment to pain.[2]
- Aspects of the social environment may interact with an individual's coping style; catastrophizing may activate the social environment so the patient gains support from others.[17] It is not known how well these efforts work.

Assessment
- Any interview should include a structured or unstructured assessment of the patient's perception of others' responses to pain behavior.
- If a family member is present for some part of the evaluation, behavioral observation of interactions with the patient, the family member's level of support, and specific actions taken in response to pain behavior can be extremely useful.

Assessment Questions
- How does (the person of interest) react when you are in pain?
- How do others help when you are in pain?
- Are there ways that they make things worse?

SECONDARY GAIN

- *Primary gain* refers to the relief of distress by a bodily symptom, and *secondary gain* refers to the benefits to an individual that arise from the development of one or more symptoms.

- *Sick role* refers to a constellation of behaviors that are frequently assumed to be reinforced by one or more secondary gains.
- Many secondary gains have been identified[18]:
  ○ Financial compensation associated with injury or disability.
  ○ Conversion of a socially unacceptable disability (eg, psychiatric disorder) into a socially acceptable disability (eg, chronic physical condition).
  ○ Elicitation of care and sympathy from family and friends.
  ○ Avoidance of an unpleasant or unsatisfactory life role or activity (eg, a disliked job, undesirable family responsibilities).
  ○ Increased ease of access to desired drugs and medications.
  ○ Increased control over family members.
- There are currently no good estimates of the prevalence of secondary gain factors among chronic pain patients.

Assessment
- Assessment of secondary gain is notoriously difficult, especially in the context of brief contacts in a medical setting.
- The rate of false positives when attempting to identify individuals in whom secondary gain is prominent is probably unacceptably high.

Assessment Questions
- Do you have any litigation pending at this time?
- If so, when do you think this will be resolved?
- What do you hope to get from any settlement?
- What would things be like if you no longer had pain?

PSYCHOLOGICAL ASPECTS OF PATIENT–PROVIDER INTERACTIONS

- Listening carefully, answering questions, encouraging dialogue, and making clear statements are among the key components of good patient–provider communication.[19] Benefits include improved patient compliance with medical regimens, reduced likelihood of litigation, and improved patient satisfaction with care.
- Research has targeted improving physician–patient relationships as a way of reducing health care utilization. Merely providing patients with a regular source of care does not generally reduce their emergency room usage,[20] although improved communication and patient education seem to be effective.
- Self-management programs, in which patients take an active role in their own health care and focus on adaptive efforts to manage symptoms, improve symptoms, reduce utilization, and improve communication.

- High users of medical services are often characterized by dissonance between themselves and their physician. This dissonance is characterized by such factors as poor patient understanding of the condition, lack of agreement about diagnosis and/or treatment goals, and unclear follow-up plans.
- Relying on patient reports of satisfaction with pain management may lead to overestimates of the quality of care, as many patients report "very good" care even when experiencing inadequate pain relief.
- Patient satisfaction does not correlate with pain ratings at admission or discharge or with change in pain over the course of a hospital stay.[21]

POTENTIAL BIASES ON THE PART OF HEALTH CARE PROVIDERS

- Health care providers often underestimate the pain and disability levels of their patients, and this bias is strongest when the patients are elderly or are members of an ethnic minority group.
- There is little evidence for the validity of expert judgments regarding a chronic pain patient's likely prognosis. For example, among back pain patients followed longitudinally, no relationship was observed between providers' estimates of patients' rehabilitation potential and actual rehabilitation outcomes.[22]
- While some patients may inspire suspicion that their reports of pain are exaggerated or feigned, no accepted methodology exists for detecting malingering. Individuals instructed to simulate or "fake" pain produce higher scores on measures of pain, distress, and impairment than actual pain patients, but cutoff scores with acceptable sensitivity and specificity have not been identified.
- The prevalence of opioid abuse and dependence among patients with chronic pain is consistently overestimated by health care providers.

RECOMMENDATIONS FOR HEALTH CARE PROVIDERS

- Develop standardized assessments of psychosocial factors, such as mood, coping, and social relationships, even if they are as brief as single questions.
- If time and resources are available, assessment of psychosocial factors should include an interview, behavioral observations, and one or more standardized instruments.
- Disability is often not strongly related to pain; assessment of other factors that may contribute to disability (eg, depression) may help with treatment plans.

- Familiarity with local resources, such as support groups and community mental health centers, can facilitate treatment of patients with pain.
- When feasible, involving a spouse or significant other may enhance the effectiveness of behavioral interventions (ie, coping skills training, exercise programs).
- True malingering is probably rare in chronic pain patients, and the impact of secondary gain issues is not well understood; the grounds for disbelieving a patient's report of pain are rarely tenable.
- To whatever extent possible, encourage patients to be "self-managers" of their pain. That is, provide them with one or more concrete strategies or goals (eg, 5 minutes per day of stretching exercises, simple relaxation techniques, leaving the house at least once a day) to pursue on their own.
- Assess your communication skills: How well do you educate patients about their condition? How well do you listen when they speak? How much input do your patients have regarding treatment decisions? How clearly do you describe treatment goals?

REFERENCES

1. **Picavet HS, Vlaeyen JW, Schouten JS.** Pain catastrophizing and kinesophobia: Predictors of chronic low back pain. *Am J Epidemiol.* 2002;156:1028.
2. **Keefe FJ, Lumley M, Anderson T, et al.** Pain and emotion: New research directions. *J Clin Psychol.* 2001;57:587.
3. **Turk DC, Okifuji A.** Psychological factors in chronic pain: Evolution and revolution. *J Consult Clin Psychol.* 2002; 70:678.
4. **Ehde DM, Jensen MP, Engel JM, et al.** Chronic pain secondary to disability: A review. *Clin J Pain.* 2003;19:3.
5. **Vowles KE, Gross RT.** Work-related beliefs about injury and physical capability for work in individuals with chronic pain. *Pain.* 2003;101:291.
6. **Asghari A, Nicholas MK.** Pain self-efficacy beliefs and pain behaviour: A prospective study. *Pain.* 2001;94:85.
7. **Jensen MP, Turner JA, Romano JM.** Changes in beliefs, catastrophizing, and coping are associated with improvement in multidisciplinary pain treatment. *J Consult Clin Psychol.* 2001;69:655.
8. **Wilson KG, Eriksson MY, D'Eon JL, et al.** Major depression and insomnia in chronic pain. *Clin J Pain.* 2002;18:77.
9. **Nielson WR, Weir R.** Biopsychosocial approaches to the treatment of chronic pain. *Clin J Pain.* 2001;17:S114.
10. **Weir R, Nielson WR.** Interventions for disability management. *Clin J Pain.* 2001;17:S128.
11. **Burke P, Elliott M, Fleissner R.** Irritable bowel syndrome and recurrent abdominal pain: A comparative review. *Psychosomatics.* 1999;40:277.

12. **Fillingim RB, Edwards RR, Powell T.** Sex-dependent effects of reported familial pain history on recent pain complaints and experimental pain responses. *Pain.* 2000;86:87.

13. **Whitehead WE, Palsson O, Jones KR.** Systematic review of the comorbidity of irritable bowel syndrome with other disorders: What are the causes and implications? *Gastroenterology.* 2002;122:1140.

14. **Alonso C, Coe CL.** Disruptions of social relationships accentuate the association between emotional distress and menstrual pain in young women. *Health Psychol.* 2001;20:411.

15. **Flor H, Knost B, Birbaumer N.** The role of operant conditioning in chronic pain: An experimental investigation. *Pain.* 2002;95:111.

16. **Flor H, Turk DC, Scholz OB.** Impact of chronic pain on the spouse: Marital, emotional and physical consequences. *J Psychosom Res.* 1987;31(1):63–71.

17. **Sullivan MJ, Thorn B, Haythornthwaite JA, et al.** Theoretical perspectives on the relation between catastrophizing and pain. *Clin J Pain.* 2001;17:52.

18. **Ferrari R, Kwan O.** The no-fault flavor of disability syndromes. *Med Hypotheses.* 2001;56:77.

19. **Sarver JH, Cydulka RK, Baker DW.** Usual source of care and nonurgent emergency department use. *Acad Emerg Med.* 2002;9:916.

20. **Boushy D, Dubinsky I.** Primary care physician and patient factors that result in patients seeking emergency care in a hospital setting: The patient's perspective. *J Emerg Med.* 1999;17:405.

21. **Kelly AM.** Patient satisfaction with pain management does not correlate with initial or discharge VAS pain score, verbal pain rating at discharge, or change in VAS score in the emergency department. *J Emerg Med.* 2000;19:113.

22. **Jensen IB, Bodin L, Ljungqvist T, et al.** Assessing the needs of patients in pain: A matter of opinion? *Spine.* 2000; 25:2816.

9 TOPICAL AGENTS

Bradley S. Galer, MD
Arnold R. Gammaitoni, PharmD

RATIONALE FOR USE

- Peripheral mechanisms of pain are inherent in most chronic pain states including peripheral neuropathies, rheumatologic conditions, and musculoskeletal conditions. These mechanisms are believed to be clinically relevant sources of pain and, thus, appropriate targets for drug therapy.[1]
- Targeted peripheral (or topically applied) analgesics (TPAs), by definition, produce their pharmacologic action solely by local activity in the peripheral tissues, nerves, and/or soft tissues, without producing clinically significant serum drug levels.[2] Unlike transdermal agents, which are specifically formulated to produce a systemic effect (eg, the fentanyl patch), TPAs have a reduced risk of producing systemic side effects or drug–drug interactions.[3] This is particularly advantageous in patients with chronic pain conditions who are often receiving numerous systemic medications for multiple medical conditions.
- Three TPAs are currently available in the United States: lidocaine patch 5% (Lidoderm, Endo Pharmaceuticals Inc., Chadds Ford, Pa); capsaicin cream or lotion (Zostrix, GenDerm, Scottsdale, Ariz); and eutectic mixture of lidocaine 2.5% and prilocaine 2.5% (EMLA, AstraZeneca Pharmaceuticals LP, Wilmington, Del). In Europe, nonsteroidal anti-inflammatory drugs (NSAIDs) delivered topically in patches and gels are also available. This review focuses on the aforementioned three TPAs that are currently prescribed in the United States.

LIDOCAINE PATCH 5%

FORMULATION

- The lidocaine patch 5% is a 10×14-cm topical patch composed of an adhesive material containing 5% lidocaine (700 mg) in an aqueous base, which is applied to a nonwoven polyester felt backing and covered with a polyethylene terephthalate film-release liner. The release liner is removed prior to application.[4]

MECHANISM OF ACTION

- Lidocaine blocks abnormal activity in neuronal sodium channels,[5] which are believed to play a critical role in the etiology of many types of pain, in both its initiation and its maintenance.[6]
- In neuropathic pain, animal models have demonstrated an upregulation of abnormal sodium channels on the damaged sensory peripheral nerve.[6,7]
- In inflammatory conditions, such as osteoarthritis, animal studies have reported clinically active abnormal sodium channels, which, when antagonized, reduce spontaneous nociceptive activity and alleviate pain behaviors of the rodent[8] and, therefore, provide a novel target for the lidocaine patch 5%.
- Lidocaine has also been shown to inhibit the expression of nitric oxide and subsequent release of pro-inflammatory cytokines from T cells and, thus, provides another potential analgesic mechanism for the lidocaine patch in the treatment of inflammatory pain conditions.[9]
- In addition to its sodium channel–blocking activity, the lidocaine patch acts as a protective barrier against cutaneous stimuli for patients with allodynia.[1,7]

- Importantly and uniquely, the novel formulation of the lidocaine patch delivers sufficient levels of lidocaine to the local tissues to produce an analgesic effect (pain relief) without anesthesia (sensory deficits, ie, "numbness").[2]

EFFICACY

- Table 9–1 summarizes clinical studies of the lidocaine patch 5%.

NEUROPATHIC PAIN

Postherpetic Neuralgia
- The lidocaine patch is the first drug ever approved by the US Food and Drug Administration (FDA) for a neuropathic pain disorder, that is, postherpetic neuralgia (PHN).[4]

- The lidocaine patch has been confirmed in several randomized controlled studies to be of benefit in PHN.[7,10,11]
- In patients with PHN and moderate allodynia, the lidocaine patch significantly reduces pain intensity compared with observation or a vehicle patch. Most patients experience at least moderate pain relief. In one study of refractory PHN, 24 of 35 patients reported slight or better pain relief (averaging scores at 4 and 6 hours), and 10 patients reported moderate or better relief.[7]
- In an enriched enrollment study of 32 patients with PHN who were known responders to the lidocaine patch, the lidocaine patch provided significantly more pain relief than a vehicle patch, using "time to exit" as the primary endpoint.[10]
- The lidocaine patch was superior to a vehicle patch in reducing all common pain qualities associated with

TABLE 9–1 Lidocaine Patch 5% Evidence Base

POPULATION	DESIGN	RESULTS
PHN[7]	Randomized, double-blind, crossover controlled study: $N=35$; four single sessions (12 h): 2 with lidocaine patch, 1 with vehicle patch (double-blind), and 1 with observation only	Reduced pain intensity significantly vs vehicle (at 4, 6, 9, and 12 h; $P<0.05$) and observation (at all time points from 30 min to 12 h; $P<0.05$)
PHN (responders to lidocaine patch >1 mo before trial)[10]	Randomized, double-blind, placebo-controlled, enriched enrollment study: $N=32$; patients randomized to lidocaine patch or vehicle, then switched to other Tx after maximum of 14 d or when pain relief worsened by ≥2 categories on 2 consecutive days	Median time to exit >14 d vs 3.8 d with vehicle ($P<0.001$)
PHN[11]	Randomized, double-blind, parallel-design study: $N=96$; 3-wk duration	Significant improvement in all common neuropathic pain qualities ($P<0.05$); potential benefit for nonallodynic pain states
PHN[12]	Open-label, nonrandomized, effectiveness study: $N=332$; 28-d duration	Statistically significant reductions in pain intensity and pain interference with quality of life ($P=0.001$); approximately 60% of patients reported moderate to complete pain relief
Peripheral neuropathic pain conditions[13]	Randomized, double-blind, controlled trial: $N=58$; 1-wk duration	Significant reduction in pain vs placebo ($P≤0.05$)
Refractory neuropathic pain with allodynia[14]	Open-label prospective study: $N=16$; mean duration 6.2 wk for 15 patients (1 patient dropped out after 4 d due to lack of relief)	13 patients (87%) experienced moderate or better pain relief with lidocaine patch
Diabetic neuropathy[15]	Nonrandomized, open-label, pilot study: $N=56$; 3-wk therapy	Significant reductions in overall pain intensity ($P<0.001$), and improvements in common pain qualities ($P<0.05$) and functional outcomes ($P<0.005$)
HIV peripheral neuropathy[16]	Nonrandomized, open-label, pilot study: $N=16$; 4-wk therapy	Significant reductions in pain intensity ($P<0.05$), and improvements in common pain qualities ($P≤0.001$) and functional outcomes ($P<0.05$)
Low back pain of varying duration from acute through chronic[17]	Nonrandomized, open-label, pilot study: $N=129$; 2-wk therapy	Significant reductions in overall pain intensity, and improvements in common pain qualities and functional outcomes ($P<0.0001$)
Myofascial pain, moderate to severe intensity, with identifiable trigger points; 66.6% had low-back pain[19]	Nonrandomized, open-label study: $N=27$; 28-d duration	Significant improvements in average pain intensity, walking, ability to work, and sleep ($P<0.05$); 30% of patients experienced moderate/better relief
Osteoarthritis pain of 1 or both knees[20]	Nonrandomized, open-label, pilot study: $N=167$; 135 patients with lidocaine patch as add-on therapy and 32 as monotherapy; 2-wk duration	Significant reductions in overall pain intensity and improvements in functional outcomes and QOL ($P<0.0001$)

PHN, postherpetic neuralgia; QOL, quality of life.

neuropathic pain (eg, "burning," "dull," "deep," "superficial," and "sharp" pains) in a 3-week, prospective, randomized, controlled trial of 96 patients with PHN.[11]
- Statistically significant reductions in pain interference with quality of life were noted with the lidocaine patch in a large (*N* = 332), open-label, effectiveness study.[12]

Peripheral Neuropathic Pain (other than PHN)
- A randomized, controlled trial demonstrated significant benefit of the lidocaine patch over placebo in patients with diverse peripheral neuropathic pain conditions (ie, PHN, diabetic neuropathy, stump neuralgia, postsurgical neuralgia, meralgia paresthetica).[13]
- In an open-label trial, the lidocaine patch improved pain in patients with a variety of refractory neuropathic conditions with allodynia, including postthoracotomy pain, stump neuroma pain, intercostal neuralgia, painful diabetic polyneuropathy, meralgia paresthetica, complex regional pain syndrome, radiculopathy, and postmastectomy pain[14]: 13 of 16 patients reported moderate or better pain relief with the lidocaine patch.

Painful Diabetic Neuropathy
- The lidocaine patch may have clinical utility in the treatment of painful diabetic neuropathy. Data from a multicenter, open-label, pilot study indicate that the lidocaine patch significantly reduces overall pain intensity, improves commonly reported pain qualities, and results in improved functional outcomes in patients with painful diabetic neuropathy with and without allodynia.[15]

HIV-Associated Neuropathy
- In a multicenter, open-label, pilot study reported the lidocaine patch significantly reduced overall pain intensity, improved common pain qualities, and resulted in improved functional outcomes in patients with painful HIV-associated neuropathy.[16]

Erythromelalgia
- According to a recently published case report, the lidocaine patch significantly relieved the pain of erythromelalgia of the feet in a 15-year-old girl.[17]

OTHER PAIN STATES

Low Back Pain
- Several clinical reports have described successful treatment of chronic low back pain patients with the addition of the lidocaine patch to analgesic regimens, with patches applied directly over the painful back region.[18,19]
- In a multicenter, prospective, open-label study, the lidocaine patch significantly improved all common pain qualities and functionality in 129 patients with acute, subacute, and chronic low back pain.[18]

Myofascial Pain
- A prospective, single-site, open-label trial has reported successful treatment of regional, chronic, refractory, myofascial pain with the lidocaine patch. Statistically significant mean improvements were noted for average daily pain intensity and pain interference with general activity, walking, ability to work, relationships, sleep, and enjoyment of life.[20]

Osteoarthritis
- Both a large, multicenter, prospective, open-label trial and a Letter to the Editor from a practicing rheumatologist have reported significant clinical benefit from the lidocaine patch in the treatment of osteoarthritis (OA).[21]
- A large prospective trial of 167 patients with osteoarthritis demonstrated that placing the lidocaine patch directly on the skin of an osteoarthritic knee results in statistically significant improvements in the pain, stiffness, physical function, and composite indices measured by the validated Western Ontario and McMaster Universities Osteoarthritis Index.[21]
- Additional randomized, controlled trials are needed to further validate the efficacy and safety of the lidocaine patch in conditions other than PHN.

SIDE EFFECTS

- A major clinical advantage to all TPAs, such as the lidocaine patch 5%, is their lack of clinically significant systemic activity.[2]
- Only a small amount (ie, 3±2%) of lidocaine has been found to be absorbed in healthy subjects treated with the lidocaine patch.[2,4,5]
- Side effects appear to be limited to mild skin irritation at the lidocaine patch application site.[2,4,5]
- The most common adverse reactions are local, in the skin region directly underlying the patch, and generally tend to be mild, resolving without the need for intervention.[2,15,18,21]
  ○ Application site burning: 1.8%
  ○ Dermatitis: 1.8%
  ○ Pruritis: 1.1%
  ○ Rash: <1%
- No serious systemic adverse events have been related to treatment with the lidocaine patch in six recent clinical trials to date.[2,15,18,21] Of the 450 patients

studied in these trials, the most frequently reported systemic adverse event was mild to moderate headache (1.8%). Other less common systemic adverse events included dizziness and somnolence (<1%).

DOSAGE AND ADMINISTRATION

- The current FDA-approved labeling recommends that patients apply up to three lidocaine patches to the most painful areas of intact skin and wear them no longer than 12 hours in a 24-hour period.[4] Patients should be instructed to cover as much of the painful area as possible.
- Increasing the dosage to four lidocaine patches applied either once daily for 24 hours or twice daily every 12 hours for 3 consecutive days was shown to be safe and well-tolerated in a pharmacokinetic study of 20 normal subjects. Plasma lidocaine levels were approximately 14.3% of those associated with cardiac activity and 4% of those typically associated with toxicity. Continuous 24-hour application of up to four lidocaine patches was safe and well-tolerated in recent studies of patients with low back pain and osteoarthritis.[18,21]
- A regimen of four lidocaine patches worn 18 h/d for 3 consecutive days also was shown to be well-tolerated in 20 normal subjects.[2] This "18-hours-on, 6-hours-off" regimen with a maximum of four lidocaine patches was used successfully in a trial of patients with diabetic neuropathy ($N=56$).[15]
- The lidocaine patch 5% should be used with caution in patients with severe hepatic disease and in those receiving antiarrhythmic or local anesthetic drugs.[4]
- One to two weeks of therapy with the lidocaine patch may be required to determine whether a patient will experience satisfactory relief. However, one study reported that a small subgroup of patients with PHN required up to 4 weeks of treatment with the lidocaine patch to obtain maximal benefit.[15] No dose escalation is necessary and tolerance does not develop with the lidocaine patch.[10,22]

TOPICAL CAPSAICIN

FORMULATION

- Capsaicin (*trans*-8-methyl-*N*-vanillyl-6-nonenamide), a naturally occurring substance, is a component of the red chili pepper.
- For many centuries, even prior to the advent of clinical study, the contents of the chili pepper have been compounded into topical mixtures for the treatment of a variety of pains.

- Capsaicin is available in the United States without prescription as a cream or lotion in strengths of 0.025% and 0.075%.[23]
- Medicinally available capsaicin is a natural mixture of several different active chemicals and has not actually obtained a full FDA new drug application approval.

MECHANISM OF ACTION

- Several different potential analgesic mechanisms of action have been postulated for topically applied capsaicin.

SUBSTANCE P DEPLETION
- One theory of the analgesic effect of capsaicin is the depletion of substance P from presynaptic terminals, which depresses the function of type C nociceptive fibers (substance P is one of the principal mediators of pain).[24]

NEURODEGENERATION
- Recent animal and human studies have demonstrated that topical application of capsaicin to the skin results in damage to the underlying nociceptive peripheral nerves.[25,26] One study found that application of capsaicin cream 0.075% to human skin four times daily for 3 weeks results in a reduction in the average number of epidermal nerve fibers by 82% compared with pretreatment values.[26] Epidermal innervation recovered gradually to nearly 83% of normal at 6 weeks after discontinuing capsaicin usage. The investigators concluded that neurodegeneration may account for the pain relief associated with capsaicin.

EFFICACY

- Table 9–2 summarizes clinical trials of capsaicin cream.

NEUROPATHIC PAIN

Postherpetic Neuralgia
- Two randomized, controlled studies reported statistically significant pain reduction with capsaicin in patients with PHN.[27,28] In one trial, 54% of patients treated with capsaicin and 6% of control subjects reported ≥40% pain relief after 6 weeks of therapy ($P=0.02$); however, it should be noted that this trial failed to use an intent-to-treat efficacy analysis.[27]

Chronic Neuropathic Pain
- One randomized, controlled study demonstrated the efficacy of capsaicin compared with placebo for the treatment of a variety of neuropathic conditions.[29]

TABLE 9–2 Capsaicin Evidence Base

POPULATION	DESIGN	RESULTS
PHN >12 mo[27]	Randomized, double-blind, vehicle-controlled: N=32; capsaicin cream 0.075% or vehicle applied 3–4 times/d for 6 wk	Significant decrease in pain with capsaicin vs control (P<0.05)
PHN >6 mo[28]	Randomized, double-blind, vehicle-controlled: N=131; capsaicin cream 0.075% or vehicle applied 4 times/d for 6 wk	Significant improvements in pain with capsaicin vs vehicle (P<0.05)
Chronic neuropathic pain[29]	Randomized, double-blind, placebo-controlled: N=200; placebo cream, doxepin 3.3%/capsaicin 0.025% cream, or doxepin 3.3%/capsaicin 0.025% cream 3 times/d for 4 wk	Significant reductions in overall pain scores in all 3 treatment groups (P<0.001); overall pain relief was similar among groups
Postmastectomy pain >5 mo[30]	Randomized, parallel, double-blind, vehicle-controlled trial: N=25; capsaicin cream 0.075% or vehicle applied 4 times/d for 6 wk	Significantly greater improvement in jabbing pain and pain relief with capsaicin than with vehicle (P<0.05)
Diabetic neuropathy and radiculopathy[31]	Randomized, double-blind, vehicle-controlled trial: N=252; capsaicin cream 0.075% or vehicle applied 4 times/d for 8 wk	Significantly greater pain relief and improvement in pain intensity (P<0.05)
Diabetic neuropathy[32]	Randomized, double-blind, vehicle-controlled trial: N=22; capsaicin cream 0.075% or vehicle applied 4 times/d for 8 wk	Significantly more capsaicin patients had overall improvement (P<0.05)
Variety of painful polyneuropathies[33]	Randomized, double-blind, placebo-controlled study	No improvement vs placebo
HIV-associated peripheral neuropathy[34]	Randomized, double-masked, controlled, multicenter trial: N=26; capsaicin cream 0.075% or vehicle applied 4 times/d for 4 wk	Current pain scores were worse at 1 wk with capsaicin patients vs vehicle (P<0.05); no other statistically significant differences in pain measures; dropout rate was significantly higher with capsaicin
OA and RA, moderate to very severe knee pain[35]	Randomized, double-blind, vehicle-controlled: N=70 (OA) and N=31 (RA); capsaicin cream 0.025% or vehicle applied 4 times/d for 4 wk	Significantly greater reduction in pain scores vs placebo (OA: P<0.05; RA: P=0.003)
OA[36]	Randomized, double-blind, vehicle-controlled: N=200; patients randomized to vehicle, capsaicin cream 0.025%, glyceryl trinitrate 1.33%, or capsaicin cream 0.025% +glyceryl trinitrate cream 1.33% for 6 wk	Capsaicin+glyceryl trinitrate was more effective than either agent alone in reducing pain scores (P<0.05); each agent alone and combination significantly reduced pain vs baseline (P<0.05)

OA, osteoarthritis; PHN, postherpetic neuralgia; RA, rheumatoid arthritis.

Postmastectomy Pain
- A randomized, controlled study found capsaicin to be efficacious compared with placebo in the treatment of postmastectomy pain: 46% of patients receiving capsaicin were satisfied with the pain relief and tolerability of this agent.[30]

Painful Diabetic Neuropathy
- Two randomized trials reported that capsaicin produced significant pain relief in patients with painful diabetic neuropathy.[31,32]

Painful Polyneuropathy
- A randomized, double-blind, placebo-controlled study from the Mayo Clinic reported negative results in patients with chronic distal painful polyneuropathy treated with capsaicin cream.[33]

HIV-Associated Neuropathy
- Capsaicin failed to demonstrate benefit in HIV-associated peripheral neuropathy.[34]

OTHER PAIN STATES

Osteoarthritis and Rheumatoid Arthritis
- In a randomized, double-blind, controlled trial, capsaicin was significantly superior to vehicle in reducing pain scores compared with baseline for patients with osteoarthritis or rheumatoid arthritis.[35]
- In another randomized, double-blind, controlled trial, the combination of glyceryl trinitrate cream 1.33% and topical capsaicin 0.025% was more effective in osteoarthritis than either agent alone.[36] Because pain relief was not immediate, it was concluded that capsaicin cream is more appropriate treatment for background pain than for acute flares.

Periocular and Facial Pain
- Case reports have indicated that capsaicin has some benefit in periocular or facial pain (if patients can describe a trigger point and have a history of nerve damage).[24]

Neurogenic Residual Limb Pain
- Case reports have described relief in neurogenic residual limb pain with capsaicin treatment.[37]

SIDE EFFECTS

- A major clinical advantage to all TPAs, such as capsaicin, is their lack of clinically significant systemic activity. Thus, minimal systemic side effects or drug–drug interactions have been demonstrated with appropriate use of capsaicin.

BURNING SENSATION AT APPLICATION SITE
- A major clinically significant side effect associated with topical capsaicin is a burning or stinging sensation at the application site.
- From 30%[27] to 92%[30] of patients experience a burning or stinging sensation after application of capsaicin. This reaction usually diminishes with time (after 3 days to 2 weeks of regular use),[27,30] but also seriously limits patient compliance with treatment.[22] Capsaicin cream 0.025% may be more tolerable than the 0.075% preparation.[22]
- Combining capsaicin with topical doxepin 3.3%, a tricyclic antidepressant,[29] or glyceryl trinitrate cream 1.33%[36] has been reported to attenuate the burning effect of capsaicin.
- The burning sensation associated with capsaicin complicates the blinding of clinical trials.

BURNING SENSATION IN OTHER BODILY REGIONS
- Patients must be instructed to wash their hands immediately following capsaicin application. Failure to do so with subsequent touching of sensitive bodily regions (eg, eyes, mucous membranes, broken or irritated skin, genitalia) can result in an immediate severe burning sensation.[23]

SNEEZING AND COUGHING
- If inhaled, capsaicin can be an irritant to the nose and lungs. Sneezing and coughing, therefore, are observed occasionally with capsaicin treatment.[30,31]

DOSAGE AND ADMINISTRATION

- Topical capsaicin cream generally is applied three or four times daily.[23]
- Topical capsaicin should be applied in a well-ventilated area and thinly enough to prevent formation of a layered or caked residue.[31] Patients should consider wearing a plastic glove or using a cotton applicator to apply the medication.[23]

- The treated area should not be washed for at least 1 hour after application.[36]
- Pain relief usually is noted within 2–6 weeks,[27,38] although one trial in patients with osteoarthritis or rheumatoid arthritis recorded significant relief at 1 week.[35]

EUTECTIC MIXTURE OF LOCAL ANESTHETICS

FORMULATION

- Eutectic mixture of local anesthetics (EMLA) cream (lidocaine 2.5% and prilocaine 2.5%) generally is applied to intact skin under an occlusive dressing.[39]
- EMLA is indicated as a topical anesthetic for use on normal intact skin for local analgesia and on genital mucous membranes for superficial minor surgery and as pretreatment for infiltration anesthesia.[40]

MECHANISM OF ACTION

- EMLA causes an anesthetic effect (sensory loss) in the skin area to which it is applied by producing an absolute sodium channel blockade of sensory nerves, resulting in a dense anesthesia. (Note: This is in contradistinction to the lidocaine patch 5%, which does not produce anesthesia, but only analgesia.)[39]
- The onset of skin anesthesia depends primarily on the amount of cream applied. Skin anesthesia increases for 2–3 hours under an occlusive dressing and persists for 1–2 hours after removal. EMLA should be used with caution in patients receiving class 1 antiarrhythmic agents.[39]

EFFICACY

- Table 9–3 summarizes clinical studies of EMLA cream.

POSTOPERATIVE PAIN SKIN ANESTHESIA
- Multiple randomized controlled studies have demonstrated the clinical efficacy of EMLA for its approved skin anesthetic indication.[40]

POSTHERPETIC NEURALGIA
- In one small study (*N*=12), EMLA cream 5% applied for 24-hour periods significantly improved mean pain intensity 6 hours after application as measured by a visual analog scale.[41]

TABLE 9–3 EMLA Evidence Base

POPULATION	DESIGN	RESULTS
Refractory PHN[41]	Open-label study: $N=12$; EMLA cream 5% applied for 24-h periods	Significant decrease in pain intensity after 6 h ($P<0.05$)
PHN, spontaneous and evoked pain[37]	Open-label study: $N=11$; EMLA cream 5% applied daily for 5 h/d for 6 d	No significant reduction in ongoing pain intensity and mechanical allodynia, but repeated applications significantly reduced paroxysmal pain ($P<0.05$) and dynamic and static mechanical hyperalgesia ($P<0.01$); significant improvements in spontaneous ongoing pain were seen only in patients with mechanical allodynia
Postoperative pain (acute/chronic)[43]	Double-blind, randomized, placebo-controlled study: $N=45$; EMLA cream 5% or placebo applied preoperatively and then daily for 4 d postoperatively	No significant reduction in acute pain at rest or with movement; time to first analgesic requirement ($P=0.04$) and analgesic consumption on days 2–5 ($P<0.01$) significantly better for EMLA vs placebo; 3 mo postoperatively, pain in chest wall and axilla, and total incidence and intensity of chronic pain were significantly less in EMLA group ($P=0.004$, $P=0.025$, $P=0.002$, and $P=0.003$, respectively)

PHN, postherpetic neuralgia.

• In another small study ($N=11$), 5% EMLA cream applied daily under an adhesive occlusive dressing for 5 h/d for 6 days had no significant effect on mean ongoing pain intensity as measured by a visual analog scale.[42] However, eight patients reported that the number of painful attacks decreased by $\geq50\%$. EMLA had significant benefit in a subset of eight patients with tactile allodynia.

ACUTE AND CHRONIC POSTSURGICAL PAIN

• In one double-blind, randomized study of women undergoing breast surgery for cancer ($N=45$), EMLA cream 5% or placebo was applied 5 minutes prior to surgery and daily for 4 days during the postsurgical period. Acute pain at rest and with movement in the chest wall, axilla, and/or medial upper arm was assessed by visual analog scale. Acute pain at rest and with movement did not differ between the EMLA and control groups, and the analgesics consumed during the first 24 hours were the same. However, time to the first analgesia requirement was longer and analgesic consumption during the second to fifth days was less in the EMLA group. Three months postoperatively, pain in the chest wall and axilla and total incidence and intensity of chronic pain were significantly less in the EMLA group than the control group. Use of analgesics at home and abnormal sensations did not differ between the two groups.[43]

SIDE EFFECTS

• A major clinical advantage to all TPAs, such as EMLA, is their lack of clinically significant systemic activity. Thus, minimal systemic side effects or drug–drug interactions have been noted with appropriate use of EMLA.[40]
• The peak blood levels of lidocaine and prilocaine absorbed with the application of EMLA 60 g to 400 cm² are well below systemic toxicity levels.[40]
• Treatment with EMLA results in localized reactions in 56% of patients. These reactions are usually mild and transient, resolving spontaneously within 1–2 hours.[40]
• The most commonly reported local adverse reactions include[40]:
  ○ Pallor/blanching: 37%
  ○ Erythema: 30%
  ○ Temperature sensation alteration: 7%
  ○ Edema: 6%
  ○ Itching: 2%
  ○ Rash: <1%
• EMLA should not be used in patients with congenital or idiopathic methemoglobinemia or in those taking drugs associated with drug-induced methemoglobinemia.[40]

DOSAGE AND ADMINISTRATION

• A thick layer of EMLA should be applied to intact skin and covered with an occlusive dressing.[40]
• Dermal analgesia can be expected to increase for up to 3 hours and continue for 1–2 hours after removal of EMLA.[40]
• Although the incidence of systemic adverse events with EMLA is very low, caution should be used, especially when applying it over large areas of skin and leaving it on longer than >3 hours.[40]

TOPICAL NONSTEROIDAL ANTI-INFLAMMATORY DRUGS

FORMULATIONS

• Topical NSAIDs are not currently available in the United States. A topical diclofenac patch preparation is in phase 3 trials for the treatment of acute minor sports injury pain. In Europe and Asia, multiple topical NSAIDs are available as patches, gels, and creams.

EFFICACY

• In Europe and Asia, topical NSAIDs have several approved registration indications, including sports injury and osteoarthritis pains.
• Based on an extensive scientific review of the literature, the Cochrane Study Group reported that topical NSAIDs have proven short-term efficacy for the treatment of lateral elbow pain.[44]
• A quantitative review concluded that at least one in three patients who use a topical NSAID (eg, ibuprofen, ketoprofen, felbinac, piroxicam) achieve a successful outcome compared with those treated with placebo.[45] Forty trials of topical NSAIDs in acute pain (eg, recent soft tissue injuries, sprains, strains, trauma) and 13 in chronic rheumatologic conditions were reviewed.

SIDE EFFECTS

• A major clinical advantage of all TPAs such as NSAIDs is their lack of clinically significant systemic activity. Thus, minimal systemic side effects or drug–drug interactions have been demonstrated with appropriate use of topical NSAIDs.[44,45]
• According to a review article on topical NSAIDs, local skin reactions were rare (3.6%), as were systemic effects (<0.5%).[45]

REFERENCES

1. **Galer BS.** Topical drugs for the treatment of pain. In: Loeser JD, ed. *Bonica's Managment of Pain.* 3rd ed. Hagerstown, Md: Lippincott Williams & Wilkins; 2001:2.

2. **Gammaitoni AR, Davis MW.** Pharmacokinetics and tolerability of lidocaine patch 5% with extended dosing. *Ann Pharmacother.* 2002:36;236–240.

3. **Argoff CE.** New analgesics for neuropathic pain: The lidocaine patch. *Clin J Pain.* 2000;16(2, suppl):S62–66.

4. **Lidoderm®** (Lidocaine Patch 5%) [package insert]. Chadds Ford, Pa: Endo Pharmaceuticals Inc; 2002.

5. **Comer AM, Lamb HM.** Lidocaine patch 5%. *Drugs.* 2000;59:245–249.

6. **Waxman SG.** The molecular pathophysiology of pain: Abnormal expression of sodium channel genes and its contribution to hyperexcitability of primary sensory neurons. *Pain.* 1999;6:S133–S140.

7. **Rowbotham MC, Davies PS, Verkempinck C, Galer BS.** Lidocaine patch: Double-blind controlled study of a new treatment method for post-herpetic neuralgia. *Pain.* 1996; 65:39–44.

8. **Khasar SG, Gold MS, Levine JD.** A tetrodotoxin-resistant sodium current mediates inflammatory pain in the rat. *Neurosci Lett.* 1998;256:17–20.

9. **Saito I, Koshino T, Nakashima K, Uesugi M, Saito T.** Increased cellular infiltrate in inflammatory synovia of osteoarthritic knees. *Osteoarthritis Cartilage.* 2002;10: 156–162.

10. **Galer BS, Rowbotham MC, Perander J, Friedman E.** Topical lidocaine patch relieves postherpetic neuralgia more effectively than a vehicle topical patch: Results of an enriched enrollment study. *Pain.* 1999;80:533–538.

11. **Galer BS, Jensen MP, Ma T, Davies PS, Rowbotham MC.** The lidocaine patch 5% effectively treats all neuropathic pain qualities: Results of a randomized, double-blind, vehicle-controlled, 3-week efficacy study with use of the neuropathic pain scale. *Clin J Pain.* 2002; 18:297–301.

12. **Katz NP, Gammaitoni AR, Davis MW, Dworkin RH, and the Lidoderm Patch Study Group.** Lidocaine patch 5% reduces pain intensity and interference with quality of life in patients with postherpetic neuralgia: An effectiveness trial. *Pain Med.* In press.

13. **Meier T, Baron R, Faust M, et al.** Efficacy of the lidocaine patch 5% in the treatment of focal peripheral neuropathic pain syndromes: A randomized, double-blind, placebo-controlled study. *Pain.* 2003;106:151–158.

14. **Devers A, Galer BS.** Topical lidocaine patch relieves a variety of neuropathic pain conditions: An open-label study. *Clin J Pain.* 2000;16:205–208.

15. **Galer BS, Hart-Gouleau S, Dworkin RH, Domingos J, Gammaitoni A.** Effectiveness and safety of the lidocaine patch 5% in patients with painful diabetic neuropathy: A prospective, open-label pilot study. Paper presented at: 5th International Conference on the Mechanisms and Treatment of Neuropathic Pain; November 21–23, 2002; Southampton, Bermuda.

16. **Berman SM, Justis JC, Ho MI, Ing M, Eldridge D, Gammaitoni AR.** Lidocaine patch 5% (Lidoderm®) improves common pain qualities reported by patients with

HIV-associated painful peripheral neuropathy: An open-label pilot study using the Neuropathic Pain Scale. Paper presented at: 10th World Congress of Pain; August 17–22, 2002; San Diego, Calif.

17. **Davis MD, Sandroni P.** Lidocaine patch for pain of erythromelalgia. *Arch Dermatol.* 2002;138:17–19.

18. **Gimbel, J, Moskowitz M, Hines R, et al.** Lidocaine patch 5% effectively treats common pain qualities reported by patients with acute, subacute, and chronic low back pain. Paper presented at: 5th International Conference on the Mechanisms and Treatment of Neuropathic Pain; November 21–23, 2002; Southampton, Bermuda.

19. **Hines R, Keaney D, Moskowitz MH, Prakken S.** Use of lidocaine patch 5% for chronic low back pain: A report of four cases. *Pain Med.* In press.

20. **Lipman AG, Dalpiaz AS, Lordon SP.** Topical lidocaine patch therapy for myfascial pain. Paper presented at: American Pain Society 21st Annual Scientific Meeting; March 15, 2002; Baltimore, Md.

21. **Burch F, Codding C, Patel N, et al.** Effectiveness and safety of the lidocaine patch 5% as add-on or monotherapy in patients with pain from osteoarthritis: A prospective, open-label, multicenter study. Paper presented at: 5th International Conference on the Mechanisms and Treatment of Neuropathic Pain; November 21–23, 2002; Southampton, Bermuda.

22. **Kanazi GE, Johnson RW, Dworkin RH.** Treatment of postherpetic neuralgia: An update. *Drugs.* 2000;59:1113–1126.

23. *Drug Facts and Comparisons 2002.* 56th ed. St. Louis, Mo: Wolters Kluwer; 2002:1792.

24. **Lincoff NS, Rath PP, Hirano M.** The treatment of periocular and facial pain with topical capsaicin. *J Neuro-ophthalmol.* 1998;18:17–20.

25. **Mannion RJ, Doubell TP, Coggeshall RE, Woolf CJ.** Collateral sprouting of uninjured primary afferent A-fibers into the superficial dorsal horn of the adult rat spinal cord after topical capsaicin treatment to the sciatic nerve. *J Neurosci.* 1996;16:5189–5195.

26. **Nolano M, Simone DA, Wendelschafer-Crabb G, Johnson T, Hazen E, Kennedy WR.** Topical capsaicin in humans: Parallel loss of epidermal nerve fibers and pain sensation. *Pain.* 1999;81:135–145.

27. **Bernstein JE, Korman NJ, Bickers DR, Dahl MV, Millikan LE.** Topical capsaicin treatment of chronic postherpetic neuralgia. *J Am Acad Dermatol.* 1989;21: 265–270.

28. **Watson CP, Tyler KI, Bickers DR, Millikan LE, Smith S, Coleman E.** A randomized vehicle-controlled trial of topical capsaicin in the treatment of postherpetic neuralgia. *Clin Ther.* 1993;15:510–526.

29. **McCleane G.** Topical capsaicin of doxepin hydrochloride, capsaicin and a combination of both produces analgesia in chronic human neuropathic pain: A randomized, double-blind, placebo-controlled study. *Br J Clin Pharmacol.* 2000;49:574–579.

30. **Watson CP, Evans RJ.** The postmastectomy pain syndrome and topical capsaicin: A randomized trial. *Pain.* 1992; 51:375–379.

31. **The Capsaicin Study Group.** Treatment of painful diabetic neuropathy with topical capsaicin: A multicenter, double-blind, vehicle-controlled study. *Arch Intern Med.* 1991; 151:2225–2229.

32. **Tandan R, Lewis GA, Krusinski PB, Badger GB, Fries TJ.** Topical capsaicin in painful diabetic neuropathy: Controlled study with long-term follow-up. *Diabetes Care.* 1992;15:8–14.

33. **Low PA, Opfer-Gehrking TL, Dyck PJ, Litchy WJ, O'Brien PC.** Double-blind, placebo-controlled study of the application of capsaicin cream in chronic distal painful polyneuropathy. *Pain.* 1995;62:163–168.

34. **Paice JA, Ferrans CE, Lashley FR, Shott S, Vizgirda V, Pitrak D.** Topical capsaicin in the management of HIV-associated peripheral neuropathy. *J Pain Symptom Manage.* 2000; 19:45–52.

35. **Deal CL, Schnitzer TJ, Lipstein E, et al.** Treatment of arthritis with topical capsaicin: A double-blind trial. *Clin Ther.* 1991;13:383–395.

36. **McCleane G.** The analgesic efficacy of topical capsaicin is enhanced by glyceryl trinitrate in painful osteoarthritis: A randomized, double blind, placebo controlled study. *Eur J Pain.* 2000;4:355–360.

37. **Cannon DT, Wu Y.** Topical capsaicin as an adjuvant analgesic for the treatment of traumatic amputee neurogenic residual limb pain. *Arch Phys Med Rehabil.* 1998; 79:591–593.

38. **Watson CP.** Topical capsaicin as an adjuvant analgesic. *J Pain Symptom Manage.* 1994;9:425–433.

39. **Louis J.** EMLA Cream. International Center for the Control of Pain in Children and Adults. Available at: *http://www. nursing.uiowa.edu/sites/adultpain/Topicals/emlatt.htm.* Accessed July 3, 2002.

40. EMLA® Cream (lidocaine 2.5% and prilocaine 2.5%) [package insert]. Wilmington, Del: AstraZeneca LP; 2002.

41. **Stow PJ, Glynn CJ, Minor B.** EMLA cream in the treatment of post-herpetic neuralgia: Efficacy and pharmacokinetic profile. *Pain.* 1989;39:301–305.

42. **Attal N, Brasseur L, Chauvin M, Bouhassira D.** Effects of single and repeated applications of a eutectic mixture of local anesthetic (EMLA) cream on spontaneous and evoked pain in postherpetic neuralgia. *Pain.* 1999; 81:203–209.

43. **Fassoulaki A, Sarantopoulos C, Melemeni A, Hogan Q.** EMLA reduces acute and chronic pain after breast surgery for cancer. *Reg Anesth Pain Med.* 2000;25: 350–355.

44. **Green S, Buchbinder R, Barnsley L, et al.** Non-steroidal anti-inflammatory drugs (NSAIDs) for treating lateral elbow pain in adults. *Cochrane Database Syst Rev.* 2002: CD003686.

45. **Moore RA, Tramer MR, Carroll D, Wiffen PJ, McQuay HJ.** Quantitative systematic review of topically applied non-steroidal anti-inflammatory drugs. *BMJ.* 1998; 316:333–338.

10 ACETAMINOPHEN AND NONSTEROIDAL ANTI-INFLAMMATORY DRUGS

Michael W. Loes, MD

ACETAMINOPHEN

- Acetaminophen, an atypical, short-acting analgesic with a plasma half-life of 2–3 hours, is a synthetic agent derived from *p*-aminophenol, the major metabolite of phenacetin, an analgesic widely used in Europe but banned in the United States because of an association with analgesic nephropathy, which pathologically presents as either acute papillary necrosis or interstitial nephritis.[1]
- The analgesic mechanism of action of acetaminophen is primarily through the spinal cord and cerebral cortex, but it also causes a weak central inhibition of prostaglandin synthetase.[2]
- Acetaminophen is arguably the most commonly used analgesic and is considered first-step pharmacotherapy for controlling the pain of osteoarthritis in doses up to 4000 mg/d.[3]
- The drug is frequently used in combination with opioid analgesics, such as codeine, hydrocodone, oxycodone, propoxyphene, and pentazocine. The result is enhanced analgesic effect and less likelihood of abuse because combination products cannot easily be altered for use in ways other than intended. A combination product with tramadol is also available, and multiple products contain aspirin.
- Acetaminophen is also an effective antipyretic. Because of its ability to lower fever, it is extensively used in preparations to treat upper respiratory infections, kidney and bladder problems, and any clinical state where fever or pain may be present. Combination products for flu, sinus congestion, menstrual cramps, and insomnia fill the shelves of pharmacies and grocery stores. It behooves physicians to question their patients regarding these products, especially when prescribing 3 or 4 g/d for arthritis, because many patients are taking products that they do not realize contain acetaminophen. The result can be inadvertent overdose and toxicity.
- Acetaminophen is metabolized by the microsomal enzyme system of the liver as are many other analgesics, anticonvulsants, antibiotics, antifungal agents, and other drugs. Thus, this common pathway can be overwhelmed. Intentional or accidental overdoses of acetaminophen are common, and every emergency room has protocols in place to treat these potentially

fatal ingestions, most commonly using acetylcysteine (Mucomyst). While recognition and treatment have improved, these overdoses can be fatal. Acetaminophen toxicity is one of the most common causes of drug-associated death in children and adolescents.
- For analgesia, the conventional dose for older children or adults is 325–650 mg every 4–6 hours until pain is relieved. For younger children, a single dose should not exceed 60–120 mg depending on age and weight and should not be administered for more than 10 days. See chapter 38 for more information on pediatric pain management. Extended-release tablets are available that release 325 mg immediately from the outer shell, with a matrix core releasing an additional 325 mg during an 8-hour period. In equal doses, the degree of analgesia and antipyresis is similar to that produced by aspirin.

NONSTEROIDAL ANTI-INFLAMMATORY DRUGS (NSAIDs)

ASPIRIN: A BALANCED VIEW

- Aspirin, a nonsteroidal anti-inflammatory drug (NSAID), is a tried and tested analgesic. Rapid acting and extremely effective for common headaches and short-term pain problems, aspirin is the most frequently purchased over-the-counter pain reliever worldwide and with good reason: It works.
- Aspirin is a broad-spectrum inhibitor of prostaglandins, a family of fatty acids so ubiquitous in the human body they are detected in almost every tissue and body fluid. First discovered in the 1930s, prostaglandins produce a wide range of effects, notably the sensitization of nociceptors.
- Yet aspirin therapy is not without significant risks. A select group of patients—those with asthma, nasal polyps, and/or urticaria (known as Franklin's triad)—are at significant risk of anaphylaxis leading to rapid bronchial constriction, laryngeal edema, hypotension, and, often, death. Another important precaution regarding aspirin is that it should never be given to children under the age of 2 years who are suffering from a cold, flu, or chicken pox because of the risk of Reye's syndrome, a potentially fatal pediatric illness.
- Cross-reacting aspirin sensitivity is rare in asthmatic patients under age 10 in the absence of Franklin's triad. In adults, cross-reactivity is estimated at about 20% among those who are sensitive to aspirin. In patients with Franklin's triad, cross-reactivity is extremely high (approximately 85%).

- The idiosyncratic reactions in sensitive individuals to particular NSAIDs apart from those specific to aspirin are structure specific. For example, celecoxib is contraindicated in patients with allergy to sulfa drugs. In this situation, a rash should not preclude the choice of another NSAID. Piroxicam (Feldene) and sulindac (Clinoril) are two agents where macular popular rashes are reasonably common. When the offending agent is stopped, the rash goes away and another can be chosen.
- While aspirin is recognized primarily as preventive therapy for heart attacks and strokes, a 6-year randomized trial conducted among 5139 apparently healthy male doctors found that those taking 500 mg aspirin daily had significantly fewer migraines than the non-aspirin users.[4]
- The FDA has approved the use of aspirin to reduce the risk of heart attack and stroke in men and women who have suffered a heart attack or an ischemic stroke or who are at high risk. (Aspirin prophylaxis, however, is not a universal recommendation for these conditions, and the risk/benefit ratio needs to be seriously considered.)

OTHER NONSTEROIDAL ANTI-INFLAMMATORY DRUGS

- NSAIDs are an important component in balanced analgesia in the management of acute and chronic pain.
- The starting doses of available NSAIDs are listed in Table 10–1, and the elimination half-lives in Table 10–2.
- All NSAIDs are highly protein bound.
- NSAIDs are contraindicated only in individuals with Franklin's triad (syndrome of nasal polyps, angioedema, and urticaria) in whom anaphylactoid reactions have occurred.
- Unless contraindicated, NSAIDs should be considered along with standard therapy in the inpatient and outpatient settings.
- NSAIDs have a direct action on spinal nociceptive processing with a relative order of potency that correlates with their capacity to inhibit cyclooxygenase (COX) activity.
- The two isoforms of cyclooxygenase, COX-1 and COX-2, are genetically distinct, with COX-1 located on chromosome 7 and COX-2 on chromosome 1.
- COX-1 is considered constitutive or part of the basic constitutional homeostasis, while COX-2 is inducible; that is, it responds to specific insult.
- Various NSAIDs inhibit the isoforms differentially. The goal is to inhibit COX-2 while preserving

TABLE 10–1 Conservative Adult Starting Doses of NSAIDs for Pain

NSAID	STARTING DOSE
Celecoxib (Celebrex)	100 mg qd
Choline magnesium salicylate (Trilisate)	750 mg bid
Diclofenac sodium (Voltaren)	50 mg bid
Diclofenac potassium: immediate release	50 mg tid
Diflunisal (Dolobid)	500 mg bid
Etodolac (Lodine)	400 mg bid
Fenoprofen (Nalfon)	200 mg qid
Ibuprofen (Motrin, Advil, Nuprin)	200 mg qid
Indomethacin (Indocin)	25 mg bid
Ketorolac (Toradol)	10 mg bid
Ketoprofen tromethamine (Orudis, Oruvail)	75 mg bid
Meclofenamate (Meclofen)	50 mg tid
Mefenamic acid (Ponstel)	250 mg qd
Meloxicam (Mobic)	7.5 mg qd
Nabumetone (Relafen)	1000 mg qd
Naproxen (Naprosyn)	250 mg bid
Naproxen sodium (Anaprox)	275 mg tid
Oxyaprozin (Daypro)	600 mg qd
Piroxicam (Feldene)	20 mg qd
Rofecoxib (Vioxx)	12.5 mg qd
Salsalate (Disalcid)	750 mg bid
Sulindac (Clinoril)	150 mg bid
Tolmetin (Tolectin)	400 mg tid
Valdecoxib (Bextra)	10 mg qd

COX-1 because gastric problems are reduced by protecting the constitutional homeostasis of the COX-1 system. Quantification tables exist for the relative inhibition of COX-1/COX-2 by various NSAIDs, but introduction of the relatively selective agents (celecoxib, rofecoxib, and valdecoxib), more commonly referred to as "coxibs," has rendered these data obsolete.
- Etodolac (Lodine), nabumetone (Relafen), and meloxicam (Mobic) remain in use because they are relatively more selective than the first NSAIDs produced and less expensive than the coxibs.
- Although NSAIDs act primarily through their effects on peripheral prostaglandin synthetase, additional

TABLE 10–2 Elimination Half-Lives of NSAIDs

NSAID	ELIMINATION HALF-LIFE (h)
Celecoxib	8
Diclofenac	1–2
Fenoprofen	3
Ibuprofen	1–2
Ketoprofen	2
Ketorolac	4–6
Nabumetone (6NMA)	24
Naproxen	14
Oxaprozin	40
Rofecoxib	17
Piroxicam	50
Tolmetin	5
Valdecoxib	8–11

central mechanisms for their action have also been demonstrated.

- Clinically, NSAIDs have an important role as adjuvants to other analgesics and have an opioid-sparing effect in the range of 20–35%. Combining an optimal dose of an NSAID with an opioid produces an additive analgesic effect known as *synergy* that is greater than that obtained alone by doubling the dose of either drug.

- Elimination kinetics and degree of protein binding vary widely among NSAIDs. Hence, drug displacement occurs when NSAIDs are combined with other highly protein-bound drugs, including warfarin (Coumadin) and lithium salts (Eskalith); caution is advised in such cases because the increased levels affect clotting time and the potential for lithium toxicity. The protein binding of all NSAIDs except aspirin to platelet cyclooxygenase is reversible. Thus, coagulation is affected by aspirin as long as that platelet is alive and circulating, approximately 3 weeks. If a patient is on daily aspirin and is scheduled for major surgery, especially cardiovascular surgery, it is prudent to substitute a shorter-acting NSAID with an equally short effect on coagulation, such as ibuprofen (Advil, Motrin), 2 to 3 weeks prior to surgery.

- Only ketorolac is available in both oral and parenteral formulations. The parenteral form of ketorolac (Toradol)) has been successfully used to manage postoperative pain either by intermittent intravenous boluses or by patient-controlled devices.

- Indomethacin (Indocin) and aspirin are available in oral form and also as suppositories.

- Choline magnesium trisalicylate (Trilisate) and ibuprofen (Motrin) come in liquid forms.

- The rapidly dissolving NSAID formulations are useful for acute pain but are not indicated for the treatment of osteoarthritis or rheumatoid arthritis. These include diclofenac sodium (Voltaren), naprosyn sodium (Anaprox), and ketorolac (Toradol).

- The following nonsteroidal agents with anti-inflammatory effects are not considered NSAIDs: acetaminophen, colchicine, methotrexate (Immunex), hydroxychloroquine (Plaquenil), penicillamine (Cuprimine, Depen), gold salts (Thiomalate), etanercept (Enbrel), infliximab (Remicade, Centocor), leflunomide (Arava), mycophenolate mofetil (Cell Cept), and cyclosporin (Neoral). Acetaminophen is a *para*-aminophenol derivative with analgesic and antipyretic properties that appears to be equipotent to aspirin in inhibiting central prostaglandin synthesis but does not inhibit peripheral prostaglandin synthetase. Colchicine is not an analgesic and is generally effective only when used to treat acute gouty arthritis, although some investigators have found it

effective in low back pain syndromes. The major mechanisms for these agents are immunologic.

PAIN

- In the American Pain Society's March 2002 guidelines for the management of pain in osteoarthritis, rheumatoid arthritis, and juvenile chronic arthritis, acetaminophen was recommended for mild pain associated with osteoarthritis and a selective COX-2 inhibitor for moderate to severe pain and inflammation.[5]

- A dilemma exists regarding the long-term use for pain of COX-2-specific inhibitors, specifically rofecoxib (Vioxx) 50 mg/d compared with naproxen (1000 mg/d). Data gathered during the 1-year "VIGOR" study of this comparison showed that rofecoxib was associated both with a significantly lower incidence of serious upper gastrointestinal events and with a significantly higher incidence of serious cardiovascular events. Various authors have suggested that this effect is likely due to naproxen's ability to inhibit platelet aggregation; rofecoxib does not have this effect.[6–9] Rofecoxib for pain at the 50-mg/d dose has not been studied for more than 5 days and, hence, is not recommended for chronic use.

- Although COX-2 inhibitors are worthwhile analgesics and have both an improved gastrointestinal side effect profile and reduced or absent platelet inhibition activity compared with nonselective NSAIDs, the consensus of the International COX-2 Study Group was that the rates of hypertension and edema with coxibs are similar to those observed with nonselective NSAIDs.

STRUCTURE AND FUNCTION

- Chemical structure determines metabolism, absorption, volume of distribution, protein binding, and elimination pathways.

- NSAIDs have varying chemical structures and are in different classes. Some clinicians have advocated trying an agent from another class if the first choice does not work. Although this view has not been well supported, switching classes may be of value in patients who experience problematic side effects.

- Drug interactions and effects on platelet function may differ among NSAIDs.

- Receptor affinity differs, and there may be other subtle differences in pharmacodynamics.

- Table 10–3 displays the structural classification of NSAIDs.

TABLE 10–3   NSAID Structural Classification

Proprionic acid derivatives	Pyranocarboxylic acid
Fenoprofen calcium (Nalfon)	Etodolac (Lodine)
Flurbiprofen (Ansaid)	
Ibuprofen (multiple trade names)	Salicylates
Ketoprofen (Orudis)	Acetylsalicylic (aspirin)
Naproxen sodium (Naprelan,	Salsalate (various)
Naprosyn)	Magnesium salicylate
Naproxen sodium (Aleve,	Diflunisal (Dolobid)
Anaprox)	
Oxaprozin (Daypro)	Naphthylalkanone
	Nabumetone (Relafen)
Fenamates	
Mefenamic acid (Ponstel)	Oxicam
Meclofenamate sodium	Piroxicam (Feldene)
(Meclomen)	
	Pyrazole derivatives
Indoles	Phenylbutazone (Butazolidin)
Indomethacin (Indocin)	Oxyphenbutazone (Tandearil)
Sulindac (Clinoril)	
Tolmetin sodium (Tolectin)	Pyrrolo
	Ketorolac tromethamine
Phenylacetic acids	(Toradol)
Diclofenac sodium (Voltaren)	
Diclofenac potassium (Cataflam)	Coxibs
	Celecoxib (Celebrex)
Benzylacetic acid	Rofecoxib (Vioxx)
Bromfenac sodium (Duract)	Valdecoxib (Bextra)

TABLE 10–4   Comparative NSAID Toxicity Scores*

Salsalate	1.00
Ibuprofen	1.25
Diclofenac	3.57
Fenoprofen	3.57
Sulindac	4.75
Naproxen	5.20
Ketoprofen	6.00
Indomethacin	6.25
Piroxicam	8.00
Tolmetin	8.73
Meclofenamate	9.00

*Serious reactions per million prescriptions; based on data from (1) the Committee on Safety of Medicine: *Br Med J.* 1986;292:614 and 1986; 292:1190; (2) Griffin MR, et al. *Ann Intern Med.* 1991;114:257; and (3) Fries, et al. *Arthritis Rheumatol.* 1991;34:1353.

CAUTIONS AND ADVERSE EFFECTS

GASTROINTESTINAL

- Gastrointestinal (GI) tract complications associated with NSAIDs are the most common and are often serious.
- Endoscopic studies have shown that within 1 week of starting NSAID therapy, more than 30% of patients develop gastric erosions or ulcers, and within 1 year, approximately 3–6% have significant GI bleeding. NSAID-associated gastropathy accounts for at least 2600 deaths and 20,000 hospitalizations each year in the United States in patients with rheumatoid arthritis alone. Across-the-board data show that 200,000–400,000 hospitalizations are caused by GI complications (bleeding and perforation). The cost of these hospitalizations is $0.8 to $1.6 billion per year.
- A prospective study of the rate of GI complications in patients with rheumatoid arthritis demonstrated that approximately 6% per year experience a significant GI side effect from NSAIDs, and approximately 1.3% of these require hospitalization.
- The duration of NSAID therapy appears to be the single most important factor predicting GI bleeding. Patients on NSAIDs for 5 years have a five times greater risk of GI bleeding than those on NSAIDs for 1 year, and the risk at 1 year is four times greater than it is at 3 months. Most of these patients did not

have preceding GI problems, and prophylactic treatment with antacids and H2 blockers was of marginal value for duodenal ulcers and of no value for gastric ulcers.
- The relative risk of a GI-provoked hospitalization was more than five times greater in patients taking NSAIDs. A toxicity index in patients with rheumatoid arthritis revealed that salsalate and ibuprofen are the least toxic and tolmetin sodium, meclofenamate, and indomethacin the most toxic (see Table 10–4 for comparative NSAID toxicity scores).

RENAL

- NSAID-associated kidney problems are common because more than 17 million Americans take these drugs.
- The most common renal problem associated with NSAID usage is reversible depression of renal function.
- Fenoprofen and indomethacin are associated with the highest incidence of renal dysfunction, and nonacetylated salicylates with the lowest.
- Fenoprofen has been implicated in the development of interstitial nephritis. Specific risk factors for renal toxicity include congestive heart failure, coexistent liver failure, and consumption of diuretics.
- Renal problems are most common in patients taking aspirin and ibuprofen, not because these drugs are the most toxic, but because so many people take them. It has been estimated that aspirin and ibuprofen cause renal dysfunction in 13–18% of users.
- The elderly are at highest risk because, by age 65, they have usually already lost 25–40% of normal renal function. In a sensitive individual, significant adverse changes in kidney function can occur within 3–7 days. The result can be acute renal failure, dialysis, and/or death if the complication is not recognized. Subtle alternations in creatinine clearance are common and frequently overlooked. In one study, aspirin reduced creatinine clearance by as much as 58% in patients with lupus nephritis.

- Another renal adverse event is "analgesic nephropathy," which occurs when large quantities of combination over-the-counter analgesics, most often acetaminophen, aspirin, and caffeine, are consumed.
- Phenacetin, which is also associated with renal failure, remains in wide use from international sources.

HEPATIC

- The most common hepatic problem with NSAIDs is mild elevations of hepatic enzymes, estimated at 2–5%. This elevation is higher in patients with rheumatoid arthritis, congestive heart failure, renal failure, and concurrent acetaminophen use and in those who are alcohol drinkers or of advanced age.
- Diclofenac (Voltaren) has been associated with more hepatic problems than other agents.
- In 1998, bromfenac sodium (Duract) was pulled off the market because of hepatic toxicity.
- Acute NSAID-associated hepatic injury, primarily cholestatic injury, leads to 5 in 100,000 Medicare hospitalizations.
- Liver toxicity is more likely to be dose-related than idiosyncratic. For diclofenac (Voltaren) or diclofenac potassium (Cataflam), the base incidence doubles for every doubling of dose.
- Because elevations in liver function tests are the first warning of more problems to come, checking and following liver profiles when patients are on NSAIDs is advisable.

CARDIAC

- The elderly taking NSAIDs daily have an increased risk of heart problems, especially in the presence of congestive heart failure. NSAIDs inhibit prostaglandins in the kidney and, in doing so, often cause salt retention and edema.
- The 2–4% incidence of edema from NSAIDs has not appreciably changed with the introduction of the coxibs.
- Patients with a history of congestive heart failure have a twofold increase in exacerbation of this condition, resulting in hospitalization when they are placed on an NSAID.
- The Warfarin Aspirin Study of Heart Failure (WASH) randomized 279 congestive heart failure patients to receive either aspirin 300 mg/d, warfarin to a target international ratio of 2.5, or no antithrombotic therapy. During a mean follow-up of 27 months, 64% in the aspirin group required hospitalization compared with 47% in the warfarin group and 48% in the control group. The increased incidence of hospitalization in the aspirin group was for worsening heart failure. The combined endpoint of death, nonfatal myocardial infarction, or stroke occurred in 32% of the aspirin patients compared with 26% in the other two groups.

- NSAIDs, especially indomethacin, piroxicam, and naproxen, also cause an average increase in mean blood pressure of 10 mm Hg.

CUTANEOUS

- Between 5 and 10% of patients on NSAIDs develop a rash or pruritus. This most commonly occurs with use of piroxicam, sulindac, or meclofenamate.
- Urticaria alone most commonly occurs with aspirin, indomethacin, and ibuprofen, while photosensitivity is most often seen with piroxicam.

CENTRAL NERVOUS SYSTEM

- Severe headache is the most frequent central nervous system (CNS) toxic effect reported, though others include cognitive dysfunction, dizziness, sleeplessness, irritability, syncope, and, rarely, seizures. Indomethacin (Indocin) is the worst offender here, with 10–25% of patients reporting headache.
- Elderly patients using NSAIDs, especially naproxen and ibuprofen, are the most likely to report confusion.

MISCELLANEOUS TOXIC EFFECTS

- Tinnitus is most commonly seen with aspirin use, although nonacetylated salicylates can also cause this condition.
- Anaphylactoid reactions are more common with tolmetin and aspirin than with other NSAIDs.
- Hematologic effects are common with all NSAIDs because these pharmaceuticals decrease platelet adhesiveness. The most serious hematologic adverse event, aplastic anemia, has been reported with use of phenylbutazone, which is no longer available in the United States but is still available internationally.
- Indomethacin and diclofenac have also been associated with anemia more often than other NSAIDs.
- Aspirin is associated with Reye's syndrome and not advised in children with febrile viral syndromes.
- The single doses and maximal daily doses of NSAIDs for children are listed in Table 10–5.

PLATELETS

- NSAIDs prevent platelet aggregation. Only salsalate (Disalcid) and choline magnesium trisalicylate

TABLE 10–5 NSAIDs in the Pediatric Population

	SINGLE DOSE (mg/kg)	MAXIMAL DAILY DOSE(mg/kg)
Aspirin	10–15	60
Diclofenac	1.0–2.0	No information
Ibuprofen	10	40
Indomethacin	1	3
Ketoprofen	2.5	5
Naproxen	7	15

TABLE 10–6   Interactions of Other Pharmaceuticals with NSAIDs

Antacids	May decrease the absorption of NSAIDs.
Anticoagulants	NSAIDs are highly protein bound (99%), and, when given with anticoagulants, some displacement of Coumadin will potentiate the effect of warfarin. NSAIDs also reversibly inhibit platelet aggregation (except for aspirin where the effect is irreversible). The effect parallels the drug elimination time. Hence, for drugs with long elimination times (piroxicam and oxaprozin) the effect lasts days. Giving NSAIDs to patients who are anticoagulated is not contraindicated but caution is advised! Because nonacetylated NSAIDs, such as salsalate and choline magnesium salicylate, do not directly affect platelet function, they are safer but can still potentiate Coumadin by displacing protein-bound drug.
Antirheumatic agents	Many drugs used in rheumatoid arthritis (azathioprine [Imuran], penicillamine [Depen, Cuprimine], gold compounds, and methotrexate) can cause bone marrow toxicity, including decreased white blood cells and platelets. NSAIDs may potentiate this toxic effect.
Corticosteroids	Patients who take corticosteroids concurrently are at higher risk for NSAID-induced gastropathy.
Diuretics	The action of diuretics may be potentiated with concurrent use of NSAIDs.
Lithium	The pharmacologic activity of lithium is heightened in patients taking NSAIDs. One proposed mechanism is decreased renal clearance because of decreased renal prostaglandin synthesis.
Oral hypoglycemic agents	Several NSAIDs potentiate oral hypoglycemic agents (fenoprofen, naproxen, and piroxicam) primarily by displacing sulfonylureas from plasma protein binding sites.
Phenytoin	The effect of phenytoin may be potentiated, again because NSAIDs have a high affinity for protein binding sites and can displace it. This effect has been shown with the same agents noted to displace sulfonylureas, most notably fenoprofen, naproxen, and piroxicam.
Probenecid	This agent increases plasma levels of indomethacin, naproxen, ketoprofen, and meclofenamate. Hence, lower dosages of these NSAIDs are advised when given with probenecid.

(Trilisate) lack this property. Because NSAIDs are highly protein bound, all have the potential of displacing warfarin (Coumadin) and potentiating its anticoagulant effect.

DRUG INTERACTIONS
• See Table 10–6.

INFLUENCE IN TRAUMATIC, OPERATIVE, AND POSTOPERATIVE SETTINGS

• As NSAIDs affect the arachidonic pathway involved in the response to injury, they affect the surgical stress response. In the acute postoperative model, most of these effects are favorable and have led to increased usage.
• Likely because of their analgesic, antipyretic, and sodium-retaining effects, NSAIDs attenuate endocrine metabolic effects.
• NSAIDS reduce opioid requirements, fevers, and, perhaps, fluid loss.
• On the negative side is the concern regarding the effect of NSAIDs on platelet adhesion and the potential of NSAIDs to cause postoperative bleeding, a concern that ended with the introduction of selective COX-2 agents that do not appreciably affect bleeding times.
• Parameters under dispute are those concerning post-traumatic immunosuppression, nitrogen balance, and acute-phase reactant proteins. With the controversy still current, evidence of fewer or more infectious complications is lacking.[10–18]

REFERENCES

1. **Perneger TV, Whelton PK, Klag MJ.** Risk of kidney failure associated with the use of acetaminophen, aspirin and nonsteroidal anti-inflammatory drugs. *N Engl J Med.* 1994; 331:1675.
2. **Malmberg AB, Yaksh TL.** Hyperalgesia mediated by spinal glutamate or substance P receptor blocked by spinal cyclooxygenase inhibition. *Science.* 1992;257:1276.
3. **Hochberg MC, Altman RS, Brandt KD, et al.** Guidelines for the medical management of osteoarthritis. *Arthritis Rheum.* 1995;38:1535.
4. *Is Aspirin Therapy Right for You?* [booklet]. Bayer.
5. *Guideline for Management of Pain in Osteoarthritis, Rheumatoid Arthritis and Juvenile Chronic Arthritis.* Glenview, Ill: American Pain Society; 2002:54.
6. **Ray WA, Stein CM, Hall K, et al.** Non-steroidal anti-inflammatory drugs and the risk of serious coronary heart disease: An observational cohort study. *Lancet.* 2002;359:118.
7. **Rahme E, Pilote L, LeLorier J.** Association between naproxen use and protection against acute myocardial infarction. *Arch Intern Med.* 2002;162:1111.
8. **Solomon DH, Glynn RJ, Levin R, et al.** Nonsteroidal anti-inflammatory drug use and acute myocardial infarction. *Arch Intern Med.* 2002;162:1099.
9. **Watson DJ, Rhodes T, Cai B, et al.** Lower risk of thromboembolic cardiovascular events with naproxen among patients with rheumatoid arthritis. *Arch Intern Med.* 2002;162:1105.
10. **Revhaug A, Michie HR, Manson JM, et al.** Inhibition of cyclooxygenase attenuates the metabolic response to endotoxin in humans. *Arch Surg.* 1988;123:162.
11. **Michie HR, Majzoub JA, O'Dwyer ST, et al.** Both cyclooxygenase dependent and cyclooxygenase independent

pathways mediate the neuroendocrine response in humans. *Surgery*. 1990;108:54.

12. **Hulton NR, Johnson DJ, Evans A, et al.** Inhibition of prostaglandin synthesis improves postoperative nitrogen balance *Clin Nutr*. 1988;7:81.

13. **Lalonde C, Knox J, Daryani R, et al.** Topical flurbiprofen decreases burn wound induced hypermetabolism and systemic lipid peroxidation. *Surgery*. 1991;109:645.

14. **Faist E, Ertel W, Cohnert T, et al.** Immunoprotective effects of cyclooxygenase inhibition in patients with major surgical trauma. *Trauma*. 1990;30:8.

15. **Haupt MT, Jastremiski MS, Clemmer TP, et al.** Effect of ibuprofen in patents with severe sepsis: A randomized double blind multicenter study. *Crit Care Med*. 1991;19:1339.

16. **Engel C, Dristensen SS, Axel C, et al.** Indomethacin and the stress response to hysterectomy. *Acta Anaesthesiol Scand*. 1989;33:540.

17. **Claeys MA, Camu F, Maes V.** Prophylactic diclofenac infusions in major orthopedic surgery: Effects of analgesia and acute phase proteins. *Acta Anaesthesiol Scand*. 1992;36:270.

18. **Varassi G, Panella L, Piroli A, et al.** The effects of perioperative ketorolac infusion on postoperative pain an endocrine metabolic response. *Anesth Analg*. 1994;78:514.

11 ANTIDEPRESSANTS

Michael R. Clark, MD, MPH

INTRODUCTION

ANTIDEPRESSANTS AND PAIN

- Since the first report of imipramine use for trigeminal neuralgia was published in 1960, antidepressants, particularly tricyclic antidepressants (TCAs), have been commonly prescribed for the treatment of many chronic pain syndromes, especially those involving neuropathic pain, including diabetic neuropathy, postherpetic neuralgia, central pain, poststroke pain, tension-type headache, migraine, and oral–facial pain.[1–6]
- The analgesic effects of antidepressants are independent of the presence of depression or improvement in mood.[7]
- Antidepressants improve both brief lancinating pain and constant burning pain.[8]
- Analgesia usually occurs at lower doses and with earlier onset of action than expected for the treatment of depression.

CLASSIFICATION SYSTEMS

- Neuropathic pain has been classified according to underlying pathology, such as diabetes mellitus, herpes zoster, and ischemia due to vascular occlusion.

- Linking possible mechanisms of pain (sympathetic hyperactivity, C-fiber mechanosensitivity, spontaneous activity in dorsal root ganglion cells) to specific features of pain phenomenology could improve treatment selection.[7]

PHARMACOLOGIC MECHANISMS OF ANTINOCICEPTION

DESCENDING INHIBITION

- Research suggests that the analgesic effect of antidepressants is mediated primarily by the blockade of reuptake of norepinephrine and serotonin. The resulting increase in the levels of these neurotransmitters enhances the activation of descending inhibitory neurons.
- Antidepressants, however, may produce antinociceptive effects through a variety of pharmacologic mechanisms, including other types of monoamine modulation; interactions with opioid receptors; and inhibition of ion channel activity and of *N*-methyl-D-aspartate (NMDA), histamine, and cholinergic receptors.[1,9,10]

MONOAMINE MODULATION

- Investigations have demonstrated differential effects of monoamine receptor subtypes in antidepressant-induced antinociception in the rat formalin test. The effects of antidepressants with varying degrees of norepinephrine and serotonin reuptake inhibition as well as those of their antagonists indicate that α_1 adrenoceptors and several serotonin receptor subtypes (5-HT2, 5-HT3, and 5-HT4) contribute to antinociception.
- The antinociceptive activity of a variety of antidepressants irrespective of the propensity for inhibiting reuptake of norepinephrine and/or serotonin is blocked by an α_2 but not by an α_1 adrenoceptor in the mouse abdominal constriction assay, and β adrenoceptors mediate the analgesic effects of desipramine and nortriptyline.

OPIOID INTERACTIONS

MONOAMINE RECEPTORS
- Because they interact with opioids or their antagonists, antidepressants may interact with opioid receptors or stimulate endogenous opioid peptide release.
- Studies of hot plate analgesia in mice found that the antinociceptive effect of trazodone involves mu-1 and

mu-2 opioid receptor subtypes combined with the serotonergic receptor.

- Similar studies with venlafaxine showed that antinociception is partly mediated by mu, kappa-1, kappa-3, and delta opioid receptor subtypes as well as by the α_2 adrenergic receptor.
- In contrast, mirtazapine-induced antinociception involves primarily kappa-3 opioid receptors in conjunction with serotonergic and noradrenergic receptors.

SYNERGISTIC EFFECTS

- In the rat tail-flick model, the antinociception produced by individual intrathecal administration of serotonin, desipramine, and morphine can be achieved with subthreshold doses of combinations of these agents.
- In the rat formalin test, the fluoxetine-induced antinociception that potentiates morphine analgesia is blocked by naloxone. Similar results for fluoxetine have been found in mice using acetic acid-induced writhing, tail-flick, and hot plate assays.
- Using the acetic acid-induced abdominal constriction assay in mice, investigators found that naloxone and naltrindole shift the antidepressant dose–response relationships to the right.
- These data in conjunction with findings that only naloxone displaces morphine antinociception and neither opioid antagonist affects aspirin antinociception support the role of the delta opioid receptor, as well as of endogenous opioids, in antidepressant-induced antinociception.

MISCELLANEOUS MECHANISMS

ADENOSINE

- Studies of imipramine demonstrated differential hypoalgesic effects depending on the experimental paradigm used to assess pain. For example, TCAs may reduce hyperalgesia but not tactile allodynia because different neuronal mechanisms underlie different manifestations of neuropathic pain.
- The blocking by caffeine of this effect induced with amitriptyline indicates a role for endogenous adenosine systems.

ION CHANNELS

- The opening of voltage-gated and Ca^{2+}-gated K^+ channels has been implicated in the central antinociception induced by amitriptyline and clomipramine in the mouse hot plate test. Intravenous amitriptyline impairs the function of tetrodotoxin-resistant Na^+ channels in rat dorsal root ganglia, particularly in conditions of repetitive firing and depolarizing membrane potential, which may reduce firing frequency in ectopic sites of damaged nociceptive fibers.

RELATIONSHIP TO INFLAMMATION

- Amitriptyline and desipramine, but not fluoxetine, have peripheral antinociceptive action in inflammatory and neuropathic rat models. In contrast, systemic and spinal administration of antidepressants produce analgesic effects in the rat formalin model that are not due to anti-inflammatory actions.

CLINICAL APPLICATIONS

SEROTONIN AND NOREPINEPHRINE

- Antidepressants are typically characterized according to the specificity of their neurotransmitter reuptake (Table 11–1).[10]
- The presence of noradrenergic activity is often associated with better analgesic effect than is serotonergic activity alone.
- Antidepressants with a 5-HT (serotonin)/NE (norepinephrine) ratio of less than 1 (noradrenergic) include

TABLE 11–1   Commonly Used Antidepressant Medications

GENERIC (BRAND) NAME	DAILY DOSE	PRIMARY MECHANISM
HETEROCYCLIC TERTIARY AMINES (TCAs)		
Amitriptyline (Elavil)	50–300 mg	Mixed NE and 5-HT reuptake inhibition
Imipramine (Tofranil)	50–300 mg	
Doxepin (Sinequan)	50–300 mg	
HETEROCYCLIC SECONDARY AMINES (TCAs)		
Nortriptyline (Pamelor)	50–150 mg	NE>5-HT reuptake inhibition
Desipramine (Norpramin)	75–300 mg	
SELECTIVE SEROTONIN REUPTAKE INHIBITORS (SSRIs)		
Fluoxetine (Prozac)	10–80 mg	5-HT>>NE reuptake inhibition
Sertraline (Zoloft)	50–200 mg	
Paroxetine (Paxil)	10–40 mg	
Fluvoxamine (Luvox)	100–300 mg	
Citalopram (Celexa)	20–40 mg	
ATYPICAL ANTIDEPRESSANTS		
Venlafaxine (Effexor)	75–450 mg	5-HT>NE>>DA reuptake inhibition (dose dependent)
Nefazodone (Serzone)	100–600 mg	5-HT>NE reuptake inhibition with 5-HT2 receptor blockade
Trazodone (Desyrel)	100–600 mg	
Bupropion (Wellbutrin)	100–450 mg	DA and NE reuptake inhibition
Mirtazapine (Remeron)	15–90 mg	α_2-NE and 5-HT2 presynaptic agonist with 5-HT2/3 receptor blockade

amitriptyline, imipramine, bupropion, doxepin, nortriptyline, desipramine, and maprotiline.
- Antidepressants with a 5-HT/NE ratio of more than 1 (serotonergic) include venlafaxine, nefazodone, trazodone, clomipramine, fluoxetine, fluvoxamine, paroxetine, sertraline, and citalopram.

TRICYCLIC ANTIDEPRESSANTS

UTILIZATION
- A study of TCA use found that 25% of patients in a multidisciplinary pain center were prescribed these medications. The fact that 73% of treated patients were prescribed the equivalent of 50 mg or less of amitriptyline, however, suggests there is a potential for additional pain relief with higher doses.[11]
- The cost of TCAs for pain treatment is generally much lower (less than $5.00 per month) than the cost of other antidepressants and medications with analgesic activity.
- The results of investigations to determine drug concentrations needed for pain relief support higher serum levels but are contradictory; thus, no clear guidelines have been established.[5,8,12]

TERTIARY VERSUS SECONDARY
- Generally, the tertiary TCAs with balanced effects on 5-HT and NE reuptake (imipramine, amitriptyline, doxepin) are considered more effective analgesic agents than the secondary TCAs with more selective NE reuptake inhibition (desipramine, nortriptyline, maprotiline).
- Although tertiary amines have been used most commonly, they are metabolized to secondary amines that are associated with fewer side effects, such as decreased gastrointestinal motility and urinary retention. The fact that desipramine and nortriptyline had significantly fewer side effects led to less frequent discontinuation of the drug than seen with clomipramine, amitriptyline, and doxepin. Nortriptyline, the major metabolite of amitriptyline, causes less sedation, orthostatic hypotension, and falls than does imipramine and is as effective as amitriptyline in treating chronic pain.[1,5]
- Randomized controlled trials, however, have not demonstrated consistent differences among TCAs.[5,8,12]

EFFICACY
- TCAs have been most effective in relieving neuropathic pain and headache syndromes.[5,8,9,12,13] The findings in a number of these studies have been challenged, however, because of poor study design and variable protocol criteria.

- Placebo-controlled, double-blind, randomized, clinical trials for chronic low back pain in patients without depression demonstrated significant reduction in pain intensity scores for patients treated with nortriptyline or maprotiline but not paroxetine.
- A review of 59 randomized, placebo-controlled trials concludes that high-quality research supports only the TCAs as effective analgesics.[6]
- Newer antidepressants offer different mechanisms of action, fewer side effects, and less toxicity but have not been rigorously studied in the treatment of chronic pain.[1]

SELECTIVE SEROTONIN REUPTAKE INHIBITORS

- Many studies have investigated the potential role of serotonin receptor subtypes in both nociceptive and hyperalgesic mechanisms of pain, but no definitive conclusions have been drawn.
- Selective serotonin reuptake inhibitors (SSRIs) produce weak antinociceptive effects in animal models of acute pain. This antinociception is blocked by serotonin receptor antagonists and enhanced by opioid receptor agonists.
- In human clinical trials, the efficacy of SSRIs in chronic pain syndromes has been variable and inconsistent:[14]
  - Desipramine was superior to fluoxetine in the treatment of painful diabetic peripheral neuropathy.
  - Paroxetine and citalopram were beneficial in patients with diabetic neuropathy.[8,12]
  - Fluoxetine significantly reduced pain in patients with rheumatoid arthritis and was comparable to amitriptyline. A 12-week course of fluoxetine also improved a variety of self-reported outcome measures in women with fibromyalgia.
  - The SSRIs were well tolerated and effective in the treatment of headache, especially migraine.
  - In a study of chronic tension-type headache, amitriptyline significantly reduced the duration of headache, headache frequency, and the intake of analgesics, but citalopram, an SSRI, did not.
- Until the results with SSRIs are more consistent, they are not recommended as first-choice medications unless a specific contraindication exists for TCAs.[15]

VENLAFAXINE

- The neurobiology of pain suggests a potential efficacy for all antidepressants, despite their different pharmacologic actions, in the treatment of chronic pain.[1,6]

- Venlafaxine inhibits the presynaptic reuptake of both serotonin and norepinephrine and, to a lesser extent, of dopamine, with fewer side effects than TCAs and SSRIs.
- In an animal model of neuropathic pain, venlafaxine reversed hyperalgesia and prevented its development.
- In humans, venlafaxine increased thresholds for pain tolerance to single electrical sural nerve stimulation and pain summation but had no effect on thresholds for pain detection to sural nerve stimulation, pressure pain, or pain experienced during a cold pressor test.
- Average pain relief and maximum pain intensity were significantly lower with venlafaxine than with placebo in a group of 13 patients with neuropathic pain following treatment of breast cancer. Additional analyses suggested that response improved with higher doses of venlafaxine.

NEWER ANTIDEPRESSANTS

- Norepinephrine and dopamine reuptake inhibitors, such as bupropion, produced antinociception in studies of thermal nociception. In a randomized, double-blind, placebo-controlled, crossover study of patients with neuropathic pain but without depression, bupropion SR (sustained-release) decreased pain intensity and interference of pain in quality of life.
- Nefazodone possesses the actions of analgesia and the potentiation of opioid analgesia in the mouse hot plate assay. In an open-label trial of diabetic neuropathy in 10 men, nefazodone significantly reduced self-ratings of pain, paresthesias, and numbness.
- Mirtazapine enhances postsynaptic noradrenergic and 5-HT1A-mediated serotonergic neurotransmission through antagonism of central α-auto- and hetero-adrenoreceptors. No controlled trials have been performed on the efficacy of mirtazapine in the treatment

of pain. Studies of mianserin, an older analog of mirtazapine, produced mixed results.[1]
- Monoamine oxidase inhibitors decrease the frequency and severity of migraine headaches.[8]
- Buspirone is effective in the prophylaxis of chronic tension-type headache; however, buspirone-treated patients used more rescue analgesics for acute treatment of headache than did patients treated with amitriptyline.
- Compared with placebo, protriptyline decreased chronic tension-type headache frequency by 86% in women.
- Trazodone did not decrease pain in a double-blind, placebo-controlled study of patients with chronic low back pain.[6,15]

FUTURE ANTIDEPRESSANTS

- Reboxetine is a selective noradrenaline reuptake inhibitor not yet available in the United States. In a placebo-controlled study of laser-evoked somatosensory potentials in healthy humans, reboxetine reduced N1 and P2 amplitudes along with subjective pain feelings and measurements, suggesting central and peripheral mechanisms of antinociception.
- Duloxetine, soon to be released in the United States, more potently blocks 5-HT and norepinephrine transporters in vitro and in vivo than does venlafaxine.[16] Studies of duloxetine for the treatment of depression as well as neuropathic pain are underway.

COMPARISONS

- Comparing the relative efficacy of antidepressants and other pharmacologic agents used in the treatment of pain is difficult.

TABLE 11–2 Numbers Needed to Treat for Antidepressants and Chronic Pain Conditions*

ANTIDEPRESSANT	DIABETIC NEUROPATHY	POSTHERPETIC NEURALGIA	PERIPHERAL NERVE INJURY	CENTRAL PAIN	ALL CONDITIONS
All types	3.0 (2.4–4.0)* 3.4 (2.6–4.7)[†]	2.3 (1.7–3.3)* 2.1 (1.7–3.0)[†]	2.5 (1.4–10.6)*	1.7 (1.1–3.0)*	2.9 (2.4–3.7)[†]
TCA (pooled)	2.4 (2.0–3.0)*	2.3 (1.7–3.3)*	2.5 (1.4–10.6)*	1.7 (1.1–3.0)*	2.6 (2.2–3.3)[‡] 3.5 (2.5–5.6)[†]
TCA (5-HT/NE)	2.0 (1.7–2.5)*	2.4 (1.8–3.9)*	2.5 (1.4–10.6)*	1.7 (1.1–3.0)*	2.7[†]
TCA (NE)	3.4 (2.3–6.6)*	1.9 (1.3–3.7)*	No data	No data	2.5[‡]
TCA (5-HT/NE with optimal dosing)	1.4 (1.1–1.9)*	No data	No data	No data	
SSRI	6.7 (3.4–435)*	No data	No data	Inactive*	

*From Sindrup and Jensen.[8]
[†]From Collins et al.[5]
[‡]From Sindrup and Jensen.[12]

• Several investigators suggest calculating the number needed to treat (NNT) to determine which medications are most likely to improve pain. The NNT is defined as how many patients would need to receive the specific treatment for one patient to achieve at least 50% pain relief. The formula for NNT is the inverse of the difference between the fractional response in the active treatment group and that in the placebo group. The NNT for the antidepressants used in the treatment of several types of neuropathic pain is approximately 2.5 and improves with higher serum levels (Table 11–2).[5,8,12,13] The NNT varies across studies due to differences in criteria for the calculation and definition of 50% pain relief.

• Only the effectiveness of the TCAs used to treat diabetic neuropathy and postherpetic neuralgia is supported with a variety of experimental studies that include a large number of patients.

CONCLUSION

• The effectiveness of antidepressants for the treatment of major depression is well-documented; however, the analgesic properties of this class of medication are underappreciated.[17]

• The complexity of chronic pain requires an extensive knowledge of the potential actions of many pharmacologic agents.

• It is important for the patient to understand the reason an antidepressant is being prescribed.

• It is even more important that the physician understand that one medication may be treating both pain and depression in a patient with chronic pain.

• The physician should always consider the innovative application of medications regardless of how they are traditionally classified.

REFERENCES

1. **Ansari A.** The efficacy of newer antidepressants in the treatment of chronic pain: A review of current literature. *Harvard Rev Psychiatry.* 2000;7:257–277.
2. **Clark MR.** Pain. In: Coffey CE, Cummings JL, eds. *Textbook of Geriatric Neuropsychiatry.* Washington, DC: American Psychiatric Press; 2000:415.
3. **Clark MR.** Pharmacological treatments for chronic nonmalignant pain. *Int Rev Psychiatry.* 2000;12:148.
4. **Clark MR, Cox TS.** Refractory chronic pain. *Psychiatr Clin North Am.* 2002;25:71.
5. **Collins SL, Moore RA, McQuay HJ, et al.** Antidepressants and anticonvulsants for diabetic neuropathy and postherpetic neuralgia: A quantitative systematic review. *J Pain Symptom Manage.* 2000;20:449.
6. **Lynch ME.** Antidepressants as analgesics: A review of randomized controlled trials. *J Psychiatry Neurosci.* 2001;26:30.
7. **Woolf CJ, Mannion RJ.** Neuropathic pain: Aetiology, symptoms, mechanisms, and management. *Lancet.* 1999;353:1959.
8. **Sindrup SH, Jensen TS.** Efficacy of pharmacological treatments of neuropathic pain: An update and effect related to mechanism of drug action. *Pain.* 1999;83:389.
9. **Carter GT, Sullivan MD.** Antidepressants in pain management. *Curr Opin Invest Drugs.* 2002;3:454.
10. **Feighner JP.** Mechanism of action of antidepressant medications. *J Clin Psychiatry.* 1999;60(suppl 4):4.
11. **Richeimer SH, Bajwa ZH, Kahraman SS, et al.** Utilization patterns of tricyclic antidepressants in a multidisciplinary pain clinic: A survey. *Clin J Pain.* 1997;13:324.
12. **Sindrup SH, Jensen TS.** Pharmacologic treatment of pain in polyneuropathy. *Neurology.* 2000;55:915.
13. **McQuay HJ, Tramer M, Nye BA, et al.** A systematic review of antidepressants in neuropathic pain. *Pain.* 1996;68:217.
14. **Jung AC, Staiger T, Sullivan M.** The efficacy of selective serotonin reuptake inhibitors for the management of chronic pain. *J Gen Intern Med.* 1997;12:384.
15. **Mattia C, Paoletti F, Coluzzi F, et al.** New antidepressants in the treatment of neuropathic pain: A review. *Minerva Anestesiol.* 2002;68:105.
16. **Bymaster FP, Dreshfield-Ahmad LJ, Threlkeld PG, et al.** Comparative affinity of duloxetine and venlafaxine for serotonin and norepinephrine transporters in vitro and in vivo, human serotonin receptor subtypes, and other neuronal receptors. *Neuropsychopharmacology.* 2001;25:871.
17. **Barkin RL, Fawcett J.** The management challenges of chronic pain: The role of antidepressants. *Am J Ther.* 2000;7:31.

12 ANTICONVULSANT DRUGS

Misha-Miroslav Backonja, MD

INTRODUCTION

• The category *neuropathic pain* includes a number of painful disorders of the nervous system, such as posttraumatic neuralgia and causalgia, painful diabetic neuropathy (PDN), postherpetic neuralgia (PHN), and lumbar and cervical radiculopathy.

• Neuropathic pain is clinically manifested by a spectrum of symptoms and signs that can vary in number and severity, regardless of the etiology of the disease. These symptoms and signs are important elements of pain assessment, which is used to develop a treatment plan and monitor neuropathic pain therapy.

- Multiple biochemical and pathophysiologic processes (peripheral and central sensitization) are involved in the genesis and maintenance of neuropathic pain, and the involvement of many receptors and neurotransmitter systems offers an opportunity to alleviate various manifestations of neuropathic pain with agents, such as anticonvulsant drugs (ACDs), that act on those mechanisms in specific ways.[1]

- ACDs used to treat neuropathic pain provide relief for the duration of drug administration, during which sensitization processes are presumably modulated, so these drugs may be considered neuromodulators.[2]

- Neuropathic pain frequently requires treatment with more than one medication, and each medication should have a different mode of action. Thus, systemic and rational administration allows these medications to affect multiple mechanisms involved in peripheral and central sensitization. Many pain experts refer to this approach as *rational polypharmacy* and follow the principles of sequential treatment trials by administering one medication at the time, monitoring its effects and side effects, and continuing only those that provide clinically meaningful pain relief with minimal side effects.[3]

ANTICONVULSANTS: EFFICACY DEMONSTRATED IN RANDOMIZED CLINICAL TRIALS

- Despite the availability of many ACDs, investigators have conducted randomized, clinical trials to demonstrate the efficacy of carbamazepine, gabapentin, and lamotrigine for the relief of neuropathic pain.[4]

- The clinical profiles of these agents are presented below, and those of other agents are summarized in Table 12–1.[5]

CARBAMAZEPINE

- Carbamazepine blocks ionic conductance of frequency-dependent neuronal activity without affecting normal nerve conduction suppressing spontaneous $A\delta$ and C-fiber activity, which is implicated in the genesis of pain.

- Carbamazepine was the first ACD used in clinical trials to treat a neuropathic painful disorder. In trigeminal neuralgia (TN) patients, the number needed to treat (NNT) to achieve pain relief was 2.6 (range, 2.2–3.3).[6] Carbamazepine was also efficacious in relieving PDN, with an NNT of 3.3 (range 2 to 9.4).[6] Doses in these studies ranged from 300 to 2400 mg/d

in divided doses, with a recommended serum level of between 4 and 12 ng/mL.

- Common side effects included somnolence, dizziness, and gait disturbance; previous studies raised a concern about hematopoietic effects, and it is advisable to monitor this possible complication of carbamazepine therapy.

- Despite evidence from randomized, clinical trials that carbamazepine is effective, clinical experience does not match these results, and the medication is difficult to administer because its use requires a great deal of skill in monitoring adverse effects.

GABAPENTIN

- Gabapentin was developed as a structural GABA analog, but gabapentin does not have direct GABAergic action nor does it affect GABA uptake or metabolism; thus, gabapentin's mechanism of action likely arises from its modulation of the α_2–δ subunit of N-type Ca^{2+} channels.

- Gabapentin has demonstrated its efficacy in relieving pain for patients with PDN with a NNT of 3.8 (2.4–8.7), PHN with a NNT of 3.2 (2.4–5.0), and other types of neuralgia.[7–9] In these studies, three divided doses of 900 to 3600 mg/d demonstrated efficacy in relieving neuropathic pain, and patients should receive at least 1800 mg/d before a treatment trial is considered to have failed.

- Gabapentin is well-tolerated and does not significantly differ from placebo with respect to adverse effects, the most common of which are well-tolerated and include dizziness, somnolence, ataxia, and swollen legs.

- Ease of use, good tolerability, no significant interaction with other medications, and a safe side effect profile make gabapentin the first choice for most physicians treating patients with any type of neuropathic pain.

LAMOTRIGINE

- Lamotrigine is a phenyltriazine derivative that blocks voltage-dependent Na^+ channels and inhibits glutamate release.

- In doses of 50 to 400 mg/d, lamotrigine has demonstrated efficacy in relieving pain in patients with TN refractory to other treatments (with a NNT of 2.1 [range, 1.3–6.1]), HIV neuropathy,[10] and central poststroke pain.[11] Lamotrigine also has demonstrated analgesic effect in PDN and in patients with incomplete spinal cord injury,[12] and it appears that doses of

TABLE 12–1 Neuromodulators for Analgesia

GENERIC	BRAND	MECHANISM OF ACTION	USE (FDA APPROVED)	DOSE TITRATION AND DOSE RANGE*	SERUM LEVEL	LABORATORY MONITORING	DRUG INTERACTIONS	DISCONTINUATION	SIDE EFFECTS†
Gabapentin	Neurontin	Ca²⁺ channel	Seizures, postherpetic neuralgia	100–4800 mg/d (in 3 or 4 divided doses and PRN—this is the only neuromodulator that can be also given PRN)	5–20‖	Baseline serum creatinine	Minimal	May stop abruptly; no rebound and no withdrawals related to pain symptoms	Sedation; ataxia; dizziness; nausea; vomiting; diplopia; edema; most disturbing is "feeling totally out of it"; most side effects transient (2–4 wk)
Carbamazepine‡,§	Tegretol, Carbatrol	Na⁺ channel	Seizures, trigeminal neuralgia	400–1800 mg/d (in 2 or 3 divided doses); start low (100 mg bid), increase weekly; extended release available	4–12	CBC, platelets, electrolytes (Na⁺)	VPA, LMT erythromycin, Ca²⁺ blockers	Titrate down by 25%/wk	Nausea most common; sedation; ataxia; vomiting; diplopia; rash: Stevens–Johnson; rare but serious blood dyscrasias (aplastic anemia, agranulocytosis)
Lamotrigine‡	Lamictal	Na⁺ channel	Seizures	25–600 mg/d; start low (25 mg qd), go **very** slowly, and follow package insert table	4–20‖	NA	VPA	Titrate down by 25%/wk	Sedation; ataxia; dizziness; nausea; vomiting; diplopia; rash: Stevens–Johnson life threatening especially if on valproic acid and risk higher if dose accelerated faster than package insert recommendation
Oxcarbazepine‡,§	Trileptal	Na⁺ channel	Seizures	600–2400 mg/d (in 2 divided doses); start low (150 mg bid), go slowly, increase weekly	NA	Electrolytes (Na⁺)	Minimal	Titrate down by 25%/wk	Sedation; ataxia; nausea; vomiting; diplopia; hyponatremia more often as compared with carbamazepine
Tiagabine‡	Gabitril	GABA	Seizures	8–64 mg/d (in 2–4 divided doses with food); start low (2 mg/d), go **very** slowly increase weekly	NA	NA	Minimal	Titrate down by 25%/wk	Asthenia; sedation; memory impairment; dizziness; ataxia; give with food to decrease peak related side effects
Valproic acid‡	Depakote, Depacon IV	GABA	Seizures, migraine, bipolar disorder	750–3000 mg/d (in 2 or 3 divided doses); extended-release tab also; start low (250mg bid), go **very** slow, increase weekly	50–125	AST, platelets	Everything	Titrate down by 25%/wk	Sedation; dizziness; memory impairment; weight gain; hair loss¶
Topiramate‡,§	Topamax	Mixed Na⁺ and Ca²⁺	Seizures	15–800 mg/d (in 2 divided doses); start low (15 mg bid), go **very** slowly, increase weekly	NA	Baseline serum creatinine	Minimal	Titrate down by 25%/wk	Cognitive dysfunction; dizziness; fatigue; weight loss; nephrolithiasis; paresthesias
Zonisamide‡	Zonegran	Mixed Na⁺ and Ca²⁺	Seizures	200–600 mg/d; start low (100 mg qod), go **very** slowly, increase every other week by 100 mg	10–40‖	Baseline serum creatinine	Mixed Na⁺ and Ca²⁺	Titrate down by 25%/wk	Nephrolithiasis; anemia; leukopenia; weight loss; somnolence; asthenia; cognitive dysfunction; rash; paresthesias
Levetiracetam	Keppra	Unknown	Seizures	1000–4000 mg/d (in 2 or 3 divided doses); start low (250 mg bid), go slowly, increase weekly	NA	Baseline serum creatinine	Minimal	Titrate down by 25%/wk	Somnolence; asthenia; cognitive dysfunction; behavioral abnormalities including irritability and mood changes

*In the elderly, always start with the lowest dose possible!
†All of these drugs are CNS-active and toxic effects are frequently related to the CNS!
‡Clearance increased by inducers of P450 enzymes.
§Potential birth control failure.
‖Therapeutic range not established.
¶There is no evidence that VPA works for pain disorder other than headaches.

200 mg/d relieve neuropathic pain, including that associated with HIV/AIDS. Common adverse effects relate to the central nervous system and include dizziness, ataxia, constipation, nausea, somnolence, and diplopia.
- A serious side effect is rash, which is as common as with administration of carbamazepine and can, in rare instances, progress into Stevens–Johnson syndrome. The chance of this occurring is drastically decreased when lamotrigine is titrated slowly. The adverse effects of lamotrigine are more likely to occur if patients are taking valproate at the same time, a situation that is common in epilepsy but rare in the treatment of neuropathic pain, as valproate does not have a proven record in treatment of neuropathic pain.

SUMMARY

- Evidence supports the use of carbamazepine for treatment of TN and of gabapentin for treatment of PHN and PDN. Evidence of the efficacy of lamotrigine is not robust, but the results of a number of studies for a variety of neuropathic pain disorders, including central pain syndromes, are encouraging.
- The first lesson learned from a randomized clinical trial is that ACDs are the first choice for treatment of neuropathic pain. Another lesson is that doses of these medications have to be appropriate; for example, doses should be at least 1800 mg/d in three divided doses for gabapentin and more than 200 mg/d for lamotrigine.
- It is also important to measure secondary outcomes, particularly those related to quality of life, as was done in the gabapentin trial.
- With their safe side effect profile, newer ACDs have become an important component of rational polypharmacy, but this concept needs to be further developed. Most of the newer anticonvulsants have a very wide dosing range, and that property should be explored and used.

REFERENCES

1. **Tremont-Lukats IW, Megeff C, Backonja MM.** Anticonvulsants for neuropathic pain syndromes: Mechanisms of action and place in therapy. *Drugs.* 2001; 60: 1029–1052.
2. **Wiffen P, McQuay H, Carroll D, et al.** Anticonvulsant drugs for acute and chronic pain. *Cochrane Database Syst Rev.* 2000;CD001133.
3. **Sindrup SH, Jensen TS.** Efficacy of pharmacological treatments of neuropathic pain: An update and effect related to mechanism of drug action. *Pain.* 1999;83:389–400.
4. **Kingery W.** A critical review of controlled clinical trials for peripheral neuropathic pain and complex regional pain syndrome. *Pain.* 1997;73:123–139.
5. **White HS.** Comparative anticonvulsant and mechanistic profile of the established and newer antiepileptic drugs. *Epilepsia.* 1999;40(suppl 5):S2–S10.
6. **Backonja MM.** Use of anticonvulsants for treatment of neuropathic pain. *Neurology.* 2002;10;59(5, suppl 2):S14.
7. **Backonja M, Beydoun A, Edwards KR, et al.** Gabapentin for the symptomatic treatment of painful neuropathy in patients with diabetes mellitus: A randomized controlled trial. *JAMA.* 1998;280:1831–1836.
8. **Rowbotham M, Harden N, Stacey B, et al.** Gabapentin for the treatment of postherpetic neuralgia: A randomized controlled trial. *JAMA.* 1998;280:1837–1842.
9. **Rice AS, Maton S.** Postherpetic Neuralgia Study Group. Gabapentin in postherpetic neuralgia: A randomized, double blind, placebo controlled study. *Pain.* 2001;94:215–224.
10. **Simpson DM, Olney R, McArthur JC, et al.** A placebo-controlled trial of lamotrigine for painful HIV-associated neuropathy. *Neurology.* 2000;54:2115–2119.
11. **Vestergaard K, Andersen G, Gottrup H, et al.** Lamotrigine for central poststroke pain: A randomized controlled trial. *Neurology.* 2001;56:184–190.
12. **Finnerup NB, Sindrup SH, Bach FW, et al.** Lamotrigine in spinal cord injury pain: A randomized controlled trial. *Pain.* 2002;96:375–383.

13 SODIUM AND CALCIUM CHANNEL ANTAGONISTS

Mark S. Wallace, MD

INTRODUCTION

- Several lines of evidence suggest that both spontaneous pain and evoked pain are mediated in part by voltage-sensitive sodium and calcium channels.[1]
- Sodium and calcium channel antagonists used in clinical practice are of the voltage-dependent type in that the neurons must remain depolarized for a significant period for maximal blocking action to occur.
- Both the central and peripheral nervous systems have an abundance of sodium and calcium channels.

SODIUM CHANNEL ANTAGONISTS

MECHANISM OF ACTION

- Many subtypes of sodium channels are expressed throughout the nervous system.
- Blockade of the sodium channel prevents the upstroke of the axonal action potential. If this blockade occurs

in pain-sensitive sensory neurons, pain relief may result.

- At least seven different sodium channels have been isolated, all with important biophysical and pharmacologic differences resulting in differing sensitivities to sodium channel blockers.
- Sodium channels are classified by their sensitivity to tetrodotoxin (TTX), a potent sodium channel blocker. TTX-sensitive (TTXs) sodium channels are blocked by small concentrations of TTX, whereas TTX-resistant (TTXr) sodium channels are not blocked even when exposed to high concentrations of TTX. The role of TTXs and TTXr sodium channels in nociception is controversial; however, as described above it is clear that after nerve injury and during inflammation, there are dynamic and expression changes that occur in both TTXs and TTXr sodium channels.
- Proponents for the TTXr sodium channel as being important in nociception argue that because of their different voltage sensitivities of activation and inactivation, TTXr channels are still capable of generating impulses at depolarized potentials (which characterize the chronically damaged nerve fibers), whereas TTXs channels are inactivated and cannot contribute to excitability. For example, PN3 is a subclass of the TTXr sodium channels that is located only in the peripheral nervous system on small neurons in the dorsal root ganglion and is thought to be specific to pain transmission.[2]
- The development of the spontaneous and evoked pain after nervous system injury is thought to be due not only to a change in the number of sodium channels but also a change in the distribution and type of sodium channels. These sodium channels display marked pharmacologic differences from the uninjured state.
- It is speculated that in the presence of injury, sodium channels on C fibers display an exaggerated response to sodium channel blockade as opposed to the uninjured state; therefore, it has been suggested that neuropathic pain is more responsive to sodium channel blockade than nociceptive pain.[3]
- The exact site of action of the sodium channel antagonists is unclear. However, systemic lidocaine and mexiletine decrease the flare response after intradermal capsaicin, suggesting a peripheral site of action.[4]

EFFICACY

- Systemic sodium channel antagonists have little to no effect on acute thermal and mechanical thresholds (both painful and nonpainful).[4]
- The systemic delivery of sodium channel antagonists has been shown to decrease postoperative pain and analgesic requirements.

- Studies on the systemic delivery of sodium channel antagonists for the treatment of neuropathic pain have had conflicting results. Overall, there appears to be an effect on neuropathic pain, but there is a difference in efficacy between agents due mainly to dose-limiting side effects (see below).

INDIVIDUAL DRUGS

LIDOCAINE

- Lidocaine has been extensively studied in experimental, postoperative, and neuropathic pain states.
- At maximally tolerable doses ($3 \mu g/mL$ plasma level), intravenous lidocaine has little effect on human experimental pain.[4]
- At doses below $3 \mu g/mL$ plasma level, intravenous lidocaine reduces postoperative and neuropathic pain.[5]
- When examined in patients reporting significant pain secondary to a variety of neuropathic states, subanesthetic doses of systemic lidocaine produce clinically relevant relief in diabetes, nerve injury pain states, and cancer.[6–9]
- The lidocaine dose is 2 mg/kg over 20 minutes followed by 1–3 mg/kg/h titrated to effect.
- The correlation between plasma levels and side effects has been studied the most with intravenous lidocaine (Table 13–1).

MEXILETINE

- Mexiletine is an oral bioavailable analog of lidocaine.
- At plasma concentrations up to $0.5 \mu g/mL$ plasma level, there is no effect on human experimental pain.[10]
- Mexiletine has been reported to be effective in a variety of neuropathic pain syndromes including diabetic neuropathy, alcoholic neuropathy, peripheral nerve injury, and thalamic pain. However, more recent reports question the efficacy of oral mexiletine in neuropathic pain, making it difficult to draw conclusions on efficacy.[11–17]

TABLE 13–1 Intravenous Lidocaine Side Effects versus Plasma Level

SIDE EFFECT	PLASMA LEVEL ($\mu g/mL$)
Lightheadedness	1–2
Periorbital numbness	2
Metallic taste	2–3
Tinnitus	5–6
Blurred vision	6
Muscular twitching	8
Convulsions	10
Cardiac depression	20–25

- It appears that oral mexiletine is a poor choice for the management of neuropathic pain. The exact therapeutic plasma concentration for analgesia is yet to be determined, but it appears that dose-limiting side effects occur at a lower plasma concentration than analgesia.
- It appears that the maximum tolerable dose of mexiletine is between 800 and 900 mg/d.[10,18] However, it is questionable if this dose results in analgesic plasma levels. The highest tolerated plasma mexiletine level is about 0.5 µg/mL, which is below the analgesic level.

LAMOTRIGINE

- Lamotrigine is a sodium channel antagonist with activity at glutaminergic sites resulting in anticonvulsant activity.
- It has been shown to decrease acute pain induced by the cold pressor test.
- Lamotrigine significantly reduces the analgesic requirements of postoperative pain.[19]
- Studies on the efficacy of lamotrigine for neuropathic pain have produced conflicting results likely due to differences in total daily doses. Doses below 200 mg/d are likely not efficacious. Doses between 200 and 400 mg/d appear to be efficacious in neuropathic pain.[20–22]
- Lamotrigine appears to be well tolerated with few side effects.

PROCAINE

- Procaine was one of the first local anesthetics to be used systemically for the treatment of pain.
- An advantage of procaine is its extremely low toxicity when administered systemically. A disadvantage is the extremely short half-life due to ester hydrolysis by plasma pseudocholinesterases and red cell esterases.
- The earliest uses of procaine were to supplement general anesthesia and to treat chronic musculoskeletal disorders.[23]
- It has also been shown anecdotally to be effective in the treatment of postherpetic neuralgia.[24]
- There is one controlled study using procaine 4–6.5 mg/kg that shows efficacy in postoperative pain.[25]

FLECAINIDE

- Systemic flecainide has been demonstrated to suppress ectopic nerve discharge in neuropathic rats.[26]
- The clinical use of flecainide has been mixed.
- In postherpetic neuralgia, flecainide was effective in 15 of 20 patients.[27]
- Flecainide was ineffective in a pilot study in cancer pain.[15]

CALCIUM CHANNEL ANTAGONISTS

MECHANISM OF ACTION

- Six unique types of calcium channels are expressed throughout the nervous system (designated L, N, P, Q, R, and T).
- Voltage-sensitive calcium channels of the N type exist in the superficial laminae of the dorsal horn and are thought to modulate nociceptive processing by a central mechanism.
- Blockade of the N-type calcium channel in the superficial dorsal horn modulates membrane excitability and inhibits neurotransmitter release, resulting in pain relief.

EFFICACY

- The N-type calcium channel antagonists have the most analgesic efficacy. L-type antagonists have moderate analgesic efficacy and the P/Q type have minimal analgesic efficacy.
- Unlike the systemic sodium channel antagonists, animal studies suggest that only the N-type calcium channel antagonists have an effect on acute thermal and mechanical thresholds (both painful and nonpainful). This suggests a greater analgesic potency than for the sodium channel blockers.
- Phase III trials have shown that the epidural and intrathecal delivery of the N-type calcium channel antagonist (ziconotide) decreases postoperative pain.[28]
- Rigorous phase III trials have demonstrated that intrathecal delivery of the N-type calcium channel antagonist (ziconotide) is effective in the treatment of neuropathic pain.[29]

INDIVIDUAL DRUGS

ZICONOTIDE

- Ziconotide is a 25-amino-acid peptide that is a synthetic version of a naturally occurring peptide found in the venom of the marine snail, *Conus magus*.
- It specifically and selectively binds to N-type voltage-sensitive calcium channels.
- It is the first and only N-type calcium channel antagonist to enter clinical development.
- A recent study on intrathecally administered ziconotide for neuropathic pain reported the following side effects: dizziness, nausea, nystagmus, gait imbalance, confusion, constipation, and urinary retention. These side effects are dose related and rapidly reversible on decreasing or stopping the drug.[29]

- It appears that spinally delivered ziconotide has a narrow therapeutic window. When this therapeutic window is achieved, analgesia is possible without unacceptable side effects.
- The therapeutic dose is in the range 1–3 µg/d.

L-TYPE CALCIUM CHANNEL ANTAGONISTS (NIMODIPINE, VERAPAMIL)

- Nimodipine has been shown to decrease postoperative opioid requirements.[30]
- There are numerous reports on the efficacy of L-type calcium channel antagonists for the prevention and treatment of migraine and chronic daily headaches.[31]
- Nimodipine has been shown to significantly reduce morphine requirements in cancer patients requiring morphine dose escalation.[32]

REFERENCES

1. **Cummins TR, Waxman SG.** Down regulation of tetrodotoxin-resistant sodium currents and upregulation of a rapidly repriming tetrodotoxin-sensitive sodium current in small spinal sensory neurons after nerve injury. *Neuroscience.* 1997;17:3503–3514.
2. **Tanaka M, Cummins TR, Ishikawa K, et al.** SNS sodium channel expression increases in dorsal root ganglion neurons in the carrageenan inflammatory pain model. *NeuroReport.* 1998;9:967–972.
3. **Chaplan SR, Bach FW, Yaksh TL.** Systemic use of local anesthetics in pain states. In Yaksh TL, Lynch C, Zapol WM, Maze M, Biebuyck JF, Saidman LJ (eds). *Anesthesia: Biologic Foundations.* Philadelphia: Lippincott–Raven; 1997:977–986.
4. **Wallace MS, Laitin S, Licht D, Yaksh TL.** Concentration–effect relations for intravenous lidocaine infusions in human volunteers: Effect on acute sensory thresholds and capsaicin-evoked hyperpathia. *Anesthesiology.* 1997; 86:1262–1272.
5. **Cassuto J, Wallin G, Hogstrom S, Faxen A, Rimback G.** Inhibition of postoperative pain by continuous low-dose intravenous infusion of lidocaine. *Anesth Analg.* 1985; 64:971–974.
6. **Kastrup J, Petersen P, Dejgard A, Angeo HR, Hilsted J.** Intravenous lidocaine infusion: A new treatment of chronic painful diabetic neuropathy? *Pain.* 1987;28:69–75.
7. **Marchettini P, Lacerenza M, Marangoni C, Pellegata G, Sotgiu ML, Smirne S.** Lidocaine test in neuralgia. *Pain.* 1992;48:S63–S66.
8. **Rowbotham M, Reisner-Keller L, Fields H.** Both intravenous lidocaine and morphine reduce the pain of postherpetic neuralgia. *Neurology.* 1991;41:1024–1028.
9. **Attal N, Gaude V, Brasseur L, Dupuy M, Guirimand F, Parker F, Bouhassira D.** Intravenous lidocaine in central pain: A double-blind, placebo-controlled, psychophysical study. *Neurology.* 2000;54:564–574.
10. **Ando K, Wallace MS, Schulteis G, Braun J.** Neurosensory finding after oral mexiletine in healthy volunteers. *Reg Anesth Pain Med.* 2000;25:468–474.
11. **Stracke H, Meyer UE.** Mexiletine in the treatment of diabetic neuropathy. *Diabetes Care.* 1992;15:1550–1555.
12. **Nishiyama K, Sakuta M.** Mexiletine for painful alcoholic neuropathy. *Intern Med.* 1995;34:577–579.
13. **Davis RW.** Successful treatment for phantom pain. *Orthopedics.* 1993;16:691–695.
14. **Awerbuch G, Sandyk R.** Mexiletine for thalamic pain syndrome. *Int J Neurosci.* 1990;55:129–133.
15. **Chong SF, Bretscher ME, Maillard JA.** Pilot study evaluating local anesthetics administered systemically for treatment of pain in patients with advanced cancer. *J Pain Symp Manage.* 1997;13:112–117.
16. **Wright JM, Oki JC, Graves L.** Mexiletine in the symptomatic treatment of diabetic peripheral neuropathy. *Ann Pharmacother.* 1997;31:29–34.
17. **Chiou-Tan F, Tuel S, Johnson J.** Effect of mexiletine on spinal cord injury dysesthetic pain. *Am J Phys Med Rehab.* 1996;75:84–87.
18. **Wallace MS, Magnuson S, Ridgeway B.** Oral mexiletine in the treatment of neuropathic pain. *Reg Anesth Pain Med.* 2000;25:459–467.
19. **Bonicalzi V, Canavero S, Cerutti F, Piazza M, Clemente M, Chio A.** Lamotrigine reduces total postoperative analgesic requirement: A randomized double-blind placebo-controlled pilot study. *Surgery.* 1997;122:567–570.
20. **Zakrzewska JM, Chaudhry Z, Nurmikko TJ, Patton DW, Mullens EL.** Lamotrigine (lamictal) in refractory trigeminal neuralgia: Results from a double-blind placebo controlled crossover trial. *Pain.* 1997;73:223–230.
21. **Simpson DM, Olney R, McArthur JC, Khan A, Godbold J, Ebel-Frommer K.** A placebo-controlled trial of lamotrigine for painful HIV-associated neuropathy. *Neurology.* 2000;54:2115–2119.
22. **McCleane G.** 200 mg daily of lamotrigine has no analgesic effect in neuropathic pain: A randomized, double-blind, placebo controlled trial. *Pain.* 1999;83:105–107.
23. **Edmonds GW, Comer WH, Kennedy JD, Taylor IB.** Intravenous use of procaine in general anesthesia. *JAMA.* 1949;141:761–765.
24. **Shanbrom E.** Treatment of herpetic pain and postherpetic neuralgia with intravenous procaine. *JAMA.* 1961; 176: 1041–1043.
25. **Keats AS, D'Alessandro GL, Beecher HK.** A controlled study of pain relief by intravenous procaine. *JAMA.* 1951; 147:1761–1763.
26. **Dunlop R, Davies RJ, Hockley J, Turner P.** Analgesic effects of oral flecainide. *Lancet.* 1988;1:420–421.
27. **Ichimata M, Ikebe H, Yoshitake S, Hattori S, Iwasaka H, Noguchi T.** Analgesic effects of flecainide on postherpetic neuralgia. *Int J Clin Pharmacol Res.* 2001;21:15–19.
28. **Atanassoff PG, Hartmannsgruber MW, Thrasher J, et al.** Ziconotide, a new N-type calcium channel blocker, administered intrathecally for acute postoperative pain. *Reg Anesth Pain Med.* 2000;25:274–278.

29. **Presley R, Charapata S, Perrar-Brechner T, et al.** Chronic, opioid-resistant, neuropathic pain: Marked analgesic efficacy of intrathecal ziconotide. Paper presented at: 1998 Annual American Pain Society; San Diego, CA; 1998; Abstract A894.

30. **Lehmann KA, Ribbert N, Horrichs-Haermeyer G.** Postoperative patient-controlled analgesia with alfentanil: Analgesic efficacy and minimum effective concentrations. *J Pain Symp Manage.* 1990;5:249–258.

31. **Micieli D, Piazza D, Sinforiani E, et al.** Antimigraine drugs in the management of daily chronic headaches: Clinical profiles of responsive patients. *Cephalgia.* 1985;Suppl 2:219–224.

32. **Santillán R, Hurlé M, Armijo J, de los Mozos R, Flórez J.** Nimodipine-enhanced opiate analgesia in cancer patients requiring morphine dose escalation: A double-blind, placebo-controlled study. *Pain.* 1998;76:17–26.

14 TRAMADOL

Michelle Stern, MD
Kevin Sperber, MD
Marco Pappagallo, MD

INTRODUCTION

- Tramadol was introduced into the United States market in 1995 after being widely used around the world for approximately 20 years.
- When introduced in the United States it was with the expectation that it would offer an alternative to nonsteroidal anti-inflammatory drugs (NSAIDs) and opioids for moderate to moderately severe pain.
- Tramadol is considered a more potent analgesic than oral NSAIDs, with fewer gastrointestinal, renal, and cardiac side effects.[1]
- Compared with traditional opioids, tramadol offers analgesia with reduced risk of abuse, physical dependence, sedation, and constipation.
- Although it can be administered via the epidural, intravenous, rectal, or oral route (immediate- and sustained-release) in other countries, in the United States it is currently available only in the immediate-release oral formulation.
- The oral formulation is available in two forms: a 50-mg tramadol tablet and a 325-mg/37.5-mg acetminophen/tramadol combination. It is marketed under the brand names Ultram and Ultracet, respectively (Ortho–McNeil).
- An extended-release formulation (Tramadol ER) is currently undergoing Food and Drug Administration (FDA) trials and is being tested in strengths ranging from 100 to 400 mg daily.

- The Drug Enforcement Agency (DEA) has currently classified the drug as a nonscheduled analgesic.

MECHANISM OF ACTION

- Tramadol is a synthetic 4-phenyl-piperidine analog of codeine.[2]
- Its mode of action is not yet completely understood, but it is thought to work primarily in the central nervous system.
- It differs from traditional opioids because tramadol-induced analgesia is only partially blocked by the opiate antagonist naloxone. This suggests an additional nonopioid component for the pain relief.
- Laboratory studies have provided insight into the possible dual mode of action: It binds weakly to μ-opioid receptor sites and inhibits the reuptake of norepinephrine and serotonin. Its affinity for the μ-opioid receptor compared with morphine and codeine is 1/6000 and 1/10, respectively.
- The α_2-adrenoceptor antagonist yohimbine has been shown to reduce the analgesic effects of tramadol, further supporting the nonopioid component for pain relief.

PHARMACODYNAMICS

- The chemical name is *cis*-2-[(dimethylamino)methyl]-1-(3-methoxyphenyl) cyclohexanol hydrochloride.
- The parent compound is a racemic drug and both its (+) and (−) forms play an important role in its mechanism. The (+) enantiomer has a higher affinity for the μ receptor and increases serotonin levels by inhibiting its uptake and enhancing its release. The (−) enantiomer increases norepinephrine levels by stimulating α_2-adrenergic receptors, which inhibit norepinephrine reuptake.
- Tramadol is extensively metabolized by the liver, with the major pathways being N- and O-demethylation (phase 1) and glucuronidation or sulfation. The drug and its metabolites are eliminated primarily through the kidneys, with 30% being excreted unchanged.
- Twenty-three metabolites are currently identified (11 phase 1 metabolites and 12 conjugates), but only one has been shown to play a significant role in tramadol's analgesic properties, M1.
- The M1 metabolite is the O-demethylated form of tramadol, with the (+) form having the greater potential for analgesic effect. An isoenzyme of cytochrome P450, CYP2D6, is responsible for conversion to the M1 metabolite.
- Seven percent of the Caucasian population do not have this isoenzyme and therefore are poor metabolizers of

this drug. This population has shown decreased analgesia with tramadol.

- The analgesic potency of the M1 metabolite is 6 times greater than that of its parent drug, owing to its 200 times greater affinity to the µ-opioid binding site.
- Bioavailability after oral administration is 75%, with only 20% found bound to plasma proteins.
- The average dose for a healthy adult is 50–100 mg every 6 hours.
- Times to peak plasma and half-life levels after a single 100-mg dose are 1.6 and 6.3 hours for the parent drug and 3 and 7.4 hours for the M1 metabolite, respectively.
- The analgesic benefit peaks 2 hours after the initial dose and lasts approximately 6 hours, with steady state occurring after 48 hours.
- When tramadol is given with food, the percentage absorbed and peak plasma concentration are unaffected, but the time to peak plasma concentration is increased by 35 minutes.
- Dosage adjustment is recommended in the elderly and in patients with renal and liver disease.

DOSAGE

HEALTHY ADULTS

- Tramadol is typically prescribed to healthy adults in dosages of 50–100 mg, three to four times a day. It can be used for both acute and chronic pain.
- The maximum dose recommended by the manufacturer is 400 mg in a 24-hour period secondary to the increased risk of side effects with higher doses; however, there have been limited clinical reports of the use of up to 600 mg/d in carefully selected patients.
- For Ultracet the dose recommended by the manufacturer is 2 tablets every 4 to 6 hours as needed for pain, with a duration of use not to exceed 5 days with a maximum daily dose of 8 tablets (300 mg of tramadol and 2.6 g of acetaminophen)[14]; however, these authors have found it efficacious to use in patients with chronic pain.
- A carbamazepine dose of 800 mg daily has been shown to increase the metabolism of tramadol and this may necessitate a dosage adjustment.[3]
- Ondansetron, a serotonin 5-HT-3 receptor antagonist, has also been reported to inhibit the analgesic effects of tramadol.[4,5]
- Tramadol can also have a synergistic effect with other sedating medication which may necessitate a dosage adjustment.

SPECIAL POPULATIONS

ELDERLY AND PATIENTS WITH LIVER OR RENAL DISEASE

- There are three categories of people who require an adjustment of the usual dosage for tramadol: the elderly and patients with liver or renal disease.
- Because of the increase in the elimination time of the drug in the elderly (75 years and older), their dosage should not exceed 300 mg/d.
- Advanced liver disease prolongs the drug's half–life and requires dosage reduction to 50 mg every 12 hours (maximum daily dose, 100 mg/d).
- As tramadol is excreted primarily through the kidneys, in patients with a creatinine clearance less than 30 mL/min, the rate and extent of excretion are significantly reduced, and a dosage adjustment of 50–100 mg every 12 hours (maximum daily dose, 200 mg/d) is required.
- Only 7% of tramadol and its metabolites is cleared by a 4-hour dialysis. Dialysis patients can receive their dose on dialysis day.
- For Ultracet, 2 tablets every 12 hours is the dosage recommendation for patients with a creatinine clearance less than 30 mL/min.
- Ultracet is not currently recommended for use in patients with liver disease.[6]

CHILDREN AND PREGNANT AND NURSING MOTHERS

- The safety of tramadol use in the pediatric population and pregnant and nursing mothers has not yet been established and therefore tramadol is not currently recommended in the United States, but it has been investigated in research abroad.
- Multiple pediatric studies have been performed to evaluate the use of tramadol for acute pain in children as young as 1 month and these studies consistently reported a 1–2-mg/kg single dose as safe and effective.[7]
- Tramadol is currently classified by FDA as pregnancy risk factor C. One percent of the drug dose is transferred via the placenta and 0.1% is identified in breast milk.
- A few studies that used tramadol in labor showed that it provided adequate analgesia with no significant respiratory depression in the newborn.
- There is a potential for neonatal withdrawal after chronic use during pregnancy, as demonstrated in a single case report.[8]

INDICATIONS FOR USE

- The World Health Organization (WHO) recommends tramadol as a step 2 analgesic agent for a variety of painful conditions.

- It has been used successfully for malignant pain, osteoarthritic pain, low back pain, diabetic neuropathy, fibromyalgia, restless leg syndrome, postherpetic neuralgia, pain from surgical and dental procedures, and with NSAIDs to help control breakthrough pain.[9–14]

SIDE EFFECT PROFILE

- Twenty to thirty percent of patients discontinue tramadol use secondary to intolerable side effects.
- Dizziness, lethargy, nausea, vomiting, and constipation are some of the common complaints after the first week of use.
- Complaints of nausea and vomiting decrease with continued use, while the incidence of other side effects such as dizziness, lethargy, headache, and constipation failed to significantly improve.
- The incidence of side effects may appear daunting initially, but in the authors' clinical experience, it is similar to many other opioids.[12]

TITRATION SCHEDULE

- A slow titration schedule has been shown to improve the patient's tolerance of the medication (Table 14–1); while slow titration is not desirable for treatment of acute pain, it may be useful in treatment of the patient with chronic pain who has a history of poor tolerance of medication or is at increased risk of falls. A balance

must be struck between maximizing tolerance to the drug and achieving timely pain relief for the patient.
- Two of the suggested regimens in the literature for a slow titration are a 10-day schedule and a 16-day schedule.
  - In the 10-day titration, 50 mg of tramadol daily is started and increased by 50 mg every 3 days until the target of 200 mg/d is reached.
  - A slower titration schedule for those high-risk elderly patients starts with 25 mg of tramadol daily and increases by 25 mg every 3 days until a dose of 25 mg qid is achieved. Then, the total daily dose is increased by 50 mg every 3 days until a dosage of 50 mg qid or 200 mg/d is reached. After titration, the dosage can be increased to the maximum recommended dosage for the patient.
- In the authors' experience, most patients will tolerate a slightly more aggressive titration schedule. We initiate treatment with 25 mg every 8 hours or 50 mg every 12 hours. If this dose is adequately tolerated after 3 days, we increase to 50 mg every 8 hours. The dose is titrated upward by 50–75 mg every 3–5 days until adequate analgesia is obtained or the maximum safe dosage is reached.
- If significant side effects develop, tramadol is titrated downward to a previously tolerated dose and more time is allowed before further titration is attempted.
- Patients are instructed to take the initial dose and all subsequent increased dosages of this medication in the evening and warned of the potential psychomotor effects of the medication.

TABLE 14–1   Titration Schedule

TITRATION PROTOCOL	INITIAL DOSE	TITRATION SCHEDULE	RECOMMENDED FOR
10-day titration	50 mg qd for 3 days	50 mg bid for 3 days Then increase to 50 mg tid for 3 days. Then continue at 50 mg qid May increase further until analgesic effect or recommended therapeutic dosage is reached	Elderly Fall risks Medication sensitivity

16-day titration	25 mg qd for 3 days	25 mg bid for 3 days
		Then increase to 25 mg tid for
		  3 days
		Then increase to 25 mg qid for
		  3 days
		Then increase to 50 mg bid and 25 mg
		  bid for 3 days
		Then increase to 50 mg qid
		May increase until analgesic effect or
		  recommended therapeutic dosage is achieved
			Elderly
			Fall risks
			Medication sensitivity

Author's rapid titration recommendation	75 mg daily divided into 25 mg tid with first dose at bedtime or 100 mg daily divided into 50 mg bid with first at bedtime dose	Increase by 50 or 75 mg every 3–5 days
		  until analgesic effect or recommended
		  therapeutic dosage
			Medication sensitivity
			Mild to moderate fall risks

- Written instructions may improve compliance.
- The recently introduced generic tramadol is a 50-mg tablet that is not scored, unlike Ultram, and this may complicate the gradual titration schedule using a 25-mg dosage. In this case, the alternate titration schedule starting with 50 mg bid may be preferred.

DRUG–DRUG INTERACTIONS OR THE PROBLEM WITH POLYPHARMACY

- Although tramadol has been associated with many possible side effects, the two most striking side effects are seizures and the serotonin syndrome.

SEIZURES

- There have been reports of seizures in patients taking tramadol both alone and in conjunction with other medications, although some studies have suggested that the risk of seizures with tramadol use alone was comparable to that of other centrally acting analgesics.
- The risk of seizures is increased with tramadol overdose and as the number and dosage of other psychoactive medications are increased. The psychoactive medications most commonly cited in the literature to increase the risk are antidepressants (monoamine oxidase inhibitors [MAOIs], tricyclic antidepressants, and selective serotonin reuptake inhibitors [SSRIs]), neuroleptics, and other opioids. If it is essential to use these medications in combination, caution is required and the risks versus benefits of this treatment plan should be discussed with the patient in advance.
- In one large retrospective study, seizures were reported to occur in less than 1% of tramadol users. Patients with spontaneous seizures with tramadol alone have been postulated to be individuals who are poor metabolizers of the drug.
- It is prudent to avoid the co-administration of tramadol with any medication that may lower the seizure threshold as well as in patients with a history of seizures/epilepsy, head trauma, alcohol and drug withdrawal, and any other insult to the central nervous system.
- Any protective effect of co-administration of anticonvulsant medication with tramadol has not been established.
- A seizure associated with tramadol should be treated with benzodiazepines or barbituates.[15,16]
- In tramadol overdose, coma and respiratory depression occurred only at 800 mg and higher doses, whereas seizure, tachycardia, and hypertension occurred at doses starting at 500 mg.

- It is important to note that naloxone reversed only some of the cardiorespiratory effects of the drug and its use was associated with an increase risk of seizure activity.

SEROTONIN SYNDROME

- Another severe complication, the serotonin syndrome, is associated with the use of tramadol and other agents that can increase central nervous system serotonin levels such as SSRIs and MAOIs.
- Serotonin syndrome should be suspected in patients who develop an abrupt change in mental status accompanied by autonomic symptoms and other neurologic changes. Fever, shivering, diaphoresis, nausea, vomiting, and diarrhea are potential autonomic symptoms. Increase in muscle tone, myoclonus, tremor, and ataxia may be additional neurologic findings. There have also been reports of agitation, hypomania, and hallucinations.
- Treatment includes cessation of the medication, symptom management, and antiserotonergic drugs such as cyproheptadine.[17–19]

WHY USE TRAMADOL?

- The benefits of using tramadol instead of traditional opioids include lower abuse potential and physical dependence as well as reduced incidence of such side effects as constipation, respiratory depression, and sedation.
- The rate of abuse with tramadol has been reported at less than 1 case per 100,000 patients. In 97% of the abuse cases there was a history of alcohol or drug dependence; therefore, it should be used with caution in this patient population.
- When the drug is withdrawn abruptly, development of an abstinence syndrome similar to that observed with other opioids is possible, but the rate is 1 per month per 100,000 cases. The abstinence syndrome of tramadol can be treated by reinstitution of tramadol and gradual downward titration of the dose.
- Methadone has also been shown to be effective in treating abstinence syndrome secondary to abrupt discontinuation of tramadol.
- Patients with a history of a true allergic reaction to codeine or morphine should use tramadol with caution as there is the potential for cross-reactivity since tramadol is a codeine analog.[20–22]

SUMMARY

- Tramadol's mechanism of action is not completely understood. It works both at the μ-opioid receptors and by inhibiting the reuptake of norepinephrine and serotonin in the central nervous system. Tramadol has proven effective for moderate to moderately severe pain.

- It does not affect the prostaglandin cycle, like NSAIDs, and is associated with a lower incidence of dependence and physical abuse than traditional opioids.
- Tramadol has been described as one-fifth as potent as oral morphine.
- While the efficacy of both morphine and tramadol increases with the size of the dose, dose-related toxicity limits the maximum potential of tramadol.

REFERENCES

1. **Hernandez-Diaz S, Garcia-Rodriguez LA.** Epidemiologic assessment of the safety of conventional nonsteroidal antiinflammatory drugs. *Am J Med.* 2000;110 (Suppl 3A): 20S–27S.
2. **Shipton E.** Tramadol-Present and future. *Anaesth Intensive Care.* 2000;28:4.
3. Ultracet (tramadol hydrochloride/acetaminophen) [package insert]. Raritan, NJ: Ortho–McNeil Pharmaceutical; 2001.
4. **Arcioni R, Della Rocca M, Romano S, et al.** Ondansetron inhibits the analgesic effects of tramadol: A possible 5-HT(3) spinal receptor involvement in acute pain in humans. *Anesth Analg.* 2002;94:1553–1557.
5. **De Witte J, Schoenmaekers B, Sessler D, et al.** The analgesic efficacy of tramadol is impaired by concurrent administration of ondansetron. *Anesth Analg.* 2001;92:1319–1321.
6. Ultracet (tramadol hydrochloride) [package insert]. Raritan, NJ: Ortho–McNeil Pharmaceutical; 1998.
7. **Finkel JC, Rose JB, Schmitz ML, et al.** An evaluation of the efficacy and tolerability of oral tramadol hydrochloride tablets for the treatment of postsurgical pain in children. *Anesth Analg.* 2002;94:1469–1473.
8. **Meyer FP, Rimasch H, Blaha B, et al.** Tramadol withdrawal in a neonate. *Eur J Clin Pharmacol.* 1997;53:159–160.
9. **Schnitzer TJ, Kamin M, Olson WH.** Tramadol allows reduction of naproxen dose among patients with naproxen-responsive osteoarthritis pain: A randomized, double-blind, placebo-controlled study. *Arthritis Rheum.* 1999;42:1370–1377.
10. **Mehlisch DR.** The efficacy of combination analgesic therapy in relieving dental pain. *J Am Dent Assoc.* 2002;133:861–871.
11. **Reig E.** Tramadol in musculoskeletal pain: A survey. *Clin Rheumatol.* 21 Suppl 1:S9-11; discussion S11-2, 2002.
12. **Silverfield JC, Kamin M, Wu SC, et al** for the CAPSS-105 Study Group. Tramadol/acetaminophen combination tablets for the treatment of osteoarthritis flare pain: A multicenter, outpatient, randomized, double-blind, placebo-controlled, parallel-group, add-on study. *Clin Ther.* 2002; 24:282–297.
13. **Schnitzer T, Gray W, Paster R, et al.** Efficacy of tramadol in treatment of chronic low back pain. *J Rheumatol.* 2000;27:772–778.
14. **Harati Y, Gooch C, Swenson M, et al.** Maintenance of the long-term effectiveness of tramadol in treatment of the pain of diabetic neuropathy. *J Diabetes Complications.* 2000; 14(2):65–70.
15. **Gardner JS, Blough D, Drinkard CR, et al.** Tramadol and seizures: A surveillance study in a managed care population. *Pharmacotherapy.* 2000;20:1423–1431.
16. **Gasse C, Derby L, Vasilakis-Scaramozza C, et al.** Incidence of first-time idiopathic seizures in users of tramadol. *Pharmacotherapy.* 2000;20:629–634.
17. **Lange-Asschenfeldt C, Weigmann H, Hiemke C, et al.** Serotonin syndrome as a result of fluoxetine in a patient with tramadol abuse: Plasma level-correlated symptomatology. *J Clin Psychopharmacol.* 2002;22:440–441.
18. **Duggal HS, Fetchko J.** Serotonin syndrome and atypical antipsychotics. *Am J Psychiatry.* 2002;159:672–673.
19. **Ripple MG, Pestaner JP, Levine BS, et al.** Lethal combination of tramadol and multiple drugs affecting serotonin. *Am J Forensic Med Pathol.* 2000;21:370–374.
20. **Freye E, Levy J.** Acute abstinence syndrome following abrupt cessation of long-term use of tramadol (Ultram): A case study. *Eur J Pain.* 2000; 4:307–311.
21. **Rodriguez JC, Albaladejo C, Sanchez A, et al.** Withdrawal syndrome after long-term treatment with tramadol. *Br J Gen Pract.* 2000;50:406.
22. **Leo R, Narendran R, DeGuiseppe B.** Methadone detoxification of tramadol dependence. *J Substance Abuse Treat.* 2000;19:297–299.

15 OPIOIDS

Tony L. Yaksh, PhD

Among the remedies which it has pleased Almighty God to give to man to relieve his sufferings, none is so universal and so efficacious as opium.

Sydenham, 1680

INTRODUCTION

- Opioids, originally represented by the extracts of the poppy, have historically been known to produce a powerful and selective reduction in the human and animal response to a strong and otherwise noxious stimulus.
- Early work by the German pharmaceutical chemist Serterner led to the extraction and purification of morphine.
- This, in conjunction with the development of the hollow needle and syringe, must be considered a landmark in the development of therapeutics.

- There is little doubt that morphine and its congeners have been among the most important elements in the therapeutic armamentarium employed for the management of pain.
- The issue that concerns this chapter is by what mechanisms does this therapeutically important effect occur.
- The answer consists of four parts: (1) With what membrane structures do these molecules interact? (2) What are the effects of the opiate receptor interactions on neuronal function? (3) With what neuraxial systems are these receptors associated? (4) By what mechanisms does this interaction alter pain behavior?

PHARMACOLOGIC DEFINITION OF THE OPIOID RECEPTOR FAMILY

- Families of agents structurally related to morphine were uniformly observed to have similar physiologic effects: sedation, respiratory depression, block of pain (analgesia), and constipation.
- Importantly, the overall body of data suggested that the ordering of activity of the numerous structural congeners on one endpoint reflected that on another endpoint. This structure–activity relationship pointed to a specific pharmacologically defined membrane site, a receptor.

MULTIPLE OPIATE RECEPTORS

- In the early 1970s targeted pharmacologic investigations provided defining data supporting the hypothesis that there were several subtypes of opiate receptors.
- Historic work by Martin et al in 1979 in large animal models and in humans, using pharmacologic criteria (the activity relationship ranging from full agonists to antagonists for different structurally related congeners of morphine and differential cross-tolerance), led to the postulation of three receptors, mu, kappa, and sigma, the first two being responsible for the antagonist-reversible analgesia produced by different opioid alkaloids.[1,2]
- Subsequent pharmacologic studies by Hans Kosterlitz and colleagues carried out after their identification of the endogenous opioid peptides met and leu enkephalin led to identification of the delta opioid receptor.[3]
- As indicated in Table 15–1, a variety of specific agents are believed to reflect the specific activation of the several respective receptors.

TABLE 15–1   Summary of Opioid Receptor Pharmacology

RECEPTOR	BIOASSAY	AGONISTS	ANTAGONISTS
Mu	Guinea pig ileum	Morphine	Naloxone
		Sufentanil	Naltrexone
		Meperidine	ß-Funaltrexamine
		Methadone	
		DAMGO	
Delta	Mouse vas deferens	DPDPE	Naloxone
		Deltorphin	Naltrindole
Kappa	Rabbit vas deferens	Butorphanol	Naloxone
		Bremazocine	Nor BNI
		Spiradoline	

DAMGO: [D-Ala(2), N-MePhe(4), Gly-ol(5)]enkephalin
DPDPE: Tyr-D-Pen-Gly-Phe-D-Pen-OH

RECEPTOR SUBTYPE SUBCLASSES

- In subsequent years, additional studies on opioid pharmacology suggested the possibility that there were multiple subclasses of each of the receptors.
- It should be stressed that the definition of receptor subclasses may hinge on small differential potencies of the agonists and antagonists.
- Moreover, many studies employ noncompetitive antagonists and the use of such agents in defining multiple receptor subtypes can be misleading. Still, the proposed subtype subclasses based on pharmacology are presented here for completeness.
  - *Mu subclasses:* Pasternak and colleagues proposed the existence of mu1/mu2 sites in the early 1980s based on the differential antagonism by a noncompetitive ligand (naloxonazine). Though still considered relevant by some, no specific agents have in fact been found for the proposed sites.[4,5]
  - *Delta receptor subclasses:* Porrecca and his colleagues have proposed two subtypes ($\partial1$ and $\partial2$) based on the differential effects of several agonists and antagonists.[6]
  - *Kappa receptor subclasses:* Based on the effects of the differential pharmacology of several agonists and antagonists, up to five receptor subclasses have been hypothesized.[7]

CLONING AND DEFINITION OF THE OPIOID RECEPTOR FAMILY

- The mu, delta, and kappa opioid receptors have all been cloned and sequenced.
- For each receptor, a single gene has been identified.[8]
- Splice variants have been identified for several of these receptors.
- Thus, to the degree that there are opioid receptor subclasses (eg, $\mu1/\mu2$; $\partial1/\partial2$), these distinct sites may

represent splice variants, products of posttranslational processing, or some membrane combination of distinct receptors (eg, dimerization).[9]
- Splice variants have indeed been identified for all of these receptors, though their role as receptor subclasses is not known at this time.[8]

STRUCTURAL PROPERTIES OF OPIOID RECEPTORS

- Extensive work characterizing the sequence and functionality of these receptors has revealed that the three receptors are members of the G protein-coupled superfamily of receptors.
- All three opioid receptors exert their cellular effects via a pertussis toxin-sensitive activation of heterotrimeric G proteins.
- The principal coupling appears to be mediated though Go/i proteins.[10]
- These receptors range in length from 371 (delta) to 398 (mu) amino acids and are organized with seven hydrophobic transmembrane spanning regions.
- A significant degree of sequence homology exists among the receptors, with the mu receptor, for example, having 75% amino acid homology with the delta and kappa opioid receptors.[7]

RECEPTOR COUPLING

- Agonist occupancy of opioid receptors typically leads to a wide variety of events which typically serve to inhibit the activation of the neuron.
- As indicated above, these effects are blocked by the addition of pertussis toxin, indicating that they are mediated though a G protein.[10]
- Of the several events initiated by the opioid receptor occupancy, the overall effects on system excitability often appear to be mediated by (1) membrane hyperpolarization through activation of an inwardly rectifying K^+ channel, and (2) inhibition of the opening of voltage-sensitive Ca^{2+} channels which will subsequently depress release of neurotransmitter from the terminal (see Figure 15–1).
- These joint actions often lead to powerful, receptor-mediated inhibition of neuronal excitability.[11]
- Persistent agonist activation of families of G protein-coupled receptors often results in a progressive, time-dependent loss of effect, otherwise referred to as tolerance.
- The mechanisms of tolerance are uncertain.
- At one level it has been argued that there may be a downregulation in receptor number or a persistent uncoupling of the receptor from the G protein.

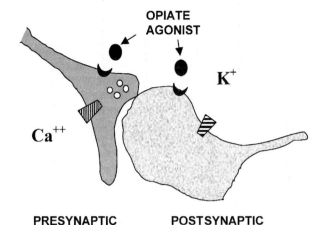

FIGURE 15–1 Summary of the effects that presynaptic opiates have on terminal excitability by preventing the opening of voltage-sensitive Ca channels to attenuate transmitter release and a post-synaptic effect that is associated with hyperpolarization through an opening of potassium channels.

- It should be noted that receptor internalization is a common property of G protein-coupled receptors with agonist occupancy.
- The internalization is believed to be driven by phosphorylation of the receptor and activation of the internalization process.
- Although internalization removes the receptor from the membrane, this activity is in fact believed to serve as a means of rapidly uncoupling the receptor and allowing it to externalize for subsequent activation.[12]

OPIOID SITES OF ACTION IN ANALGESIA

- Opiates given systemically produce a potent dose-dependent analgesia which is reversed by naloxone.
- These observations suggest an effect mediated by an opioid receptor.
- The essential question is: Where in the organism do opiates act to alter pain transmission?
- Defining the location of opiate action in producing analgesia involves assessing the effects of drugs delivered into specific brain sites and assessing the effects of the local drug action on behavior, for example, the response to a strong stimulus, such as a thermal stimulus applied to the paw of the rat.
- This induces a "pain behavior," namely, withdrawal of the stimulated paw.

SUPRASPINAL OPIATE ACTION

Microinjections and Behavioral Effects

- Examining the effects of opiates microinjected into specific sites using chronically implanted microinjection guides has shown that injections into some brain regions produce a well-defined analgesia.
- Importantly, it can be shown that the effects of the injected agonist have a pharmacology that resembles that of one or more opiate receptors (see Figure 15–2).
- Each region can have a distinct opioid receptor pharmacology.[13]

Brain Mapping for Analgesically Coupled Opioid Receptors

- Direct injection of opiates into the brain has shown that opioid receptors that modulate pain behavior are found in several restricted brain regions.
- The location of these sites as defined in the rat is summarized schematically in Figure 15–3.
- The best characterized of these sites so identified is the mesencephalic periaqueductal gray (PAG).
- Microinjections of morphine into this region block, in a naloxone-reversible fashion, nociceptive responses in the unanesthetized rat, rabbit, cat, dog, and primate.[14]

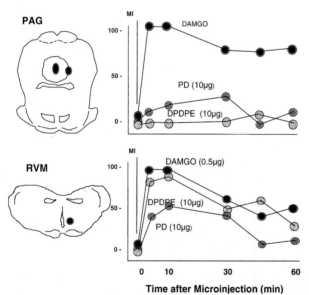

FIGURE 15–2 Effects of the microinjection (0.25–0.5 µL) of receptor selective agents DAMGO (mu), PD (kappa), and DPDPE (delta) into the mesencephalic periaqueductal gray (PAG) (top) or medulla (bottom) of an unanesthetized rat at the site indicated by the black spot and the effects on hot plate response latency. As indicated, DAMGO produces a time-dependent increase in the response latency, eg, produces analgesia in both PAG and medulla, but DPDPE and PD work only in the medulla. These effects are dose dependent and reversed by local or systemic naloxone. RVM, rostral ventral medulla

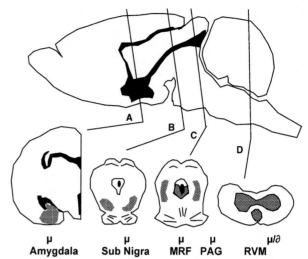

μ | μ | μ | μ | μ/∂
Amygdala | Sub Nigra | MRF | PAG | RVM

FIGURE 15–3 Summary of sites within the neuraxis at which opiate injections will result in a prominent increase in the nociceptive threshold. The approximate planes of section at which the coronal sections are taken are indicated. Darkened regions indicate the cerebral aqueductal location. Light shading indicates the active regions. (A) Diencephalic: active regions within the basolateral amygdala. (B) Mesecephalic: active sites within the substantia nigra (Sub Nigra). (C) Mesencephalic: lateral regions are the mesencephalic reticular formation (MRF); the medial region is the periaqueductal gray (PAG). (D) Medulla: site indicated is the rostral ventral medulla (RVM) with the midline structure corresponding to the raphe magnus. The receptor types that result in antinociception when delivered into that region (see text for details) are indicated.

- This local effect serves to block not only spinally mediated reflexes (such as the tail flick) but also the supraspinally organized response.

Mesencephalic Mechanisms

- In the diversity of sites, it is unlikely that all of the mechanisms whereby opiates act within the brain to alter nociceptive transmission are identical.
- Even within a single brain region, it appears that multiple mechanisms may exist for altering pain transmission.
- Several mechanisms exist whereby opiates may act to alter nociceptive transmission. Thus if we consider only the PAG, there are at least five mechanisms (see Figure 15–4).
  - PAG projection to the medulla, which serves to activate bulbospinal projections releasing serotonin and/or noradrenaline at the spinal level. Currrent thinking is that excitatory projections from the PAG are under the tonic inhibitory control of GABAergic interneurons. These neurons are inhibited by mu opiates, leading to a disinhibition and a net excitatory drive into the bulbospinal nuclei.[15] The spinal delivery of adrenergic and serotonergic

antagonists reverses the PAG morphine-induced inhibition of spinal nociceptive processing.[16]

○ PAG outflow to the medulla, where local inhibitory interaction results in inhibition of ascending medullary projections to higher centers.[17]

○ Opiate binding within the PAG may be preterminal on the ascending spinofugal projection. This preterminal action would inhibit input into the medullary core and mesencephalic core.[18]

○ Outflow from the PAG can serve to act to modulate excitability of dorsal raphe and locus coeruleus, from which ascending serotonergic and noradrenergic projections originate to project to limbic/forebrain. Considerable evidence emphasizes the importance of these forebrain projections in modulating emotionality and may thus account for the affective actions of opiates.[19]

SPINAL ACTION

- The local action of opiates in the spinal cord will selectively depress the discharge of spinal dorsal horn neurons activated by small (high-threshold) but not large (low-threshold) afferents (Figure 15–5).[20]

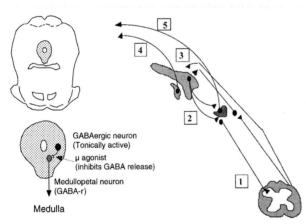

FIGURE 15–4 Upper left: Mesencephalic periaqueductal gray (PAG). Lower left: Organization of opiate action within the periaqueductal gray. In this schema, mu opiate actions block the release of GABA from tonically active systems that otherwise inhibit the excitatory projections to the medulla leading to activation of PAG outflow. Right: Overall organization of the mechanisms whereby a PAG mu opiate agonist can alter nociceptive processing: (1) PAG projection to the medulla which serves to activate bulbospinal projections releasing serotonin and/or noradrenaline at the spinal level. (2) PAG outflow to the medulla, where local inhibitory interaction results in an inhibition of ascending projections. (3) Opiate binding on the ascending spinofugal projection inhibits input into the medullary core and mesencephalic core. (4, 5) Outflow from the PAG can serve to act to modulate excitability of dorsal raphe and locus coeruleus from which ascending serotonergic and noradrenergic projections originate to project to limbic/forebrain (see text for details).

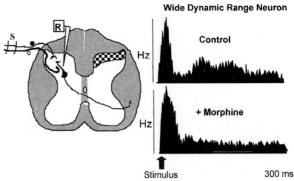

FIGURE 15–5 Model for electrically activating large and small afferents while recording using single-unit microelectrodes of the activity in a single dorsal horn wide-dynamic-range neuron. As indicated on the right (showing the response over a 300-ms time trace), this brief electrical stimulus leads to an initial burst of activity reflecting the activation of the neurons by the rapidly conducting large (low-threshold) afferents followed by the activity evoked by the more slowly conducting (higher-threshold A∂ and C fibers). As indicated (bottom) the application of morphine results in a selective depression of the later discharge.

- Intrathecal administration of opioids reliably attenuates the response of the animal to a variety of unconditioned somatic and visceral stimuli that otherwise evoke an organized escape behavior in all species thus far examined.[21]
- The mechanism of this is considered below.
  - ○ Receptor autoradiography with opiate ligands has revealed that binding is limited for the most part to the substantia gelatinosa, the region in which small afferents show their principal termination.[22]
  - ○ Dorsal rhizotomies result in a significant reduction in dorsal horn opiate binding, suggesting that a significant proportion is associated with the primary afferents.[23]
  - ○ Confirmation of the presynaptic action is provided by the observation that opiates reduce the release of primary afferent peptide transmitters such as substance P contained in small primary afferents.[24]
  - ○ The presynaptic action corresponds to the ability of opiates to prevent the opening of voltage-sensitive Ca^{2+} channels, thereby preventing release.
  - ○ A postsynaptic action was demonstrated by the ability of opiates to block the excitation of dorsal horn neurons evoked by glutamate, reflecting a direct activation of the dorsal horn.
  - ○ The activation of potassium channels leading to a hyperpolarization was consistent with the direct postsynaptic inhibition.
- The joint ability of spinal opiates to reduce the release of excitatory neurotransmitters from C fibers as well as decrease the excitability of dorsal horn neurons is believed to account for the powerful and selective

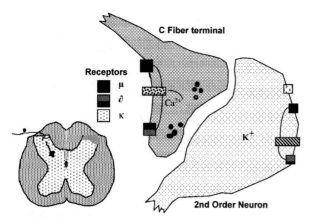

FIGURE 15–6 Summary of the anticipated organization of opiate receptors in the dorsal horn regulating nociceptive processing. As indicated, mu (μ), delta (∂), and kappa (κ) binding are high in the dorsal horn, particularly in the region associated with the termination of small unmyelinated afferents (C fibers). A significant proportion of these sites are located on the terminals of the small afferent as suggested by the loss of such binding after rhizotomy. In addition, there is a postafferent terminal localization of these sites that is apparently coupled through Gi protein to K^+ channels, leading to hyperpolarization of the neuron. Occupancy of the presynaptic mu and delta sites reduces the release of sP and/or CGRP in part by inhibition of the opening of voltage-sensitive calcium channels (see text for further discussion).

these sites are coupled to mechanisms governing the excitability of the membrane; thus the effects are not naloxone-reversible.

- High doses of agents such as sufentanil can block the compound action potential, but this is not naloxone-reversible and is thought to reflect on a "local anesthetic" action of the lipid-soluble agent.
- It is certain that opiate receptors exist on the distant periphery.
- Models in which peripheral opiates appear to work are those that possess a significant degree of inflammation and are characterized by a hyperalgesic component.
- Previous work has indeed demonstrated that local opiates in the knee joint and in the skin can reduce the firing of spontaneously active afferents observed when these tissues are inflamed[26] (Figure 15–7).
- The mechanisms of the antihyperalgesic effects of opiates applied to inflamed regions (as in the knee joint) are at present unexplained.
- It is possible, for example, that the opiates may act on inflammatory cells that are present and are releasing cytokines and products that activate or sensitize the nerve terminal.[27]

effect on spinal nociceptive processing (see Figure 15–6).

PERIPHERAL ACTION

- It has been a principal tenet of opiate action that these agents are "centrally" acting.
- Direct application of opiates to the peripheral nerve can in fact produce a local anesthetic-like action at high concentrations, but this is not naloxone-reversible and is believed to reflect a "nonspecific" action.
- Moreover, in pain models examining normal animals, it can be readily demonstrated that if the agent does not readily penetrate the brain, its opiate actions are limited.
- Alternately, studies employing the direct injection of these agents into peripheral sites have demonstrated that under conditions of inflammation where there is a "hyperalgesia," the local action of opiates can be demonstrated to exert a normalizing effect on the exaggerated thresholds.
- This has been demonstrated for the response to mechanical stimulation applied to inflamed paw or inflamed knee joints.[25]
- While opiate "binding" sites are being transported in the peripheral sensory axon, there is no evidence that

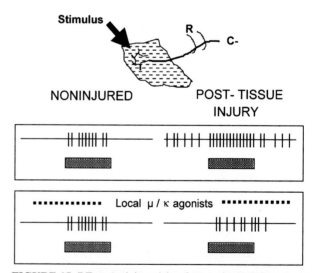

FIGURE 15–7 Top: Activity arising from a single C fiber that is innervating a patch of uninjured (left) and injured (right) skin in the presence of a strong mechanical stimulus applied to the receptive field (as indicated by the horizontal bar). Note spontaneous activity and enhanced response in C fiber innervating injured skin. Similar observations are made in a variety of injury models such as in the knee joint and cornea. Bottom: The application of opioid agonists to the tissue results in suppression of the spontaneous activity otherwise noted in the C fiber. The opioids will not block activity evoked by an otherwise adequate mechanical or thermal stimulus. These effects are naloxone-reversible (see text for further discussion).

OPIATE MECHANISMS IN HUMANS

SUPRASPINAL

- In humans it is not feasible to routinely assess the site of action within the brain where opiates may act to alter nociceptive transmission.
- Intracerebroventricular opioids, however, have been employed for pain relief in cancer patients.
- An important characteristic of this action is that the time of onset is relatively rapid for even the water-soluble agent morphine.
- Gamma scans of human brain have shown that morphine, even 1 hour after injection, remains close to the ventricular lumen.[28]
- Accordingly, it seems probable that the site of opiate action in the human must lie close to the ventricular lumen.
- In this regard, preclinical studies in species such as the primate have emphasized the importance of the periaqueductal sites.

SPINAL

- There is an extensive literature indicating that opiates delivered spinally can induce powerful analgesia in humans.
- The pharmacology of this action has been relatively widely studied and it appears certain that mu, delta, and, to a lesser degree, kappa agonists are effective after intrathecal or epidural delivery.
- The effects of spinal opiates are reversed by low doses of systemic naloxone. Importantly, the activity of spinally delivered agents in modulating acute nociception in animal models, such as for the rodent hot plate, reveals an ordering of activity that closely resembles that observed in humans for controlling clinical pain states.[29]

PERIPHERAL

- It was shown that intraarticular morphine injections have a powerful sparing effect on subsequent analgesics.
- The appropriate controls emphasize that the effects are indeed mediated by a local action and not by a CNS redistribution.
- A wide variety of studies have been undertaken to indicate that there is a modest antihyperalgesic effect of opiates reflecting a peripheral effect.[30]

SUMMARY

- Opiates produce a potent modulatory effect on nociceptive transmission by an action on specific receptors that reflects a modulation of afferent input at both the spinal and supraspinal levels.

- In addition, these agents have strong influence over the affective component of pain by mechanisms that reflect on actions mediated at the supraspinal level though forebrain systems mediating emotionality.
- These joint effects on neuraxial function provide an important key to defining the analgesic actions exerted by these classes of receptor agonists.

REFERENCES

1. **Martin WR, Eades CG, Thompson JA, Huppler RE, Gilbert PE.** The effects of morphine- and nalorphine-like drugs in the nondependent and morphine-dependent chronic spinal dog. *J Pharmacol Exp Ther.* 1976;197:517–532.
2. **Martin WR.** History and development of mixed opioid agonists, partial agonists and antagonists. *Br J Clin Pharmacol.* 1979;7(Suppl 3):273S–279S.
3. **Lord JA, Waterfield AA, Hughes J, Kosterlitz HW.** Endogenous opioid peptides: Multiple agonists and receptors. *Nature.* 1977;267:495–499.
4. **Pasternak GW.** Studies of multiple morphine and enkephalin receptors: Evidence for mu1 receptors. *Adv Exp Med Biol.* 1988;236:81–93.
5. **Pasternak GW.** The pharmacology of mu analgesics: From patients to genes. *Neuroscientist.* 2001;7:220–231.
6. **Burkey TH, Ehlert FJ, Hosohata Y, et al.** The efficacy of delta-opioid receptor-selective drugs. *Life Sci.* 1998;62:1531.
7. **Minami M, Satoh M.** Molecular biology of the opioid receptors: Structures, functions and distributions. *Neurosci Res.* 1995;23:121–145.
8. **Wei LN, Loh HH.** Regulation of opioid receptor expression. *Curr Opin Pharmacol.* 2002;2:69–75.
9. **Levac BA, O'Dowd BF, George SR.** Oligomerization of opioid receptors: Generation of novel signaling units. *Curr Opin Pharmacol.* 2002;2:76–81.
10. **Connor M, Christie MD.** Opioid receptor signalling mechanisms. *Clin Exp Pharmacol Physiol.* 1999;26:493–499.
11. **Grudt TJ, Williams JT.** Opioid receptors and the regulation of ion conductances. *Rev Neurosci.* 1995;6:279–286.
12. **Alvarez VA, Arttamangkul S, Dang V, et al.** Mu-opioid receptors: Ligand-dependent activation of potassium conductance, desensitization, and internalization. *J Neurosci.* 2002;22:5769–5776.
13. **Yaksh TL, Rudy TA.** Narcotic analgesics: CNS sites and mechanisms of action as revealed by intracerebral injection techniques. *Pain.* 1978;4:299–359.
14. **Nunes-de-Souza RL, Graeff FG, Siegfried B.** Strain-dependent effects of morphine injected into the periaqueductal gray area of mice. *Braz J Med Biol Res.* 1991;24:291–299.
15. **Fields HL.** Pain modulation: Expectation, opioid analgesia and virtual pain. *Prog Brain Res.* 2000;122:245–253.
16. **Yaksh TL.** Direct evidence that spinal serotonin and noradrenaline terminals mediate the spinal antinociceptive

effects of morphine in the periaqueductal gray. *Brain Res.* 1979;160:180–185.

17. **Wang WH, Lovick TA.** The inhibitory effect of the ventrolateral periaqueductal grey matter on neurones in the rostral ventrolateral medulla involves a relay in the medullary raphe nuclei. *Exp Brain Res.* 1993;94:295–300.

18. **Ramberg DA, Yaksh TL.** Effects of cervical spinal hemisection on dihydromorphine binding in brainstem and spinal cord in cat. *Brain Res.* 1989;483:61–67.

19. **Kent JM, Mathew SJ, Gorman JM.** Molecular targets in the treatment of anxiety. *Biol Psychiatry.* 2002;52:1008–1030.

20. **Yaksh TL.** Inhibition by etorphine of the discharge of dorsal horn neurons: Effects on the neuronal response to both high- and low-threshold sensory input in the decerebrate spinal cat. *Exp Neurol.* 1978;60:23–40.

21. **Yaksh TL.** Spinal opiate analgesia: Characteristics and principles of action. *Pain.* 1981;11:293–346.

22. **Ninkovic M, Hunt SP, Kelly JS.** Effect of dorsal rhizotomy on the autoradiographic distribution of opiate and neurotensin receptors and neurotensin-like immunoreactivity within the rat spinal cord. *Brain Res.* 1981;230:111–119.

23. **Abbadie C, Lombard MC, Besson JM, Trafton JA, Basbaum AI.** Mu and delta opioid receptor-like immunoreactivity in the cervical spinal cord of the rat after dorsal rhizotomy or neonatal capsaicin: An analysis of pre- and postsynaptic receptor distributions. *Brain Res.* 2002;930:150–162.

24. **Aimone LD, Yaksh TL.** Opioid modulation of capsaicin-evoked release of substance P from rat spinal cord in vivo. *Peptides.* 1989;10:1127–1131.

25. **Stein C.** Peripheral mechanisms of opioid analgesia. *Anesth Analg.* 1993;76:182–191.

26. **Andreev N, Urban L, Dray A.** Opioids suppress spontaneous activity of polymodal nociceptors in rat paw skin induced by ultraviolet irradiation. *Neuroscience.* 1994;58:793–798.

27. **Stein C, Machelska H, Binder W, Schafer M.** Peripheral opioid analgesia. *Curr Opin Pharmacol.* 2001;1:62–65.

28. **Lazorthes YR, Sallerin BA, Verdie JC.** Intracerebroventricular administration of morphine for control of irreducible cancer pain. *Neurosurgery.* 1995;37:422–428.

29. **Wallace M, Yaksh TL.** Long-term spinal analgesic delivery: A review of the preclinical and clinical literature. *Reg Anesth Pain Med.* 2000;25:117–157.

30. **Dionne RA, Lepinski AM, Gordon SM, Jaber L, Brahim JS, Hargreaves KM.** Analgesic effects of peripherally administered opioids in clinical models of acute and chronic inflammation. *Clin Pharmacol Ther.* 2001;70:66–73.

16   MISCELLANEOUS DRUGS

Mark S. Wallace, MD

INTRODUCTION

- Some drugs are known to result in analgesia in certain pain syndromes.

- The co-administration of these agents with traditional analgesics such as the opioids, NSAIDs, and acetaminophen may enhance analgesic efficacy.[1]

PHENOTHIAZINES

- The use of the phenothiazines in pain management is controversial; therefore, they should be reserved for selected cases when more established therapies have failed.
- Analgesic efficacy is not well established.
- They are most commonly co-administered with the opioids and antidepressants.
- Most of the efficacy studies have been in postoperative pain with mixed results. Methotrimeprazine has been shown to be the most efficacious.[2,3]
- A few studies have indicated efficacy in diabetic peripheral neuropathy and postherpetic neuralgia.[1,4,5]
- Side effects include sedation, hypotension, and extrapyramidal symptoms.

BENZODIAZEPINES

- Benzodiazepines are frequently used as an adjuvant in the treatment of acute pain; however, their use in chronic pain is controversial. The exception is clonazepam, which has anticonvulsant activity and is used in the treatment of neuropathic pain. Diazepam also has anticonvulsant properties.[1]
- Analgesic efficacy is not well established, but these agents appear to alter the unpleasantness of the pain experience.[6]
- Benzodiazepines have muscle relaxant properties and may be used as a muscle relaxant and antispasmodic (see below).

ANTIHISTAMINES

- Hydroxyzine, phenyltoloxamine, and orphenadrine have been shown to be efficacious in a variety of pain syndromes including headache, low back pain, postoperative pain, and cancer pain.[7–10]
- It is unclear whether the mechanism of action is through block of peripheral or central histamine receptors. Histamine can activate C fibers; therefore, histamine receptor blockade may result in analgesia. Analgesia may also be the result of the sedative and muscle relaxant properties of these agents
- Hydroxyzine is the most widely used agent and is the only antihistamine that has been proven to have intrinsic analgesic activity.

- Antihistamines are most commonly co-administered with the opioids in the treatment of postoperative pain.

CNS STIMULANTS

AMPHETAMINES

- Amphetamines are often co-administered with the opioids to treat opioid-induced sedation.
- Amphetamines may also be used to treat depression.
- The amphetamines enhance the analgesic effect of the opioids.[11]
- There are reports of efficacy of the amphetamines in the treatment of neuropathic pain.
- The mechanism of amphetamine potentiation of opioid analgesia is unknown. Amphetamines stimulate the release of catecholamines in the central nervous system, which may result in analgesia.

CAFFEINE

- Caffeine enhances the analgesic effect of aspirin and acetaminophen.
- It is used in a variety of pain syndromes including cancer, headache, and postoperative pain.[12]
- The mechanism of its action is unclear.

CORTICOSTEROIDS

- The corticosteroids have been proven efficacious in advanced cancer pain including diffuse bony metastasis, tumor infiltration of neural structures, and spinal cord compression.
- The pain relief may be the result of a direct analgesic action and tumor size reduction.
- Corticosteroids improve appetite and mood.
- The dosing is empirical and should be individualized.

MUSCLE RELAXANTS

- The use of the muscle relaxants is usually limited to the treatment of acute muscle problems, with placebo-controlled studies showing efficacy in low back pain.[13]
- Because of abuse potential and dependence, long-term use of the muscle relaxants for chronic pain is controversial and the efficacy studies are less convincing.

- *Site of Action*: Muscle relaxants act at several sites important to muscle tone:
  - Direct effect on skeletal muscle fiber (dantrolene, methocarbamol)
  - Polysynaptic reflexes (benzodiazepines, baclofen, tizanidine, other muscle relaxants)
  - Descending facilitory systems (benzodiazepines, other muscle relaxants)

BACLOFEN

- The antispasmodic effect of baclofen is thought to be secondary to GABA-B activity at the spinal cord level, which inhibits evoked release of excitatory amino acids.
- It is indicated for the treatment of spasticity secondary to spinal cord injury.
- There exists anecdotal evidence that baclofen may have intrinsic analgesic efficacy.

DANTROLENE

- Dantrolene is a potent antispasmodic that dissociates the excitation–contractioin coupling mechanism of skeletal muscle by interfering with the release of calcium from the sarcoplasmic reticulum.
- Fatal and nonfatal liver disorders may occur with dantrolene; therefore, this drug should be used in selected cases only. Therapy should be stopped if benefit is not evident by 45 days.
- Dantrolene is indicated for the treatment of spasticity secondary to spinal cord injury.

BENZODIAZEPINES

- The antispasmodic effect of benzodiazepines is thought to be secondary to GABA-A activity at the spinal cord level.
- Long-term use for chronic pain is controversial due to disturbances in REM sleep, possible tolerance and habituation, and difficulties in withdrawing the drug.
- Because long-term use is controversial, diazepam should be used in selected cases only.

QUININE SULFATE

- Quinine sulfate has a direct effect (curare-like) on muscle. It decreases excitability of the motor endplate. It also affects the distribution of calcium within muscle fibers.

- Quinine sulfate is used for the treatment of nocturnal leg cramps although well-controlled studies on efficacy for this condition are lacking.

TIZANIDINE

- Tizanidine is a centrally acting α_2-adrenergic agonist that reduces spasticity by increasing presynaptic inhibition of motor neurons in the spinal cord.
- Similar in structure to clonidine, it has 1/50th of the potency of clonidine in lowering blood pressure.
- Tizanidine is indicated for the treatment of spasticity secondary to spinal cord injury and multiple sclerosis.
- It may have intrinsic analgesic activity secondary to the α_2-adrenergic agonism.

OTHER SKELETAL MUSCLE RELAXANTS

- Examples of centrally acting muscle relaxants include carisoprodol, chlorphenesin carbamate, chlorzoxazone, cyclobenzaprine hydrochloride, methocarbamol, and orphenadrine citrate.
- Many of these are available in combination with certain other drugs.
- There is no evidence that any one muscle relaxant is more efficacious than the others.
- Cyclobenzaprine is structurally similar to the tricyclic antidepressants.
- Side effect is sedation and long-term use should be limited to bedtime dosing only.
- Long-term bedtime dosing may be beneficial in the treatment of fibromyalgia.

NMDA RECEPTOR ANTAGONISTS

- The *N*-methyl-D-aspartate (NMDA) ionophore is located on postsynaptic neurons in the dorsal horn.
- The release of glutamate from the presynaptic terminal activates the NMDA ionophore channel causing an influx of calcium, which initiates a cascade of effects resulting in spinal "windup."
- Binding sites that influence the influx of calcium include:
  - A magnesium binding site within the channel that when occupied inhibits channel opening
  - A glycine binding site that must be occupied for the channel to open

  - A polyamine site that regulates NMDA ionophore excitability
- The channel may be blocked in a noncompetitive use-dependent fashion with agents such as ketamine, dextromethorphan, memantine, and MK801.
- Because of the minimal literature on the clinical use of NMDA antagonists, it is difficult to provide guidelines.[14,15]

REFERENCES

1. **Fields H.** *Pain*. New York: McGraw–Hill; 1987.
2. **Lasagna L, DeKornfeld, TJ.** Methotrimepraxine: A new phenothiazine derivative with analgesic properties. *JAMA*. 1961;178:119–122.
3. **McGee JL, Alexander, MR.** Phenothiazine analgesia—fact or fantasy? *Am J Hosp Pharm*. 1979;36:633–640.
4. **Farber GA, Burks JW.** Chlorprothixene therapy for herpes zoster neuralgia. *South Med J*. 1974;67:808–812.
5. **Nathan PW.** Chlorprothixene in post-herpetic neuralgia and other severe chronic pain. *Pain*. 1978;5:367-371.
6. **Graceley RH, McGrath P, Dubner R.** Validity and sensitivity of ratio scales of sensory and affective verbal pain descriptors: Manipulation of affect by diazepam. *Pain*. 1978; 5:19–29.
7. **Beaver WJ, Freise G.** Comparison of the analgesic effect of morphine, hydroxyzine and their combinations in patients with postoperative pain. *Adv Pain Res Ther*. 1976;1:553–557.
8. **Stambaugh JE, Lane C.** Analgesic efficacy and pharmakinetic evaluation of meperidine and hydroxyzine, alone and in combination. *Cancer Invest*. 1983;1:111–117.
9. **Gold RH.** Treatment of low back syndrome with oral orphenadrine citrate. *Curr Ther Res*. 1978;23:271–276.
10. **Gilbert MM.** Analgesic/calmative effects of acetaminophen and pheynyltoloxamine in treatment of simple nervous tension accompanied by headache. *Curr Ther Res*. 1976; 20:53–58.
11. **Forrest WH, Brown BW, Brown CR, et al.** Dextroamphetamine with morphine for the treatment of postoperative pain. *N Engl J Med*. 1977;296:712–715.
12. **Laska EM, Sunshine A, Mueller F, et al.** Caffeine as an adjuvant analgesic. *JAMA*. 1986;251:45–50.
13. **Max MB, Gilron IH.** Antidepressants, muscle relaxants, and *N*-methyl-D-aspartate receptor antagonists. In: Loesser J, ed. *Bonica's Management of Pain*. Philadelphia: Lippincott, Williams & Wilkins; 2001:1710–1726.
14. **Wallace MS.** Pharmacologic treatment of neuropathic pain. *Curr Pain Headache Rep*. 2001;5:138–150.
15. **Irving G, Wallace M.** *Pain Management for the Practicing Physician*. New York: WB Saunders; 1996:37–47.

17 INTRAVENOUS AND SUBCUTANEOUS PATIENT-CONTROLLED ANALGESIA

Anne M. Savarese, MD

INTRODUCTION

- Patient-controlled analgesia (PCA) is a method of pain relief that allows patients to self-administer small doses of opioids on demand, accompanied by the option of a continuous infusion, using a programmable infusion device.
- Versatile routes and pharmacologic agents exist for PCA administration; this chapter focuses on intravenous and subcutaneous routes of opioid analgesia.

RATIONALE

- After initial loading doses establish effective analgesia, frequent small doses of self-administered opioid maintain a patient's plasma opioid concentration above the minimal effective analgesic concentration (MEAC), and below higher concentrations at which unwanted side effects occur.
- Analgesic administration is simplified so that patients self-select when and how much medication they receive to achieve optimal pain relief.
- Immediate access, avoidance of injections, independence from nursing requests, better pain relief, fewer unpleasant side effects, and a sense of control contribute to patient acceptance and satisfaction with this technique.
- PCA technology permits flexible titration and efficiently adjusts to the wide interindividual variability

in analgesic requirements between patients and even within patients.
- Variability in patient-specific opioid requirements during PCA therapy results from differences in pharmacokinetics, pharmacodynamics, pain intensity, psychological makeup, anxiety, and previous painful experiences.
- Programmable features and PCA device engineering contribute to the excellent overall patient safety and efficacy of this technique.

ADVANTAGES

- Painless routes of administration (intravenous or subcutaneous/clysis)
- Avoids peaks, valleys, fluctuations, and delays in pain relief
- Provides prompt and lasting comfort
- Flexible, titratable, and individualized therapy
- Facilitates rapid establishment of analgesia and equianalgesic transitions
- Potential for fewer opioid-related side effects compared with intermittent bolus administration
- Enhanced sense of control over the pain experience
- Decreased nursing burden compared with conventional methods

DISADVANTAGES

- Requires specialized equipment (the PCA infusor device or "pump")
- Requires patient self-awareness and cognitive understanding of the principles of PCA therapy for safe and effective use
- Potential for operator and/or mechanical errors in programming or delivery

INDICATIONS

- Relief of moderate to severe acute pain
- Postoperative pain
- Burns/trauma
- Sickle cell crisis/pancreatitis/painful medical conditions
- Cancer pain/painful conditions related to cancer treatment

CONTRAINDICATIONS

- History of device tampering with prior PCA use/opioid diversion
- Developmental disability/cognitive impairment which limits understanding of PCA therapy or limits successful interface with the pump
- Patient or parent/family refusal

INTRAVENOUS OPIOID PCA: "HOW TO DO IT"

THE PCA PRESCRIPTION

- The clinician selects an opioid analgesic in a standard concentration and then programs the PCA pump parameters, including the clinician loading dose, the PCA or patient demand/bolus dose, the dosing interval or "lock-out," the time-based cumulative dose limit, and the optional "background" continuous/basal infusion.
- Efficacy and safety of IV PCA are probably more significantly related to these prescribed parameters than the choice of any particular opioid analgesic.
- The PCA microprocessor programs, stores, and retrieves data, so that the patient's pattern of analgesic use and cumulative consumption can be reviewed. Suggested prescriptions for IV PCA are found in Table 17–1.

CHOICE OF OPIOID

- The ideal agent for IV PCA should be rapid in onset, be intermediate in duration, be lacking in potentially toxic metabolites, have a broad safety margin, and be readily available, inexpensive, and stable in solution.
- Clinicians typically choose morphine, hydromorphone, and fentanyl for IV PCA.
- Use of meperidine is discouraged for PCA of more than 48 hours' duration because of the risk of normeperidine accumulation and CNS toxicity with repetitive administration.
- Initial choice of opioid is influenced by practitioner familiarity and preference, as well as patient factors such as prior drug responses, clinical status, comorbid conditions, and expected clinical course.
- As individual patient's responses vary, the clinician must be prepared to switch agents on an equi-analgesic basis if the patient fails to achieve adequate relief or if dose-limiting or intolerable side effects occur.
- Opioids for IV PCA should be compounded in standard concentrations, preferably equi-analgesic on a volume basis, to facilitate safe and convenient conversions during PCA therapy.

CLINICIAN LOADING DOSE

- Successful PCA therapy requires that an analgesic plasma level be established by one or more loading doses before the patient begins to maintain this level by self-administering smaller PCA demand doses.
- During ongoing PCA therapy, some patients with large or fluctuating analgesic requirements may need upward titration of their PCA prescription preceded by reloading.
- The clinician loading dose feature allows initial and subsequent loading doses to be administered via the PCA device, rather than by separate syringe boluses.
- This facilitates convenient and rapid titration to effective analgesia, and records all administered opioid doses in the PCA history software, thereby improving patient safety, limiting diversion, and simplifying opioid tracking.

TABLE 17–1   Suggested Intravenous PCA Prescriptions for Opioid-Naïve Adult Patients

DRUG	STOCK SOLUTION (mg/mL)	LOADING DOSE (mg)	PCA DOSE (mg)	LOCKOUT (min)	BASAL RATE (mg/h)	1-H LIMIT (mg)
Morphine	1	2–5	0.5–2.5	6–10	0.5–1	8–15
Hydromorphone	0.2	0.4–0.8	0.1–0.4	6–10	0.1–0.2	1.2–2.4
Meperidine	10	10–50	8–15	8–15	0–5	30–40 (≤ 750/24°)
Fentanyl	0.020	0.020–0.050	0.020–0.040	6–10	0.010–0.030	0.080–0.200

PCA DEMAND OR BOLUS DOSE

- The optimal PCA dose should provide measurable and satisfactory pain relief with minimal side effects.
- The patient must "feel" the effect of an adequate dose to encourage patient interaction and prevent frustration with the PCA device.
- Too large of a dose will lead to unpleasant (nausea, pruritus, dysphoria) or even potentially dangerous (sedation, confusion, respiratory depression) side effects, which may inhibit the patient from interacting with the PCA device or necessitate interruption or discontinuation of PCA therapy.
- Decreased starting doses are suggested for patients with advanced age, hepatic or renal insufficiency, pre-existing respiratory or neurologic impairment, morbid obesity, or sleep apnea.
- Increased starting doses are appropriate for opioid-tolerant patients and those using opioids to control preexisting pain.
- In general, if the patient consistently receives more than three to four PCA doses per hour, PCA "demands" significantly exceed delivered doses, and pain scores remain unacceptable, then an upward titration of 25–50% in the PCA dose is indicated.

DOSING INTERVAL OR "LOCK-OUT"

- The lock-out is the programmed delay between the last delivered dose and the next possible dose, despite the number of demands made by the patient to the PCA device.
- The dosing interval should reflect the time to peak effect for the prescribed opioid, so that successive doses are not administered before the patient "feels" the effect of the preceding self-administered dose.
- This is a critical programming feature affecting both safety and efficacy of PCA.
- The lock-out interval protects the patient from repetitive doses (despite demands) over too short a period, while permitting an adequate interval for successive doses to be successfully delivered so that an effective analgesic plasma concentration is achieved, especially during active periods with increased analgesic requirements.

TIME-BASED CUMULATIVE DOSE LIMIT

- This parameter allows the clinician to restrict the patient's cumulative opioid consumption to a time-based limit, typically 1 or 4 hours.

- This feature permits the flexibility of a "generous" PCA dose and "short" lock-out, while still protecting the patient from an excessive cumulative dose over the specified period.
- This is particularly useful when prescribing for patients with expected periods of increased analgesic requirements, such as physical therapy and dressing changes.

BACKGROUND CONTINUOUS/ BASAL INFUSION

- For most adult patients the routine use of a background or concurrent opioid infusion is not recommended, as it results in increased opioid consumption, increased side effects, increased risk for respiratory depression, and no real improvement in sleep, quality of pain relief, or patient satisfaction.
- Therapy must be individualized, and clinical experience suggests that some adult patients benefit from a continuous infusion.
- Children and adolescents may benefit more from background infusions than adults.
- In general, for acute pain patients the basal should provide about one-third of the expected total hourly opioid requirement, while for chronic or cancer pain patients the reverse ratio is suggested, and the basal should provide about two-thirds of the expected total hourly opioid requirement.

INTRAVENOUS OPIOID PCA: TIPS FOR SUCCESS

- PCA technology facilitates on-demand analgesia tailored to the individual patient's needs, but it is not to be mistaken for a "one size fits all" or "set it and forget it" therapy. The success, efficacy, and safety of PCA are enhanced by:
  - Management by a dedicated acute pain service (APS)
  - Prescribing of PCA, as well as supplemental analgesics, sedatives, and transition analgesics, restricted to one team only, ideally an APS
  - Establishment of institutional policies, standardization of opioid formulations, preprinted PCA order sets, and management guidelines to ensure consistent clinical practice
  - Staff education about PCA and pain management in general
  - Patient/family education about PCA therapy (see Table 17–2)

TABLE 17–2   PCA Teaching Tips for Patients and Families

1. Demonstrate how to use the pump to give pain medication, and have the patient return the demonstration.
2. Instruct the patient in the use of an appropriate assessment tool (pain scale).
3. Inform the patient that the goal of PCA therapy is a resting pain score (PS) of 0 to 3, and a dynamic PS of ≤ 5 on a 0–10 pain scale, where 0 = no pain and 10 = the worst pain possible.
4. Instruct the patient and family members that only the patient is to activate the PCA demand button.
5. Explain that the lock-out interval is set so that the patient cannot receive additional medication until the last dose has had some effect, regardless of how often the demand button is pressed.
6. Instruct the patient to "premedicate" by activating the PCA demand button once or twice about 10 to 15 min before engaging in activities such as getting out of bed, ambulating, coughing, using incentive spirometry, and participating in physical therapy or dressing changes.
7. Instruct the patient to notify the nurse for unrelieved pain despite using the PCA pump, nausea/vomiting, itching, dysphoria/confusion, and difficulty passing urine or stool.
8. Instruct the patient to notify the nurse of any unexpected change in the site, severity, or quality of the pain being treated, as this may represent a new medical or surgical condition requiring investigation or treatment.
9. Instruct the patient and family members to notify the nurse if the pump alarms. Be sure the patient can correctly identify the "normal" sound the pump makes when delivering medication.
10. Refute common myths about opioid-based acute pain management; ie, inform the patient and family that the risk for addiction is negligible, that overdose is unlikely given the pump's safety features, and that inadequate analgesia or unpleasant side effects will be aggressively managed.
11. Counsel the patient that concurrent use of unprescribed medications, such as street drugs and alcohol, increases the risk for serious side effects, and may disqualify the patient from receiving PCA therapy.

○ Proactive side effect management, especially for common "nuisance" side effects such as pruritus and nausea (see Table 17–3)
○ Standardized and frequent assessment/monitoring of vital signs, pain scores, sedation levels, side effects, patient responses to interventions, and pump prescription/programming verification
○ "Built-in" PCA delivery system safety features, such as locked drug reservoirs, tamper resistance, security locks and programming access codes, anti-syphon valves, antireflux valves, and user-friendly interfaces to diminish the risks for operator programming errors
○ Ongoing institutional quality management and improvement

DISCONTINUING PCA THERAPY

• Adult postoperative patients are usually ready to transition from IV PCA to oral analgesics when normal gastrointestinal function is restored and opioid con-

TABLE 17–3   Opioid-Related Side Effect Management for Adult Patients on PCA Therapy

SIDE EFFECT	INTERVENTION
Nausea/vomiting	Reduce the dose of opioid
	Ondansetron 4–8 mg IV q6h
	or
	Dolasetron 12.5–25 mg IV q12h
	or
	Prochlorperazine 10–25 mg IV q6h
	or
	Metoclopramide 10–20 mg IV q6h
	or
	Droperidol 0.625–1.25 mg IV q6h
	Switch opioid
Pruritus	Reduce the dose of opioid
	Diphenhydramine 25–50 mg IV q6h
	or
	Hydroxyzine 25–50 mg PO q6h
	Switch opioid
	Naloxone 0.5 μg/kg/h IV continuous infusion
Urinary retention	Reduce the dose of opioid
	Bladder catheterization
	Naloxone 100-μg IV push × 1
	Bethanecol 0.05 mg/kg SC × 1
Constipation	Stool softener and stimulant laxative in combination, eg, Senokot
Respiratory depression	Stop any background continuous/basal infusion
	Remove the PCA button from the patient's reach
	Stimulate the patient and call for help
	Remain with the patient and continue frequent assessments
	Provide supplemental oxygen
	Assess airway patency, respiratory effort, and Spo₂
	Provide airway management as appropriate
	Administer naloxone 100 mcg IVP q3–5 min
	Consider naloxone IV infusion 0.5–3 μg/kg/h
	Avoid co-administration of any other respiratory depressants (eg, sedative/hypnotics)
	Depending on episode severity and patient response, consider resuming PCA at a decreased dose without basal or, alternatively, moving patient to a monitored setting

sumption is about 50 mg parenteral morphine equivalents over the preceding 24 hours.
• For patients with mild to moderate pain, conventional fixed combination agents (eg, acetaminophen/oxycodone) are usually sufficient.
• The first dose of oral analgesic is given while the patient still has access to the PCA pump; if at the time of peak effect for the oral agent the patient is comfortable, the pump is discontinued, and the transition oral analgesics are continued.
• For patients with more severe pain or documented higher opioid requirements, long-acting or sustained-release oral opioids (eg, methadone, morphine [MS

Contin], oxycodone hydrochloride [Oxycontin]) should be considered.

- Patients with significant ongoing opioid requirements who are otherwise ready to transition but still cannot take enteral medications are candidates for long-acting transdermal fentanyl (Duragesic).
- The long-acting agent is begun, the background continuous/basal infusion is stopped, and the patient is allowed access to PCA demand doses for about another 18–24 hours.
- Ultimately an equi-analgesic conversion is made so that about two-thirds to three-fourths of the expected 24-hour requirement is achieved by the long-acting agent, with the remainder provided in immediate-release or short-acting opioids.

SUBCUTANEOUS (CLYSIS) OPIOID PCA

- Clysis administration of opioid analgesics is conceptually similar to intravenous analgesia when provided in a continuous plus demand paradigm (ie, basal plus PCA mode).
- It provides more rapid and reliable absorption, as well as essentially painless administration, when compared with intramuscular injections.
- It finds application in patients with limited intravenous access who, in all other respects, meet eligibility criteria for opioid PCA.
- Typical patients for clysis opioid PCA are pediatric, elderly, debilitated, or in hospice, with significant acute pain superimposed on chronic pain, such as that from malignancy or end-stage medical conditions.
- The only real contraindication is localized infection at the site for placement of the indwelling subcutaneous needle, and because there are multiple suitable skin sites, this contraindication is an infrequent impediment.
- The key differences compared with intravenous PCA are:
  - Clysis cannot accommodate rapid titration or dose adjustments like the intravenous route; clysis does provide adequate prolonged analgesia
  - The rate-limiting step in prescribing clysis is the amount of fluid volume the subcutaneous tissue depot can absorb; in general, volumes greater than 1.0 mL/h are not recommended.
  - Compounding the opioid analgesic solution must account for this hourly volume restriction; in general, opioids are concentrated to about 10 times what would be used for conventional IV PCA analgesia; most often morphine and hydromorphone are used.
  - Many patients managed with clysis opioid analgesia are opioid tolerant, so double-check that the solution and programming will deliver appropriate individualized doses while respecting the hourly volume restriction.
- Preferred sites are the infraclavicular area, abdomen, lateral aspect of the thigh, or flexor aspect of the forearm, as these provide easy inspection for site "healthiness," minimize needle motion/dislodgement, and allow adequate patient mobility after attachment to PCA pump tubing.
- Be sure to choose sites away from scars, wounds, or ostomy sites.
- The skin is topically anesthetized with EMLA and aseptically prepared with chlorhexidine or povidone, a preflushed sterile 25- or 27-gauge steel butterfly or specialty subcutaneous needle is inserted, and then a sterile transparent dressing is applied with benzoin adhesive.
- The pump prescription should provide almost all the expected hourly requirement as the basal, with only a few PCA demand doses per day for incident pain.
- Sites may be rotated electively at about 5 days, or sooner if redness, irritation, or leakage occurs.
- Side effect management is similar to that for intravenous opioid PCA.

FURTHER READING

American Society of Anesthesiologists Task Force on Pain Management. Practice guidelines for acute pain management in the perioperative setting: A report by the American Society of Anesthesiologists Task Force on Pain Management, Acute Pain Section. *Anesthesiology*. 1995;82:1071–1081.

Chumbley GM, Hall GM, & Salmon P. Why do patients feel positive about patient-controlled analgesia? *Anaesthesia*. 1999;54:386–389.

Macintyre PE. Safety and efficacy of patient-controlled analgesia. *Br J Anaesth*. 2001;87:36–46.

Walder B, Schafer M, Henzi I, & Tramer MR. Efficacy and safety of patient-controlled opioid analgesia for acute post-operative pain. A quantitative systematic review. *Acta Anaesthesiologica Scandinavica*. 2001; 45:795–804.

Werner MU, Soholm L, Rotbell-Nielsen P, & Kehlet H. Does an acute pain service improve postoperative outcome? *Anesth Analg*. 2002;95:1361–1372.

18 EPIDURAL ANALGESIA

Jeffrey M. Gilfor, MD
Eugene R. Viscusi, MD

BACKGROUND AND HISTORY

- Epidural analgesia has become a cornerstone of acute pain management.
- Since 1901, when Corning described the epidural space, and through the pioneering efforts of Edwards, Hingson, Pages, Dogliotti, Tuohy, and Bromage, epidurals have become a standard modality for anesthesia. In the United States, Dr. Brian Ready has been a driving force behind the establishment of epidural analgesia as the modality of choice for postoperative pain control.
- Improvements in technique, equipment, and pharmacologic science have made the technique one of the most widely used in the anesthesiologist's arsenal.

ANATOMY

- The epidural space exists between the dura and the ligamentum flavum. Because the dura and ligamentum flavum adhere to one another, the epidural space is a "potential" space that surrounds the dural sac (see Figure 18–1 and Table 18–1):
  - Anteriorly, it is bounded by the posterior longitudinal ligament.
  - Posteriorly, it is bounded by the ligamentum flavum and the periosteum of the laminae.
  - Laterally, the intervertebral foramina containing their neural elements abut the epidural space.
  - The epidural space is continuous with the paravertebral space via the intervertebral foramina.
  - Superiorly, the space is anatomically closed at the foramen magnum where the spinal dura attaches to the dura of the cranium.
  - Caudally, the epidural space ends at the sacral hiatus and is closed by the sacrococcygeal ligament.
- The epidural space contains areolar connective tissue, fat, lymphatics, arteries, veins, and the spinal nerve roots as they exit the dural sac and pass through the intervertebral foramina.
- Posteriorly, the epidural space is entered by passing through the skin and thin subcutaneous tissue between the vertebral spinous processes, piercing the two relatively soft supraspinous and interspinous ligaments, and entering the often leathery tough ligamentum flavum that posteriorly bounds the epidural space. Especially in the elderly, the ligamentum flavum can be calcified (making it difficult to distinguish from bone) or uncharacteristically soft.
- Lacunae in the midline (especially in the thoracic region) may result in false loss of resistance when placing an epidural.

EPIDURAL MEDICATIONS

GENERAL COMMENTS REGARDING EPIDURAL MEDICATIONS

- All medications placed in the epidural space must be free of preservatives.

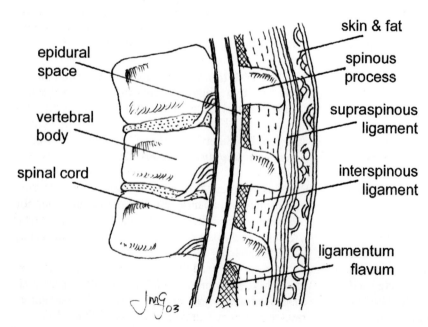

FIGURE 18–1 Anatomy of the epidural space.

TABLE 18–1 Main Features of Spinal Anatomy

Cervical region	Very thin ligamentum flavum
	C7 and T1 have almost horizontal spinous processes
	C7 is the most prominent cervical spine (vertebra prominens)
	Lamina are shaped like narrow rectangles
	Usually exhibits marked negative pressure (especially if seated)
Thoracic region	Very narrow lateral epidural space
	Ligamentum flavum is thicker than in cervical region, but thinner than midlumbar
	T5 through T9 spinous processes are the most angulated, making midline approach difficult
	Spinal cord is narrowest in the thoracic region
	Usually exhibits negative pressure (especially when seated)
Lumbar region	Widest epidural space
	Spinal cord ends at about L1–2 (in adults)
	Ligamentum flavum is the thickest
	Spinous processes have the least angulation
	Lumbar region has very prominent lateral epidural veins

- It is of utmost importance to maintain sterility when preparing epidural infusions or when drawing up bolus drugs.
- The incidence of contamination or medication error is lower when infusions are prepared centrally by the hospital pharmacy. Standard concentrations and additives should be established with the pharmacy.
- Standardization of epidural analgesic medications for the institution may reduce costs and minimize waste by allowing batch preparation.
- Epidural medications must be appropriately labeled (see Figure 18–2).
- Epidural catheters must be readily identifiable by medical and nursing staff to prevent unintended injection or infusion of inappropriate agents. Brightly colored flag-type labels near the injection port end of the catheter work well for this purpose (see Figure 18–3).

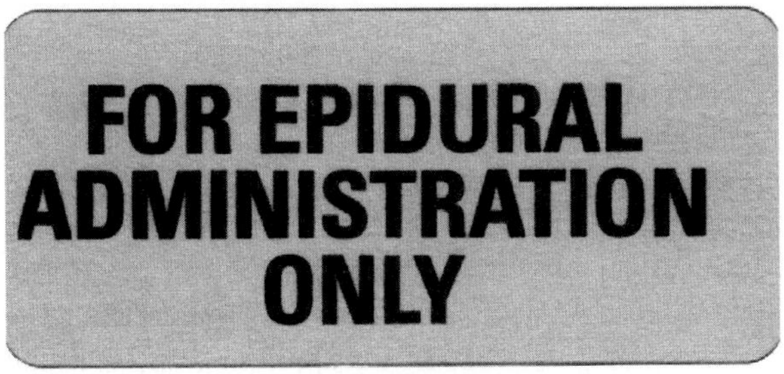

FIGURE 18–2 Typical epidural medication label.

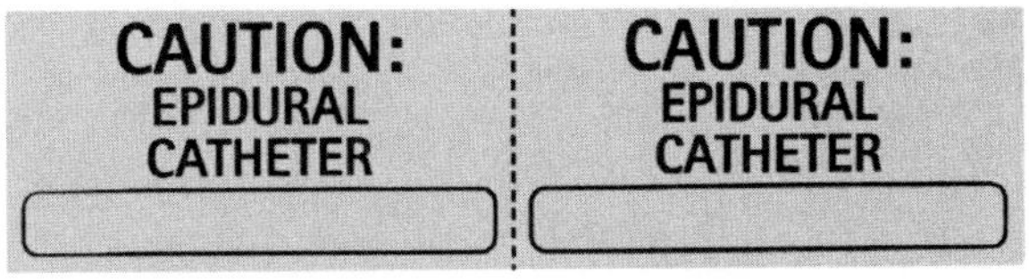

FIGURE 18–3 Typical epidural catheter label.

DELIVERY METHODS

- In the past, epidural medications were delivered as single-shot boluses, on an as-needed basis. This practice, however, inevitably leads to periods of inadequate analgesia and increased severity of unwanted side effects resulting from high peak medication levels.
- Newer methods employ continuous and patient-controlled epidural analgesia (PCEA) infusions to alleviate the shortcomings of periodic bolus dosing.
- The PCEA method allows for a continuous level of epidural analgesia, with small boluses initiated by the patient to cover periods of increased discomfort (eg, transfers or physical therapy).
- Continuous versus intermittent bolus dosing provides superior analgesia with lower incidence and severity of side effects.
- Several types of delivery devices are available for use in delivering epidural medications.
  - *Syringe pumps*: Deliver contents of the syringe during a specified period (minutes, hour, or days). Typically, however, these pumps cannot accommodate the quantities of medication in the concentrations usual for epidural analgesia. Syringe pumps are best used for intrathecal drug delivery and pediatric acute pain management.
  - *Peristaltic pumps*: Deliver medications from a flexible reservoir via tubing that is squeezed between rollers that create a positive displacement of a given volume of fluid with each cycle. Peristaltic pumps can accommodate larger volumes (50–1000 mL) than are possible with syringe pumps and are typically employed for epidural analgesia. Peristaltic pumps permit various flow rates and more PCEA options.
  - *Elastomeric reservoir pumps*: Force fluid from an elastomeric pressurized medication reservoir through a flow regulator. These devices are not well-suited for in-hospital epidural drug administration because the flow rate is specific for the regulator installed in the pump mechanism and, therefore, is not adjustable.
- Delivery rates for adult epidural analgesic solutions are usually between 4 and 20 mL/h. The lower rates are used for thoracic epidural infusions; the higher rates are used for lumbar infusions (Table 18–2).

TABLE 18–2 Common Infusion Rates of Epidural Solutions

Thoracic catheter	4–10 mL/h
Lumbar catheter	10–18 mL/h

LOCAL ANESTHETICS

- Local anesthetics play the central role in epidural analgesia.
- The major sites of action for epidural local anesthetics are the spinal nerve roots and dural cuff regions, where there is a relatively thin dural cover. Only a small fraction of local anesthetic diffuses into the subarachnoid space.
- In epidural analgesic applications, as opposed to spinal and epidural anesthesia, selection of the local anesthetic is typically not dependent on the drug's onset time or duration of action. The particular local anesthetic is chosen primarily because for its block density and side effect profile.
- The local anesthetics used most frequently for epidural analgesic purposes are bupivacaine and ropivacaine.
- Bupivacaine, the most widely studied local anesthetic, has been associated with significant cardiotoxicity and motor (versus sensory) blockade.
- Commercially available bupivacaine is a racemic mixture of the *R* and *S* isomers. The *R* isomer is more toxic than the *S* moiety.
- Ropivacaine, the *S* isomer of the propyl analog of bupivacaine, has a safer cardiotoxic profile than the bupivacaine enantomers.
- The most common side effects associated with epidural local anesthetics are hypotension, numbness, and motor block. These effects can be managed by decreasing the infusion rate or concentration of local anesthetic.
  - Hypotension, resulting from epidural-induced sympathectomy, can be minimized or reversed by repleting intravascular volume with crystalloid or colloid. This hypotension can be difficult to treat in thoracic surgery patients, who are often maintained on the "dry side" by the surgical service. Treatment with boluses of adrenergic agents (phenylephrine and ephedrine) may be used as a temporizing measure until fluid volume can be increased. If a continuous infusion is required, dopamine is the drug of choice. Inotropic agents are preferred over "afterload" agents that might trigger the Bezold–Jarish reflex.
  - Sensory block, to some degree, is an obvious result of epidural local anesthetics.
  - Some patients may be disturbed by numbness to light touch in certain areas. Reducing the concen-

tration of local anesthetic in the epidural infusion may reduce the level of sensory blockade at the expense of pain relief.
  - Using ropivacaine instead of bupivacaine may reduce the motor block component while maintaining adequate sensory analgesia.
  - Motor block is less likely to be an issue with an epidural placed in the thoracic region. A thoracic epidural catheter can provide adequate pain relief after most surgical procedures (except those in the lower extremity).

OPIOIDS

- Opioids have played a significant role in epidural analgesia. Nearly every available preservative-free opioid preparation has been used.
- Opioids may be used alone or, more commonly, as an adjunct to local anesthetic analgesia.
- Although the various opioids differ slightly in pharmacokinetics, they share side effects to varying degrees. When adding opioids to epidural analgesia, always increase monitoring for respiratory depression and sedation and administer, as needed, medications to treat nausea, pruritus, sedation, and respiratory depression.
  - *Nausea*: Treat with ondansetron, prochlorperazine, or low-dose naloxone.
  - *Pruritus*: Treat with an antihistamine, such as diphenhydramine, low-dose naloxone, or a small dose of oral naltrexone.
  - *Respiratory depression*: Although rare at the typically low opioid concentrations used in epidural analgesia, respiratory depression can be reversed with naloxone. Naloxone should be administered in 40-µg boluses, until the desired effect is reached. Excessive naloxone administration can result in acute withdrawal syndrome consisting of tachycardia, tachypnea, hypertension, and severe pain. Naloxone-induced acute withdrawal syndrome can result in stroke, myocardial ischemia, or myocardial infarction.
  - *Sedation*: Although less problematic in the in-hospital setting, sedation can also be reversed with naloxone.
  - *Neuraxial effects*: An agonist–antagonist may be used to treat neuraxial opioid side effects but may cause dysphoric reactions.
- Epidural morphine and hydromorphone produce a local analgesic effect, followed by redistribution to the central compartment cerebrospinal fluid (CSF). The efficacy of epidural morphine and hydromorphone is enhanced by placement of the epidural catheter at the correct interspace (center of surgical manipulation).

TABLE 18–3 Typical Concentrations for Epidural Opioids

Morphine	0.025–0.05 mg/mL
Hydromorphone	5–10 µg/mL
Fentanyl	2–5 µg/mL
Sufentanyl	1–2 µg/mL

- Epidural infusions with a local anesthetic (with or without opioid) reduce postoperative pain and shorten postoperative ileus after abdominal surgery. The best effects are found with the catheter tip located at the interspace at the center of surgical manipulation (Table 18–3).

OTHER ADDITIVES

- Agents may be added to epidural preparations to enhance efficacy. Although many preservative-free agents are used in the epidural space, few are approved for this purpose.
- Any medication used in the epidural space MUST be free of preservatives.
- Epinephrine and clonidine may enhance epidural analgesia.
  - Clonidine stimulates postsynaptic α_2 receptors in the dorsal horn interneurons, producing analgesia.
  - The recommended starting dose for epidural clonidine infusion is 30 µg/h. Data for doses above 40 mg/h are lacking.
  - Side effects of epidural clonidine include decreased heart rate and blood pressure. Patients receiving epidural clonidine should be closely monitored during the first 24 hours of treatment for hypotension, bradycardia, and excess sedation.
  - Epinephrine (in concentrations of 2–3 µg/mL) may enhance epidural analgesia, possibly by a mechanism of action similar to that of clonidine, without causing bradycardia or hypotension.

OTHER ADDITIVES UNDER INVESTIGATION

- Many agents have been suggested for use as additives to enhance epidural analgesia. None has been approved for this purpose, and most are not available in a preservative-free form in the United States. They are included here for completeness.
- A variety of α_2 agonists (other than clonidine and epinephrine) may enhance epidural analgesia and may warrant additional study.
  - Epidural dexmetotomidine acts as an α_2 agonist with a mechanism of action and analgesic effect almost identical to those of clonidine.
  - Tizanidine, a newer α_2 agonist, is an analog of clonidine that has minimal cardiovascular effects.
- Ketamine (an NMDA receptor antagonist) may increase analgesia and prolong blockade when combined with epidural morphine.
- Tramadol (not available in parenteral form in the United States) is a weak mu receptor agonist and serotonin/norepinephrine reuptake inhibitor that may provide some analgesia in epidural use, but data thus far are equivocal.
- Ketorolac (a nonsteroidal anti-inflammatory drug) has been used to enhance epidural analgesia and duration.
- Epidural neostigmine produces analgesia, but its use has been limited by its tendency to cause nausea.

ADJUNCTS TO EPIDURAL ANALGESIA

- Acute pain management is best served using multimodal therapy.
- Intravenous patient-controlled analgesia (PCA) infusions may be safely used in conjunction with epidural local anesthetics.
- Opioids can be used either in the epidural or intravenous PCA; avoid simultaneous use in both.
- Anxiety can be an important component of postoperative pain. Some patients benefit from addition of anxiolytic medication to their analgesic therapy.
- Care must be taken when using benzodiazepines with opioids due to resulting synergy in producing respiratory depression and decreased level of consciousness.
- Muscle spasm can complicate analgesia and may not respond well to systemic opioids or epidural analgesia. Small doses of benzodiazepines (eg, diazepam 2.5–5 mg) may relieve spasms. As stated above, the additive effects of these agents on sedation and respiratory depression must be considered.

EPIDURAL ANALGESIA FOR THE CHRONIC PAIN PATIENT WITH ACUTE PAIN

- Patients who chronically take pain medications at home pose a challenge with respect to management of acute postoperative pain.
  - Chronic pain may cause neurologic changes that sensitize the response to noxious stimuli.
  - Chronic pain patients on opioids often require higher doses of opioids because of tolerance.
  - Patients chronically taking opioids require opioid medication equivalent to their baseline dosage, as a minimum, to prevent acute withdrawal.
  - Parenteral opioids administered using intravenous PCA only (without a basal rate) may be insufficient

to control pain. A basal opioid infusion (equivalent to baseline opioid requirements) may be necessary.

◦ Chronic pain patients who use a fentanyl transdermal patch should continue using the patch throughout the perioperative period (it is neither necessary nor desirable to discontinue the patch preoperatively).

◦ Chronic pain patients who use extended-release pain medications at home should be restarted on their at-home medication as soon as possible postoperatively.

• Nonsteroidal medications (eg, ketorolac) and the newer COX-2 inhibitors may be used as an adjunct to epidural analgesia.

• Oral or transdermal clonidine may be a helpful adjunct for the chronic pain patient with acute pain.

EQUIPMENT

• Epidurals must be performed in an area designed for cardiovascular monitoring and airway and cardiopulmonary support, such as a dedicated block room or the operating room. The procedure may also be done in a separate area of the patient holding room as long as monitoring and emergency equipment and drugs are available.

• Sterile epidural kits are prepackaged with all the necessary equipment and medications for performing the procedure. Most kits are disposable.

• Most epidural catheters have a "dead space" equal to approximately 0.3 mL.

• Epidural catheters are manufactured in 16–21 gauge and are approximately 100 cm in length. Most are made of polyamide nylon. Modern catheters have centimeter markers and a radiopaque distal tip.

• On removing an epidural catheter, visually inspect and record that the tip is intact.

• In studies of obstetric patients, lateral-hole epidural catheters have demonstrated the best block spread.

• Common epidural catheters include the single-terminal-opening and the three-lateral-opening types. The three-holed design may have arisen from a desire to produce lateral full-bore equivalent flow with the minimum number of holes while at the same time maintaining catheter tensile strength. As manufacturing techniques improved, the holes were moved closer to the end, thereby minimizing the probability of a multicompartment block.

• "Successful" test dosing of a multiport epidural catheter may not rule out intrathecal or intravascular placement. One port can be intrathecal, while others are epidural. Fluid pressure exerted during test dosing is greater than that during continuous pump infusion. This difference may result in unequal flow distribution between the ports such that all or most of the test dose exits an epidural port.

PLACING THE EPIDURAL

• Because the epidural is a "potential" space between the ligamentum flavum and the dura, take care to stop advancing the needle as soon as the tip exits the ligamentum flavum, or the dura may be punctured.

• Select an interspace for epidural placement, such that the catheter tip will rest in the approximate center of stimulus.

• The epidural may be placed using the midline or paramedian approach.

◦ The midline approach is favored in the lumbar region, where the spinous processes are nearly horizontal in the seated patient.

◦ A paramedian approach may be advisable when placing a thoracic epidural, especially between T5 and T9, where the spinous processes almost overlap. When placing a thoracic epidural using the midline approach, angle the needle 50°–60° (up from the back plane) to pass between the two adjacent spines (see Figure 18–4).

• Once the tip of the epidural needle is situated in the epidural space, thread the epidural catheter 3–5 cm.

◦ Never withdraw the catheter from the needle once it has passed the tip. Doing so could shear the catheter tip, leaving it in the epidural space. Withdraw the entire assembly (needle and catheter) and reinsert after inspection of the catheter and replacement of the needle stylet.

◦ The catheter should advance easily into the epidural space. Ease in advancing the catheter into the epidural space provides another confirmation of correct placement.

◦ Without fluoroscopic guidance, the epidural catheter cannot reliably be directed one way or the other once it leaves the tip of the epidural needle.

◦ Advancing the catheter more than 5 cm increases the potential for knotting or could place the catheter tip too far from the intended center of epidural action to allow for adequate analgesia.

◦ Catheters placed 3 cm or less into the epidural space have a tendency to come out.

ACTIVATING THE EPIDURAL

• Before the epidural catheter can be used for infusion of analgesic medication, confirm that the tip lies within the epidural space and not within an epidural vein or the intrathecal space.

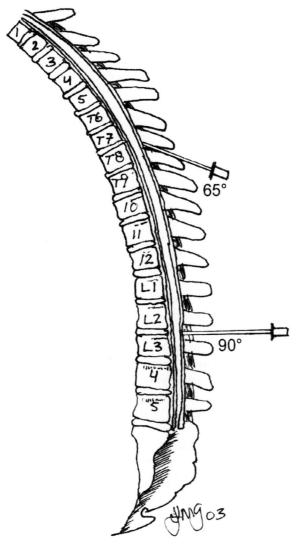

FIGURE 18–4 Epidural "angle of attack."

- A small dose of lidocaine containing epinephrine is used as a "test dose":
  - About 3 cc of 1.5 or 2% lidocaine (45–60 mg) with epinephrine (5–10 μg) is used for this purpose.
  - If the catheter tip rests intravascularly, the 5 or 10 μg of epinephrine should cause an increase in heart rate (15–20 bpm) easily seen on the monitor.
  - If the catheter tip rests intrathecally, the test dose will result in a wide dense block (sensory and motor). The dose is small enough not to result in a high spinal.
- A "negative" test dose does not eliminate the possibility of intrathecal or intravascular catheter placement. Constant vigilance is required whenever epidural analgesia is used.
  - Elderly patients and those taking beta-blocking medication may not display a significant heart rate

increase from intravascular injection of the few micrograms of epinephrine in the test dose.
  - It may take 10 minutes or more for the full manifestations of an intrathecal test dose to be seen. Profound hypotension and bradycardia may be early signs.
  - As stated previously, multiport catheters may allow one or more ports to be intrathecal, while others are within the epidural space. Test dosing may inject medication preferentially through some (but not other) ports.
- Treat every epidural catheter bolus dose as potentially intrathecal or intravascular. Bolus epidural medications incrementally rather than all at once.
- Although it has become standard practice, negative aspiration of the epidural catheter does not rule out intravascular or intrathecal placement.
- If the test dose is positive for intravascular or intrathecal placement, the catheter can be withdrawn 1 cm and retested. This can be repeated several times as long as a sufficient length of catheter remains in the epidural space (at least 1 cm). Often it is easier simply to remove the epidural catheter and reinsert it one interspace above or below.

EPIDURAL COMPLICATIONS

- Complications of epidural analgesia include inadequate analgesia, excessive blockade, unintentional intrathecal or intravascular injection and its sequelae, and the potentially more serious infections or hematomas that can lead to neurologic damage (Table 18–4).
- A study of more than 1000 patients who had postoperative epidural analgesia showed a 20% incidence of inadequate analgesia resulting from catheter dislodgement. There was 1 subarachnoid catheter migration, 3 intravascular migrations, 40 catheter leaks, 57 catheter site inflammations, and 5 catheter infections requiring antibiotic treatment.
- Early recognition and management are the keys to minimizing poor outcome.
- The complication rate for serious neurologic injury resulting from epidural placement has been quoted as anywhere from 1/11,000 to fewer than 1/100,000. Most of these complications were attributed to detergent contamination or toxic drug injection through the needle, causing ascending arachnoiditis.
- Epidural infection is a rare complication of epidural anesthesia. Usually the source of infection arises from bloodborne spread secondary to infection elsewhere in the body. In a review of 39 cases of epidural abscess over a period of 27 years, only one case was

TABLE 18–4   Epidural Complications

COMPLICATION	COMMENTS	TREATMENT
Headache	May be result of dural puncture (incidence 1–2%) Usually self-limiting	Analgesia Bed rest Hydration Blood patch if prolonged
Backache	At insertion site Usually transient	Analgesics and reassurance With fever or neurologic deficit—requires careful attention
Sympathetic blockade High blockade	May cause significant hypotension Respiratory distress (intercostal block) Bradycardia (high thoracic block) Unconsciousness (total spinal block) Dermatome block higher than T4 Numbness or tingling in fingers or arms Horner's syndrome	Hydration Vasopressors Resuscitation Cease epidural infusion
Nerve damage	Rare and usually transient	Investigation Neurology consult

associated with epidural anesthesia. A 1985 review of spinal and epidural abscesses indicated that the incidence of epidural abscess did not rise from 1965 to 1985, despite the increased use of epidural anesthesia/analgesia during that period. Relative contraindications to epidural placement include local infection at the intended insertion site and sepsis (Table 18–5).

EPIDURAL ANALGESIA MANAGEMENT

- The primary goals of an acute pain management service are to offer a wide variety of services in addition to epidural postoperative pain management. These services must be seamlessly integrated into the hospital infrastructure to be effective.
- Establishing a well-coordinated and effective acute pain management service requires strong institutional support and collaboration among anesthesiologists, surgeons, nurses, pharmacists, and administrators. In our experience, once established, an effective acute pain management service becomes an expected part of perioperative patient care.
- Optimal analgesia requires therapeutic fine-tuning to maximize benefits with minimal side effects. This can be accomplished only with close patient surveillance. A nurse-based acute pain management service is the most effective way to provide this level of service.

- With appropriate training and well-designed protocols, nurses and nurse clinicians can be empowered to assess pain and side effects and to adjust therapy at "the point of care."
- Physicians maintain the role of deciding in what circumstances epidural analgesia is appropriate and perform the procedure.
- Nurses manage the epidural when patients are returned to "the floor," using physician-determined protocols.
- Carefully designed plans or protocols may include epidural analgesia, traditional NSAIDs, COX-2 inhibitors, and opioids.
- Standard physician orders facilitate a uniform approach to epidural and adjunct analgesia management. Although standard orders should allow for some degree of customization to accommodate individual patient needs, the vast majority of situations can be managed using standardized orders. An example of such standardized epidural orders is provided in Figure 18–5.
- The appropriate level of epidural analgesia surveillance "on the floor" requires cooperation from floor nurses, who must be trained to recognize and record the most common problems of epidural analgesia (eg,

TABLE 18–5   Epidural Abscess versus Hematoma

	ABSCESS	HEMATOMA
Time course	Insidious and slow Hours to days	Acute and abrupt Minutes to hours
Typical symptoms	Starts with local back pain and tenderness percussion	Starts with local back pain and tenderness to percussion
	Weakness progresses over hours or days, often abruptly ending in a cauda equina syndrome, paraplegic or quadriplegic pattern	Weakness progresses very rapidly to cauda equina syndrome or paresis
		Bowel and bladder dysfunction often occurs with lumbar lesions
	Fever and leukocytosis are usual Bowel and bladder dysfunction often occurs with lumbar lesions Sepsis Mental status changes	
Diagnosis	MRI with gadolinium is the study of choice	MRI with gadolinium is the study of choice
Treatment	Surgical decompression, with medical treatment reserved for early/mild cases or those not fit for surgery	Surgical decompression

Thomas Jefferson University Hospital

🍎 *Jefferson Health System*

‖‖‖‖‖‖‖‖‖‖‖‖‖‖‖‖‖‖‖‖‖
⋆ 0 1 9 4 0 0   0 1 0 2 ⋆

MR#

LW Acct#

Name

Department of Anesthesia

Epidural / Intrathecal Analgesia Order Form

Complete or Imprint with Address-O-Plate

No administration (po, subq, IM or IV) of any narcotics, sedatives, hypnotics, tranquilizers, antiemetics or antihistamines unless part of this protocol or ordered by anesthesiology.

Allergies _____

1. This patient has ☐ Epidural catheter ☐ Intrathecal catheter ☐ Neither

2. This patient's primary mode of therapy is either *(choose a or b):*

   a. Continuous infusion of

   ☐ **Bupivacaine** _____ % (final concentration) ☐ **Ropivacaine** _____ % (final concentration)

   ☐ **Fentanyl** _____ mcg / ml (final concentration) ☐ **Morphine** _____ mg / ml (final concentration)

   ☐ **Hydromorphone** _____ mcg/ml (final concentration) ☐ **Epinephrine** _____

   Total volume _____ mls (qs using preservative free normal saline)
   to infuse at _____ **ml / hr** (Basal Rate).

   ☐ **Patient controlled epidural** **PCA Dose** _____ ml.
   Lockout interval _____ min.
   Hourly Limit _____ ml.

   b. Single shot ☐ **EPIDURAL** ☐ **INTRATHECAL** injection

   Medication _____ Dose _____ Time _____

3. Have naloxone 0.4mg available at bedside. Prior to administration, qs naloxone 0.4mg to 10ml with 0.9% NaCl and notify APMS service

4. Heparin lock or IV at all times.

5. Please label patient's door and medication cardex **"Intraspinal Analgesia."**

6. For solutions containing narcotics, monitor resp. rate and sedation level as follows:

   Infusions q _____ hr x _____, then q _____ hr for duration of therapy.

   Following Bolus Resp. rate q 15 min. x 2.

7. For infusions containing local anestetic, monitor motor score, B.P., and HR as follows:

   Infusions q 4 hr. for duration of therapy.

   Following Bolus q 5 min. x 4.

8. Monitor pain score q 4 hr.

9. **Treatment of side effects**

   Itching Diphenhydramine Hydrochloride (Benadryl) 25–50 mg IVPB / IM q 4 hr. prn.

   Nausea/Vomiting _____

   Urinary Retention Straight cath. q 8hr. prn; may place foley cath if patient requires second straight cath.

10. For sleep *(if resp. rate > 12 / min. and patient is easily arousable)*: Benadryl (diphenhydramine) 25–50 mg IVPB / IM / PO, qHS pm.

11. Call _____ pain service at beeper _____ for following:

    a. Resp. rate < 10. In the event of **severe** respiratory depression (RR<5), house officer or nurse may administer naloxone diluted to 10ml with 0.9% NaCl for final concentration of 0.04mg/ml. Administer 1ml (0.04mg) slowly over 1 minute, repeating 1ml doses as needed, up to 3ml over 3 minutes.

    b. Altered mental status or patient becomes difficult to arouse.

    c. Inadequate analgesia.

    d. Pruritus or Nausea and Vomiting not controlled by above measures.

    e. Problems with Intraspinal catheter.

    f. Increasing motor block.

12. Other _____

APMS RNs Only

☐ Follow thoracic epidural protocol

☐ Follow lumbar epidural protocol

☐ Alternate plans

  ☐ Epidural local and IV
    PCA opioid

☐ Other _____

_____

_____

_____

_____

_____

IMPORTANT: DO NOT WRITE IN MARGINS

Signature	Date Ordered	Time Ordered

Form 0194-00 (Rev. 1/02)   White: Chart Copy • Yellow: Pharmacy Copy   MJUG 01.4265

FIGURE 18–5 Example of standardized epidural orders.

pain, pruritus, respiratory depression, sedation, and excessive motor blockade). A standardized flowsheet for recording epidural (and other analgesic) parameters can be used.

FURTHER READING

Acute Pain Management Guideline Panel. Acute pain management in adults: Operative procedures, quick reference guide for clinicians. *J Pharm Care in Pain and Symptom Control.* 1993;1(1):63–84.

ASRA Consensus Statement. Regional anesthesia in the anticoagulated patient defining the risks. www.ASRA.com

Correll DJ, Viscusi ER, Grunwald Z, et al. Epidural analgesia with intravenous morphine patient-controlled analgesia: Postoperative outcomes measures after mastectomy with immediate TRAM flap breast reconstruction. *Reg Anesth Pain Med.* 2001;26:444–449.

De Leon-Casasola OA, Lema MJ. Postoperative epidural opioid analgesia: What are the choices? *Anesth Analg.* 1996;83:867–875.

Eisenach JC, DeKock M, Klimscha W. Alpha2-adrenergic agonists for regional anesthesia. A clinical review of clonidine (1984–1995). *Anesthesiology.* 1996;85: 655–674.

Fink B. History of Neural Blockade. In: Cousins MJ, Bridenbaugh PO (eds). *Neural Blockade.* Philadelphia: Lippincott; 1988.

Geibler RM, Scherer RV, Peters J. Incidence of neurologic complications related to thoracic epidural catheterization. *Anesthesiology.* 1997;86:55–63.

Gottschalk A, Smith DS, Jobes DR, et al. Preemptive epidural analgesia and recovery from radical prostatectomy: A randomized controlled trial. *JAMA.* 1998;279:107–108.

Liu S, Carpenter RL, Neal JM. Epidural anesthesia and analgesia. Their role in postoperative outcome. *Anesthesiology.* 1995;82:1474–1506.

Liu SS, Carpenter RL, Mackey DC. Effects of perioperative analgesic technique on rate of recovery after colon surgery. *Anesthesiology.* 1995;83:757–765.

Rawal N, Berggren L. Organization of acute pain services: A low-cost model. *Pain.* 1994;57:117–123.

Ready LB. Development for an anesthesiology-based postoperative pain management service. *Anesthesiology.* 1988;68:100–106.

Steinbrook R. Epidural anesthesia and gastrointestinal motility. *Anesth Analg.* 1998;86:837–844.

Tuman KJ, McCarthy RJ, March RJ. Effects of epidural anesthesia and analgesia on coagulation and outcome after major vascular surgery. *Anesth Analg.* 1991; 73:696–704.

Viscusi ER, Jan R, Warshawsky D. An acute pain management service with regional anesthesia: How to make it work. *Techniques in Reg Anesth and Pain Man.* 2002;6(2):40–49.

Yeager MP, Class DD, Neff RK. Epidural anesthesia and analgesia in high-risk surgical patients. *Anesthesiology.* 1987;66:729–736.

---

19 INTRATHECAL THERAPY FOR CANCER PAIN

Peter S. Staats, MD
Frederick W. Luthardt, MA

INTRODUCTION

- Just as a superhighway provides discrete travel lanes for a host of different vehicles, the spinal cord contains various pathways along which a host of receptors and compounds travel to transmit information, including pain signals, to the brain.
- We can reduce or eliminate pain by directly injecting into the intrathecal space agents that can interfere with the transmission of these signals. Despite our expanding knowledge of the receptors and compounds that govern these signals and the increasing sophistication of the technology at our disposal, we have not identified the ideal agent or combination of agents for intrathecal analgesia.
- Our delivery methods are also less than ideal, and, despite nearly a quarter century of experience, use of intrathecal therapy remains in its infancy.

• Indications for intrathecal analgesia include failed back surgery syndrome, chronic regional pain syndrome, postherpetic neuralgia, peripheral nerve injury, and cancer pain.

INTRATHECAL AGENTS

MORPHINE

• Preservative-free morphine is the only agent approved by the US Food and Drug Administration and by manufacturers of pumps for intrathecal delivery to treat pain and is the most widely used intrathecal agent for pain.
• The recommended daily starting dose is 0.5 mg/d, and the maximum recommended dose is 20 mg/d. These numbers should be modified according to clinical practice.
• We lack crucial information on the long-term effects of intrathecal morphine, however, especially on the ability of increasing doses to deal with the loss of efficacy that accompanies the development of tolerance as well as on the factors that influence the formation of granulomas (see below).

OTHER AGENTS IN USE

• In an attempt to improve analgesia and reduce side effects and despite the lack of standard practice guidelines that would provide important information on neurotoxicity, drug stability, pump compatibility, and drug efficacy, clinicians are also administering the following analgesics intrathecally (Figure 19–1).
  ○ *μ opioids*: hydromorphone, methadone, fentanyl (100 times more potent than morphine), and sufentanil (1000 times more potent than morphine)
  ○ *GABA-A agonist*: midazolam hydrochloride (Versed) (rarely used in the United States)
  ○ *α_2-Adrenergic agonist*: clonidine (persisting side effects include low blood pressure, lethargy, malaise, and headache)
  ○ *N-Methyl D-aspartate receptor antagonist*: ketamine
  ○ *Cyclooxygenase inhibitor*: aspirin, ketorolac (experimental)

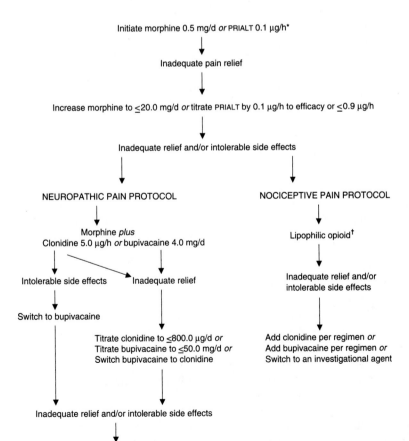

FIGURE 19–1 Intrathecal analgesic algorithm. *Under US Food and Drug Administration evaluation. †Hydromorphone, fentanyl, sufentanil.

○ *GABA-B agonist*: baclofen
○ *N-type (neuronal-specific) calcium channel blocker*: PRIALT

- Prior to using novel drugs, physicians should be familiar with associated spinal cord toxicity, drug efficacy, and safety concerns.
- Some of these agents are lipophilic (eg, hydromorphone, fentanyl, sufentanil, methadone), as opposed to morphine, which is hydrophilic. Clonidine is moderately lipophilic. The degree of lipophilicity determines how readily a compound dissolves into fat and veins and, thus, how rapidly it is transported and dispersed in the intrathecal space.

COMBINING AGENTS

- Clinicians are also combining analgesics with opioids for intrathecal delivery in an attempt to improve pain scores without increasing opioid dose (see Figure 19–1).
- Combinations include:
  ○ Bupivacaine or clonidine with morphine, hydromorphone, fentanyl, sufentanil, methadone, or meperidine.
  ○ Intrathecal meperidine may erode pumps but offers combination opioid/local anesthetic relief, intermediate solubility, and high-concentration stability.
  ○ Intrathecal bupivacaine may cause seizures, cauda equina syndromes, or prolonged sensory deficits.[1]

AGENTS UNDER INVESTIGATION

INTRATHECAL STEROIDS

- Intrathecal steroids were used in the 1980s to treat neuropathic pain arising from lumbosacral radiculitis until lawsuits alleged the agent or the polyethylene glycol vehicle caused arachnoiditis.
- Taking another look at intrathecal steroids, investigators randomized 277 patients with postherpetic neuralgia to receive intrathecal placebo, local anesthetics, or local anesthetics plus methylprednisolone once a week for 4 weeks. At 1 year, the steroid group had marked reduction in pain.[2]
- A double-blind, controlled, prospective study found more rapid reduction of residual neuropathic pain with intrathecal administration of β-methasone than with placebo.[3]
- A comparison of epidural versus intrathecal administration of local anesthetic plus steroid revealed a significant advantage for intrathecal administration in reducing pain and allodynia.[4]

- These results must be replicated prior to routine use of intrathecal steroids.

CALCIUM CHANNEL BLOCKERS

- PRIALT, the agent formerly known as SNX-111 and as ziconotide, is a neurotoxin synthesized to duplicate the chemical structure of a component of the venom of the Philippine marine snail, *Conus magus*.
- PRIALT is under investigation for treatment of neuropathic and cancer pain.
- Gradually titrating the dose of PRIALT from a low starting point allows management of the adverse events that occur after blocking the N-type calcium channel.
- Clinical studies indicate that PRIALT is a safe and effective treatment for refractory pain.[5]

ADDITIONAL AGENTS UNDER INVESTIGATION

- The somatostatin analogs octreotide and vapreotide have received attention as promising intrathecal agents, but commercial development seems unlikely.[6]
- Acetylcholinesterase inhibitors, such as neostigmine.
- Tricyclic antidepressants.
- Nitric oxide synthase inhibitors.

EFFECT OF SPINAL OPIOIDS

GENERAL EFFECTS

- No change in response to light touch
- No change in autonomic outflow
- No change in voluntary motor function
- Dose-dependent analgesia
- Stereospecificity
- Antagonized in dose-dependent manner by naloxone
- High levels of binding in substantia gelatinosa (where most small primary afferent fibers terminate)

POTENTIAL SIDE EFFECTS

- Pruritus (tolerance can develop)
- Edema
- Itching
- Dysphoria
- Nausea, vomiting (tolerance can develop)
- Histamine release
- Sedation
- Respiratory depression
- Gastrointestinal hypomotility/constipation
- Urinary hesitancy/retention

- Sexual impotence (reductions have been noted in production of sex hormones)
- Abnormal body temperature regulation
- Headache
- Anaphylaxis
- Agitation
- Seizures
- Somnolence

OUTCOMES

- Approximately 5–10% of cancer patients are appropriate candidates for intrathecal analgesia, which is the most effective way to deliver opioids to treat cancer pain.[7]
- Long-term dosing is generally stable for cancer patients.[8]
- A randomized trial comparing the impact of adding intrathecal analgesic treatment to medical management with that of medical management alone in 200 patients with refractory cancer pain found that intrathecal therapy[9]:
  - Improved pain scores
  - Reduced the incidence of drug-related toxicity
  - Reduced reliance on systemic analgesics
  - Improved the quality of life for patients and caregivers
  - Improved survival rates

DRUG DELIVERY SYSTEMS

- For treatment lasting ≤ 3 months, use of an external pump with a percutaneously placed intrathecal catheter:
  - Reduces the cost of treatment
  - Is minimally invasive because it does not involve implanting a pump
  - Carries a low risk of infection (the risk of infection increases over time)

CONSTANT-FLOW-RATE PUMP

- This implanted titanium pump has two hollow chambers divided by a bellows:
  - Freon is sealed in one chamber; the other is filled percutaneously with the pharmaceutical via a self-sealing septum.
  - When the drug reservoir is full, the Freon is compressed into a liquid state.

- Body temperature causes the Freon to vaporize in the chamber, expanding and exerting pressure on the drug reservoir that forces the drug through an outlet filter into a flow-restricting capillary tube to a silicone rubber delivery tube.
- The result is a constant flow of the drug if body temperature and pressure remain constant.
- Increasing or decreasing the drug dose requires altering the concentration of the drug in the reservoir (draining and replacing the infusate).
- The service life of this delivery system is limited only by the tolerance of the refill septum to puncture.
- Constant-flow-rate pumps are generally used when stable dosing is required or when the drugs are not compatible with other types of pumps.
- Several brands of constant-flow-rate pumps are available.

PROGRAMMABLE PUMP

- This pump has an expandable/collapsible reservoir with a self-sealing septum for percutaneous injection, a battery module, a microprocessor programming module, a 0.22-μm retention filter for contaminants, and a peristaltic pump motor that uses compressed internal tubing to draw infusate from the reservoir through an extension catheter to the intraspinal catheter.
- The rate of infusion is determined by the rate of revolution of the pump rotor.
- External programming of medication delivery relies on a computer, printer, and programming head that uses radiofrequency as a link.
- Telemetric interrogation of pump status allows clinicians to troubleshoot or change drug delivery parameters and algorithms.
- This apparatus is ideal for chronic pain patients.

THE CLINIC

- The clinic's basic resources must include:
  - A health care professional whose work is dedicated to implant coordination, patient education, and guiding the patient through the process. This person has a role in:
    - The preoperative screening trial
    - Surgical implantation
    - Pump programming
    - Pump refills
    - Long-term patient management
    - Dealing with adverse events
  - Multispecialty access (including psychological consultations) for appropriate patient selection.

PATIENT SELECTION

NATURE OF THE PAIN

- Patients must have chronic pain, which is defined as pain:
  ○ Of more than 3–4 months' duration
  ○ Extending more than a month beyond the expected duration for a normal healing process
  ○ Expected to last beyond 3 months (eg, cancer pain)
- The pain must not be relieved by optimum medical management (inadequate pain relief or adequate pain relief but intolerable side effects).
- Those with neuropathic pain (caused by damage to the nervous system and described as burning, tingling, shooting, etc) are less likely to gain relief from intrathecal opioids than patients with nociceptive pain (mediated by dispersed receptors in cutaneous tissue, bone, muscle, connective tissue, vessels, and viscera).

INCLUSION CRITERIA

- The patient should have progressed through an accepted pain treatment continuum (ie, the World Health Organization ladder).
- The pain is likely to respond to treatment.
- The patient responds to opioids.
- No untreated psychopathology exists to impede treatment success.
- A screening trial was successful.

ABSOLUTE EXCLUSION CRITERIA

- Aplastic anemia
- Systemic infection
- Known allergy to implant material
- Known allergy to medication
- Active intravenous drug abuser
- Physical impairment to pump or catheter implantation
- Psychosis or dementia

RELATIVE EXCLUSION CRITERIA

- Emaciation
- Ongoing anticoagulation therapy
- Child awaiting fusion of epiphyses
- Possibility of occult infection
- Recovering drug addict
- Nonresponsiveness to opioids (may consider other pharmaceuticals)
- Lack of family or social support

- Socioeconomic problems
- Lack of access to medical care

ASSESSMENT AND SCREENING

THE PSYCHOLOGICAL ASSESSMENT

- The clinician should not ask if the patient is a candidate for implantable therapy, but should seek to uncover, assess, and treat, if possible[10]:
  ○ A predominantly psychological origin of the pain
  ○ A major psychopathology
  ○ A mood disorder
  ○ The potential for self-harm
  ○ Dementia
  ○ Anxiety
  ○ Catastrophizing
  ○ An unusually high degree of distress
  ○ Addictive issues
  ○ Sleep disturbances
  ○ Conflicting motives and expectations

SCREENING TRIALS

- Involve acute administration of spinal opioids
- The goals of screening trials are to determine:
  ○ If the therapy is likely to lead to adequate pain relief
  ○ The existence of side effects that would preclude long-term therapy

SCREENING TECHNIQUES

SINGLE BOLUS DOSE
- Screening with a single intrathecal bolus dose administered by lumbar puncture may maximize the incidence of nausea and urinary retention.
- Pain can be relieved for as long as 24 hours, but relief generally peaks in the first few hours.
- Single bolus screening may invoke a placebo response (but this does not mean that the patient will not do well with intrathecal analgesia).

EPIDURAL DRUG DELIVERY
- Screening with epidural infusion involves a tunneled or percutaneously placed epidural catheter and permits a trial to extend for days or weeks.
  ○ Dosing is 10 times higher than used for intrathecal administration.
  ○ Epidural infusion screening provides information on efficacy but not on the side effects of intrathecal administration.

INTRATHECAL DRUG DELIVERY

- Screening with a tunneled or percutaneously placed intrathecal catheter is optimum for achieving screening goals and permits sequential trials of pharmaceuticals.
- The disadvantage of the percutaneous approach is that proceeding to pump implantation would require a second procedure.

Percutaneous Approach

- The STAATS (Simple Tunneling Approach and Technique Securing Catheters) method (see Figure 19–2 for an illustrated description of this technique).
- The advantages of this method are:
  - Reduction in rate of infection
  - No incision pain to confuse results
  - Ease of removal
  - Reduction in incidence of catheter migration

Surgical Approach

- Prepare the patient's back in an operating room equipped with fluoroscopy.
- Square off the area with sterile towels and apply a "chest–breast" drape with a wide opening.
- Make a 1- to 2-inch incision and paraspinous intrathecal puncture with the appropriate needle.
- Introduce the catheter under fluoroscopic guidance to the desired level.
- Tunnel a disposable extension catheter with a malleable cardiac pacemaker tunneling trocar to the flank opposite the surgeon from the back skin incision.
- Connect this catheter to the intrathecal catheter, tie it with 2-O silk, and anchor it to lumbar fascia with 2-O silk in figure-8 fashion.

Step 1: Insertion of first needle and catheter
- Prepare sterile surgical site.
- Apply local anesthetic.
- Using fluoroscopic guidance, advance a 17-gauge Tuohy needle into the intrathecal space.
- Thread catheter through the Tuohy to the appropriate depth.
- Confirm with clear cerebrospinal fluid flow.

Step 2: Insertion of stylet
- Remove the stylet from another 17-gauge Tuohy needle.
- Insert stylet next to the first Tuohy needle.
- Advance the stylet along the first needle 2–3 mm subcutaneously.
- Press on the skin, turn the stylet, and advance the stylet laterally 5–7 cm.
- Allow the tip of the stylet to puncture the surface of the skin.

Step 3: Placement of second needle and removal of first needle.
- Insert the emerging end of the stylet into the barrel of a second 17-gauge Tuohy needle.
- Advance the second Tuohy needle back into the tunnel created by the stylet (it will surround the stylet).
- Advance the second Tuohy out the first puncture point next to the catheter.
- Remove the first Tuohy needle (the catheter stays).

Step 4: Securing the Catheter
- Thread the external end of the catheter (that will eventually connect to the pump) through the second Tuohy so the catheter emerges from the skin at the second puncture point, and now curves under the skin at the first puncture point and is secured by the skin.
- Connect the free end of the catheter to the external intrathecal pump.

FIGURE 19–2 Intrathecal catheter placement using the Simple Tunneling Approach and Securing Catheters (STAATS) method. Copyright Peter S. Staats; reproduced with permission.

- Suture the wound with an interrupted inverted layer of 3-O absorbable suture and sterile tape or staples.
- Bandage the catheter exit point (eg, with a Biopatch impregnated with Hibiclens).
- If the catheter type permits, fit it with a Luer-lock connection for mating with the infusion catheter.
- The advantage is that no second procedure is needed to implant the catheter.

MANAGING SYSTEMIC OPIOID USE DURING SCREENING

- Complete withdrawal can cause discomfort or abstinence syndrome.
- One protocol suggests converting half of the oral dose to its intrathecal equivalent and replacing 20% of the remaining oral dose each day with an equivalent dose of intrathecal analgesic.[11]

LENGTH AND SUCCESS OF SCREENING TRIAL

- These may be important for ensuring adequate screening (and improving the likelihood of a successful outcome).
- Tunneled catheter patients may remain hospitalized for 3 days.
- Outpatient trials may extend for a week or longer.
- The trial is successful if the patient achieves a 50% reduction in pain with no intolerable side effects.

IMPLANT PROCEDURE

PUMP PREPARATION

- To cut time and cost, have an implant assistant prepare the pump while the surgeon prepares the patient.

CONSTANT-FLOW-RATE PUMP
- Check the preset flow rate.
- Fill the pump with the pharmaceutical.
- Place the pump in a body-temperature saline bath.
- Cut the attached catheter, and monitor for flow.

PROGRAMMABLE PUMP
- Note the pump model number, reservoir size, and presence of a catheter access port.
- Do not remove from the packaging until cerebrospinal fluid has been accessed.
- Interrogate the pump in its container to ensure that the calibration constant matches that recorded on the

packaging and to determine how much factory-filled fluid needs to be removed.
- Warm the pump to 35°–40°C.
- With the pump in its sterile container, purge all fluid and air from reservoir with a Huber-type needle and light aspiration if necessary.
- If the volume removed differs by 20% from the packaging information, the pump may be faulty.
- If the fluid does not flow out, submerge the pump in warm saline to verify the presence of bubbles from the catheter port.
- Place the pump in saline until internal purge is complete—about 15 minutes.
- Fill the reservoir with only 10 cc of the drug to avoid overpressurization (refills can be up to 18 cc).
- Do not allow air to enter the reservoir.

PATIENT PREPARATION AND IMPLANT TECHNIQUE

- Spend time discussing the location of the pump with the patient (right or left lower abdominal quadrant). The iliac crest, symphysis pubis, ilioinguinal ligament, and costal margin should not contact the pump when the patient is seated.
- Anesthesia may be general (deferring the use of muscle relaxants until the catheter is threaded into intrathecal space) or local, which is preferred in an outpatient setting.
- If necessary, implant the catheter, clamp it to the drape to prevent loss of cerebrospinal fluid, and pack the incision with antibiotic sponge.
- If using an existing catheter, place the patient in a lateral decubitus position, implant side up, and disconnect and remove the disposable extension catheter. Then, clamp the catheter to prevent the loss of cerebrospinal fluid.
- Make a 10-cm incision in the lower abdomen to the fat layer, and fashion a subcutaneous pocket large enough for the pump (enough space to insert four fingers). The upper side of the incision should be the width of the pump (approximately 2.5 cm). Keep the pocket tight enough to prevent pump rotation. The depth should allow reliable telemetry (no more than 2.5 cm). Maintain meticulous hemostasis to avoid hematoma. Pack the pocket with an antibiotic sponge.
- Position the pump in the pocket so that the refill port is easy to locate and will not be obscured by the scar.
- Tunnel the extension catheter from the pump pocket to the incision in the patient's back with a malleable tunneling device (such as a cardiac pacemaker or shunt tool or the system included with the programmable pump).

- For the programmable pump, attach the extension catheter (for the constant-flow-rate pump, the catheter is attached at the factory).
- Connect the extension and internal catheters with the titanium or plastic tubing provided by the pump manufacturer. To prevent migration, anchor the connection with 2-O nonabsorbable braided tie and anchor the resulting construct to the underlying muscle fascia in figure-8 fashion.
- Pumps with an attached catheter must be placed in the pocket before tunneling. Programmable pumps go in the pocket after tunneling.
- Pumps with Dacron pouches do not require suturing; pumps with anchor loops require at least two nonabsorbable stitches in tissue that will not quickly necrose to prevent rotation and a third to prevent flipping. Place stitches in the pocket first, then through the pump loops; then place the pump in the pocket and tie the sutures. It is possible, however (especially in thin patients), to place a pump without a Dacron pocket in a pouch successfully without suturing.
- Close the incision with an interrupted, inverted layer of 2-O absorbable suture in the abdomen and 3-O in the back. Finish by applying steritape or surgical staples.

POTENTIAL COMPLICATIONS

POSTOPERATIVE HEMATOMA

- Perioperative bleeding resulting in hematoma is troublesome but preventable by meticulous pocket creation and by lightly binding a wrap (eg, an Ace bandage) around the abdomen to compress the pump pocket for 24–48 hours postprocedure.

EPIDURAL AND INTRATHECAL HEMORRHAGE

- Hemorrhage can cause neurologic damage and can be fended off by preoperatively discontinuing nonsteroidal anti-inflammatory agents and reversing anticoagulation therapy.
- Hemorrhage requires immediate MRI or CT/myelogram to determine the necessity of neurosurgical intervention.
- Signs of hemorrhage include:
  ○ A sudden increase in focal back pain with associated tenderness
  ○ Progressive lower-extremity numbness and/or weakness
  ○ Loss of bowel and/or bladder control signaled by retention/constipation or incontinence

WOUND INFECTION

- Efforts to prevent infection include administration of prophylactic antibiotics, such as intravenous cephalosporin, 1 hour before the procedure; intraoperative antibiotic irrigation; and, in the case of a screening trial, daily prophylaxis.
- All but superficial wound infections require system removal to avoid the possibility of epidural abscess or meningitis.

NEUROLOGIC INJURY

- Nerve root injury is possible because fluoroscopy does not reveal intraspinal neural structures during needle placement.
- To some extent, the possibility of injuring nerve roots can be reduced by placing the catheter with the patient under local anesthesia, which allows the patient to report radiating electric shock-like or burning sensations.
- If a patient reports sensations indicating involvement of a nerve root, remove the needle immediately and consider placement at a different level.

SPINAL CORD INJURY

- Catheter placement puts the spinal cord at risk.
- To minimize this risk, do not force entry or advancement of spring-wound or internally stiffened catheters (this action could bury the tip in an intramedullary location).
- Penetration of the spinal cord often produces dysesthesias or a nondermatomal, burning, stinging pain below the entry point. Neurologic signs may not be noticeable, however, until the drug is infused.
- Neurologic signs call for immediate radiographic assessment and appropriate neurosurgical intervention.

CEREBROSPINAL FLUID LEAKAGE

- Placing catheters in the subarachnoid space can lead to cerebrospinal fluid leaks because the opening created by the needle in the dura mater is larger than the catheter. Often, however, the dura mater is elastic enough to seal this opening.
- If a leak leads to spinal headache or subdermal collection of cerebrospinal fluid, inject a 10- to 20-cc patch of autologous venous blood at or one level above the catheter entry point under fluoroscopic guidance.

FORMATION OF AN INFLAMMATORY CATHETER-TIP MASS (GRANULOMA)

- Granuloma formation is likely related to long-term administration of opioids and to be dose- or concentration-related.[12,13]
- Suspect this complication when any of these conditions occur:
  - The expected and measured residual pump volume varies more than 20%
  - An increase in pain indicates a loss of analgesia.
  - The patient exhibits new and progressive signs of neurologic deficit.
- First evaluate the catheter with soft tissue radiography for suspected migration, kinks, or separation.
- To check for obstruction, inject nonionic contrast material in the injection side port, if present. To avoid a possible drug overdose caused by release of a large bolus of medication directly into the subarachnoid space, try to aspirate the catheter before injecting contrast medium. For a catheter without a side port, evaluate obstruction by emptying the pump and injecting a radioisotope (eg, indium). Depending on pump type, program a bolus dose or wait an appropriate time before scanning the catheter.
- Catheter tip obstruction may require catheter revision or replacement.

CATHETER FAILURE

- Catheter failure is the most common device complication.
- The development of reinforced catheters has reduced catheter problems.
- If the catheter is simply disconnected, it may be possible to reconnect it under local anesthesia without removal.
- Failed catheters, on the other hand, generally require removal and replacement.

PUMP COMPLICATIONS

- Overpressurization from overfilling (constant-flow-rate pump) can impede the delivery of predictable amounts of the drug or cause system failure. (Overpressurization in the programmable pump simply activates the reservoir valve and prevents infusion.)

- As constant-flow-rate pumps approach refill time, drug delivery may slow slightly as the Freon reaches its maximum volume. If this causes problems for the patient, refill can be scheduled sooner.
- Potential complications with programmable pumps include:
  - Battery failure (lifetime is 3–5 years), which requires pump replacement.
  - Rotor stalling, confirmed radiographically by imaging the rotor, programming a bolus dose, and repeating the image after 15 minutes. If the rotor has not turned 90°, the pump must be replaced.
  - Failure of the telemetry or electric module renders the pump nonprogrammable. Pump replacement depends on the need to change the programming.
- Pump movement (rotation or flipping) can cause the catheter to dislodge or coil. This may require pump revision and anchoring. Patients are generally aware that a pump has flipped.

INFUSATE COMPLICATIONS

- Errors in type of drug or drug concentration delivered can be life-threatening (overdose).
- Avoid these errors by keeping meticulous records initially and at each drug refill on the type of system, drug, drug concentration, dead space in system, and programmed delivery.
- Take special care when administering more than one drug.
- Unless they have a fenestrated screen that will not admit the standard refill needle, systems with side ports carry the risk of direct injection of a drug overdose.
  - Because injecting a dose into the side port also forces the residual drug in the catheter into the intrathecal space, carefully note the concentration and volume of drug in the catheter before using a side port for bolus dosing or troubleshooting.
  - It is best to aspirate the side port before using it for injection.
  - The risk of overdose may outweigh any troubleshooting advantages offered by a side port.
  - To treat overdose:
    - Immediately remove cerebrospinal fluid and replace it with preservative-free saline.
    - Place an intravenous line and admit the patient to intensive care with monitoring for respiratory depression.
    - Use naloxone to treat respiratory depression, and monitor for hypertension.
    - Manage overdose-related neurotoxicity and seizure symptomatically.

ROADBLOCKS TO CLINICAL USE OF INTRATHECAL ANALGESIA

- The general reluctance of US physicians to treat pain
- The failure to assess the long-term cost–benefit of this initially expensive therapy
- Discomfort with implanting such a large delivery device
- The refusal of many pharmaceutical manufacturers to gain US Food and Drug Administration approval for additional intrathecal drugs

THE FUTURE OF INTRATHECAL THERAPY

- Adaptation for indications beyond pain and spasticity
- Development of alternate drug delivery systems, such as injecting sustained-release formulations of local anesthetics, injecting allographed catecholamine-producing cells,[14] and using an adenovirus to deliver a β-endorphin gene

REFERENCES

1. **Hassenbusch SJ, Stanton-Hicks M, Covington E, et al.** Long-term intraspinal infusions of opioids in the treatment of neuropathic pain. *J Pain Symptom Manage.* 1995;10:527.
2. **Kotani N, Kushikata T, Hashimoto H, et al.** Intrathecal methylprednisolone for intractable postherpetic neuralgia. *N Engl J Med.* 2000;343:1514.
3. **Langmayr JJ, Obwegeser AA, Schwarz AB, et al.** Intrathecal steroids to reduce pain after lumbar disc surgery: A double-blind, placebo-controlled prospective study. *Pain.* 1995;62:357.
4. **Kikuchi A, Kotani N, Sato T, et al.** Comparative therapeutic evaluation of intrathecal versus epidural methylprednisolone for long-term analgesia in patients with intractable postherpetic neuralgia. *Reg Anesth Pain Med.* 1999; 24:287.
5. **Staats PS, Luthardt F, Shipley J, et al.** Long-term intrathecal ziconotide therapy: A case study and discussion. *Neuromodulation.* 2001;4:121.
6. **Mollenholt P, Rawal N, Gordh T Jr, et al.** Intrathecal and epidural somatostatin for patients with cancer: Analgesic effects and postmorten neuropathologic investigations of spinal cord and nerve roots. *Anesthesiology.* 1994;81:534.
7. **Paice JA, Penn RD, Shott S.** Intraspinal morphine for chronic pain: A retrospective multicenter study. *J Pain Symptom Manage.* 1996;11:71.
8. **Schultheiss R, Schramm J, Neidlhardt J.** Dose changes in long-term and median-term intrathecal morphine therapy of cancer pain. *Neurosurgery.* 1992;31:664.
9. **Smith TJ, Staats PS, Deer T, et al.** Randomized clinical trial of an implantable drug delivery system compared with

comprehensive medical management for refractory cancer pain: Impact on pain, drug-related toxicity, and survival. *J Clin Oncol.* 2002;20:4040.

10. **Olson K.** *An Approach to Psychological Assessment of Chronic Pain Patients.* Minneapolis, Minn: NCS Assessments; 1992.

11. **Krames ES.** Intrathecal infusion therapies for intractable pain: Patient management guidelines. *J Pain Symptom Manage.* 1993;8:36.

12. **Yaksh RL, Hassenbusch S, Burchiel K, et al.** Inflammatory masses associated with intrathecal drug infusion: A review of preclinical evidence and human data. *Pain Med.* 2002;3:300.

13. **Hassenbusch S, Burchiel K, Coffey RJ, et al.** Management of intrathecal catheter-tip inflammatory masses: A consensus statement. *Pain Med.* 2002;3:313.

14. **Pappas GD, Lazorthes Y, Bes JC, et al.** Relief of intractable cancer pain by human chromaffin cell transplants: Experience at two medical centers. *Neurol Res.* 1997;19:71.

20 INTERPLEURAL ANALGESIA

Michael D. McBeth, MD

INDICATIONS

- Placement of an interpleural catheter should be considered when unilateral relief of pain is needed.
- An interpleural catheter for acute pain is usually limited for use in subcostal surgical procedures,[1,2] trauma, and thoracic-abdominal cancer pain.[3,4]
- Interpleural catheters have been placed for long duration in the treatment of chronic pain where more conventional therapies have proved ineffective (see Table 20–1).
- Multiple studies have shown interpleural analgesia to be ineffective in relieving postthoracotomy pain or improving pulmonary function.[5–8]

CONTRAINDICATIONS

- Contraindications include conditions that can increase the incidence of significant morbidity or decrease the effectiveness of the procedure.
- Systemic anticoagulation and low platelet disorders can increase the incidence of hemothorax and frank hemorrhage.[6]
- Sepsis can influence the risk of infection of the pleural space, as well as exacerbate the systemic side effects of the local anesthetic.
- Placement of a catheter while using positive-pressure ventilation can be difficult and raise the risk of pneumothorax.[9]

TABLE 20–1 Indications for Use of Interpleural Anesthesia

DURATION OF PAIN	LOCATION
Acute pain	
Postoperative	Upper extremity
	Thoracic (breast)
	Upper abdominal
	Renal
	Gastric fundoplication
	Open cholecystectomy
	Percutaneous transhepatic biliary procedures
Trauma	Thoracic contusion
	Rib fractures
	Chest drainage after pneumothorax
Chronic pain	
Postherpetic neuralgia	Chest, abdomen
Complex regional pain syndrome	Upper extremity
Chronic pancreatitis	Abdomen
Cancer pain	
Esophageal	Thorax
Lung	Thorax
Pancreatic	Abdomen
Breast	Thorax

- Pleural effusion (congestive heart failure, malignant) and hemothorax can also create difficulty in evaluating the placement of the catheter in the subpleural space, as well as affect the diffusion properties of the local anesthetic.
- Pulmonary infection and inflammatory conditions may affect catheter placement and absorption, diffusion, and effectiveness of local anesthetic.
- Systemic toxicity may result from rapid uptake through inflamed tissue.
- Trauma patients with resultant closed head injury may not be good candidates due to incidence of Horner's syndrome (pupillary constriction).

ANATOMY

- The posterior thorax is covered with large muscle groups, including trapezius muscle, which is superior and medial to the catheter entry zone. The serratus anterior and serratus posterior muscles lie laterally and erector spinae muscle medially. The latissimus dorsi muscle lies inferiorly. The level of catheter placement (T8) is approximately at the inferior border of the scapula and at the lower one-third of the lung field. Deep to the large muscles lay the external, internal, and innermost intercostal muscles, with an external and internal intercostal member adherent to the adjacent rib.
- The costal pleura is the innermost covering of the thoracic cage, with the subpleural space providing separation between the lung's parietal pleura. This is the

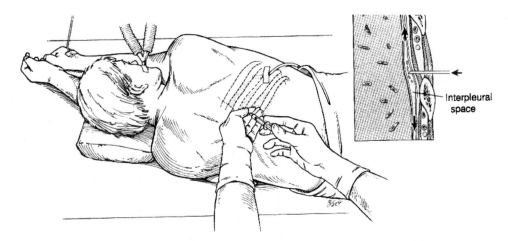

FIGURE 20–1 Insertion of a Tuohy needle into the sub-pleural space providing separation between the lung's parietal pleura. (From Raj PP. *Clinical Practice of Regional Anesthesia.* New York: Churchill Livingstone; 1991:303.)

space into which the catheter is inserted via a Tuohy needle (see inset, Figure 20–1).

- The intercostal neurovascular bundle exits the spine and follows along the inferior aspect of the rib, with the vein superior and the intercostal nerve inferior. The spinal nerve's dorsal ramus exits posteriorly and innervates the erector spinae and other dorsal muscle groups. The ventral ramus travels between the innermost and internal intercostal muscle to the anterior chest wall. The ventral ramus has two cutaneous branches, the lateral cutaneous branch (which innervates the posterior lateral chest wall) and the anterior branch (which innervates the anterior chest wall).
- The sympathetic trunk is positioned on either side, lateral (approximately) midbody to the thoracic vertebra. The origins of the greater, lesser, and least splanchnic nerves begin at the midthoracic spine and end at the lower thoracic vertebra.
- Infusion of local anesthetic has been shown to provide local anesthetic blockade of the intercostal nerves[10,11] and possibly ipsilateral phrenic nerve[12] secondary to diffusion. Due to the proximity of the thoracic sympathetic chain, diffusion of local anesthetic may also provide unilateral sympathetic blockade, which may account for the analgesic effects in the treatment of cancer and complex regional pain syndrome,[13] as well as the side effects (ie, Horner's syndrome).

TECHNIQUE

PLACEMENT

- The patient is placed in the lateral decubitus position, with the target side up (Figure 20–1).
- Location of catheter placement should be marked, approximately 8–10 cm from midline, between the

seventh and eighth ribs, usually counting superiorly from T12.

- The skin is anesthetized at the superior aspect of the eighth rib. A Tuohy needle is then advanced perpendicularly to the superior portion of the rib, until bony contact is made. The Tuohy needle is directed slightly superior and "walked" off over the top of the rib for approximately 3–4 mm. Using a glass syringe with saline or air, the Tuohy needle is advanced until a negative pressure is experienced, signifying entry into the subpleral space.[14] The syringe is removed, and a flexible catheter is inserted to a depth of 8–10 cm (care must be taken to cover the hub of the needle with a finger until the catheter is threaded). The Tuohy needle bevel should be directed medially so the catheter will travel medially to reside at the costovertebral junction. Once the catheter is placed, the needle is removed with care to prevent backing out of the catheter. The catheter is then secured.
- Tunneling the catheter should be considered if prolonged use is anticipated.
- The catheter is then aspirated, and a test dose of lidocaine is injected to evaluate possible intravascular placement.
- A chest radiograph (PA and lateral) should be checked prior to infusion to evaluate placement and degree of pneumothorax.

DRUG

- Bupivacaine has been the most evaluated drug, and has a history of safety and efficacy.
- *For Bolus Infusion:* A standard solution of 20 mL of 0.5% bupivacaine has a mean duration of 7–10 hours (three injections/24 hours), with a mean peak plasma level of 1.868 μg/mL[15] compared with a level of

TABLE 20–2   Complications of Interpleural Anesthesia

Placement
  Pneumothorax
  Pleural effusion
  Hemothorax
  Intrabronchial placement
  Brachial plexus blockade
  Empyema
Local anesthetic effects
  Seizure
  Local anesthetic toxicity (systemic)
  Phrenic nerve paralysis (evident on chest radiograph)
  Bronchospasm
  Horner's syndrome*

*Pupillary constriction, ptosis of upper eyelid, slight elevation of lower lid, sinking of eyeball, narrowing of palpebral fissure, and nasal stuffiness associated with anhidrosis and flushing of affected side of the face.

3.03 µg/mL with 20 mL of bupivacaine 0.5% plus epinephrine (5 µg/mL) at an interval of 4 hours.[16] Interpleural spread (T3 to L1) of the bolus is similar in the supine and lateral positions, usually within an hour of infusion.[17]

• *For Continuous Infusion*: Bupivacaine 0.25% at the rate of 5 to 10 mL/h (0.125 mL/kg/h) has been shown to be adequate in pain relief after surgery ranging from cholecystectomy to lateral flank incisions. Addition of opioid to infusion or bolus does not add significant benefit over intravenous delivery.

COMPLICATIONS

• Complications arise mainly from catheter placement and local anesthetic effects.[9]
• A pneumothorax (most common)[18] is difficult to prevent, but limiting the amount of entrained air at needle or catheter placement should be a priority. The air should be reabsorbed within 24–48 hours and is rarely clinically significant.
• Painstaking sterility with catheter placement and infusion setup will limit the incidence of infection.
• The use of a soft-tip catheter may help to reduce trauma to the lung and bronchial structures.
• Monitoring of blood levels for local anesthetic may provide early detection of elevated levels and minimize systemic side effects (see Table 20–2).

REFERENCES

1. **Razzaq R, England RE, Martin DF.** Techniques for providing analgesia during percutaneous biliary interventional procedures. *Clin Radiol.* 2000;55:131.

2. **Rademaker BM, Sih IL, Kalkman CJ.** Effects of interpleurally administered bupivicaine 0.5% on opioid analgesic requirements and endocrine response during and after cholecystectomy: A randomized, double blind, controlled study. *Acta Anaesthesiol Scand.* 1991;35:108.

3. **Myers D, Lema MJ, deLeon-Casasola OA, Bacon DR.** Interpleural analgesia for the treatment of severe cancer pain in terminally ill patients. *J Pain Symptom Manage.* 1993; 8:505.

4. **Amesbury B, O'Riordan J, Dolin S.** The use of interpleural analgesia using bupivicaine for pain relief in advanced cancer. *Palliat Med.* 1999;13:153.

5. **Richardson J, Sabanathan S, Shah R.** Post-thoracotomy spirometric lung function: The effect of analgesia. A review. *J Cardiovasc Surg.* 1999;40:445.

6. **Savage C, McQuitty C, Wang D, Zwischenberger JB.** Postthoracotomy pain management. *Chest Surg Clin North Am.* 2002;12:251.

7. **Elman A, Debaene B, Magny-Metrot C, Murciano G.** Interpleural analgesia with bupivicaine following thoracotomy: Ineffective results of a controlled study and pharmacokinetics. *J Clin Anesth.* 1993;5:118.

8. **Silomon M, Claus T, Huwer H, Biedler A, Larsen R, Molter G.** Interpleural analgesia does not influence postthoracotomy pain. *Anesth Analg.* 2000;91:44.

9. **Gomez MN, Symreng T, Rossi NP, Chiang CK.** Interpleural bupivicaine for intraoperative analgesia: A dangerous technique? *Anesth Analg.* 1988;67:578.

10. **Juruki I.** Diffusion of bupivicaine into the intercostal muscles following interpleural analgesia. *Masui—Jpn J Anesthesiol.* 1997;46:1299.

11. **Pettersson N, Perbeck L, Brismar B, Hahn RG.** Sensory and sympathetic block during interpleural analgesia. *Reg Anesth.* 1997;22:313.

12. **Kowalski SE, Bradley BD, Greengrass RA, Freedman J, Younes MK.** Effects of interpleural bupivicaine (0.5%) on canine diaphragmatic function. *Anesth Analg.* 1992; 75:400.

13. **Ramojoli F, DeAmici D.** Is there a bilateral block of the thoracic sympathetic chain after unilateral intrapleural analgesia? *Anesth Analg.* 1998;87:360.

14. **Ben-David B, Lee E.** The falling column: A new technique for interpleural catheter placement. *Anesth Analg.* 1993; 76:1159.

15. **Kaukinen S, Kaukinen L, Kataja J, Karkkainen S, Heikkinen A.** Interpleural analgesia for postoperative pain relief in renal surgery patients. *Scand J Urol Nephrol.* 1994;28:39.

16. **Lee A, Boon D, Bagshaw P, Kempthorne P.** A randomized double-blind study of interpleural analgesia after cholecystectomy. *Anaesthesia.* 1990;45:1028.

17. **Stromskage KE, Hauge O, Steen PA.** Distribution of local anesthetics injected in the interpleural space, studied by computerized tomography. *Acta Anaesthesiol Scand.* 1990;34:323.

18. **Stromskage KE, Minor B, Steen PA.** Side effects and complications related to interpleural analgesia: An update. *Acta Anaesthesiol Scand.* 1990;34:473.

21 PERIPHERAL NERVE BLOCKS AND CONTINUOUS CATHETERS

Eric Rey Amador, MD
Sean Mackey, MD

GENERAL PRINCIPLES

- Peripheral nerve blocks and/or continuous perineural catheters can be used in the management of both acute and chronic pain. They are especially effective in the perioperative period when a balanced, multimodal therapeutic approach is used. Perioperative techniques can be used as the sole anesthetic or in conjunction with general anesthesia.
- Because of technologic and pharmacologic advances in recent years, the use of nerve blocks for both inpatient and outpatient pain management has dramatically increased.

BENEFITS AND RISKS

- Peripheral nerve blockade for acute pain management is associated with significantly improved postoperative pain control, decreased incidence of postoperative nausea and vomiting, improved hemodynamic stability, and a reduced time to discharge.[1]
- Contraindications to peripheral nerve blockade include patient refusal and localized infection, with relative contraindications being preexisting neurologic deficit, coagulopathy, and bacteremia.
- Risks associated with peripheral nerve blockade include local anesthetic toxicity, persistent paresthesias, bleeding, infection, and failed/inadequate block. Specific nerve blocks also carry site-specific risks.
- Local anesthetic toxicity initially manifests neurologically with perioral numbness and tinnitus with risk of progression to seizure.
- Local anesthetics are also cardiotoxic and can result in arrhythmias. Evidence suggests that bupivacaine is significantly more arrhythmogenic than other local anesthetics.[2] Newer agents such as ropivacaine and levobupivacaine have a duration of action similar to that of bupivacaine with less arrhythmogenic potential.
- Persistent paresthesias are rare and, if they do occur, normally resolve within 6 weeks.

METHODS

- Peripheral nerve blocks should be performed only by practitioners who have a thorough understanding of the relevant functional neuroanatomy, surrounding anatomic landmarks, and the resources and skills to handle potential complications. Blocks should be performed in a monitored setting with resuscitation equipment readily available.
- Most practitioners use mild to moderate sedation during block placement with a combination of anxiolytic and analgesic medications. If a paresthesia technique is being used, mild sedation is preferred. Except in pediatric or unusual cases, nerve blockade should not be performed under general anesthesia.
- Local anesthetic selection is dependent on the practitioner's desired onset time and duration of action:
  - 2% lidocaine and 1.5% mepivacaine have rapid onset coupled with a short duration of action.
  - 0.5% bupivacaine, 0.75% ropivacaine, and 0.5% levobupivacaine have an extended duration of action but a slower onset time.
- Administration of local anesthetic solutions should always begin with a 1-cc test dose (to rule out intraneural injection) followed by incremental dosing with close monitoring of the patient.
- Patients should be advised as to the expected duration of sensory and motor blockade. If a short-acting local anesthetic is given for a case expected to result in significant postoperative pain, then a plan should be devised to address the patient's pain control when the block wears off.
- Additional agents can be added to the solution to achieve desired effects[1] (Table 21–1).

TABLE 21–1   Effects of Additives on Neural Blockade

MEDICATION	DOSE	EFFECT	COMMENT
Epinephrine	1/200,000–1/400,000	Marker of intravascular injection Increases block duration	Increased duration of action with lidocaine or mepivacaine
Sodium bicarbonate	1 cc in 10 cc	Decreases onset time	Precipitates with bupivicaine, ropivicaine, and levobupivicaine
Clonidine	0.5 µg/kg	Improves block quality and increases duration	Higher doses have increased side effects
Opioids	Numerous	Improves block quality	Evidence lacking

- Nerve localization can be performed based on anatomic location or paresthesia or with a nerve stimulator. When a nerve stimulator is used, continued twitches at a current of <0.5 mA indicate appropriate needle placement.

UPPER EXTREMITY

- The brachial plexus is composed of the nerve roots C5 to T1, which combine to form the superior, middle, and inferior trunks. These trunks further divide to form the lateral, medial, and posterior cords, which then give off the peripheral nerves of the upper extremity (Table 21–2).
- Rescue blocks can be performed at the level of the midhumerus, elbow, and wrist for inadequate blocks.

INTERSCALENE BLOCK

- The interscalene block is performed predominantly for shoulder surgery. Interscalene blocks generally do not provide adequate coverage of the arm due to only partially blocking the median nerve and essentially no blocking of the ulnar nerve. The interscalene groove, formed by the bodies of the anterior and middle scalene muscles, is palpated at the level of C6 or the cricoid cartilage. A needle is directed medially and caudally until localization is confirmed.
- Either paresthesia or nerve stimulation can be used to determine proper needle placement. If nerve stimulation is used, diaphragmatic movement indicates stimulation of the phrenic nerve and therefore the needle should be readjusted posteriorly. Likewise, rhomboid/trapezius movement demonstrates a needle directed too far posteriorly.
- Typical doses of local anesthetic range from 30 to 40 cc.
- Site-specific consequences of this block include a high percentage of ipsilateral diaphragmatic paralysis and Horner's syndrome. These are expected with an interscalene block. Rarely, this block is associated with complications such as pneumothorax, seizures (due to intra-arterial injection), and epidural/intrathecal injection resulting in a high spinal.[3]

SUPRACLAVICULAR AND INFRACLAVICULAR BLOCKS

- Performed at the level of the cords of the brachial plexus, these blocks are excellent for surgeries distal to the midhumeral level. Utilization of a nerve stimulator is preferred. Both blocks are associated with the potential risk of pneumothorax, although it is generally accepted that the supraclavicular block has a higher incidence of pneumothorax compared with the more recent approaches to the infraclavicular block.
- Several approaches have been described to the supraclavicular block. One approach is to locate the subclavian artery at the level of the midclavicle by palpating or using ultrasound guidance. The needle is then directed parallel to the neck until motor response distal to the wrist is consistently obtained.
- The popularity of the infraclavicular block has increased with the recent description of the lateral coracoid approach. The needle entry site is 2 cm medial and 2 cm caudal from the coracoid process with the needle directed perpendicular to all planes. A nerve stimulator is used to achieve motor response distal to the wrist.
- Local anesthetic solution of 20–40 cc is the typical dose.
- These techniques may prove to be superior to the axillary block because of better patient tolerance, decreased tourniquet pain, lower incidence of incomplete block, and they can be performed with the patient's arm at the side.

AXILLARY BLOCK

- The axillary block is frequently performed for surgeries distal to the elbow. Once the axillary artery is identified, several techniques can be performed to locate the nerves: perivascular, transarterial, paresthesia, or nerve stimulation.
- Local anesthetic doses of 20–40 cc are deposited depending on the technique used. Pressure on the arm distal to the injection site may be helpful in promoting proximal spread.
- Tourniquet pain is better tolerated if a ring block is performed to anesthetize the intercostal brachial and medial brachial cutaneous nerves.

TABLE 21–2 Upper Extremity Nerve Distribution

NERVE	MOTOR	SENSATION
Musculocutaneous	Arm flexion	Lateral forearm
Median	Lateral deviation of wrist and grip of thumb and index and middle fingers	Medial aspect of palm including thumb and index and middle fingers
Ulnar	Medial deviation of wrist and grip of 4th and 5th fingers	Medial forearm and lateral aspect of hand including 4th and 5th fingers
Radial	Arm, wrist, and finger extension	Extensor surfaces of arm and hand

LOWER EXTREMITY

- The neuroanatomy to the lower extremity is composed of the lumbar and lumbosacral plexuses. The lumbar plexus is derived from the ventral rami of L1 through L3 with part of L4 and occasionally contributions from T12. The lumbosacral plexus is derived from L4 through S3. Whereas it is common to provide complete upper extremity anesthesia with a single injection at the brachial plexus, regional anesthesia approaches in the lower extremity often require two separate injections—one for each component of the lumbar and sacral plexuses (Table 21–3).
- All blocks use 20–30 cc of local anesthetic and are performed best with a nerve stimulator.

SCIATIC NERVE BLOCK

- The sciatic nerve can be approached several ways. Blocks of the sciatic nerve have the slowest onset times and the longest durations of the peripheral nerve blocks.
- The sciatic nerve divides into the common peroneal nerve and tibial nerves typically within the popliteal fossa.
- The tibial nerve provides sensation to the heel and plantar aspect of the foot and performs plantar flexion and inversion. The common peroneal nerve provides sensation to the lateral lower leg and dorsal aspect of the foot and performs dorsiflexion and eversion.
- The most popular techniques are the classic posterior approach with the patient in Sim's position (lateral decubitus with operative leg up and bent at the knee with nonoperative leg straight), anterior approach with the patient supine, posterior popliteal approach with the patient prone, and lateral popliteal approach with the patient supine.
- For the posterior approach, a line is drawn from the greater trochanter to the posterior superior iliac spine.

TABLE 21–3 Lower Extremity Nerve Distribution

NERVE	MOTOR	SENSATION
Femoral	Leg extension	Anterior thigh and knee Medial aspect of lower leg by saphenous nerve
Lateral femoral cutaneous	None	Lateral thigh
Obturator	Adductors	Medial thigh
Tibial	Plantar flexion and inversion of foot	Heel and plantar aspect of foot
Common peroneal	Dorsiflexion and eversion of foot	Lateral lower leg and dorsal aspect of foot

A second line is drawn from the greater trochanter to the sacral hiatus. From the midpoint of the first line a third line is drawn perpendicular and where this line intersects the second line is the location of needle placement.[4]
- The posterior popliteal approach is performed for ankle and foot surgery. With the patient prone and the leg supported at the ankle, the needle is inserted at a 30°–45° angle 8 cm above the popliteal skin crease and 1 cm lateral to the midline. Because the sciatic nerve may have split into its two components at this level, some practitioners search for both the common peroneal and tibial nerves and anesthetize them individually.
- In patients who are unable to move from the supine position, the sciatic nerve can be reached by both the anterior approach and the lateral popliteal approach.
- Both Beck and Chelly have described anatomic bony landmarks for the anterior approach. An additional technique helpful in obese patients is to place the needle 2.5 cm distal to the inguinal crease and 2.5 cm medial to the femoral artery. The needle is then directed 10°–15° from the vertical plane with the leg externally rotated.[5]
- The lateral popliteal nerve block is performed with needle insertion perpendicular to the vertical plane 7 cm above the lateral femoral epicondyle between biceps femoris and vastus lateralis. Once femur contact is made the needle is grasped 2 cm above the skin. The needle is redirected 30°–45° posteriorly and advanced approximately 2 cm beyond the depth required to make femur contact. The degree of approach is adjusted until appropriate stimulation is achieved.

LUMBAR PLEXUS BLOCK

- The lumbar plexus includes the obturator, lateral femoral cutaneous, and femoral nerves.
- A psoas compartment block can be performed and will reliably block all three nerves of the lumbar plexus. A line is drawn between the iliac crests with the patient in Sim's position. Along this line, 5 cm from midline, a needle is directed perpendicular to the skin until quadriceps stimulation occurs, confirming correct placement. This block is performed for both hip and knee surgery.
- The femoral nerve block is frequently performed and well-tolerated for knee surgery. The nerve is located at the level of the inguinal crease lateral to the femoral artery. By using increased volumes and distal pressure a "3–1" block may be achieved, but the obturator nerve is often not anesthetized.

CONTINUOUS CATHETERS

- Due to significant improvement in needle and catheter design, continuous peripheral nerve catheters are being used at an increasing rate.
- All of the previously described blocks can be performed as either "one-shot" or continuous catheter placements.
- No evidence supports one type of catheter placement system over another. They can be divided into the plastic introducer catheter with stimulating guide and the insulated Tuohy needle introducer. There are also catheters with a metallic stylet that allow stimulation.
- Common postoperative regimens include 0.2% ropivicaine (6–10 cc/h), 0.125–0.25% bupivicaine (6–12 cc/h), and 0.125–0.25% levobupivicaine (6–12 cc/h).[6]
- Drug delivery systems have been developed that are now allowing patients to go home with continuous catheters in place. Ongoing studies will determine the safety and efficacy of these "ambulatory" continuous catheter systems.
- The future of continuous catheters will be significantly affected if extended-duration long-acting local anesthetics become available. A single injection technique is faster and less cumbersome than placement of a perineural catheter.[7]

REFERENCES

1. **Chelly JE.** *Peripheral Nerve Blocks—A Color Atlas.* Philadelphia: Lippincott; 1999.
2. **Groban L.** Central nervous system and cardiac effects from long-acting amide local anesthetic toxicity in the intact animal model. *Reg Anesth Pain Med.* 2003;28:3–11.
3. **Murphy DB, Chan VWS.** Upper extremity blocks for day surgery. *Techniques Reg Anesth Pain Med.* 2000;4:19–29.
4. **Brown DL.** *Atlas of Regional Anesthesia.* 2nd ed. Philadelphia: WB Saunders; 1999.
5. **Van Elstrate AC, Poey C, Lebrum T, Pastureau F.** New landmarks for the anterior approach to the sciatic nerve block: Imaging and clinical study. *Anesth Analg.* 2002; 95:214–218.
6. **Chelly JE, Casati A, Fanelli G.** *Continuous Peripheral Nerve Block Techniques.* London: Mosby; 2001.
7. **Liu SS, Salinas FV.** Continuous plexus and peripheral nerve blocks for postoperative analgesia. *Anesth Analg.* 2003; 96:263–272.

22 ABDOMINAL PAIN

Alan Millman, MD
Elliot S. Krames, MD

INTRODUCTION

- The abdomen is one of the most common sites of regional pain.
- Pain in the abdomen is usually caused by disorders of viscera in the abdominal cavity or pelvic cavity. The next most common cause of abdominal pain is referred pain from diseases of the thorax.
- The somatic and visceral nerve supplies of both regions have a common segmental distribution in the spinal cord. The physiologic mechanisms of visceral pain share similarities and differences with somatic pain mechanisms.

CLASSIFICATION

- Abdominal pain can be classified into pain caused by abdominal visceral disease, musculoskeletal pain, neuropathic pain, and other pain.[1]

ABDOMINAL VISCERAL DISEASE

- Visceral pain is:[2]
  - Not evoked from all viscera (liver, kidney, lung, and most solid viscera are not sensitive to pain)
  - Not always linked to visceral injury (cutting the intestines causes no pain, while bladder stretching is painful without any discernible injury)
  - Diffuse and poorly localized (with few "sensory" visceral afferents and extensive divergence in the central nervous system [CNS])
  - Referred to other locations (viscerosomatic convergence in the CNS)
  - Accompanied by motor and autonomic reflexes (nausea, vomiting, diaphoresis, pallor, lower back muscle tension with renal colic, etc)
- *Unreferred parietal pain* is acute, intense, sharp, localized, and aggravated by movement, and may be localized to the abdominal/thoracic wall directly over the site of inflammation/injury (eg, right lower quadrant pain in acute appendicitis).
- *Referred parietal pain* is remote from the pain generator site (eg, shoulder pain from diaphragmatic irritation).

MUSCULOSKELETAL PAIN

- Musculoskeletal pain is usually focal. Examples include, but are not limited to: rib fracture/dislocation, intercostal cartilage fracture/subluxation, trauma with secondary abdominal wall hemorrhage, and postoperative pain. Thoracic spine disorders can refer anteriorly.

NEUROPATHIC PAIN

- Spinal cord lesions or compression of the spinal cord involving lower thoracic levels cause dull, aching, poorly localized pain.
- Thoracic root inflammation/lesions cause sharp, burning pain in a segmental distribution (examples include: herpes zoster, herniated disks, and vertebral tumors).

- Intercostal neuropathy can cause anterior abdominal pain.

OTHER PAIN

- Systemic, hematologic, and endocrine disorders can cause various types of abdominal pain (examples include porphyria causing severe, episodic, deep abdominal pain).
- Vascular diseases, such as rupture of an abdominal aortic aneurysm and occlusion of the superior mesenteric artery, cause abdominal pain and/or back pain.

ANATOMY OF THE ABDOMEN

BOUNDARIES

- For descriptive purposes, the abdomen can be divided into nine regions (see Figure 22–1).[1,3]
- The abdomen is bounded:
  - Anteriorly by the rectus abdominis muscles, the aponeuroses of the external oblique, the internal oblique.
  - Laterally by the external and internal oblique muscles, the rectus abdominis, the iliac muscles, and the bones.
- Posteriorly by the lumbar vertebral column, the psoas and quadratus lumborum muscles, the diaphragmatic crura, and the posterior iliac bones.
- Superiorly by the diaphragm.
- Inferiorly by the superior aperture of the pelvis.

COMPONENTS

MUSCLES
- Anterolateral: flat muscular sheets (the external and internal obliques, the rectus abdominis).
- Posterior: psoas major/minor muscles, quadratus lumborum, and iliacus muscles.
- Diaphragm: superior boundary.

PERITONEUM
- Parietal: serous membrane lining the abdominal wall.
- Visceral: serous membrane reflected over the viscera.
- The parietal and visceral peritoneal layers are derived from the somatopleural and splanchnopleural layers of the lateral mesoderm plate.

OMENTA
- Greater omentum: a two-layer peritoneal fold that descends downward from the stomach and duodenum

in front of the small intestine, then reflects upward to the level of the transverse colon.
- Lesser omentum: the peritoneal fold extending from the stomach and first portion of the duodenum to the liver.

MESENTERIES
- The mesenteries are the collective of peritoneal folds that contain blood vessels, nerves, and lymph vessels. When stretched, the mesenteries provoke painful stimuli.

NERVES/PLEXUSES
- The parietal peritoneum derives its nerve supply from the spinal nerves, which also supply the corresponding muscles and skin.
- The visceral peritoneum derives its nerve supply from the autonomic nervous system that supplies the viscera.
- In conscious patients, pain can be elicited by chemical and thermal noxious stimuli to the parietal peritoneum but not to the viscera, which respond to mechanical noxious stimuli such as stretch and tension.
- Figure 22–2 diagrams the abdominal nervous supply.

Vagus Nerves
- Vagus nerves supply parasympathetic, preganglionic fibers, and sensory fibers to the abdominal viscera except the left half of the transverse colon and descending colon, which are supplied by the sacral parasympathetic nerves.
- Vagal efferents have parasympathetic preganglionic cell bodies located in the medulla.
- Vagal afferents have pseudounipolar sensory cells in the inferior vagal ganglion (nodose), located just caudad to the jugular foramen.

Sympathetic Nerves
- Sympathetic efferents supply the abdominal viscera with cell bodies in the T5 to L2 spinal segments.
- Axons pass through the sympathetic chains without synapsing via splanchnic nerves to end in three prevertebral ganglia: the celiac, the aorticorenal, and the inferior mesenteric ganglia. Here they synapse with postganglionic neurons.

Celiac Plexus
- The celiac plexus is the largest prevertebral plexus, with parasympathetic and sympathetic efferent and afferent fibers in the ganglia.
- It is located inferior to the diaphragm, posterior to the stomach, just anterior to the aorta at the L1/L2 vertebral body levels, and surrounding the celiac artery.

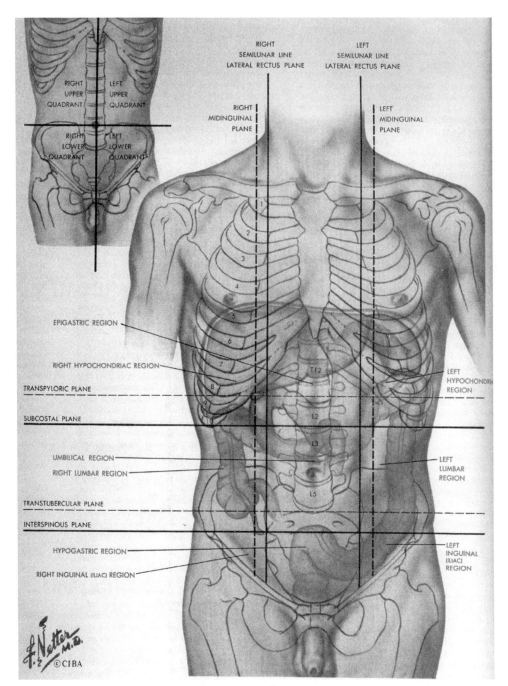

FIGURE 22–1 Regions of the abdomen. From Netter.[3]

Superior and Inferior Hypogastric Plexuses
- These plexuses are the continuation of the abdominal aortic plexus portion of the celiac plexus.
- They contribute sympathetic, parasympathetic, and afferent nerves to the pelvic viscera.
- The superior hypogastric plexus is located anterior to the S1 vertebral body, and the inferior hypogastric plexus lies on either side of the rectum within the sacral pelvis.

Intrinsic (Enteric) Nervous System
- This consists of cell bodies and short axons within the gastrointestinal tract.
- *Auerbach's plexus* lies between the longitudinal and circular muscle layers within the intestinal viscera.
- *Meissner's plexus* is in various muscle and submucosal layers within the intestinal viscera.

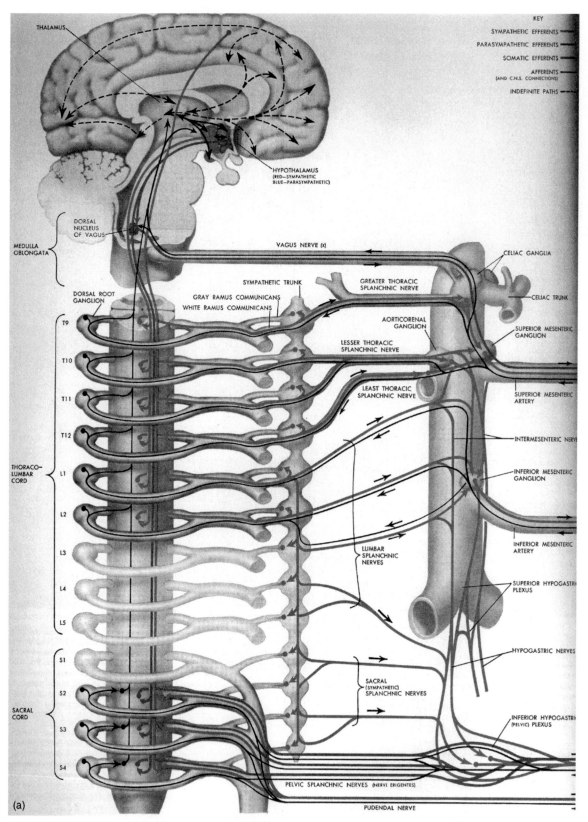

FIGURE 22–2 Diagrammatic representation of the abdominal nerves and plexuses. From Netter.[3]

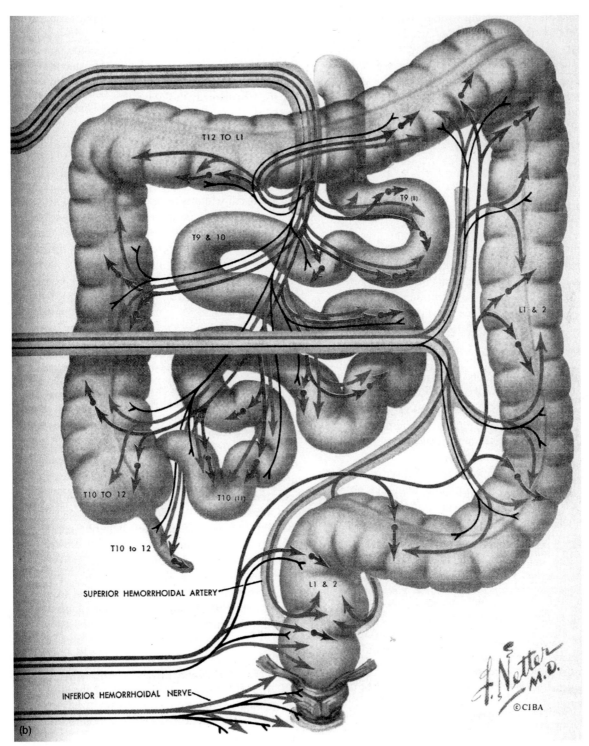

T12 TO L1

T9 (8)

T9 & 10

L1 & 2

T10 TO 12

T10 (11)

T10 to 12

SUPERIOR HEMORRHOIDAL ARTERY

L1 & 2

INFERIOR HEMORRHOIDAL NERVE

FIGURE 22–2 (*Continued*)

EVALUATION OF THE PATIENT

- Evaluation of the patient comprises elicitation of a detailed history and the physical exam.[4]

HISTORY

- What are the characteristics of the abdominal pain: its rapidity of onset, quality, intensity, location, duration, and aggravating and/or alleviating factors?

- What are the effects of: eating, swallowing, belching, deep breathing, flatus, defecation, urination, trunk movements, and supine/prone positions?
- What are any associated symptoms: nausea, vomiting, dyspnea, hematemesis, hemoptysis, melena, weakness, and/or numbness?
- Noted in detail are previous medical history, drugs taken (licit and illicit), family history, social history, toxic exposures, and patient age.

PHYSICAL EXAM

VITAL SIGNS
- Tachycardia and hypotension or orthostatic hypotension indicating hypovolemia/shock, bradycardia from acute gastric dilation, unilateral blood pressure gradient from acute aortic dissection, tachypnea with metabolic acidosis, fever indicating infection, and so on.

INSPECTION
- General appearance: Patients with renal or biliary colic may writhe in bed constantly. Patients with peritonitis lie still, avoid the slightest motion, and may draw up their legs to reduce intraabdominal pressure.
- Respiratory rate is increased in patients with peritonitis, obstruction, or hemorrhage.
- Skin: Patients with abdominal visceral disease may have jaundice, scleral icterus, or spider angiomas.
- Hands: Patients may present with muscle atrophy. Nailbed lunula are increased in patients with cirrhosis.
- Face: There may be temporal wasting with visceral disease, lip/tongue telangiectasias from Osler–Weber–Rendu syndrome, or cushingoid facies.
- Abdomen: Increased intraabdominal pressure may caused an everted umbilicus. Cachexia may be the result of severe malnutrition or cancer. Protuberance of the abdomen may result from obesity, gaseous distension, ascites, or organomegaly. Ecchymoses of abdomen or flanks might be due to hemorrhagic pancreatitis, strangulated bowel, or hemoperitoneum.
- Hernias: Valsalva maneuver may cause inguinal, umbilical, or femoral area hernias.
- Superficial veins: caput medusae from portal hypertension, cephalad draining veins from vena caval obstruction.

AUSCULTATION
- Supine: absence of bowel sounds in ileus secondary to peritonitis; borborygmi—high-pitched "tinkles"; hyperperistalsis in early obstruction.

- Succussion splash: The physician applies the stethoscope, shakes the patient side-to-side, and listens for sloshing from stomach or colon distension.
- Bruits: abdominal aorta or renal artery stenosis.
- Peritoneal friction rubs: during inspiration with hepatic or splenic pathology.

PERCUSSION
- Abdomen: tympany from gas in stomach or bowels; suprapubic dullness in bladder distention or uterine enlargement.
- Liver: 10-cm width is normal at midclavicular line.
- Spleen: The physician percusses at the lowest intercostal space at the left midaxillary line. Splenic enlargement can cause percussion changes from resonance to dullness on full inspiration.
- Ascites: shifting dullness sensitive; fluid wave specific.

PALPATION
- Palpation begins in an area away from the pain.
- For light palpation, the flat of the hand, not the fingertips, is used.
- For deep palpation to ascertain organ size, the left hand is placed over the right and steady pressure is gently applied with the left hand.
- "Guarding" refers to muscle spasm. "Involuntary guarding" occurs when the patient cannot eliminate the response. "Rigidity of the muscle" describes a tense and boardlike abdominal wall. Rigidity implies peritonitis.
- Fothergill's sign differentiates between an intraabdominal and an intramuscular cause of spasm. First, after the patient relaxes the abdominal muscles, the physician palpates the abdomen. The physician then asks the patient to contract the abdominal muscle by placing his or her head to the chest; the physician palpates the abdomen again. If tenderness is less during abdominal contraction, then the process is intraabdominal.
- Rebound: The physician performs deep, slow palpation away from the suspected area of inflammation. The palpating hand is then quickly removed. If pain is felt after release of pressure, this "rebound" suggests peritoneal inflammation on that side.
- Palpation for the liver: The physician places his or her left hand posteriorly between the 12th rib and the iliac crest; the right hand is placed in the right upper quadrant below the area of liver dullness. Enlargement of edge of the liver most likely indicates cirrhosis, hepatitis, vascular congestion, or neoplasm.
- Murphy's sign: If the patient suddenly stops inspiratory efforts during liver palpation because of

pain on inspiration, the cause may be acute cholecystitis.

- Spleen: The physician palpates during deep inspiration with the patient lying on the right side. A palpable spleen suggests congestion, tumor, or infection.
- Kidneys: Palpable kidneys with costovertebral angle tenderness suggest kidney disease.

RECTAL EXAM

- Irregularities, undue tenderness, or masses are noted.
- The physician palpates for prostate nodules or asymmetries.
- An occult blood test on residual fecal matter is performed.

TESTICULAR EXAM

- Evidence of torsion or inflammation is sought.
- Epididymitis or orchitis may present with hypogastric discomfort.

PELVIC EXAM

- A bimanual and speculum exam should be performed on all women with abdominal pain, especially on women of reproductive age.
- The patient is checked for adnexal masses (ectopic pregnancy, ovarian tumor, abscess, cyst, or torsion); cervical motion tenderness (pelvic inflammatory disease); discharge, bleeding, or tissue in vault (possible spontaneous abortion); and uterine tenderness (endometritis, fibroids, or carcinoma). Cultures for *Chlamydia trachomatis* and *Neisseria gonorrhoeae* should be taken.

SPECIAL MANEUVERS

- Iliopsoas test: The patient lies on his or her unaffected side and extends at the hip against resistance. The test is positive if the maneuver produces abdominal pain. Appendicitis will cause pain on the right side with this maneuver.
- Obturator test: The patient is placed supine with the hip flexed and knee joint bent. The hip is then rotated internally and externally. Pain occurs if there is inflammation adjacent to the obturator muscle.

DIFFERENTIAL DIAGNOSIS

INTRAABDOMINAL DISEASE

- Parietal peritoneal inflammation may be due to generalized bacterial or chemical peritonitis, localized peri-

tonitis from either pancreatitis or appendicitis, or mesenteric traction/distension from a tumor.
- Obstruction of a hollow viscus includes obstruction of the small or large intestine, obstruction of the biliary system, ureteral obstruction, or obstruction of the uterus.
- Examples of rapid capsular distension of a solid viscus include liver capsule stretching from hepatitis or common bile duct obstruction, stretching of the splenic capsule from hemorrhage or acute splenomegaly, and renal capsule stretching from pyelonephritis.
- Examples of acute ischemia include mesenteric thrombosis/embolism; splenic thrombosis/embolism; hepatic infarction/toxemia; torsion of the ovary, testicle, gallbladder, spleen, or appendix; vascular rupture; and sickle cell anemia.

EXTRAABDOMINAL DISEASE

- Thoracic viscera: pulmonary (pneumonia, pulmonary embolism), cardiac (myocardial infarction/ischemia), esophageal (rupture, spasm), and so on.
- Neuropathic disorders: spinal cord (compression, tumor), mechanical radiculopathy (herniated disk), infectious radiculopathy (herpes zoster), and so on.
- Musculoskeletal disorders: rib fracture, costal cartilage fracture, costochondritis, myofascial pain syndromes, trauma, rectus sheath hematoma, and so on.

METABOLIC DISORDERS AND TOXINS

- Exogenous: iron, lead, mercury, aspirin, arsenic, alcohols, acidic/alkali caustic compounds, black widow venom, and so on.
- Endogenous: acute intermittent porphyria, uremia, diabetes/diabetic ketoacidosis, and so on.

PSYCHOLOGICAL DISORDERS

- Anxiety, depression, hypochondriasis, somatoform disorder, conversion disorder, and irritable bowel syndrome.

DIAGNOSTIC STRATEGIES

ACUTE ABDOMINAL PAIN

- This pain is a great challenge to the primary care physician, gastroenterologist, emergency room physician,

TABLE 22–1

I. Intraabdominal disease
  A. Parietal peritoneal inflammation
    1. Generalized peritonitis
      a. Primary bacterial infection (eg, pneumococcal, streptococcal, enteric bacillus)
      b. Bacterial contamination (eg, perforated appendix, pelvic inflammatory disease, ruptured hepatic abscess)
      c. Chemical peritonitis (eg, perforated ulcer, pancreatitis, ruptured ovarian cyst, rupture of follicle)
    2. Localized peritonitis (eg, acute appendicitis, cholecystitis, peptic ulcer, colitis, regional enteritis, abdominal abscess, Meckel's diverticulltis, pancreatitis, gastroenteritis, hepatitis)
    3. Distension or traction of mesentery (eg, tumor)
  B. Mechanical obstruction of hollow viscus that leads to increased tension, stretching
    1. Obstruction of small or large intestine (eg, tumor, adhesions, hernia, volvulus, intussusception)
    2. Obstruction of biliary system (eg, gallstones, strictures, tumors)
    3. Obstruction of ureter (eg, calculi, external tumors, kinking)
    4. Obstruction of uterus (eg, tumor, childbirth)
  C. Rapid distension of capsule of solid viscus that leads to increased tension or stretching
    1. Capsule of liver (eg, toxic or viral hepatitis, rapidly growing tumor, common duct obstruction)
    2. Capsule of spleen (eg, acute splenomegaly, hemorrhage, abscess, cyst, tumor)
    3. Capsule of kidney (eg, pyelonephritis, hemorrhage, abscess, ureteral obstruction)
  D. Acute ischemia
    1. Mesenteric embolism or thrombosis
    2. Splenic embolism or thrombosis
    3. Hepatic infarction or toxemia
    4. Rapid torsion of gallbladder, spleen, ovarian cyst, testicle, appendix
    5. Vascular rupture
    6. Sickle cell anemia

II. Extraabdominal disease
  A. Thoracic visceral disease
    1. Pneumonia, pulmonary embolism, pneumothorax
    2. Acute myocardial infarction, myocarditis, angina pectoris
    3. Esophageal rupture, esophageal spasm
  B. Neuropathic and musculoskeletal disorders
    1. Diseases of the spinal cord (eg, tumor, tabes dorsalis, spinal cord compression)
    2. Infectious or mechanical radiculopathy (eg, herpes zoster, postherpetic neuralgia, compression by disorders of the spine)
    3. Fracture of lower ribs leading to neuropathy and neuralgia
    4. Fracture or dislocation of the lower costal cartilages
    5. Myofascial pain syndromes, trauma to abdominal muscles, polymyositis

III. Metabolic disorders and toxins or poisons
  A. Exogenous causes
    1. Spider bite (eg, black widow)
    2. Lead and other heavy metal poisoning
  B. Endogenous causes
    1. Uremia
    2. Porphyria
    3. Diabetes mellitus
    4. Allergic diseases

IV. Abdominal pain primarily of psychological origin
  A. Irritable bowel syndrome
  B. Anxiety states
  C. Depression
  D. Hypochondriasis
  E. Operant abdominal pain

From Bonica and Graney.[1]

surgeon, and pain physician. The history and physical examination are the foundation of the evaluation.

• Figure 22–3 shows the initial algorithm for the evaluation of a patient who is hemodynamically unstable or has a rigid abdomen. These patients may need rapid fluid resuscitation and immediate transfer to the operating room.

• Patients who are stable without a rigid abdomen are best evaluated by localizing the signs and symptoms. First, whether the pain is well or poorly localized is determined, as seen in Figure 22–4.

• A differential diagnosis might be established if the pain is well localized to the epigastrium or one of the four quadrants of the abdomen, as seen in Figure 22–5.

• It is important to realize that women of childbearing age have many possible causes of abdominal pain. Pregnancy testing and speculum and bimanual examinations should be part of the workup in this population, and pelvic ultrasound is often helpful.[5]

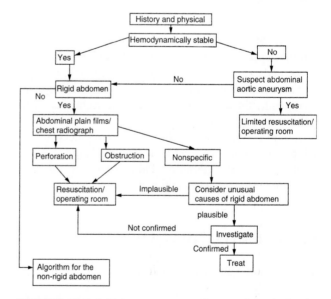

FIGURE 22–3 Initial management of acute abdominal pain. From Martin and Rossi.[5]

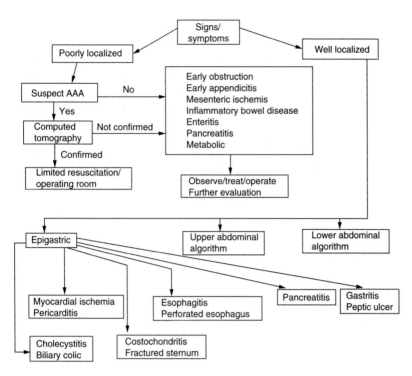

FIGURE 22–4 Acute abdominal pain: algorithm for the nonrigid abdomen. From Martin and Rossi.[5]

PEDIATRIC POPULATION

- Causes of acute abdominal pain in children are best divided on the basis of age (see Figure 22–6).
- In infants, intussusception is the most common cause of pain.
- In children, appendicitis, gastroenteritis, adenitis, pneumonia, and constipation are common.
- In adolescents, appendicitis, pelvic inflammatory disease, ovarian cysts, gastroenteritis, and urinary tract infections should be considered.[6]

GERIATRIC POPULATION

- The prevalence and frequency of abdominal aortic aneurysm (AAA), a manifestation of atherosclerosis, increases with age. Most (75%) AAAs are asymptomatic when diagnosed but can be palpated on routine exam. All older patients with backache should have an abdominal exam to rule out AAA. Abdominal, flank, or back pain may indicate imminent rupture. Syncope, hypotension, or a pulsatile tender mass may be present. Mesenteric ischemia or infarction causes abdominal distension and pain.
- Five medical conditions should always be ruled out in the elderly patient with acute abdominal pain:
  - Inferior wall myocardial infarction
  - Pneumonia or pulmonary infarct
  - Diabetic ketoacidosis
  - Pyelonephritis
  - Inflammatory bowel disease

- Other possible causes of abdominal pain in the elderly include constipation, drug-induced pain from polypharmacy (eg, NSAID-caused gastritis, erythromycin, immunosuppressants, antibiotics causing colitis), trauma (elder abuse), bowel obstruction, and peritonitis.[7]

CHRONIC ABDOMINAL PAIN

- History and physical examination form the foundation for evaluating chronic abdominal pain.[8]
- Table 22–2 notes various pertinent historical considerations, and Table 22–3 lists various physical findings.
- It is important to determine the *pattern of pain*. Chronic abdominal pain can be classified into chronic intermittent pain, chronic unrelenting pain with an identifiable cause, and chronic intractable pain. Table 22–4 is a useful guide for the differential diagnoses.
  - Chronic intermittent abdominal pain is usually explained by a discrete physiologic disorder, and often the underlying condition can be treated.
  - Chronic unrelenting abdominal pain is usually caused by a clear pathophysiologic abnormality, such as chronic pancreatitis or metastatic cancer.
  - Chronic intractable abdominal pain is present most of the time for at least 6 months. Typically, these patients have had extensive diagnostic testing and

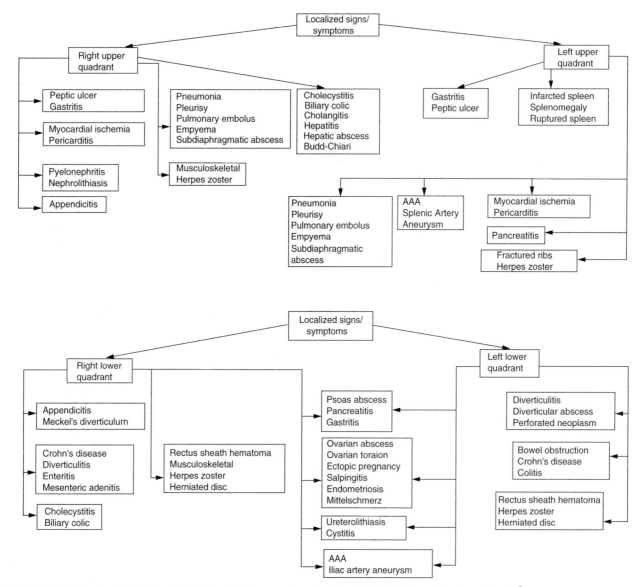

FIGURE 22–5 Acute abdominal pain: differential diagnoses based on localized pain. From Martin and Rossi.[5]

surgical procedures without definitive results. More than 50% have suffered childhood physical or sexual abuse.[8] Pain at other locations and other somatic symptoms are common.

SPECIAL CONSIDERATIONS

Acute Intermittent Porphyria
- Patients with AIP suffer from recurrent bouts of severe abdominal pain, constipation, and peripheral neuropathy; have "port wine" urine; and may have associated neuropsychiatric disorders.
- AIP is autosomal dominant with incomplete penetrance.

- The pain is usually characterized as crampy, poorly localized, and commonly precipitated by prescription and recreational drugs. Smoking may trigger an attack.
- Urinary porphobilinogens are increased and account for the "port wine" color.
- Therapy with heme albumin, hematin, or heme arginate administered intravenously may lead to rapid recovery. Opiate analgesics for pain and phenothiazines for nausea are useful.

Abdominal Migraine
- This migraine variant is associated with recurrent abdominal symptoms, usually vomiting and epigastric pain.

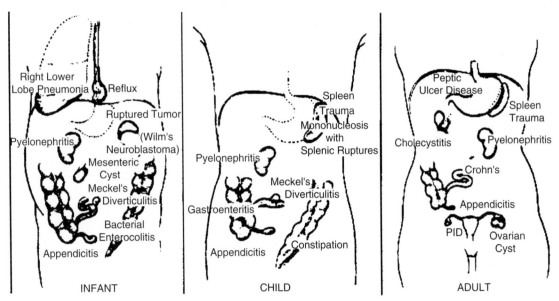

FIGURE 22–6 Differential diagnosis of acute abdominal pain in the infant, child, and adolescent. From Hatch.[6]

- Headache may or may not be present.
- Pathophysiology of this disorder remains unclear.

Abdominal Epilepsy
- This disorder is associated with paroxysmal abdominal symptoms including periumbilical and right upper quadrant pain, bloating, and diarrhea.
- All patients have neurologic symptoms including headache, blurred vision, confusion, blindness, or fatigue. Temporal lobe seizure activity is found on EEG.
- Anticonvulsants have efficacy with both abdominal and neurologic symptoms.

Familial Mediterranean Fever
- Episodic abdominal pain, fever, peritoneal signs, arthritis, and leukocytosis in patients of Mediterranean descent might be associated with this disorder.
- Autosomal recessive, it usually begins at 5 to 15 years of age.
- There are no diagnostic tests for this disorder.
- Chronic colchicine therapy reduces the number of attacks and may help during acute attacks.

TABLE 22–2

PERTINENT HISTORICAL ELEMENT	RELATED CONDITION
Follows ingestion of drugs or medications	Acute intermittent porphyria
Related to medications	Pancreatitis
Related to menstrual cycle	Endometriosis
	Mittelschmerz
Related to eating	Mesenteric ischemia
	Pancreatitis
	Biliary disease
Related to neurologic abnormalities	Abdominal migraine
	Abdominal epilepsy
	Acute intermittent porphyria
Related to body position	Nerve entrapment syndrome
	Nerve root compression
	Vertebral body fracture
	Rib tip syndrome
Fever and arthralgias	Familial Mediterranean fever

From Zackowski.[8]

TABLE 22–3

PHYSICAL FINDING	RELATED CONDITION
Jaundice	Choledocholithiasis
	Gallstone pancreatitis
Purpura or retinal cytoid bodies	Autoimmune process
Distended abdomen	Intermittent bowel obstruction
Spasm and rigidity of abdominal wall	Lead poisoning
Palpable mass	Hernia
	Neoplasm
Focal neurologic finding	Nerve root compression
	Vertebral body fracture
Anal fissure	Crohn's disease
Dark-red "port-wine" urine	Acute intermittent porphyria
Occult blood in stool	Colonic or gastric malignancy
	Crohn's disease
	Peptic ulcer disease
	Ulcerative colitis
Carnett's test positive	Abdominal wall hernia
	Cutaneous nerve entrapment
	Myofascial pain syndromes
	Rectus sheath hematoma
	Rib tip syndrome

From Zackowski.[8]

TABLE 22–4

Chronic Intermittent Abdominal Pain

Abdominal epilepsy
Abdominal migraine
Abdominal wall
    Cutaneous nerve entrapment syndromes
    Abdominal wall hernia
    Myofascial pain syndromes
    Rectus sheath hematoma
    Rib tip syndrome
Acute intermittent porphyria
Ampullary stenosis
Autoimmune disorders
Cholelithiasis
Crohn's disease
Diabetic radicutopathy
Endometriosis
Familial Mediterranean fever
Familial pancreatitis
Heavy metal poisoning
Intermittent intestinal obstruction
    Intussusception
    Internal hernia
    Abdominal wall hernia
Mesenteric ischemia
Nerve entrapment syndromes
Ovulation (ie, mittelschmerz)
Ulcerative colitis
Vertebral nerve root compression

Chronic Unrelenting Abdominal Pain with an Identifiable Cause

Autoimmune processes
Chronic pancreatitis
Intraabdominal malignancies
    Gastric or hepatic metastases
    Lymphoma
    Metastatic malignancy
    Pancreatic or biliary tree cancer
Nerve entrapment syndrome
Occult intraperitoneal abscess
Osteoporosis

Chronic Intractable Abdominal Pain

Chronic pancreatitis
Functional dyspepsia
Intraabdominal malignancies
Irritable bowel syndrome
Psychiatric disorders
    Somatization
    Psychogenic (conversion) pain
    Hypochondriasis
    Munchausen syndrome
    Malingering

From Zackowski.[8]

Functional Dyspepsia
- This may cause persistent or recurrent pain or discomfort in the epigastric or upper abdomen area. It is associated with bloating and early satiety.
- Other conditions, under the rubric of organic dyspepsia, are associated with these symptoms.
- Functional dyspepsia has no identifiable structural or biochemical abnormality.

- Antisecretory and promotility (eg, cisapride, metoclopramide) agents are useful therapies.

PATHOPHYSIOLOGY OF VISCERAL PAIN

OVERVIEW

- The neurologic mechanisms of visceral pain differ from those involved with somatic pain.[1,2,9,10]
- The perception and psychological processing of visceral pain differ from those of somatic pain. Most visceral sensations, whether from vagal or spinal afferents, do not reach consciousness.
- Gastrointestinal innervation has been categorized as parasympathetic or sympathetic, but it is more appropriate to designate the pattern by the name of the nerves involved (ex-vagus, pelvic, hypogastric nerves) (see Figure 22–7).
- Afferent fibers convey mechanical, thermal, chemical, and osmotic changes to modulating neurons in the spinal cord. Further information is sent to the brainstem, hypothalamus, limbic system, thalamus, and cerebral cortex.[1]
- More than 90% of vagal afferents are unmyelinated C-fibers; the rest are myelinated $A\delta$ and $A\beta$ fibers.
- Intrinsic afferents control and coordinate local gastrointestinal function. They contribute indirectly to visceral sensations by changes in secretomotor activity (see Figure 22–8).

NEUROPHYSIOLOGY

- The cell bodies of vagal afferents are in the nodose ganglia and those of spinal afferents are in the dorsal root ganglia. These afferents then project to the brainstem and spinal cord (see Figure 22–8).[10]
- Visceral and somatic information converge in the spinothalamic, spinoreticular, and dorsal column pathways. This "viscerosomatic convergence" can result in referred pain (see Figure 22–9).[2]
- Nerve terminals within the gastrointestinal wall convey mechanosensory information. Vagal afferents have low thresholds of activation and reach maximum responses within physiologic levels of distension. Spinal afferents can respond beyond the physiologic level and encode both physiologic and noxious levels of stimulation. Vagal afferents are involved with physiologic regulation and modulate sensory experience. Spinal afferents mediate pain.

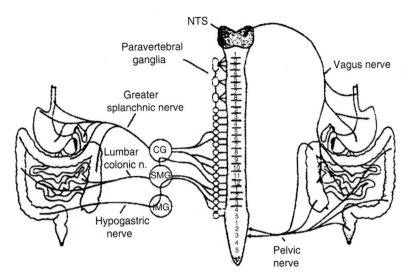

FIGURE 22–7 Representation of visceral sensory innervation of the gastrointestinal tract. The nerves that are associated with the sympathetic nervous system are on the left. These spinal visceral afferent fibers traverse both prevertebral (CG, celiac ganglion; IMG, inferior mesenteric ganglion; SMG, superior mesenteric ganglion) and paravertebral ganglia en route to the spinal cord. On the right, the pelvic and vagus nerve innervation to the sacral cord and brainstem. From Gebhart.[9]

- Afferents are thought to have collateral branches to blood vessels and enteric ganglia to modify local blood flow and reflex pathways.
- Spinal afferents use CGRP (calcitonin gene-related protein) and substance P transmitters that may contribute to inflammation.
- Visceral afferents may play a cytoprotective role by increasing mucosal blood flow.
- Mechanosensitivity: Vagal afferents branch in circular and longitudinal muscle layers that respond to tension generated from passive stretch or active contraction. However, other vagal sensory endings called IGLE surround myenteric ganglia. These fibers may respond to muscle stretch/contraction. Spinal afferents can be influenced by many chemical mediators

from injury and/or inflammation. Bradykinin and prostaglandins may potentiate each other and lead to hypersensitivity. Previously insensitive fibers may become sensitive during inflammation.

TRANSMISSION

- Traditional theory held that the viscera were innervated by separate classes of sensory receptors, some concerned with autonomic regulation and some with sensation and pain, or that a single type of receptor sent normal signals in response to low frequencies of activation (nonnoxious) but, at high frequencies, signaled pain.[2]

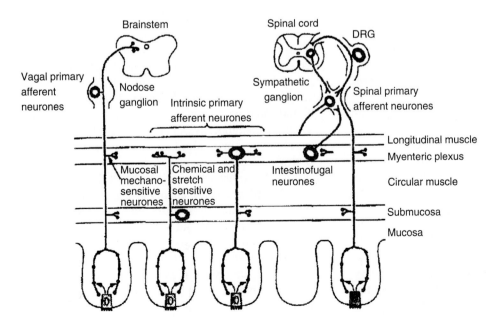

FIGURE 22–8 Arrangement of the primary afferent neurons within the intestine, and central connections. From Grundy.[10]

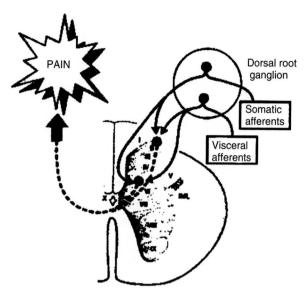

FIGURE 22–9 Viscerosomatic convergence of primary afferent fibers on neurons of lamina I and lamina V of the dorsal horn. From Cervero and Laird.[2]

- Research, however, shows that high- and low-threshold receptors are present in viscera.
- For high-threshold receptors, the relationship between stimulus intensity and nerve activity (encoding) is evoked by stimuli entirely within the noxious range.
- Low-threshold receptors are intensity-encoding receptors with a low threshold to natural stimuli and encoding that spans the range of stimulation intensity from innocuous to noxious.
- Another theory is that silent nociceptors (unresponsive afferent fibers) exist and become activated only in the presence of inflammation.
- These fibers are concerned only with tissue injury and inflammation (not with mechanical stimuli).
- The importance of these silent nociceptors has not been established.
- The strongest evidence is that both high-threshold and intensity-encoding receptors contribute to peripheral encoding of noxious stimuli.
- Brief, acute, visceral pain initially triggers high-threshold afferents. Extended visceral stimulation (ie, hypoxia and inflammation) sensitizes high-threshold receptors and activates silent nociceptors. The CNS receives a barrage of afferent stimuli, initially from the acute injury; then central mechanisms amplify and sustain the peripheral input.
- Also, damage and inflammation of the viscus alter its normal pattern of motility and secretion. This changes the environment around the nociceptor endings, which increases excitation of sensitized nociceptors and excites distant fibers. The resultant discharges may be greater in magnitude and duration than the

initial injury. Therefore, visceral pain may persist after the initial injury has begun resolving.

BIOCHEMISTRY

- Two classes of unmyelinated primary afferents innervate somatic and visceral tissues. One expresses peptide neurotransmitters, such as substance P and CGRP, and the other does not. They also terminate in different lamina of the spinal dorsal horn.
- Somatic fibers contain both classes, but visceral belong only to the peptide class. Therefore, peptides are particularly important to future therapy for visceral pain. Some preliminary data suggest that substance P may have a specific role in visceral hyperalgesia. Several receptor antagonists for substance P are being tested and may lead to new therapies for visceral pain.[2]

CENTRAL SENSITIZATION

- In somatic nociceptive systems, the frequency-dependent increase in neuronal excitability is known as "windup." Visceral nociceptor neurons do not "wind up" as somatic neurons do. Prolonged noxious stimuli evoke increased excitability of viscerosomatic neurons in the spinal cord. These highly selective changes occur only on cells driven by the conditioning visceral stimulus. This increase in excitability may be due to the properties of the activated neuronal network and/or to the release of certain transmitters. Positive feedback loops between spinal and supraspinal structures may be prominent and could be responsible for the enhanced autonomic and motor reflexes seen with visceral pain.[2,11]
- Transmission of pain was once thought to occur via crossed spinothalamic and spinoreticular pathways (ascending the contralateral side of the spinal cord after crossing the gray matter). Investigators have found three new pathways, however, that carry visceral nociception: the dorsal columns, the trigemino-parabrachio-amygdaloid, and spino-hypothalamic pathways.
- *N*-Menthyl-D-aspartate (NMDA) receptors in the spinal cord may play an important regulatory role. NMDA receptor antagonists blocked visceral pain perception in rats but did not affect painful stimuli of somatic tissues.
- Substance P and the neurokinin 1 receptor may play a role in persistent visceral pain at the spinal cord level.
- Many cerebral areas are involved in signal processing as well.

- PET and functional MRI scans show several cerebral structures activated during somatic pain, including the anterior cingulate cortex, insula, thalamus, somatosensory areas, prefrontal cortex, inferior parietal cortex, lentiform nucleus, hypothalamus, periaqueductal gray, and cerebellum. Studies of gastrointestinal distension showed a similar pattern of activity (illustrated in Figure 22–10).[12]

PERIPHERAL SENSITIZATION

- Low-threshold or intensity-encoding receptors respond within the physiologic range. They also respond to distending stimuli in the noxious range of >30 mm Hg (see Figure 22–11). The response magnitude in the noxious range is greater than that of the high-threshold fibers, which do not respond until the stimulus is at or exceeds noxious levels.
- In patients with irritable bowel syndrome (IBS), the response shifts leftward, suggesting visceral hyperalgesia (see Figure 22–12). Visceral afferent neurons should exhibit sensitization (primary hyperalgesia), therefore, and the spinal neurons on which they terminate should change their excitability (secondary hyperalgesia).

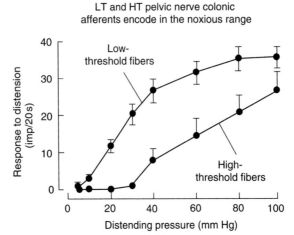

FIGURE 22–11 Mechanosensitive pelvic nerve sensory fibers that innervate the urinary bladder or distal colon have low (<5 mm Hg) or high (>30 mm Hg) thresholds for response to distension. Both low- and high-threshold fibers encode the distending pressure well into the noxious range (>40 mm Hg). From Gebhart.[9]

- Experimental inflammation of viscera awakens silent afferent fibers which become sensitive to mechanical stimuli.[9]

INFLAMMATORY AND NONINFLAMMATORY MEDIATORS

- Local tissue injury releases chemical mediators (potassium, hydrogen ions, ATP, bradykinin) and inflammatory mediators (eg, PGE_2 [prostaglandin E_2]). These substances activate nerve endings and trigger release of algesic mediators (eg, histamine, serotonin, nerve growth factor) from other cells and

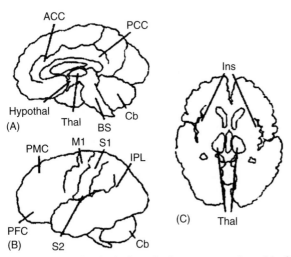

FIGURE 22–10 Principal cerebral structures activated in functional imaging studies of somatic and visceral stimulation. (A) Medial view of right hemisphere. ACC, anterior cingulated cortex; PCC, posterior cingulated cortex; Hypothal, hypothalamus; Thal, thalamus; BS, brainstem; Cb, cerebellum. (B) Lateral view of left cerebral hemisphere. PFC, prefrontal cortex; PMC, premotor cortex; M1, primary motor cortex; S1, primary somatosensory cortex; S2, secondary somatosensory cortex; IPL, inferior parietal lobule. (C) Cerebral cross-sectional view at the level of the insulae and thalami. Ins, insula. From Ladabaum et al.[12]

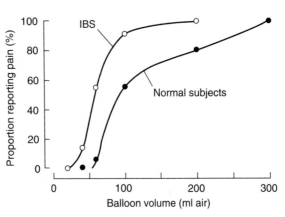

FIGURE 22–12 Illustration of the presence of visceral hyperalgesia in patients with irritable bowel syndrome. From Gebhart.[9]

afferent nerves. This sensitizes afferent nerve terminals causing an increased response to painful stimuli.
- Activation of immunocytes (ex-mast cells) and local adrenergic nerve fibers results in a state of prolonged or permanent sensitization.
- Stress alters perception of visceral pain, possibly because of increased mast cell degranulation.[13]

LABORATORY STUDIES

ACUTE ABDOMINAL PAIN

- Laboratory tests are helpful to aid in diagnosis and to assist in preparation for an operation, if needed.
  - Complete blood count (CBC) and differential
  - Liver function tests
  - Serum electrolytes
  - Serum creatinine
  - Blood urea nitrogen
  - Amylase or lipase
  - Urinalysis
  - Urine or serum pregnancy test

CHRONIC ABDOMINAL PAIN

- In chronic recurrent abdominal pain, tests may identify a discrete cause. Laboratory studies should be ordered only if their results may alter diagnosis or therapy. CBC, ESR (erythrocyte sedimentation rate), and liver function tests may lead to a diagnosis. A pregnancy test should be performed in women.[8]

IMAGING

IMAGING FOR ACUTE ABDOMEN

- X-rays: upright, KUB (kidneys, ureter, bladder), and upright chest films.
- CT scanning is the standard for detecting most causes of acute abdominal pain. It is highly sensitive for appendicitis, diverticulitis, intestinal ischemia, pancreatitis, intestinal obstruction, and perforated viscus. Helical CT reduces artifact from respiration and reduces scanning times. CT scans are enhanced greatly by the use of gastrointestinal and intravenous contrast administration. Helical CT angiography can also allow accurate assessment of thoracoabdominal vessels.
- Ultrasound is most useful in pelvic imaging. A full bladder acts as an acoustic window for pelvic images.

Vaginal ultrasound provides images of the uterus and adnexa. For suspected cholelithiasis and cholecystitis, ultrasound is the initial imaging method of choice (the liver acts as an acoustic window).
- MRI is not the modality of choice for acute abdomen due to high cost, artifact from bowel motion, patient limits of tolerance, and lack of ready availability.[14]

IMAGING FOR CHRONIC ABDOMINAL PAIN

- X-rays: Upright, KUB, and upright chest films should be performed in the patient without an obvious diagnosis. Upright x-rays during an attack may show dilated loops of bowel caused by intermittent obstructing hernia or intussusception, for example.
- Sigmoidoscopy or barium enema may show ischemic colitis or endometriosis.
- CT scan may reveal various pancreatic or biliary tract lesions, masses, or dilated bowel loops.
- Ultrasound may reveal biliary tract abnormalities.[8]

TREATMENT

THE TREATMENT OF CHRONIC PAIN SYNDROMES: INTRODUCTION

- The goals of pain therapies are to:
  - Reduce intensity of pain
  - Improve physical and emotional functioning
  - Reduce drains on health care resources
- The pain-treating physician should know and understand all of the appropriate "tools of the trade" for the treatment of chronic pain of both terminal illness and nonmalignant origin.
- These tools include all of the modalities and therapies, conservative or invasive, used for treating chronic, nonmalignant, AIDS-related, and cancer-related pain syndromes. These therapies can be broadly categorized as noninvasive and invasive (see Figure 22–13).

NONINVASIVE THERAPIES
- Cognitive and behavioral therapies to improve locus of self-control, increase awareness and understanding of the painful experience, promote activity that is not harmful or activating of the painful experience, increase relaxation time, promote behavior that is healing, and reduce behavior that perpetuates the chronic painful experience.
- Rehabilitational pain medicine.

Noninvasive Therapies	Invasive Therapies
Excercise	Pharmacologic Pain Medicine
Cognitive Behavioral Therapy	Anesthetic Blocking Techniques
Physical and Occupational Therapy	Neuromodulatory Techniques
Chiropractic Manipulation	Surgery
Nutritional Therapy	Neuroablation
Massage Therapy	
Psychotherapy	
Alternative Therapies	

FIGURE 22–13 Tools of the trade.

- Alternative pain-relieving therapies, such acupuncture, acupressure, meditation and relaxation, nutrition, Qui-gong, and so on.

INVASIVE THERAPIES
- Pharmacologic interventions:
  - Nonopioid analgesics, including centrally acting nonopioids (such as methotrimeprazine, tramadol, and acetaminophen) and peripherally and centrally active NSAIDs.
  - Opioid analgesics.
  - Adjuvant medications: agents that are labeled for other medical purpose but have analgesic or co-analgesic properties, including the heterocyclic antidepressants; serotonin-specific reuptake inhibitor (SSRI) antidepressants; membrane-stabilizing drugs, such as anticonvulsants; local anesthetic oral analogs and local anesthetics; α_1 blocking agents; β blockers; calcium channel blockers; and so on.
- Peripheral nerve blocks.
- Sympathetic nerve blocks.
- Neurodestructive procedures.
- Neuromodulatory procedures:
  - Spinal cord stimulation
  - Deep brain and motor cortex stimulation
  - Intrathecal and epidural delivery of opioid and nonopioid analgesics
  - Surgical interventions

and severe pain and recommend "tailoring" the strength and potency of pain medications to the severity of the pain syndrome.
  - Nonopioid analgesics are suggested for mild to moderate cancer pain.
  - Weak to moderate strength opioids, such as codeine and hydrocodone in combination with nonopioid and adjunctive medications, are suggested for moderately severe cancer pain.
  - Potent opioids, such as morphine, hydromorphone, and methadone, together with nonopioids and adjuvant medications, are suggested for strong and severe cancer-related pain.
  - By following these guidelines, physicians should be able to control the pain of 50–80% of patients dying of cancer.

ALGORITHM FOR CHRONIC NONMALIGNANT PAIN
- Apply the KISS principle: "Keep it sweet and simple."
- Use a "pain treatment continuum" (see Figure 22–15).
  - Use least invasive and least costly therapies first.
  - Use more costly and more invasive procedures when less costly or invasive therapies fail.
  - Use these either in a series (use one therapy at a time, abandon those that do not work, advance to more invasive therapies as in climbing a ladder) or in parallel (use more than one therapy simultaneously and advance to more costly and invasive

THINKING ALGORITHMICALLY: USING A PAIN TREATMENT CONTINUUM

ALGORITHM FOR CANCER-RELATED PAIN
- The 1980s saw the introduction of the World Health Organization Guidelines for pain management for the dying patient.[15] This attempt to simplify pain management for cancer patients underscores simple interventions that can be used by technologically advanced as well as technologically deprived societies (see Figure 22–14).
- These guidelines group cancer-related pain syndromes by severity and intensity into mild, moderate,

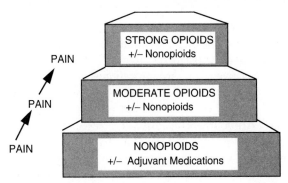

FIGURE 22–14 World Health Organization Narcotic Ladder.

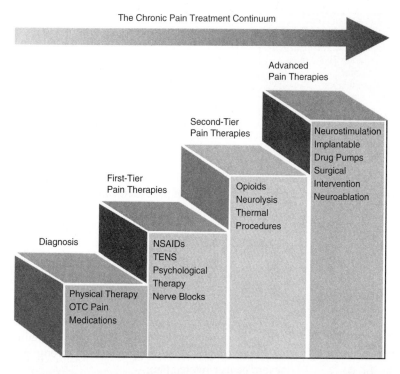

The Chronic Pain Treatment Continuum

Advanced
Pain Therapies

Second-Tier
Pain Therapies

Neurostimulation
Implantable
Drug Pumps
Surgical
Intervention
Neuroablation

First-Tier
Pain Therapies

Opioids
Neurolysis
Thermal
Procedures

Diagnosis

NSAIDs
TENS
Psychological
Therapy
Nerve Blocks

Physical Therapy
OTC Pain
Medications

FIGURE 22–15 Pain treatment continuum for chronic pain. Should be used in the treatment of chronic visceral abdominal pain.

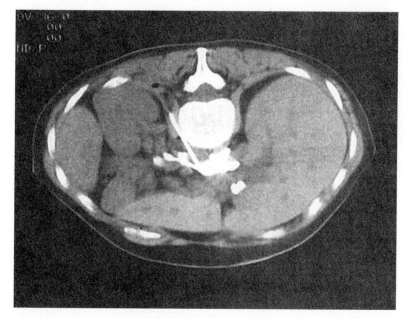

FIGURE 22–16 Transaortic celiac plexus block with local anesthetic or alcohol. CT scan at L1, axial image. Needle on right is transaortic with dye surrounding the aorta and celiac plexus.

therapies as the therapies fail to provide pain relief). The therapies listed in Figure 22–15 move from conservative to invasive procedures.

ACUTE ABDOMINAL PAIN

- Depending on the diagnosis, treatment may include acute fluid resuscitation measures, surgery, opioid analgesics, antibiotics, and other modalities.

CHRONIC ABDOMINAL PAIN

- Depending on the diagnosis, treatment of patients with chronic recurrent abdominal pain may include surgical interventions (eg, incarcerated hernias, neoplasms with hemorrhage or causing acute obstruction).
- Treatment of patients with chronic, unrelenting, abdominal pain, either cancer-related or nonmalignant, should follow a pain treatment algorithm.

- A pain treatment continuum that obeys the KISS principle should be used.
- Treatments should be performed within a multidisciplinary pain treatment center.
- Learning coping mechanisms, accepting that there may not be a diagnosis for their pain, and learning relaxation strategies are useful treatment goals for these patients.
- Appropriate interventions include:
  ○ Sympathetic blocks with local anesthetics or sympatholysis of the celiac plexus or superior hypogastric plexus with alcohol or phenols (see Figure 22–16)
  ○ Continuous epidural blockade
  ○ Intrapleural analgesia
  ○ Spinal cord stimulation
  ○ Intrathecal analgesia

REFERENCES

1. **Bonica J, Graney D.** General considerations of abdominal pain. In: Loeser J, Butler S, Chapman C, Turk D, eds. *Bonica's Management of Pain.* 3rd ed. Philadelphia: Lippincott Williams & Wilkins; 2001:1235.
2. **Cervero F, Laird JMA.** Visceral pain. *Lancet.* 1999; 353:2145.
3. **Netter F.** *The CIBA Collection of Medical Illustrations, Vol 3: Digestive System.* Part II. New York: CIBA; 1987.
4. **Swartz M.** The abdomen. In: Swartz M, ed. *Textbook of Physical Diagnosis: History and Examination.* 2nd ed. Philadelphia: WB Saunders; 1994:311.
5. **Martin RF, Rossi RL.** The acute abdomen, an overview and algorithms. *Surg Clin North Am.* 1997;77:1227.
6. **Hatch EI.** The acute abdomen in children. *Pediatr Clin North Am.* 1985;32:1151.
7. **Dang C, Aguilera P, Dang A, et al.** Acute abdominal pain: Four classifications can guide assessment and management. *Geriatrics.* 2002;57:30.
8. **Zackowski SW.** Chronic recurrent abdominal pain. *Emerg Med Clin North Am.* 1998;16:877.
9. **Gebhart GF.** Visceral pain: Peripheral sensitisation. *Gut.* 2000;47:iv56.
10. **Grundy D.** Neuroanatomy of visceral nociception: Vagal and splanchnic afferent. *Gut.* 2002;51:i2.
11. **Cervero F.** Visceral pain: Central sensitization. *Gut.* 2000;47:iv59.
12. **Ladabaum U, Minoshima S, Owyang C.** Pathobiology of visceral pain: Molecular mechanisms and therapeutic implications, V. Central nervous system processing of somatic and visceral sensory signals. *Am J Physiol Gastrointest Liver Physiol.* 2000;279:G1.
13. **Bueno L, Fioramonti J.** Visceral perception: Inflammatory and non-inflammatory mediators. *Gut.* 2002;51:i19.
14. **Gupta H, Dupuy DE.** Advances in imaging of the acute abdomen. *Surg Clin North Am.* 1997;77:1245.
15. *Cancer Pain Relief.* 2nd ed. Geneva: World Health Organization; 1989.

23   UPPER EXTREMITY PAIN

Matthew Meunier, MD

INTRODUCTION

- Upper extremity pain can be related to acute trauma, the delayed effects of trauma, degenerative changes, local and remote neurologic compromise, and vascular compromise, as well as local or systemic inflammatory disease.

NEED TO RULE OUT ACUTE TREATABLE CAUSES

- A history of recent trauma should be evaluated with plain x-rays, with a minimum of two 90° orthogonal views of the affected part.
- Special attention to fracture or subluxation should be given.
- Referral to an appropriate specialist should occur to treat the underlying injury.
- A sensation of painful "sliding in and out of joint" can be a sign of chronic instability and again should be evaluated by an appropriate specialist prior to starting any pain control regimen.
- Patients with instability may well have normal-appearing radiographs.
- Degenerative conditions in the hand, wrist, elbow, or shoulder need to be ruled out.
- Typical subjective clues include a feeling of pain at the end of range of motion, pain worsening following activity, a feeling of stiffness, and localization of discomfort to a specific location.
- Radiographs show a characteristic narrowing of the joint space with osteophytes typically present at the margins of the joint.
- Finally, all radiographs should be evaluated for the possibility of neoplastic activity, either primary or metastatic.

COMPRESSIVE NEUROPATHY

- Chronic compression of a nerve can be a cause of regional pain.

- The most commonly involved are the median nerve at the carpal tunnel and the ulnar nerve at the cubital tunnel.[1]

CARPAL TUNNEL SYNDROME

- Carpal tunnel syndrome (CTS) is compression of the median nerve under the transverse carpal ligament. (The *carpal tunnel* is defined as the space bordered by the hook of the hamate, the triquetrum and pisiform at the ulnar side, and the scaphoid, trapezium, and flexor carpi radialis sheath on the radial side. The transverse carpal ligament is the roof, and the concave arch of carpal bones is the floor. The narrowest portion is at the level of the capitate.)
- Normal pressure in the carpal tunnel is 0–5 mm Hg, can rise to 30 mm Hg at rest in CTS, and is >90 mm Hg with wrist flexion or extension in patients with CTS.
- Classic symptoms include night pain that wakes the patient from sleep, pain with maximal wrist flexion or extension, decreased grip strength, and decreased dexterity.
- The exam should include: Phalen's test (maximal wrist flexion for 30 seconds with distal subjective changes), Durkan's test (direct compression over carpal tunnel with distal subjective changes), and Tinel's test (percussion along the path of the median nerve with radiation to fingertips).
- In addition, thenar atrophy and thenar motor strength, as well as subjective sensation and two-point discrimination, should be evaluated (normally <5 mm).

CUBITAL TUNNEL SYNDROME

- The ulnar nerve can be compressed in the cubital tunnel at the elbow causing pain and numbness in the ulnar border of the forearm and hand, with, classically, numbness of the small finger.
- In addition, atrophy of the first dorsal interosseous muscle (radial border of index finger metacarpal), clawing of the small finger, weakness of small finger adduction (Wartenberg's sign), and weakness of grip and pinch are later findings of chronic ulnar nerve compromise.
- The cubital tunnel is a fibrous sheath at the level of the elbow, terminating in the proximal portion of the flexor carpi ulnaris.
- Prolonged elbow flexion, direct pressure over the medial forearm or elbow, and idiopathic causes can all result in ulnar nerve compression.

- In the exam, increased numbness and tingling in the small finger with elbow flexion (elbow flexion test) and pain and distal radiation of tingling when ulnar nerve percussion at the elbow is performed (Tinel's sign) are observed. Decreased subjective sensation in the small finger is often present. Decreased grip strength, decreased pinch strength, ulnar-sided digital clawing, and first dorsal interosseous atrophy are all later findings.

OTHER SITES OF COMPRESSION

- Other sites of compression include the median nerve in the forearm (most commonly under the pronator teres), the radial nerve in the axilla (quadrangular space syndrome) or forearm (most commonly under the supinator), and the ulnar nerve in Guyon's canal (ulnar border of carpal tunnel).
- These are all far less frequent than carpal tunnel or cubital tunnel syndrome and often present with a deep aching sensation.
- Finally, in any patient with suspected idiopathic nerve compression, cervical spine pathology needs to be ruled out.

ELECTROPHYSIOLOGIC TESTING

- Prolonged distal latency, decreased amplitude, increased area, and decreased conduction velocity can all indicate compromise of the nerve.[2]

TREATMENT

- The mainstay of treatment remains splinting in a position to decrease pressure on the affected nerve (wrist straight for the median nerve, elbow at approximately 45° for the ulnar nerve).
- Splints should be worn at the minimum at night and, preferably, as much as tolerated during the day.
- For carpal tunnel syndrome, a local anesthetic and steroid (1 cc of lidocaine or marcaine combined with 1 cc of Kenalog or similar steroid) are injected into the carpal tunnel combined with splinting or surgical release. The injection point is 1 cm proximal to the wrist flexion crease and 1 cm ulnar to the palmaris longus tendon (or approximately 1 cm radial to flexor carpi ulnaris). The needle should be oriented 45° to the long axis of the arm in both the radial–ulnar and palmar–dorsal planes, aiming distally. Injection directly into the median nerve should be avoided. If resistance is felt, repositioning should occur. Injection around the ulnar nerve at the cubital tunnel is not recommended.

POSTTRAUMA: CRUSH, NEUROMA, DYSVASCULAR CONDITIONS

- Chronic pain can be a complication following upper extremity trauma.
- The effects of residual articular incongruity can often lead to degenerative arthrosis.
- The mainstay of treatment is nonsteroidal anti-inflammatory medication; however, some patients find this is inadequate for pain control requirements.
- Surgical options include arthrodesis, allograft replacement, and total joint prosthetic replacement and should be explored prior to commencement of a complex medication regimen.

NERVE TRAUMA CAN LEAD TO CHRONIC PAIN

- An area of intense sensitivity with distal radiation of an "electric shock" particularly in the area of previous trauma should raise suspicion for a neuroma.
- Occasionally surgical treatment can be effective, typically burying the neuroma under a muscular or fat flap.
- Traumatized nerves in continuity (ie, with brachial plexus or upper extremity traction injuries) can be quite painful.
- If compression from scar or local tissues, intraneural fibrosis, and neuroma in continuity has been ruled out, then medical treatment may well be needed for control of symptoms.
- Historically the primary treatment has been neurontin (mechanism unknown); however, recent evidence suggests that antidepressants such as amitriptyline have been at least equally effective in controlling chronic nerve pain symptoms.

TRAUMA CAN LEAD TO CHRONIC ARTERIAL INSUFFICIENCY OR TO CHRONIC VENOUS CONGESTION

- Arterial insufficiency often causes a claudication-type pain, most common with increasing levels of activity, or in more severe cases, ischemic pain occurs.
- In addition, patients often complain of stress- or cold-induced symptoms.
- The most severe group may even present with vascular insufficiency ulceration distal to the level of compromise.
- Although it may sound obvious, the first line of treatment is smoking cessation, cold avoidance, and stress reduction.

- In addition, surgical evaluation for possible reconstruction or arterial sympathectomy should be considered.
- For persistent symptoms, beta blockade and calcium channel blockade can also be effective treatment.
- Sympathetic blockade with local injections can be useful in establishing the diagnosis, but is unlikely to offer long-term relief.
- Venous stasis can also be a cause of pain, most likely related to pooling of blood, increased local pressures, and deoxygenation of pooled blood.
- Treatment is directed at improving venous return and typically includes compressive garments and avoiding dependent positioning.

VASCULOPATHY: SCERODERMA, BUERGER'S DISEASE

- Chronic vaso-occlusive and vasospastic conditions can often lead to ischemic pain.[3]
- The most commonly encountered include systemic sclerosis (scleroderma and CREST), thrombangitis obliterans (TAO, or Buerger's disease), and Raynaud's phenomenon and syndrome.
- Raynaud's phenomenon is common in the early stages of almost all of the vasculopathic conditions and classically has three phases: blanching (white), cyanosis (blue), and rubor (red).
- These phases correlate with the initial vasospasm and vascular insufficiency (white), vascular pooling and deoxygenation (blue), and subsequent reactive hyperemia (red).
- The hyperemic phase is accompanied by a classic burning pain sensation. Later, cases often present with digital contracture and ulceration. Frank gangrene is unfortunately not all that uncommon.
- In all vaso-occlusive conditions the primary goal of treatment is to limit vascular spasm. Unfortunately, success is unpredictable and often of limited long-term effectiveness.
- As with posttraumatic vasculopathy, calcium channel blockade, stellate ganglion or brachial plexus blocks, or surgical sympathectomy, although not providing a cure, may allow modification of symptoms and allow digital ulcerations to heal.

COMPLEX REGIONAL PAIN SYNDROME

- Following occasionally even incidental trauma, hypersensitivity to stimuli can occur in an injured limb.[4]
- The diagnosis is suspected in patients who show allodynia (pain in a specific dermatomal distribution to

normal stimuli) and hyperesthesia (increased sensitivity to stimulation) to a normal stimulus.

- Classic findings include pain out of proportion to normal stimuli, loss of motion in the affected extremity, hyperhidrosis, shiny red skin, and increased hair growth on the affected limb.
- Diagnosis includes the use of physical exam, radiographs (osteopenia), and bonescan (increased uptake in phase three); however, the gold standard for diagnosis of sympathetic mediated complex regional pain syndrome (CRPS) is improvement of symptoms following stellate ganglion blockade.
- Prior to undergoing treatment, it is paramount that underlying causes of chronic pain, particularly compressive neuropathy, be ruled out.
- Classification is based on either the presence or absence of sympathetic mediated pain or the presence or absence of a defined nerve injury. Type I CRPS, or classic reflex sympathetic dystrophy, is not related to a defined nerve injury. In type II, a neural injury is present.[5,6]
- Treatment centers on controlling pain and improving function.
- Treatment of CRPS incorporates a multidisciplinary approach; however, current diagnostic criteria do not predict the success of specific treatment regimens.
- Aggressive, but careful, hand therapy is essential in the recovery of function.
- In addition, treatment of the underlying causes, the allodynia and hyperesthesia, and any psychologic factors is part of a potentially successful program.
- Approximately 80% of patients diagnosed and treated within 1 year of onset have an improvement or full recovery from CRPS.
- In patients with symptoms lasting longer than 1 year approximately 50% have significant impairment despite adequate treatment.

REFERENCES

1. **Gelberman RH, Eaton RG, Urbaniak JR.** Peripheral nerve compression. *Instr Course Lect.* 1994;43:31–53.
2. **Mackinnon SE.** Pathophysiology of nerve compression. *Hand Clin.* 2002;18:231–241.
3. **Troum SJ, Smith TL, Koman LA, Ruch DS.** Management of vasospastic disorders of the hand. *Clin Plast Surg.* 1997; 24:121–132.
4. **Koman LA, Poehling GG, Smith TL.** Complex regional pain syndrome: Reflex symathetic dystrophy and causalgia. In: Green DP, Hotchkiss RN, Pederson WC, eds. *Green's Operative Hand Surgery.* 4th ed. New York: Churchill Livingstone; 1999.
5. **Wilson PR.** Post-traumatic upper extremity reflex sympathetic dystrophy. *Hand Clin.* 1997;13:367–372.
6. **Cooney WP.** Somatic versus sympathetic mediated chronic limb pain: Experience and treatment options. *Hand Clin.* 1997;13:355–361.

24   LOWER EXTREMITY PAIN

William Tontz, Jr., MD
Robert Scott Meyer, MD

INTRODUCTION

- Evaluation of pain in the lower extremity can be a diagnostic challenge.
- A thorough assessment requires a precise understanding of both primary pain generators and referred pain in specific areas of the extremity.
- Questions regarding the characteristics of the pain, such as its location, onset, duration, quality, radiation, and severity, are important, and frequently a preliminary diagnosis can be made on history alone.
- A detailed physical examination is critical, and with this added information the correct diagnosis can usually be reached with confidence.
- This chapter provides a detailed differential diagnosis of lower extremity pain by region, with tips on history, exam findings, and diagnostic tests that will help determine the correct diagnosis.

SACROILIAC JOINT PAIN

- The diagnosis of sacroiliac joint pain can be difficult due to its anatomic location, and disorders of this joint are frequently underdiagnosed.
- The sacroiliac joint is commonly affected by osteoarthritis and is also a characteristic feature of patients with spondyloarthropathies such as ankylosing spondylitis and psoriatic arthritis. Patients with a history of intravenous drug use may present with a septic sacroiliac joint arthritis.
- A typical pain pattern of sacroiliac disease is the involved buttock area with referral to the low back, the posterior thigh, and, occasionally, the groin. It is very important to rule out sacroiliac joint pain and dysfunction in patients with low back pain as it may be the primary cause of the back pain in up to 20% of these patients.[1]
- The physical examination of the sacroiliac joint includes palpation of the posterior joint and several provocative maneuvers. The joint can be stressed by

distraction, compression, and rotation of the pelvis. Patrick's test or *fabere* sign (flexion, abduction, external rotation, and extension of the hip) typically reproduces the pain in the buttock area. If this test causes groin pain, the hip joint is the more likely pain generator.

- Plain radiographs, including AP and oblique views of the pelvis, may be helpful in documenting sacroiliac joint arthritis and are less expensive than a CT scan. The latter, however, is the preferred study to qualify the degree of osteoarthritis. In cases of septic arthritis, inflammatory arthritis, or other disorders where soft tissue imaging of the joint is important, MRI is the modality of choice.[2]

- An injection of anesthetic and steroid into the sacroiliac joint, along with an arthrogram for confirmation, is extremely useful in confirming the diagnosis of sacroiliac joint pain and dysfunction.

HIP PAIN

- Intra-articular causes of hip pain include osteoarthritis, inflammatory arthritis, septic arthritis, osteonecrosis,[3] labral pathology, and femoral neck stress fractures[4,5]. Common extra-articular causes of pain include greater trochancteric bursitis, snapping hip, iliopsoas bursitis/tendonitis, muscle strains about the hip, and referred pain such as facet joint arthritis of the low back, lumbar radiculitis, and sacroiliac joint pathology.[6–9]

- It is important for the patient to relate where the hip pain is located. Lateral hip pain implies greater trochanteric bursitis, whereas groin pain is typically seen with iliopsoas bursitis/tendonitis or intra-articular causes, particularly arthritis. Buttock pain can also occur with intra-articular conditions but referred pain from the back or sacroiliac joint should be considered. It is not uncommon for groin pain from intra-articular causes, particularly arthritis, to radiate down into the thigh and medial knee.

- A focused history should include exposure to risk factors for osteonecrosis such as alcohol use, corticosteroid use, clotting disorders, and previous hip trauma.[3] A history regarding overuse syndromes or amenorrhea in a young woman may lead to the diagnosis of a femoral neck stress fracture[5] or musculotendinous strain. A history of audible snapping or clicking implies the presence of etiologies such as coxa saltans (snapping hip),[8] iliopsoas bursitis, and labral pathology.[6] Patients with hip arthritis usually give a history of mechanical symptoms such as locking, clicking, and catching.

- Typical physical examination findings in patients with arthritis include limited hip range of motion, --

particularly internal rotation, hip joint contractures (positive Thomas test), limb shortening, and a positive Trendelenburg sign or gait. A Patrick or FabER test should be performed to help rule out sacroiliac pain and a strait leg raise and neurologic examination performed to rule out lumbar radiculitis. A good screening test for intra-articular hip pathology, particularly arthritis, is the Stinchfield test. The patient is asked to actively elevate a straight leg off the exam table. The examiner then adds some gentle manual resistance. The test is positive if it causes typical groin, thigh, or buttock pain, sometimes associated with yielding weakness.

- A hip apprehension test may be useful in the diagnosis of hip anterior labral pathology. In this test the patient has pain with flexion, adduction, and internal rotation of the hip joint while supine. A click may also be reproduced with this maneuver.

- Plain radiographs to look for arthritis should include an AP pelvis and AP and lateral views of the symptomatic hip. A hip stress fracture or osteonecrosis of the femoral head[2,10–12] may not be apparent on plain films and further advanced imaging such as MRI should be obtained if clinical suspicion is high. An MRI arthrogram may be useful in the diagnosis of hip labral pathology[13,14]

- Iliopsoas bursography for suspected iliopsoas bursitis with audible snapping may be useful.

- Diagnostic and/or therapeutic extra- and intra-articular injections about the hip are often very useful. Common examples include a greater trochanteric bursa injection, an intra-articular hip joint injection, an iliopsoas bursa injection, a sacroiliac joint injection, and lumbar spine injections such as facet joint and epidural injections (Table 24–1).

KNEE PAIN

- Intra-articular causes of knee pain include arthritis, articular cartilage injuries, meniscus tears, ligament

TABLE 24–1 Differential Diagnosis of Hip Pain

Extra-articular causes
  Referred pain from the lumbar spine or sacroiliac joint
  Greater trochanter bursitis
  Iliopsoas tendonitis
  Coxa saltans (snapping hip)
  Muscle strains and contusions
Intra-articular causes
  Labral pathology
  Loose bodies
  Osteonecrosis of the femoral head
  Osteoarthritis, inflammatory arthritis, septic arthritis
  Femoral neck stress fractures

tears, tendon tears, spontaneous osteonecrosis of the knee (SONK), an inflamed plica, and patellofemoral pain syndrome.[15–17] Extra-articular etiologies include iliotibial band syndrome, patellar or quadriceps tendonitis, pes anserine tendonitis, and referred pain from the hip and lumbar spine. Also in the differential diagnosis, particularly in a patient with a recent injury or surgical procedure to the knee, is reflex sympathetic dystrophy.

- It is useful to ask the patient to describe the exact location of the pain and even to point to where the pain is located. Anterior knee pain is suggestive of patellar or quadriceps tendonitis or patellofemoral pathology. Lateral knee pain may represent iliotibial band tendonitis, a lateral meniscus tear, or lateral compartment arthritis. Medial knee pain may represent pes anserine tendonitis, a medial meniscus tear, and medial compartment arthritis. Low back pain may radiate to the medial or lateral knee depending on its dermatomal distribution, and hip pain classically refers to the medial knee.
- A focused history should include questions regarding mechanical problems, such as clicking, catching, locking, and giving way. These symptoms usually point to an internal derangement such as a meniscus tear or arthritis. Questions with respect to associated injuries or surgery, along with a history of temperature and skin color changes, may lead to a diagnosis of reflex sympathetic dystrophy.
- A screening examination of the lumbar spine, along with a neurologic examination of the lower extremities, as well as a good examination of the hip, is very useful in ruling out causes of referred pain to the knee, particularly when the clinical suspicion is high.
- Useful physical examination findings for the diagnosis of meniscus tears include focal joint line tenderness and positive provocative maneuvers such as McMurray's test. A thorough exam should also include range of motion of the knee, a ligament stability exam, and competency of the patellar and quadriceps tendon. Typical exam findings in cases of arthritis include deformity of the knee, limited range of motion, and crepitus in the knee. Typical findings of reflex sympathetic dystrophy include temperature changes, skin color changes, and pain out of proportion to exam findings, and are discussed in more detail in other chapters.
- Physical examination findings for extra-articular causes of knee pain typically involve tenderness to palpation of the involved structure, such as the patellar or quadriceps tendon, pes anserine insertion, and insertion of the iliotibial band at Gerdy's tubercle.
- Plain radiographs are useful in the workup of knee pain and should always be weight bearing. Advanced

TABLE 24–2 Differential Diagnosis of Knee Pain

Extra-articular causes
  Referred pain from the lumbar spine or hip joint
  Iliotibial band syndrome
  Patellar or quadriceps tendonitis
  Pes anserine tendonitis
Intra-articular causes
  Meniscal tear
  Chondral injuries
  Osteonecrosis
  Ligament injury
  Tendon injury
  Symptomatic plica
  Patellofemoral pain syndrome
  Osteoarthritis, inflammatory arthritis, septic arthritis

imaging such as MRI can be extremely helpful for suspected meniscal, chondral, and ligament injuries and for osteonecrosis.

- As in other areas of the lower extremity, differential diagnostic injections may be quite useful. An injection of anesthetic and steroid into the pes anserine bursa, for example, may help differentiate between a medial meniscus tear and pes tendonitis/bursitis (Table 24–2).

LEG (CALF) PAIN

- There are four compartments in the leg with a specific nerve in each: anterior (deep fibular nerve), lateral (superficial fibular nerve), superficial posterior (sural nerve), and deep posterior (tibial nerve).
- Extrinsic causes of leg pain include any referred spine, hip, or knee pathology.
- Intrinsic causes include parostitis ("shin splints"), tendonitis, stress fracture, acute or chronic exertional compartment syndrome, and local infection or tumor.
- It is important to determine where knee pain is located, originates, or radiates toward. Anterior tibial pain is suggestive of parostitis, whereas specific pain over a compartment suggests tendonitis.
- The history should include questions regarding onset (acute, insidious, chronic), trauma, constitutional symptoms, radiation, or origin of pain. The patient should be asked if he or she increased specific activities such as running prior to the onset of pain. Many "overuse syndromes" are the result of increasing a particular activity.
- Associated numbness along a particular sensory nerve distribution occurring with increased physical activity is suggestive of exertional compartment syndrome.
- Physical exam findings for *extrinsic* causes of knee pain include tenderness over the patellar or quadriceps

TABLE 24–3 Differential Diagnosis of Leg Pain

Extrinsic causes
    Spine, hip, or knee pathology
Intrinsic causes
    Parostitis
    Stress fracture
    Acute or chronic exertional compartment syndrome
    Tendonitis
    Vascular claudication
    Infection/tumor

tendons with tendonitis and tightness over the iliotiibial band with snapping over the greater trochanter with hip flexion.[8] Physical exam findings for *intrinsic* pathology include joint line tenderness for meniscal or chondral lesions, tenderness in the medial parapatellar region for plica syndrome,[18] and effusion for chondral injuries or osteoarthrosis. Pain out of proportion to radiographic findings suggests SONK.[16]

- Instability of the knee in the anterior, posterior, medial, or lateral plane suggests ligamentous injury.
- Radiographs include weight-bearing AP and lateral views of the knee.
- Advanced imaging such as MRI is used for suspected meniscal/chondral pathology, SONK, or ligamentous insufficiency.
- Treatment is effective if differential diagnosis is narrowed to a short list. Physical therapy and non-steroidal anti-inflammatory drugs are used for the majority of extrinsic causes if effective. Treatment of proximal pathology such as herniated nucleus pulposus in the spine or hip pathology to diminish the referred pain in the knee can be provided.[18]
- On failure of nonoperative therapy, treatment of intrinsic causes include arthroscopy for meniscal or chondral pathology, osteotomy for limb malalignment, and intra-articular injections versus arthroplasty for symptomatic and significant osteoarthritis (Table 24–3).

REFERENCES

1. **Bernard TN, Kirkaldy-Willis WH.** Recognizing specific characteristics of nonspecific low back pain. *Clin Orthop.* 1987;217:266-280.
2. **Braun J, Sieper J, Bollow M.** Imaging of sacroiliitis. *Clin Rheumatol.* 2000;19:51–57.
3. **Lavernia CJ, Sierra RJ, Grieco FR.** Osteonecrosis of the femoral head. *J Am Acad Orthop Surg.* 1999;7:250–261.
4. **Anderson K, Strickland SM, Warren R.** Hip and groin injuries in athletes. *Am J Sports Med.* 2001;29:521–533.
5. **Teitz CC, Hu SS, Arendt EA.** The female athlete: Evaluation and treatment of sports-related problems. *J Am Acad Orthop Surg.* 1997;5:87–96.
6. **Edwards DJ, Lomas D, Villar RN.** Diagnosis of the painful hip by magnetic resonance imaging and arthroscopy. *J Bone Joint Surg Br.* 1995;77:374–376.
7. **McCarthy JC.** Hip arthroscopy: Applications and technique. *J Am Acad Orthop Surg.* 1995;3:115–122.
8. **Allen WC, Cope R.** Coxa saltans: The snapping hip revisited. *J Am Acad Orthop Surg.* 1995;3:303–308.
9. **Lyons JC, Peterson LF.** The snapping iliopsoas tendon. *Mayo Clin Proc.* 1984;59:327–329.
10. **Mankin HJ.** Nontraumatic necrosis of bone (osteonecrosis). *N Engl J Med.* 1992;326:1473–1479.
11. **Mont MA, Hungerford DS.** Non-traumatic avascular necrosis of the femoral head. *J Bone Joint Surg Am.* 1995;77:459–474.
12. **Hungerford DS.** Pathogenesis of ischemic necrosis of the femoral head. *Instr Course Lect.* 1983;32:252–260.
13. **Byrd JW.** Labral lesions: An elusive source of hip pain case reports and literature review. *Arthroscopy.* 1996;12:603–612.
14. **Hawkins RB.** Arthroscopy of the hip. *Clin Orthop.* 1989;44–47.
15. **James SL.** Running injuries to the knee. *J Am Acad Orthop Surg.* 1995;3:309–318.
16. **Ecker ML.** Spontaneous osteonecrosis of the distal femur. *Instr Course Lect.* 2001;50:495–498.
17. **Fulkerson JP.** Patellofemoral pain disorders: Evaluation and management. *J Am Acad Orthop Surg.* 1994;2:124–132.
18. **Ewing JW.** Plica: Pathologic or not? *J Am Acad Orthop Surg.* 1993;1:117–121.

25 HEADACHES

Joel R. Saper, MD, FACP, FAAN

EPIDEMIOLOGY

- Primary headache disorders are highly prevalent conditions affecting tens of millions of US citizens and hundreds of millions of individuals worldwide.[1,2]
- The lifetime prevalence of common headache disorders can be more than 78%, with migraine prevalence greater than 20% in adult women.
- The economic and quality-of-life burden of migraine alone is substantial, with the most disabled half of migraine sufferers accounting for more than 90% of migraine-related work loss.
- Barriers to successful care include failure to properly diagnose, underestimation by both the professional and public domains of the morbidity of these conditions, and denied access to appropriate treatment.

PRIMARY AND SECONDARY HEADACHES

- *Primary headaches* include those in which intrinsic dysfunction of the nervous system, often genetic in origin, predisposes to increased vulnerability to headache attacks. Examples include cluster headache and migraine.
- *Secondary headaches* are those in which the headache is secondary to an organic or physiologic process, intracranially or extracranially.[1]
- According to the International Headache Society (IHS) classification,[3] the primary headache entities include:
  1. Migraine
     a. With aura
     b. Without aura
     c. Chronic
  2. Cluster headache
  3. Tension-type headache
- Secondary headaches can arise from more than 300 conditions, among which are ischemic, metabolic, intracranial, cerebrospinal fluid (CSF) hypotension/hypertension, infectious, endocrine, and cervicogenic disorders.

MIGRAINE

- *Migraine* is a complex neurophysiologic disorder characterized by episodic and progressive forms of head pain, in association with numerous neurologic and nonneurologic (autonomic, psychophysiologic) accompaniments. These can precede, accompany, or follow the headache itself.
- Migraine is classified into three major subtypes:
  ○ *Migraine with aura*: Heralding neurologic events lasting 30 minutes to 1 hour occur before the head pain attacks (only 20% of migraine attacks).
  ○ *Migraine without aura*: Attacks of migraine and accompaniments occur without clear-cut pre-headache neurologic symptomatology.
  ○ *Chronic migraine*: In this progressive form of migraine intermittent attacks occur at increasing frequency, eventually reaching 15 or more days per month. By definition, chronic migraine occurs on a backdrop of episodic *migraine without aura*, often accompanied by comorbid neuropsychiatric phenomena. *Chronic migraine* is frequently associated with medication overuse and "rebound" (see later). Comorbid conditions associated with migraine, particularly *chronic migraine*, include depression, anxiety and panic disorders, bipolar disorder, obsessive–compulsive disorder, character disorders, and perhaps fibromyalgia.[1–3]

CLINICAL SYMPTOMATOLOGY

- Eighty to ninety percent of cases have a family history.
- The 3:1 female:male gender ratio is thought to be related primarily to the adverse influence of estrogen on migraine mechanisms.
- Attacks generally last 4–72 hours.
- Attacks are often accompanied by a wide range of autonomic and cognitive symptoms.
- In complex cases, particularly *chronic migraine*, an association with several neuropsychiatric comorbid disorders, including depression, panic/anxiety syndromes, sleep disturbance, and obsessive–compulsive disorder, is likely.
- Predisposed individuals are particularly vulnerable to provocation (triggering) by certain extrinsic and intrinsic events, including hormonal fluctuation (ie, menstrual periods, use of oral contraceptives), weather changes, certain foods, skipped meals and fasting, extra sleeping time, and stress.[1,2]

PATHOPHYSIOLOGY OF MIGRAINE

- Migraine is a brain disorder that generally renders the brain "hypersensitive" and overresponsive to a variety of internal and external stimuli.[4] Trigeminal/cervical connections and cervical activation[5] may be important phenomena in the clinical manifestations, pathogenesis, and treatment. Key features of current pathophysiologic concepts include[2,4]:
  ○ Trigeminal-mediated perivascular (neurogenic) inflammation resulting in painful vascular and meningeal tissue.
  ○ The perivascular release of vasoactive neuropeptides, particularly calcitonin gene-related peptide (CGRP).
  ○ The development of allodynia and central sensitization as attacks progress.[6]
  ○ The presence of an active "modulator zone" in the dorsal raphe nucleus of the midbrain during migraine attacks.[7]
  ○ Activation and threshold reduction of neurons in the descending trigeminal system following C2–3 cervical stimulation.[5]
  ○ The deposition of nonheme iron in the brainstem, roughly correlated to increasingly frequent attacks.[8]
  ○ A yet-to-be-defined relationship to nitrous oxide.[4]

TENSION-TYPE HEADACHE

- This controversial disorder is classified into both episodic and chronic forms.[3] Episodic forms have certain features that overlap with *migraine without aura*, although there is a general absence of throbbing pain and autonomic accompaniments. *Chronic tension-type headache* overlaps in clinical features with *chronic migraine*. Both forms of *tension-type headache* may be present in patients who have otherwise typical migraine headaches. Some authorities believe that these disorders are variant forms of migraine.

CHRONIC DAILY HEADACHE

- *Chronic daily headache* is a frequency-based descriptive term that embodies four overlapping clinical subtypes:
  - *Chronic migraine*, with or without medication overuse
  - *Chronic tension-type headache*, with or without medication overuse
  - *New daily, persistent headache*: Onset of daily, persistent head pain without the progressive features of chronic migraine but often associated with comorbid and medication misuse features
  - *Hemicrania continua*: Unilateral, generally persistent hemicranial discomfort with some features of migraine and which, in 20% of cases, appears to arise as a consequence of head trauma

REBOUND HEADACHE (MEDICATION MISUSE HEADACHE)

- Rebound headache (or medication overuse headache) is a self-sustaining headache condition characterized by persisting and recurring headache (usually migraine forms) against a background of chronic, regular use of centrally acting analgesics, ergotamine tartrate, or triptans.[9] The key features of this condition include[1]:
  - Weeks to months of excessive use of the above agents, with usage exceeding 2–3 days per week
  - Insidious increase in headache frequency
  - Dependable and predictable headache, corresponding to an irresistible escalating use of offending agents at regular, predictable intervals
  - Evidence of psychologic and/or physiologic dependency
  - Failure of alternate acute or preventive medications to control headache attacks
  - Reliable onset of headache within hours to days of the last dose of symptomatic treatment

CLUSTER HEADACHE AND ITS VARIANTS

- *Cluster headache* is a relatively rare disorder that affects more men than women in a ratio of 3:1.

Current concepts on pathophysiology suggest disturbances within the hypothalamus with relevant involvement of autonomic systems[1,2,10] and alterations in melatonin function.[11,12] Melatonin "finetunes" endogenous cerebral rhythms and homeostasis.
- Clinical features[1,2] of cluster headaches include:
  - Presence of headache cycles or bouts (clusters) lasting weeks to months, occurring one or more times per year or less, during which repetitive headache attacks occur
  - Individual attacks lasting 1–3 hours
  - Attacks associated with focal (orbital, temporal, or unilateral) facial pain, accompanied by lacrimation, nasal drainage, pupillary changes, and conjunctival injection
  - Attacks commonly occur during sleeping times or napping
  - High likelihood of blue or hazel-colored eyes; ruddy, rugged, lionized facial features; and long history of smoking and excessive alcohol intake
- Table 25–1 lists the clinical distinctions between cluster headache and migraine.
- *Cluster headache* may occur in its episodic form (bouts or cycles of recurring headaches followed by a period of no headache [interim], lasting weeks to years) or in a chronic form without an interim period, with headache attacks daily for years without interruption. Treatment differences may exist.[2]

TABLE 25–1 Clinical Features Distinguishing Between Cluster and Migraine Headaches

FEATURE	CLUSTER	MIGRAINE
Location of pain	Always unilateral, periorbital; sometimes occipital referral	Unilateral, bilateral
Age at onset (typical)	Onset 20 years or older	10–50 years (can be younger or older)
Gender difference	Majority male	Majority female in adulthood
Time of day	Frequently at night, often same time each day	Any time
Frequency of attacks	1–6 per day	1–10 per month in episodic form
Duration of pain	30–120 min	4–72 h
Prodrome	None	Often present
Nausea and vomiting	2–5%	85%
Blurring of vision	Infrequent	Frequent
Lacrimation	Frequent	Infrequent
Nasal congestion/ drainage	70%	Uncommon
Ptosis	30%	1–2%
Polyuria	2%	40%
Family history of similar headaches	7%	90%
Miosis	50%	Absent
Behavior during attack	Pacing, manic, and histrionic	Resting in quiet, dark room

From Saper et al.[1]

- In addition to *cluster headache*, several short-lasting headache entities are recognized and currently classified along with cluster headache in a category referred to as the *trigeminal autonomic cephalgias.*[13] These include:
  - Cluster headache
  - Chronic and episodic paroxysmal hemicrania
  - SUNCT syndrome (short-lasting unilateral neuralgiaform pain with conjunctival injection and tearing)
  - Cluster–tic syndrome (the association of cluster headache with trigeminal neuralgic symptomatology)
- These disorders are characterized primarily by the presence of short-lasting, variable-duration—seconds (SUNCT) to 3 hours (cluster headache)—headache attacks associated with autonomic features.

TREATMENT OF PRIMARY HEADACHES AND RELATED PHENOMENA

KEY TREATMENT PRINCIPLES

- Diagnosing the specific primary headache entity
- Determining attack frequency and severity
- Establishing the presence or absence of comorbid illnesses (psychiatric, neurological, medical, etc)
- Identifying confounding factors, including external or internal phenomena, such as:
  - Rebound
  - Psychologic, comorbid illnesses and medication factors (ie, estrogen replacement, nitroglycerine)
  - Hormonal disturbances
  - Use of or exposure to toxic substances
- Identifying previous treatment successes and failures

TREATMENT MODALITIES

- Nonpharmacologic (self-help, behavioral modification, biofeedback, etc)
- Pharmacologic
- Interventional, including:
  - Neuroblockade (nerve, facet, epidural space)
  - Radiofrequency and cryolysis procedures
  - Implantations and stimulation
- Hospital/rehabilitation programs

NONPHARMACOLOGIC TREATMENTS FOR PRIMARY HEADACHES

- A variety of factors related to health, habits, and education can assist patients with headache:
  - Education or provocation and relief
  - Reduction of medication overuse; treatment of rebound headache
  - Discontinuation of smoking
  - Regular eating and sleeping patterns (maintaining sameness)
  - Exercise
  - Biofeedback and behavioral treatment (cognitive behavioral therapy)
  - Other psychotherapeutic interventions

TREATMENT OF REBOUND HEADACHE

- Rebound headache (also called medication overuse headache) requires treatment, as continued use renders patients refractory to effective treatment. Outpatient and inpatient strategies are available, depending on the intensity of medication usage and characteristics of the case. The following principles apply:
  - Gradual discontinuation of offending agent (taper if opioid- or barbiturate-containing)
  - Aggressive treatment of resulting severe headache
  - Hydration, including intravenous fluids and support in severe cases (treat nausea, etc)
  - The development of pharmacologic prophylaxis
  - Implementation of behavioral therapies
  - Use of infusion or hospitalization techniques for advanced and severe conditions
- Rebound or medication overuse headaches, which most likely result from chronic changes to receptors, must be distinguished from headaches resulting from exposure to toxic substances or other agents or drugs. These have a direct provocative influence.[14]

PHARMACOLOGIC TREATMENT OF MIGRAINE

- Table 25–2 lists pharmacologic agents used in headache management and clinical information regarding their use.[1,2,4]
- The pharmacologic treatment of headache involves the use of *abortive (acute)* and *preventive* medications. *Abortive (acute) treatments* are used to terminate evolving or existing attacks. *Preventive treatment* is implemented to reduce the frequency of attacks and prevent overuse of acute medications. Most patients require combination treatment. *Preemptive treatment* is a short-term preventive course of therapy used in anticipation of a predictable event, such as a menstrual period or vacation-related headache.

TABLE 25–2   Selected Drugs Used in the Pharmacotherapy of Head, Neck, and Face Pain*[†]

DRUG NAME	mg/DOSE	STANDARD DAILY ADMINISTRATION	NOTES
Symptomatic drugs			
Analgesics			
Excedrin[‡]	—	Varies	Avoid more than 2 d/wk of use
NSAIDs			
Naproxen sodium (PO)[‡]	275–550	bid–tid	Avoid extended, daily use
Indomethacin (PO)	25–50	bid–tid	Avoid extended, daily use
Indocin SR (PO)	75	1 qd or bid	Avoid extended, daily use
Indomethacin (PR)	50	bid–tid	Avoid extended, daily use
Meclofenamate (PO)	50–200	bid	Avoid extended, daily use
Ibuprofen (PO)[‡]	600–800	bid–tid	Avoid extended, daily use
Ketorolac (PO)	10	qid	Avoid extended, daily use
Ketorolac (IM)	30	tid	Avoid extended, daily use; appears particularly valuable when ergot derivatives and narcotics must be avoided and parenteral therapy is necessary; no more than occasional, short-term use is advisable because of renal toxicity, most likely in predisposed patients
Special migraine drugs			
Isometheptene combinations[‡] (Midrin, etc.)	—	2 caps at onset, 1–2q30–60 min	Max 5–6 caps/day; 2 d/wk
Ergotamine tartrate (ET)[‡] Oral (Cafergot, Wigraine, etc.)	1 mg ET, 100 mg caffeine	2 tabs at onset, 1–2q30–60 min	Max 4–6/day; 2 d/wk
Suppositories (Cafergot, Wigraine)	2 mg ET, 100 mg caffeine	$\frac{1}{3}$–1 at onset; may repeat in 60 min	Max 2/d; 2 d/wk
Sublingual (Ergomar, Ergostat)	2 mg ET	1 at onset; may repeat after 15 min 0.25–1 mg SC, IM, IV tid	Max 2/d; 2 d/wk
Dihydroergotamine (DHE)[‡] IM/IV	0.25–1	0.25–1 mg SC, IM, IV tid	Can be used 2 or 3 times/d in conjunction with antinauseant, analgesic, etc; IM more effective than SC
DHE Nasal Spray[‡]	1	1 spray each nostril (2 mg/spray); repeat in 15 min (4 sprays=2 mg)	Use no more than 2 or 3 times/wk, on separate days
Sumatriptan (parenteral)[‡]	6 SC	May repeat in 1 h	
Sumatriptan (oral)	25–50	Take at HA onset; may repeat at 2 hrs; max 100 mg/day	
Sumatriptan (nasal spray)[‡]	5 or 20	1 spray in 1 nostril only; may repeat in 2 h; max 40 mg/24 h	
Zolmitriptan (oral)[‡]	2.5–5	1 at onset; may repeat in 2 h; max 10 mg/24 h	
Zolmitriptan (ZMT)[‡]	2.5–5	1 at onset; may repeat in 2 h; max 10 mg/24 h	Cannot be used within 24 h of ergotamine-related meds or other triptans; should not be used in presence of cardiovascular and/or cerebrovascular, severe hypertension, Prinzmetal angina, or peripheral vascular disorders; no more than 2 doses in 24 h; limit 2 d/wk usage
Naratriptan (oral)[‡]	2.5	1 at onset; may repeat in 4 h; max 5 mg/24 h	
Rizatriptan (oral)[‡]	5–10	1 at onset; may repeat in 2 h; max 30 mg/24 h	
Rizatriptan (MLT)[‡]	5–10	1 at onset; may repeat in 2 h; max 30 mg/24 h	
Almotriptan[‡]	12.5	1 at onset; may repeat; max 25 mg/24 h	
Frovatriptan[‡]	2.5	1 at onset; may repeat after 6–8 h; max 7.5 mg/24 h	
Eletriptan	20, 40	1 at onset; may repeat after 2 h	Avoid within 72 h of CYP3A4 inhibitors
Antinauseants/neuroleptics/antihistimines			
Chlorpromazine			
PO	25–100	bid–tid	
Supp	25–100	bid–tid	Limit 3 d/wk, except for persistent nausea; avoid extended use; monitor for hypotension and cardiac rhythm effects (QT interval)
IM	25–100	bid–tid	
IV	2.5–10	bid–tid	
Metoclopramide	10–20	tid	
(PO—tablet and syrup)			
(Parenteral)	10	tid	

Table 25–2 continues

TABLE 25–2 *(Continued)*

DRUG NAME	mg/DOSE	STANDARD DAILY ADMINISTRATION	NOTES
Promethazine			
PO	25–75	tid	Limit 3 d/wk, except for persistent nausea; avoid extended use; monitor for hypotension and cardiac rhythm effects (QT interval)
IM	25–75	tid	
Perphenazine			
PO	4–8	bid-tid	
IM	5	bid	
Diphenhydramine	25–50	tid	Anticholinergic effects
Hydroxyzine (PO, IM)	25–75	bid-tid or at hs	Can be used as a symptomatic or preventive treatment
Cyproheptadine (PO)	2–4	tid-qid	
Anticonvulsants			
Valproic acid (IV)	250–750	1000–3000 mg/day	See Anticonvulsants under Preventive drugs
Steroids			
Prednisone (PO)	40–60	in 1 or divided doses	4- to 10-d program; avoid repeated use
Preventive drugs§			
Tricyclic antidepressants			
Amitriptyline	10–150		
Nortriptyline	10–100	Divided doses or hs	Bedtime dose aids sleep disturbance
Doxepin	10–150		
Other antidepressants			
Fluoxetine	20	20–80 mg/d in divided dose	Actual efficacy for headache uncertain; administer with care to patients using lipophilic beta blockers (propranolol, metoprolol, etc) or switch to hydrophilic beta blockers such as nadolol; value for headache of numerous other antidepressants under investigation
MAO inhibitors			
Phenelzine	15–30	15–90 mg/d in divided dose	Dietary and medication restrictions mandatory
Beta adrenergic blockers			
Propranolol‡	20–50	tid-qid (standard dose)	Monitor cardiac function, BP, pulse, lipids
Atenolol	50–100	bid	
Timolol‡	10–20	bid	
Metoprolol	50–100	bid	
Nadolol	20–120	bid	
Calcium channel antagonists			
Verapamil	80–160	tid-qid	Monitor cardiac function, BP, pulse, lipids; eliminated by kidneys
Nimodipine	30–60	tid	
Diltiazem	30–90	tid	
Ergotamine derivatives			After 6 mo therapy, review cardiac, pulmonary, and retroperitoneal regions for fibrotic changes; carefully observe contraindications
Methysergide‡	1–2	tid-5 times/d	
Methylergonovine	0.2–0.4	tid-qid	
Anticonvulsants			
Valproic acid‡	125–500	1–2 g/d in divided doses	Monitor hepatic and metabolic (platelets) parameters carefully; consider dose reduction when used with antidepressants, lithium, verapamil, phenothiazines, benzodiazepines, other anticonvulsants; observe warnings carefully; avoid using with barbiturates and perhaps benzodiazepines
Valproic acid (ER)‡	250–1000	500 mg–1 g/d, once per day dosing	
Valproic acid (IV)	250–750	1000–3000 mg/d	
Carbamazepine	100–200	300–200 mg/d in divided doses	Monitor hepatic and metabolic parameters carefully; consider dose reduction when used with anticonvulsants, lithium, verapamil, phenothiazines; observe warnings carefully; *reduces oral contraceptive efficacy*
Gabapentin	100–400	1800–3600 mg/d	May cause agitation and other CNS adverse effects
Topiramate	25–50	25 mg bid, tapered slowly to 200–400 mg/d	Sedation, cognitive impairment, abdominal cramps, and risk for renal stones are limiting features; liver function disturbances, acute myopia, and closed-angle glaucoma (in 1st month) require careful monitoring and immediate discontinuation; weight loss may occur

Table 25–2 continues

TABLE 25–2 (*Continued*)

DRUG NAME	mg/DOSE	STANDARD DAILY ADMINISTRATION	NOTES
Others			
Baclofen	10–20	tid-qid	Increase and decrease dose slowly and allow tolerance to develop; taper when discontinuing
Tizanidine	2–8	2–8 mg tid or prn; max dose 32–36 mg/d	May be used as abortive or preventive agent; sedation, hypotension, liver function disturbances must be considered and monitored; careful use with other α-adrenergic agonist agents such as clonidine and hepatotoxic agents is recommended; max dose is 36 mg/d
Lithium	150–300	bid-tid	Reduce dose in conjunction with verapamil, other calcium channel antagonists, and NSAIDs; monitor metabolic parameters
Oxygen inhalation	100% O_2 with mask	7 L/min for 10–15 min	Must be used at onset of attack of cluster headache; avoid around extreme heat or flame, such as cigarettes
Stadol Nasal Spray (butorphanol)[‡]	1 mg/spray; max use 2 dose d/wk		Useful for acute migraine but important side effects; dependency and addictive potential significant; avoid in patients with addictive or obsessive drug-taking patterns or history of drug overdose; avoid in patients with daily or almost daily headache; withdrawal symptoms can be severe
Botulinum toxin	Uncertain	Uncertain	At this time controlled studies have not established efficacy in headache
Melatonin	3–15	Usually hs	Its value in cluster headache is currently tentative but promising; risks in asthma and vasoconstrictive diseases remain to be defined

*Modified with permission from Saper et al.[1]

[†]Few of the medications listed in this table are either approved specifically for headache or have been shown by controlled studies to be effective for headache. Their inclusion reflects that they have been recommended from various sources as possibly useful for the treatment of some cases of headache.

[‡]Drugs that have been approved by FDA for the treatment of migraine, cluster headache, or tension-type headache.

[§]Avoid sustained use for more than 6 months without trial reduction.

ACUTE TREATMENT OF MIGRAINE

- ○ Simple and combined analgesics (acetaminophen, Excedrin, nonsteroidal anti-inflammatory drugs [NSAIDs], and others).
- ○ Mixed analgesics (barbiturate and simple analgesics: aspirin ± acetaminophen, ± caffeine), often avoided because of the likelihood of dependency and misuse.
- ○ Ergot derivatives, including dihydroergotamine.
- ○ Use of one or several triptan medications, including sumatriptan, naratriptan, almotriptan, rizatriptan, zolmitriptan, frovatriptan, and eletriptan.
- The triptans represent narrow-spectrum, receptor-specific (serotonin [5-HT_1]) agonists that stimulate the 5-HT_1 receptors to reduce neurogenic inflammation.[2,4,15,16] The ergot derivatives are broader-spectrum agents, affecting the serotoninergic receptors and also α-adrenergic and dopamine receptors (and others). While many patients respond well to the triptans, others appear to require the broader influence of ergot derivatives. Experienced clinicians are adept at administering several of the triptans as well as the ergots. Short-acting, rapidly effective triptans include almotriptan, sumatriptan, rizatriptan, zolmitriptan, and eletriptan, while naratriptan and frovatriptan have the longest half-lives. Several delivery formats are available in addition to tablets: injection (sumatriptan), nasal spray (sumatriptan and zolmitriptan), and rapidly dissolving forms (zolmitriptan and rizatriptan).

- Patients who have not responded to less potent medications require triptans or ergots for maximum benefit.
- Acute medications are used in conjunction with antinauseants and in combination with each other for maximum efficiency (do not combine ergots and triptans). Clinicians must be familiar with important contraindications and safety warnings of each of these medication groups as well as adverse effects and influence on hepatic metabolism, particularly when these drugs are used in combination with others.
- Finally, for reasons that are not fully understood but perhaps related to the cervical/trigeminal connections, occipital nerve blocks may relieve acute migraine attacks in some individuals. This method has been historically used by anesthesiologists but is increasingly employed by neurologists and others treating headache. Long-term value is rare, but short-term relief is frequently seen.

PREVENTIVE TREATMENT OF MIGRAINE

- The following medications are useful in the prevention of migraine[1,2] (see Table 25–2):
  - Tricyclic antidepressants (particularly amitriptyline, nortriptyline, and doxepin)
  - β-Adrenergic blockers (particularly propranolol and nadolol)
  - Calcium channel blockers (verapamil)
  - Anticonvulsants (valproic acid, gabapentin, topiramate)
  - Ergot derivatives (methylergonovine and methysergide)
  - Monoamine oxidase inhibitors (MAOIs) (for refractory cases)
  - Others: selective serotonin reuptake inhibitors (SSRIs), neuroleptics, tizanidine, botulinum toxin (?)
- Tricyclic antidepressants and beta blockers are well-established, first-line medications for preventive treatment of migraine in those patients who do not have contraindications or restrictions to either medication. Calcium channel blockers are generally not as effective. The anticonvulsants have considerable value and are particularly useful in the presence of neuropsychiatric comorbidity or other conditions, such as seizures and bipolar disorders, that might accompany migraine. With the possible exception of gabapentin, adverse effects generally limit their use as first-line agents in the absence of comorbidity.
- The SSRIs are helpful for neuropsychiatric comorbid conditions, such as depression and panic and anxiety disorders, but generally do not have a strong antimigraine influence. Some patients with migraine-related headaches benefit from the antidopaminergic influence of the new neuroleptics,[17] although the potential for adverse effects limits their widespread use. Tizanidine, an α-adrenergic agonist, has been shown effective in an adjunctive, preventive role.[18] Botulinum toxin is increasingly administered for the prevention of migraine. Numerous uncontrolled studies support efficacy, but there is a paucity of control data at this time. If botulinum toxin is shown to work for migraine, it is likely to work through a central mechanism and not through a primary muscular influence.[19,20]
- The treatment of *chronic migraine* is generally similar to that of episodic migraine. Treatment is directed at both the daily or almost daily pain and periodic attacks. Because of the likely pr esence of a progressive course, medication overuse, and neuropsychiatric comorbidity in this population, a more comprehensive approach beyond medications alone[21,22] is required. This includes cognitive behavioral therapy and other forms of psychotherapy and family therapy. Organic illness must be ruled out with appropriate testing in patients with frequent or daily headache and in those with neurologic findings (see Table 25–4 later).

TREATMENT OF CLUSTER HEADACHE

- Cluster headache responds and is treated differently than migraine. Because cluster headache attacks generally occur numerous times daily (one to eight times), the use of abortive medications is limited to only a few agents that are safe for such frequent use.

ACUTE TREATMENT OF CLUSTER HEADACHE

- Oxygen inhalation (7 L/min, 100% oxygen via mask)
- Triptans/ergot (avoid more than two usage days per week)
- Indomethacin, which is occasionally useful for cluster headache[1,2] (see Table 25–2)

PREVENTIVE TREATMENT OF CLUSTER HEADACHE

- Verapamil (120–160 mg three to four times daily) (Table 25–2)
- Lithium
- Divalproex/topiramate
- Melatonin 6–15 mg at night
- Seven-day prednisone burst (steroids are generally effective for cluster headache prevention, and short-term trials can be dramatically effective, but risks limit utility) (Table 25–3)
- Ergot derivatives (methylergonovine/methysergide)
- For intractable cases, hospitalization is recommended (see below). In some cases surgical intervention is required, but surgical treatment is limited due to the likelihood of postsurgical painful sequelae. Occipital nerve injection is effective in treating some attacks, and subcutaneous occipital stimulation has recently been reported as anecdotally effective (D.W. Dodick, personal communication, 2002)

TREATMENT OF OTHER PRIMARY HEADACHE DISORDERS

- *Chronic paroxysmal hemicrania* (CPH) and *episodic paroxysmal hemicrania* (EPH), as well as hemicrania continua, are characteristically sensitive to treatment with indomethacin at a dose of 25–50 mg three times

TABLE 25–3   Recommended 7-Day Prednisone Program*

DAY	BREAKFAST (mg)	LUNCH (mg)	DINNER (mg)
1	20 (4 pills)	20	20
2	20	20	20
3	20	15 (3 pills)	15
4	15	15	10 (2 pills)
5	10	10	10
6	10	5 (1 pill)	5
7	5	5	

*Five-milligram tablets; dispense 60 tablets.

daily.[23] SUNCT syndrome may respond to lamotrigine or gabapentin.[24]

DIAGNOSTIC TESTING AND SECONDARY HEADACHE DISORDERS

- More than 300 entities may produce symptoms of headache, many of which mimic the primary headache disorders. The clinician has the burden of ruling in and ruling out potentially relevant conditions in patients with recurring or persistent headache. Diagnostic testing includes a wide range of studies, including metabolic, endocrinologic, toxic, dental, traumatic, cervical, infectious, and space-occupying. Disturbances of CSF pressure, ischemic disease, and allergic conditions must be considered. Table 25–4 lists diagnostic tests that should be considered in intractable or variant cases.
- Important specific conditions to consider include those of the temporomandibular or dental structures, sphenoid sinuses (must specifically image and evaluate for sphenoid sinus disease), carotid and vertebral dissection syndromes, and cerebral venous occlusion.
- Because of the relevance of the cervical spine to the descending trigeminal system and headache physiology (trigeminal cervical connection), disturbances at the level of the upper cervical spine and its nerves and joints have become important targets for the treatment of otherwise pharmacologically resistant headaches. Premature or excessive use of interventional procedures is unwarranted, but when selective and expertly administered, they clearly have a role in the overall spectrum of diagnosis and treatment for headache conditions. Even more advanced treatments, such as implantable stimulators, are on the horizon.

TABLE 27–4   Diagnostic Testing

Physical examination
Metabolic evaluation
  Hematologic
  ESR/CRP
  Endocrinologic
  Chemistry
  Toxicology (drug screens, etc)
Standard x-rays
Neuroimaging
  CT
  MRI/MRA/MRV
Dental and otologic exam
Lumbar puncture
Radioisotope/CT myelogram
Diagnostic blockades
Arteriography

ESR, erythrocyte sedimentation rate; CRP, C-reactive protein; MRA, magnetic resonance angiography; MRV, magnetic resonance venography.

REFERRAL AND HOSPITALIZATION

- It is advisable to refer intractable headache patients to specialists, specialized clinics, and tertiary centers. Hospitalization is required for many complex patients whose medication misuse or the presence of intractable pain and behavioral/neuropsychiatric symptomatology has reached an intensity and complexity that makes outpatient therapy no longer appropriate (see below). Aggressive and thorough diagnostic assessment is mandatory to either rule out organic, toxic, or physiologic illness or define unrecognized provocative factors.

HOSPITALIZATION

- Intractable headache patients can respond to the more aggressive therapeutic environment and milieu in specialty inpatient programs when outpatient therapy has failed to establish efficacy.[25,26] Hospitalization should be considered when:
  - Symptoms are severe and refractory to outpatient treatment.
  - Headaches are accompanied by drug overuse or toxicity not treatable as an outpatient.
  - The intensity of neuropsychiatric and behavioral comorbidity renders outpatient treatment ineffective.
  - Confounding medical illness is present.
  - The presence of treatment urgency in a desperate patient exists.
- The principles of hospitalization[1] include:
  - Interrupt daily headache pain with parenteral protocols (see below).
  - Discontinue offending analgesics if rebound is present.
  - Implement preventive pharmacotherapy.
  - Identify effective abortive therapy.
  - Treat behavioral and neuropsychiatric comorbid conditions.
  - Employ interventional modalities when indicated.
  - Provide education.
  - Provide discharge and outpatient planning.
- A variety of parenteral agents can be used during hospitalization to control attacks, particularly during rebound withdrawal:
  - Dihydroergotamine (0.25–1 mg IV or IM, three times daily)
  - Diphenhydramine (25–50 mg IV or IM, three times daily)
  - Various neuroleptics (ie, chlorpromazine 2.5–10 mg IV, three times daily)
  - Ketorolac (10 mg IV or 30 mg IM, three times daily)

- ○ Valproic acid (250–750 mg IV, three times daily)
- ○ Magnesium sulfate (1 g IV, twice daily)
- These protocols can also be used for emergency department treatment of acute episodic migraine.

WHEN TO USE OPIOIDS

- Experience and data support the avoidance of sustained opioid administration in the chronic headache population. Use in acute situations when other treatments are contraindicated remains appropriate, but dose and amounts of prescriptions should be limited and monitored carefully. Sustained opioid administration can be considered in the following limited circumstances:
  - ○ When all else fails following a full range of advanced services, including detoxification
  - ○ When contraindications to other agents exist
  - ○ In the elderly or during pregnancy
- Except in the elderly or during pregnancy, patients must be refractory to aggressive therapies before opioids are administered regularly. Nearly 75% of refractory patients placed on daily opioids fail to gain effective control.[27,28] Approximately one-half of those maintained on opioids demonstrated noncompliant drug-related behavior. Despite reports of pain reduction, a major improvement in function was not noted in a significant percentage of patients.[1,27,28]

REFERENCES

1. **Saper JR, Silberstein SD, et al.** *Handbook of Headache Management.* 2nd ed. Baltimore: Lippincott Williams & Wilkins; 1999.
2. **Silberstein SD, Lipton RB, Dalessio DJ, eds.** *Wolff's Headache and Other Head Pain.* 7th ed. New York: Oxford Univ. Press; 2001.
3. **Olesen J.** Classification and diagnostic criteria for headache disorders, cranial neuralgias, and headache pain. *Cephalalgia.* 1988;8(Supp 7):1–96.
4. **Goadsby PJ, Lipton RB, Ferrari MD.** Migraine: Current understanding and treatment. *N Engl J Med.* 2002; 246:257–270.
5. **Bartsch T, Goadsby PJ.** Stimulation of the greater occipital nerve (GON) enhances responses of dural responsive convergent neurons in the trigeminal cervical complex in the rat. *Cephalalgia.* 2001;21:401–402.
6. **Burstein RH, Cutrer FM, Yarnitsky D.** The development of cutaneous allodynia during a migraine attack. *Brain.* 2000;123:1703–1709.
7. **Weiller CA, May A, Limmroth V, et al.** Brainstem activation and spontaneous human migraine attacks. *Nat Med.* 1995;1:658–660.

8. **Welch KM, et al.** Periaqueductal gray matter dysfunction in migraine: Cause or the burden of illness. *Headache.* 2001;41:629–637.
9. **Limmroth V, Katsarav AZ, Fritsche G, et al.** Features in medication overuse headache following overuse of different acute headache drugs. *Neurology.* 2002;59:1011–1014.
10. **May A, Bahra A, Buchel C, et al.** PET and MRA findings in cluster headache and MRA in experimental pain. *Neurology.* 2000;55:1328–1535.
11. **Leone M, D'Amico D, Moschiano F, et al.** Melatonin vs. placebo in the prophylaxis of cluster headache: A double-blind pilot study with parallel groups. *Cephalalgia.* 1996;16:494–496.
12. **Peres MF, Rozen TD.** Melatonin in the preventive treatment of chronic cluster headache. *Cephalalgia.* 2001;21:993–995.
13. **Goadsby PJ.** Short-lasting primary headaches: Focus on trigeminal autonomic cephalgias and indomethacin-sensitive headaches. *Curr Opin Neurol.* 1999;12:273–277.
14. **Srikiatkhachorn A, Puanguiyom MS, Govitrapon P.** Plasticity of 5-HT^{2a} serotonin receptor in patients with analgesic-induced transformed migraine. *Headache.* 1998; 38:534–539.
15. **Ferrari MD, Roon KL, Lipton RB, et al.** Oral triptans (serotonin 5-HT$^{1b/1d}$ agonist) in acute migraine treatment: A meta-analysis of 53 trials. *Lancet.* 2001;358:1668–1675.
16. **Saper JR.** What matters is not the differences between triptans, but the differences between patients. *Arch Neurol.* 2001;58:1481–1482.
17. **Silberstein SD, Peres MF, Hopkins MM, et al.** Olanzapine in the treatment of refractory migraine and chronic daily headache. *Headache.* 2002;42:515–518.
18. **Saper JR, Lake AE III, Cantrell DT, Winner PK, White JR.** Chronic daily headache prophylaxis with tizanidine: A double-blind, placebo-controlled, multicenter outcome study. *Headache.* 2002;42:570–582.
19. **Argoff CE.** A focused review of the use of botulinum toxins for neuropathic pain. *Clin J Pain.* 2002;18:S177–S181.
20. **Nixdorf DR, Heo G, Major PW.** Randomized control trial of botulism toxin A for chronic myogenous orofacial pain. *Pain.* 2002;99:465–473.
21. **Saper JR, Lake AE III.** Borderline personality disorder and the chronic headache patient: Review and management recommendations. *Headache.* 2002;42:663–674.
22. **Saper JR.** Chronic daily headache: A clinician's perspective. *Headache.* 2002;42:538.
23. **Boes CJ, Dodick DW.** Refining the clinical spectrum of chronic paroxysmal hemicrania: A review of 74 patients. *Headache.* 2002;42:699–708.
24. **Front CJ, Dodick DW, Bosch EP.** SUNCT responsive to gabapentin. *Headache.* 2002;42:525–526.
25. **Lake AE III, Saper JR, Madden SF, Kreeger C.** Comprehensive inpatient treatment for intractable migraine: A prospective long-term outcome study. *Headache.* 1993;33:55–62.
26. **Saper JR, Lake AE III, Madden SF, Kreeger C.** Comprehensive/tertiary care for headache: A 6-month outcome study. *Headache.* 1999;39:249–263.
27. **Saper JR, Lake AE III, Hamel RL, Lutz T, Branca B, Sims D.** Long-term scheduled opioid treatment for

intractable headache: 3-year outcome report. *Cephalalgia.* 2000;20:380.

28. **Saper JR, Lake AE III, et al.** 5-year outcome for sustained opioid therapy in patients with intractable headache (in preparation).

Further Reading

Goadsby PJ, Lipton RB, Ferrari MD. Migraine: Current understanding and treatment. *N Engl J Med.* 2002;246:257–270.

Olesen J, Tfelt-Hansen P, Welch KMA, eds. *The Headaches.* 2nd ed. Philadelphia: Lippincott Williams & Wilkins; 2000.

Silberstein SD, for the U.S. Headache Consortium: Practice parameter: Evidenced-based guidelines for migraine headache (an evidence-based review): Report of the Quality Standards Subcommittee of the American Academy of Neurology. *Neurology.* 2000;55:754–762.

26 LOW BACK PAIN

Michael J. Dorsi, MD
Allan J. Belzberg, MD, FRCSC

EPIDEMIOLOGY AND RISK FACTORS

- Low back pain (LBP) is pain arising from the spinal or paraspinal structures in the lumbosacral region. LBP extends approximately from the iliac crests to the coccyx.
- Radicular leg pain, or sciatica, may accompany low back pain but should be regarded as a separate entity with a distinct pathophysiology.
- LBP is the fifth most common reason for all physician visits[1] and the second most common symptomatic reason (upper respiratory symptoms are first).
- Fifty to eighty percent of adults experience LBP.[2]
- LBP is the leading cause of disability and lost production in the United States, with associated direct and indirect costs estimated to exceed $50 billion per year.[3]
- Despite the widespread opinion that 75–90% of patients with acute LBP recover within about 6 weeks, irrespective of their treatment,[4] pain may persist in up to 72% and disability in up to 12% of patients 1 year after their first episode of LBP.
- The predictors for LBP include:
  - Poor physical fitness and comorbidity
  - Social class, occupation, and employment status
  - Increasing age up to 55 years[5]
  - Obesity[5]
  - Dimensions of spinal canal
  - Smoking
  - Substance abuse history
  - Hard physical labor
- Predictors of chronicity and disability include:
  - Radicular leg pain[6]
  - Poor self-rated health status
  - A positive straight leg test[5]
  - Reduced elasticity/flexibility of the back
  - Poor coping strategies
  - High levels of distress, depression, and somatization[7]
  - Lower activity level
  - Anxiety

ETIOLOGY AND PATHOPHYSIOLOGY

- LBP can be arbitrarily classified based on symptom duration.
- The biological basis, natural history, and response to therapy differ for each category.
- Transient pain is short-lived (a few hours) and is usually activity-related.
- Patients rarely seek medical attention for transient pain unless the frequency of painful episodes becomes intolerable.
- Acute pain, by definition, resolves within 3 months. The onset of symptoms is spontaneous in approximately half of cases, with trauma accounting for the rest.
- Chronic LBP persists without change for months to years and may develop into a chronic pain syndrome marked by personality dysfunction and psychosocial and medical comorbidities.
- The differential diagnosis for LBP includes mechanical and nonmechanical causes (Table 26–1).
- Most patients have mechanical LBP.
- The specific pathology or exact anatomic source of pain cannot be determined by physical exam or diagnostic testing in 50–80% of patients with mechanical LBP.
- A pathologic diagnosis is attainable in most patients with LBP of nonmechanical origin.
- Pain can arise from anterior structures:
  - Discs
  - Vertebral bodies

TABLE 26–1   Differential Diagnosis of Low Back Pain (LBP)*

MECHANICAL LBP	NONMECHANICAL LBP	VISCERAL DISEASE
Lumbar strain or sprain	Neoplasia	Pelvic organs
Degenerative disease	Metastatic carcinoma	Prostatitis
Disks (spondylosis)	Multiple myeloma	Endometriosis
Facet joints	Lymphoma and leukemia	Chronic pelvic inflammatory disease
Diffuse idiopathic skeletal	Spinal cord tumors	Renal disease
Hyperplasia	Retroperitoneal tumors	Nephrolithiasis
Spondylolysis	Infection	Pyelonephritis
Spondylolisthesis	Osteomyelitis	Vascular disease
Herniated disk	Septic discitis	Abdominal aortic aneurysm
Spinal stenosis	Paraspinal or epidural	Aortoiliac disease
Osteoporosis with compression fracture	Abscess	Gastrointestinal disease
Fractures	Endocarditis	Pancreatitis
Congenital disease	Inflammatory arthritis	Cholecystitis
Severe kyphosis	Ankylosing spondylitis	Perforated bowel
Severe scoliosis	Reiter's syndrome	
Paget's disease	Psoriatic spondylitis	
	Inflammatory bowel disease	
	Polymyalgia rheumatica	

*Adapted from Atlas and Deyo.[8]

-   ○ Ligaments
-   ○ Muscles (ie, psoas)
- Pain can arise from midline structures:
  - ○ Spinal cord
  - ○ Neural compress
- Pain can arise from posterior structures:
  - ○ Facets
  - ○ Ligaments
  - ○ Sacroiliac joints
  - ○ Muscles

HISTORY

- Adequate history taking is essential to determine if mechanical back pain is present and to exclude "red flag" conditions, such as tumors, fractures, infections, cauda equina syndrome, and spinal osteomyelitis, that could be life-threatening if not treated (Table 26–2).

SEVERITY

- Although LBP may be severe, it is rarely described as excruciating; severe pain might indicate a new fracture, infection, or metastatic disease.

LOCATION

- Nonspecific LBP often radiates to the buttocks, hips, groin, and thighs. Radicular pain below the knee suggests nerve root compression, especially if it follows a dermatomal pattern.

TABLE 26–2   Red Flags Requiring Immediate Attention

Recent trauma
Mild trauma or strain with a history of osteoporosis
Unexplained weight loss
History of cancer
Fever
Pain worse at night
Bowel/bladder dysfunction
Intravenous drug use
Pain not relieved in the supine position/awakes patient from sleep

TIMING

- Pain severity commonly waxes and wanes over the course of a day. Pain that is constantly severe or that peaks at night when recumbent should heighten suspicions that it has a neoplastic etiology.

ALLEVIATING/AGGRAVATING FACTORS

- Back and leg pain associated with stocking-glove sensory loss during walking that is relieved by sitting or leaning forward is suggestive of neurogenic claudication due to spinal stenosis.
- Mechanical LBP due to spondylosis is typically exacerbated by increased activity and relieved by rest. Lying supine typically offers some relief.
- Postures that maximize axial loading (erect, sitting) typically exacerbate LBP.

ASSOCIATED SYMPTOMS

- Stiffness and fatigue commonly accompany LBP.

- Muscle weakness, sensory loss, and changes in bowel and bladder function suggest nerve root compression and may warrant aggressive investigation.
- Weight loss, low-grade fever, failure to improve, age greater than 50 years, and elevated sedimentation rate should increase concerns about neoplastic disease.
- Alerting features of spinal infection include fever, new-onset neurologic deficits, diabetes, immunocompromise, previous surgical procedure, catheterization, venous puncture, intravenous drug use, and an elevated sedimentation rate.

PHYSICAL EXAMINATION

INSPECTION

- With the patient erect, assess posture, symmetry, and spinal curvature.
- Asymmetric muscle spasm may produce asymmetry at the hip level or may cause new-onset scoliosis.
- Careful inspection involves evaluating muscle bulk and checking for atrophy.

PALPATION

- Assess bony spinal and soft tissue for paraspinal tenderness and muscle spasm.
- Examine the abdomen to determine if an aneurysm is present.
- Palpate for lymphadenopathy if the history is suggestive of neoplastic or infectious etiology.
- Palpate pulses in lower extremities.

RANGE OF MOTION

- Ask the patient to flex, extend, and rotate laterally to determine range limitations.
- Assess range of motion about the hip in patients with buttock or groin symptoms.

GAIT

- Normal gait, toe walking, and/or heel walking provide a gross assessment of functional strength.
- Flexed posture when walking is commonly seen with spinal stenosis or hip joint pathology.

MOTOR STRENGTH

- Examine strength in all muscle groups.
- Motor weakness, especially when it is asymmetric, can help identify an involved nerve root (Table 26–3).

TABLE 26–3 Physical Exam Findings Associated with Specific Nerve Root Impingement

NERVE ROOT	MUSCLE (MOTION)	SENSORY	DEEP TENDON REFLEX
L2	Iliopsoas (hip flexion)	Anterior thigh, groin	None
L3	Quadriceps (leg extension)	Anterior/lateral thigh	Patellar
L4	Quadriceps, ankle dorsiflexors (heel walking)	Medial ankle/foot	Patellar
L5	Ankle dorsiflexors, extensor hallucis longus (first toe dorsiflexion)	Dorsum of foot	None
S1	Gastrocnemius (toe walking)	Lateral plantar foot	Achilles

- Weakness of plantar flexion is uncovered by repetitive toe standing.

DEEP TENDON REFLEXES

- Diminished reflexes are consistent with nerve root compression (Table 26–3).
- Hyperreflexia suggests upper motor neuron injury in the spinal cord.

SENSATION

- Light touch and pinprick sensation should be assessed in a dermatomal pattern (Table 26–3).

DIAGNOSTIC SIGNS

- Straight leg raise that reproduces back pain is nonspecific but may predict a poor prognosis.
- A positive straight leg raise is highly suggestive of nerve root compression of the L5 or S1 roots.
- Extension of the hip stretches the femoral nerve and may reproduce symptoms stemming from pathology at the L3 or L4 segment.
- A contralateral "straight leg raise" that results in ipsilateral pain suggests a free fragment disc herniation.
- Internal/external rotation of the hip may detect hip joint pathology.

IMAGING

- Many imaging modalities are available for imaging the lumbar spine. Each has its own advantages, disadvantages, and indications (Table 26–4).

TABLE 26–4   Imaging Modalities for Low Back Pain

MODALITY	DEMONSTRATES	RECOMMENDED FOR	DISADVANTAGES

Plain x-rays	Lumbar alignment
	Size of vertebral bodies,
	    discs, neural foramina
	Bone density
	Fractures
	Osteophytes
		Possible fractures
		Arthropathy
		Spondylolisthesis
		Tumors
		Infections
		Stenosis
		Congenital deformities
			Do not detect disc bulges, focal
			    herniations, intraspinal masses, or small
			    paraspinous lesions
			Radiation exposure

CT	Cross-sectional images of spine	Bony/joint pathology
		    Arthropathy
		    Fractures
		    Tumors
		Lateral disc herniation
		Stenosis
		    Spinal canal
		    Neuroforaminal
		    Lateral recess
		Contraindication to MRI
			Cost
			Contrast required to image intrathecal anatomy
			Radiation exposure

MRI	Details of spinal cord
	Cauda equina
	Discs
	Paraspinal soft tissue
		Disk herniation
		Spinal stenosis
		Osteomyelitis
		Tumors
		    Spinal cord
		    Nerve roots
		    Nerve sheath
		    Paraspinal soft tissue
		Cauda equina syndrome
			Cost
			Poor for bony anatomy

- In most cases of acute LBP, imaging studies are unnecessary.
- Imaging provides valuable anatomic information but may not be helpful in identifying the cause of a patient's pain or in guiding management.
- In general, for patients under the age of 50 with acute LBP without a history of trauma, systemic disease, or neurologic deficit, the use of imaging should be delayed at least 1 month.
- Imaging is indicated in patients with clinical history and exam findings suggestive of "red flag" conditions, history of recent trauma, or persistent pain refractory to conservatory treatment.
- Imaging studies are appropriate in patients older than 50 who are more likely to have compression fractures, degenerative changes, and spinal stenosis.
- Plain radiographs in two views, anteroposterior and lateral, should be the initial modality of choice in most patients.
- Lateral oblique, flexion, and extension views should be reserved for confirmation of findings on initial films or for use when there is prior fusion or suspicion of instability.
- Many plain film findings, such as degenerative disc disease, vertebral osteophytes, facet joint arthropathy, transitional vertebrae, Schmorl's nodes, and spina bifida occulta, are present in close to one-half of the population and asymptomatic in most.[9]
- The best study for evaluation of the lumbar spine is MRI.[10]

TABLE 26–5   Contraindications to MRI

Cardiac pacemaker
Implanted cardiac defibrillator
Aneurysm clips
Carotid artery vascular clamp
Neurostimulator
Insulin or infusion pump
Implanted drug infusion device (relative)
Bone growth/fusion stimulator
Cochlear, otologic, or ear implant
Significant claustrophobia

- For patients with previous back surgery, gadolinium enhancement helps differentiate scar tissue from recurrent disc herniation.
- CT scanning is superior for imaging bony anatomy, metastases to the spine, and trauma.
- CT-myelography is indicated for patients with a contraindication to MRI (Table 26–5) or those with spinal instrumentation. This is the most sensitive test for spinal nerve compression but carries significantly greater risk than does MRI.

MANAGEMENT

- Since 1994, 11 countries have published guidelines for diagnosis and management of LBP,[8,11] which are generally followed with individual modification.
- Appropriate management involves formulating an accurate diagnosis.

- For patients with acute, nonspecific LBP, the primary treatment emphasis should be nonoperative care, time, reassurance, and education.[8,11]

NONOPERATIVE CARE

PATIENT EDUCATION
- Reassure the patient that full recovery is expected.
- Maintain an active and educational relationship with the patient.
- Future plans, diagnostic studies, and therapies should be discussed with the patient if symptoms persist.

PATIENT COMFORT
- Pain relief and return of function are primary goals.
- Work with the patient to find an effective therapeutic regimen.

PHYSICAL ACTIVITY
- Bed rest is not effective for LBP or radiculopathy and may be harmful.[11]
- Maintaining a normal activity level may result in a faster return to work, less chronic disability, and fewer recurrent problems[12] but may have little or no beneficial effect for acute LBP or radiculopathy.[11]
- Exercise may initially cause a slight increase in symptoms but overall may prove beneficial for preventing debility and improving weight control.
- Light aerobic exercises, such as swimming, walking, and using a stationary bicycle, may begin when the patient can sit comfortably and may be increased as tolerated.
- Strenuous activities, such as heavy lifting, twisting, and sitting/standing for prolonged periods, should be avoided until symptoms have resolved.
- Specific back exercises during the acute phase are not beneficial and may worsen symptoms.[12]

ORAL MEDICATIONS
- Nonsteroidal anti-inflammatory drugs (NSAIDs) and acetaminophen are first-line medications for acute LBP.[13] No intraclass differences in efficacy have been demonstrated for NSAIDs.[13] The favorable side effect profile of acetaminophen supports its use before undergoing trials with NSAIDs.
- Addition of a muscle relaxant may benefit patients with muscle spasms or trouble sleeping.
- During the acute phase, adding opiates to NSAIDs has no demonstrated clear benefit[13] and may add troubling side effects.

- Opioid use should be limited to patients with pain refractory to NSAIDs. Long-term use of opioids to treat chronic LBP, although controversial, is becoming commonplace.
- Oral corticosteroid use is controversial; some studies demonstrate lasting benefit and others show short-lived or no benefits.[14]

OTHER CONVENTIONAL THERAPIES
- Epidural steroid injections offer no long-term benefit for the treatment of LBP,[14] but may be effective in the small subset of patients with acute lumbosacral radicular pain.
- The benefit of injecting other sites to treat chronic LBP, including facet joints, trigger points, ligaments, and acute LBP without radiculopathy remains controversial,[15] but such injections may provide transient relief during acute LBP episodes.
- Although studies deny efficacy for bracing,[16] traction, physical modalities, behavioral therapy, transcutaneous electrical nerve stimulation,[16] acupuncture,[17] or "back school,"[16] many of these therapies can provide pain relief during the approximately 6 weeks it takes to heal the underlying cause of acute LBP.

SURGICAL INTERVENTION

- Only 1% of LBP sufferers have a medical condition requiring surgical intervention.[18]
- Surgical intervention should be reserved for patients with an identifiable pathology on imaging studies that is consistent with history and physical examination findings.
- Immediate surgery is reserved for patients with identifiable and correctable pathology causing incapacitating pain, progressive neurologic deficits, impaired bowel or bladder function, cauda equina syndrome, or extremely hazardous conditions (eg, infection or neoplasm).
- In cases of new-onset mechanical LBP, delaying surgery until the patient has had at least 1 month of nonoperative treatment is appropriate in most cases.
- If the patient is improving slowly, there is no harm in delaying surgery until symptoms plateau at an unacceptable level.
- Surgery on the lumbar spine corrects two abnormalities: compression of nerve roots and spinal instability.
- The procedures most frequently performed include discectomy, laminectomy, and spinal fusion.
- Satisfactory relief of pain is achieved in 16–95% of lumbar spinal fusions,[19] with better results achieved with laminectomy and discectomy.[20]

MANAGEMENT PLAN

- Overall, the prognosis remains favorable for patients presenting with acute LBP.
- Detailed history and physical examination identify those few patients with underlying conditions that require immediate attention.
- For most patients, imaging and aggressive interventions should be delayed until the patient has undergone 4–6 weeks of nonoperative care.
- Patients should be reassured that LBP only rarely leads to disability.
- Patients should be encouraged to return to normal activity and begin light aerobic exercises immediately while avoiding strenuous activities until symptoms resolve.
- Over-the-counter analgesics, NSAIDs, and acetaminophen are the first-line medications for pain relief.
- If pain is refractory to NSAIDs, opiates may be prescribed.
- If symptoms have resolved or are improving by 4–6 weeks, there is no need for further investigation.
- If symptoms progress or stabilize at an unacceptable level, clinical reassessment and imaging are mandated.
- Plain radiographs serve as the initial imaging study. MRI follows and is considered the diagnostic imaging study of choice.
- If there is bony pathology on plain radiographs or a history of trauma, a CT scan is indicated.
- Surgical intervention is an option only for patients with identifiable pathology on imaging studies that is consistent with their clinical presentation.
- Early surgical consideration is given to patients with a neurologic deficit due to nerve root compression, incapacitating pain, or a progressive neurologic deficit.
- Evidence of a cauda equina syndrome with loss of bowel or bladder control is an indication for emergent imaging and surgical decompression.

REFERENCES

1. **Hart LG, Deyo RA, Cherkin DC.** Physician office visits for low back pain: Frequency, clinical evaluation, and treatment patterns from a U.S. national survey. *Spine.* 1995;20:11.
2. **White K, Williams F, Greenberg B.** The ecology of medical care. *N Engl J Med.* 1961;265:885.
3. **Frymoyer JW, Cats-Baril WL.** An overview of the incidences and costs of low back pain. *Orthop Clin North Am.* 1991;22:263.
4. **Deyo RA, Phillips WR.** Low back pain: A primary care challenge. *Spine.* 1996;21:2826.
5. **Battie MC, Bigos SJ, Fisher LD, et al.** Anthropometric and clinical measures as predictors of back pain complaints in industry: A prospective study. *J Spinal Disord.* 1990; 3:195.
6. **Biering-Sorensen F.** A prospective study of low back pain in a general population. II. Location, character, aggravating and relieving factors. *Scand J Rehabil Med.* 1983;15:81.
7. **Pincus T, Burton AK, Vogel S, et al.** A systematic review of psychological factors as predictors of chronicity/disability in prospective cohorts of low back pain. *Spine.* 2002; 27:E109.
8. **Atlas SJ, Deyo RA.** Evaluating and managing acute low back pain in the primary care setting. *J Gen Intern Med.* 2001;16:120.
9. **Torgerson WR, Dotter WE.** Comparative roentgenographic study of the asymptomatic and symptomatic lumbar spine. *J Bone Joint Surg Am.* 1976;58:850.
10. **Modic MT, Masaryk TJ, Ross JS, et al.** Imaging of degenerative disk disease. *Radiology.* 1988;168:177.
11. **Hagen KB, Hilde G, Jamtvedt G, et al.** Bed rest for acute low back pain and sciatica. *Cochrane Database Syst Rev.* 2000;CD001254.
12. **Rozenberg S, Delval C, Rezvani Y, et al.** Bed rest or normal activity for patients with acute low back pain: A randomized controlled trial. *Spine.* 2002;27:1487.
13. **van Tulder MW, Scholten RJ, Koes BW, et al.** Nonsteroidal anti-inflammatory drugs for low back pain: A systematic review within the framework of the Cochrane Collaboration Back Review Group. *Spine.* 2000; 25:2501.
14. **Green LN.** Dexamethasone in the management of symptoms due to herniated lumbar disc. *J Neurol Neurosurg Psychiatry.* 1975;38:1211.
15. **Koes BW, Scholten RJ, Mens JM, et al.** Efficacy of epidural steroid injections for low-back pain and sciatica: A systematic review of randomized clinical trials. *Pain* 1995;63:279.
16. **van Tulder MW, Koes BW, Bouter LM.** Conservative treatment of acute and chronic nonspecific low back pain: A systematic review of randomized controlled trials of the most common interventions. *Spine.* 1997;22:2128.
17. **van Tulder MW, Cherkin DC, Berman B, et al.** The effectiveness of acupuncture in the management of acute and chronic low back pain: A systematic review within the framework of the Cochrane Collaboration Back Review Group. *Spine.* 1999;24:1113.
18. **Taylor VM, Deyo RA, Cherkin DC, et al.** Low back pain hospitalization: Recent United States trends and regional variations. *Spine.* 1994;19:1207.
19. **Turner JA, Ersek M, Herron L, et al.** Patient outcomes after lumbar spinal fusions. *JAMA.* 1992;268:907.
20. **Hoffman RM, Wheeler KJ, Deyo RA.** Surgery for herniated lumbar discs: A literature synthesis. *J Gen Intern Med.* 1993;8:487.

27 NECK AND SHOULDER PAIN

Donlin Long, MD

INTRODUCTION

- Neck pain ranks third after headache and low back pain as a cause of disability from pain in the United States.[1]
- Neck pain is second to low back pain for physical therapy referral, pain management, and spine surgery.[2]
- Painful sequelae of acceleration/deceleration injuries of the cervical spine have a huge impact worldwide.[3]
- Because conservative care of neck pain is an enormous expenditure within health care systems of most developed countries, the evaluation and rational treatment of neck pain are extremely important.
- Thus, it is essential to understand the causes, natural history, and potential treatments for cervical pain syndromes.

CAUSES AND NATURAL HISTORY

- Neck pain problems share the categories used for lumbar pain complaints.[2]
- Patients with transient syndromes who receive no treatment are ubiquitous but have little medical impact.
- Management of acute neck pain depends on the level of neurologic deficit.
- Neck pain usually relents spontaneously with symptomatic care within a month, and nearly all patients improve within 3 months; however, pain persists more than 6 months in a small percentage of patients.
- When an acute pain syndrome is associated with a significant neurologic deficit, the treatment goal may be to eliminate or control the deficit.
- Chronic pain syndromes are those that persist longer than 6 months and have little chance of spontaneous improvement. Because symptoms usually do not worsen, treatment is dictated by severity and the degree of interference with lifestyle.
- Transient and acute syndromes without neurologic deficits are often thought to arise from inflammation of ligaments and muscles,[4] but symptoms such as muscle spasm, tenderness, and focal areas of myositis (trigger points) may be epiphenomena, and we should not pursue ineffective therapies based on imaginary pathologic explanations.
- The common causes of neck pain are:
  - Acute musculoligamentous injury
  - Cervical spondylosis
  - Cervical disc herniation
  - Traumatic disc, ligament, capsular injury
  - Rheumatologic specific disease, that is, rheumatoid arthritis, ankylosing spondylitis
  - Tumor
  - Infection
- Acute neck pain syndromes with associated neurologic deficits are generally related to:
  - Acute cervical disc herniation
  - Chronic progressive nerve root or spinal cord compression
  - Tumor or infection (rarely)
- Posttraumatic injuries are equally difficult to define.[5]
  - Occasionally tests reveal evidence of a fracture, overt ligamentous injury, or clear acute disc injury, but the nonspecific changes of spondylosis are more likely.
  - Facet capsular injury may be important in a significant number of these patients.
  - Abnormalities uncovered by diagnostic nerve blocks and imaging studies explain many posttraumatic syndromes.[6]
  - For most patients, imaging study results are normal, yet epidemiologic studies prove the existence of cases of posttraumatic, musculoskeletal complaints relating to the spine.
- Unfortunately, the medicolegal and disability systems in developed countries have so clouded epidemiologic issues that it is impossible to study the problem definitively.[7,8]

DIAGNOSIS

- As with all spinal problems, diagnosis begins with a careful history.
- The origins of the pain need to be explored because management differs if the problem resulted from trauma.
- The character of the pain and nature of any pain radiation provide important information.
- Pain severity is the key to treatment choice.[9]

PHYSICAL EXAMINATION

- Physical examination is important, not to make a definitive diagnosis, but to ascertain the neurologic status of the patient, which is a key decision-making variable in management.
- Physical examination begins with assessment of range of motion supplemented by palpation for muscle spasm and areas of focal tenderness in cervical and shoulder girdle muscles.

- The routine neurologic examination includes assessment of stretch reflexes in upper and lower extremities, assessment of strength, and evaluation of sensation.
  - Hyperreflexia, abnormal pathologic signs, and gait disturbance suggest myelopathy.
  - Complaints confined to individual nerve roots suggest radiculopathy.
  - Widespread complaints involving multiple roots suggest involvement of the brachial plexus.

IMAGING THE CERVICAL SPINE

- In the acute phase with no neurologic deficit, imaging is not required unless symptomatic management fails.
- Imaging can be considered if the history suggests trauma, infection, tumor, and so on.
- When imaging is required, plain films with AP, lateral, oblique, odontoid, and flexion–extension views are obtained first.
- Cervical MRI allows the best evaluation of soft tissue, and CT best reveals bony changes.
- Both are often required, particularly to guide surgical therapy.

IMAGING FINDINGS

- Imaging studies might show only the mild age-related changes that might be expected in asymptomatic patients.
- Generalized spondylotic changes are common.
- Imaging provides a good demonstration of bony diseases, fractures, infections, tumors, acute disc herniation, chronic spondylotic changes, and arthritic conditions, such as ankylosing spondylitis and rheumatoid arthritis.
- Correlation of the imaging studies with the clinical syndrome facilitates diagnosis and management decisions.[10]
- If needed, electrophysiologic studies of nerve and muscle function differentiate peripheral neuropathy, primary muscle disease, and radicular–myelopathic syndromes.
- Electromyography is not required in most patients but helps in confirming radicular abnormality and assessing polyneuropathy syndromes.[11]
- Most patients have nonspecific acute neck pain with nonspecific shoulder, upper thoracic, and suboccipital radiation but no neurologic complaints or findings. Range of motion is restricted, and local areas of spasm and myositis are common.
- Neck pain, however, is often complicated by shoulder radiation, nonspecific arm radiation, and/or headache.

- Diagnostic blockade (most often of zygopophyseal joints, individual cervical nerve roots, and cervical discs) might reveal repairable spinal abnormalities.[12]
  - Positive blocks carried out with placebo control have a 90% selectivity and specificity.
  - Negative blocks have no diagnostic utility.
  - The lack of placebo control reduces the reliability of the blocks.[13]
  - The hypothesis is that stimulating the pain generator temporarily exacerbates the pain, and blockade reduces that pain for the expected duration of the injected local anesthetic.
  - A concordant block first reproduces the pain and then alleviates it by anesthetization.
  - Positive responses that outlast the anesthetic effect are considered indeterminate.[14]
- "Cervical discography" was introduced to identify degenerated cervical discs based on the incorrect supposition that such degeneration is always synonymous with pain generation.[15]
- The "cervical discogram" is now used to facilitate diagnostic disc blockade by reproducing the pain experienced when the disc is entered and/or distended by injection. Theoretically, this pain should be relieved by injection of a local anesthetic into the nucleus. This technique can differentially identify painful cervical segments.
- The next logical step, demonstrating the value of surgery on these segments, has not been made. Nevertheless, the approach is intuitively correct, and the "discogram" is a standard evaluation tool for patients with indeterminate clinical and imaging correlations.

TREATMENT

- In the absence of trauma or concurrent disease, most patients recover fully within 3 months and begin improving promptly when treated symptomatically with an appropriate combination of:
  - Adequate analgesia
  - Moderate restriction of activities for no more than a week
  - Avoidance of stressors that increase the pain and of local measures, such as heat, massage, ultrasound, electrical stimulation, and restoration of range of motion
  - Lightweight (2–5 pounds), over-the-door traction for 20- to 45-minute sessions
  - A soft cervical collar to support the neck and restrict neck motion
  - Passive physical therapy measures for short-term pain relief
  - Manipulation therapy for short-term pain relief

TABLE 27–1   Treatment of Acute Neck Pain

1. History and physical examination
2. Image only if there is:
   a. A "red flag" condition!
   b. An important neurologic deficit
   c. A history of trauma
3. Symptomatic care:
   a. Adequate analgesia
   b. Short-term restriction of activity
   c. Local symptomatic measures
4. Wait a month!
5. If not improved, image the neck:
   a. MRI
   b. Plain films with flexion/extension
6. Indications for surgery (benefits only root–cord compression and instability):
   a. Intractable pain
   b. Important neurologic deficit
   c. Failure to improve, 1–3 mo, and a significant disruption of lifestyle

- Occasionally patients without added symptoms experience such severe pain that symptomatic measures are inadequate; they should be treated as if they had a neurologic deficit.
- The strategy for acute pain associated with a radicular component or myelopathy depends on the severity of the pain and the deficit.
  - If the deficit is relatively minor, the patient should be treated as if the deficit did not exist.
  - If the deficit is significant (it should not be allowed to become permanent) or the pain severe, imaging should be performed immediately and treatment based on the findings. This is particularly true if there is evidence of myelopathy.
  - Most of these patients require cervical surgery (see Table 27–1).

MANAGEMENT OF SPECIFIC CLINICAL PROBLEMS

ACUTE CERVICAL DISC HERNIATION

- Acute cervical disc herniations may be midline, where they are most likely to compress the spinal cord, or lateral, where root compression is the issue.
- In patients with acute disc herniation and no or negligible neurologic deficit, symptomatic care is employed first.
- Unless the deficit is severe, a few days or up to a month should be allowed for it to relent.
- If there is a significant neurologic deficit, particularly myelopathy, surgery is unlikely to be prevented by conservative measures, and it is usually wise to proceed with an operation.
- Surgical treatment may be by the anterior or the posterior route.

- When myelopathy is present, the standard approach is anterior discectomy with or without fusion.
- Posteriorly, the procedure may be cervical laminectomy or laminoforaminotomy; the latter suffices if a single nerve root is compressed. The disc may or may not be removed.
- Outcomes are approximately equivalent, and the choice depends on the surgeon's preference and anatomic issues.

FOCAL OR DIFFUSE CERVICAL SPONDYLOSIS

- Many patients present with neck pain with or without neurologic complaints but with single- or multilevel spondylotic changes with disc degeneration and/or spur formation, often complicated by instability with some degree of spinal stenosis (Table 27–2).
- The surgical choices are again anterior and posterior.
  - Improved techniques have made multilevel anterior fusion a satisfactory choice when up to three levels are involved.
  - Posterior decompression with and without fusion is preferable when four or more levels are involved.

NECK PAIN WITHOUT SPECIFIC IMAGING ABNORMALITIES

- Another large category of patients includes those who have failed conservative symptomatic care and have incapacitating pain (Table 27–2).
- These patients may be treated with decompression or stabilization surgery if focal abnormalities can be discovered from diagnostic blocks.
- Discography identifies specific painful segments.
- Cervical facet blocks can identify painful arthropathy and individual root blocks and may substantiate a clinical impression of which nerve roots are involved.
- The procedures may be carried out equally well through an anterior or posterior approach.

NECK PAIN FROM INFECTION, TUMOR, OR INTERCURRENT DISEASE

- These problems are readily identified by imaging.
- Infections may require only antibiotic therapy after verification of the organism.
- Tumors causing pain usually must be removed.

TABLE 27–2   Long-Term Symptomatic Care

1. Avoidance of aggravating factors
2. Exercise for neck strengthening
3. Episodic use of supportive collar
4. Episodic use of traction
5. Anti-inflammatory drugs
6. Diagnostic blocks if steps 1–5 fail
7. Surgery based on block results

NECK PAIN SECONDARY TO SYSTEMIC ARTHRITIC CONDITIONS

- Neck pain is common in patients with arthritic conditions.
- Most patients are managed symptomatically.
- Some patients require operative procedures for decompression of the spinal cord, nerve roots, or stability.

NECK PAIN AND HEADACHE FOLLOWING ACCELERATION/DECELERATION INJURY

- Many patients suffer from incapacitating upper cervical pain, usually associated with suboccipital pain and radiation into C2 and C3 dermatomes.
- This condition has been ascribed to a variety of disc and ligament injuries.
- A significant number of these patients suffer from capsular injuries to cervical zygapophyseal joints, the most common being C2–3.
  - These patients can be accurately delineated with upper cervical blockade.
  - Anesthetization of C2 and C3 or upper cervical blockade of innervation of joints at C2–3 provides immediate relief.
  - In patients with positive blocks, we have achieved a 90% improvement rate with posterior fusion of C1, C2, and/or C3, depending on the level of injury.
- At least half of these patients do not respond to the blocks, indicating the possible presence of different injuries.
- This group of patients presents a major diagnostic problem.
- Cervical rhizotomy and nonspecific cervical stimulation with implanted stimulators are suggested treatments for these patients.[16,17]
- Routine imaging studies are virtually always normal or nonspecific because the capsular injuries are outside of resolution limits.
- In the United States, these complaints often occur postinjury when litigation is a factor, and the attendant psychosocial issues have colored physicians' understanding of these patients.
- Nevertheless, in patients with chronic and disabling pain who fail symptomatic measures after at least 1 year, proceeding to diagnostic blockade and possible surgery is a reasonable choice.[3,7,8]

CONCLUSION

- Acute neck pain can usually be managed symptomatically, and most occurrences spontaneously resolve within 1 month.
- Improvement within the first week is common.

- There is no need for imaging or other diagnostic studies in such patients.
- Symptomatic measures are adequate during the first month.
- Symptoms or history suggestive of significant intercurrent disease, significant neurologic deficit, or intractable pain are indications for early imaging and therapy.
- In today's legal climate, trauma is a reasonable indication for imaging.
- Symptomatic measures include adequate analgesia, local treatments to reduce spasm and inflammation, and time.
- When patients do not improve with symptomatic treatment, imaging should include plain films, MRI, and frequently CT.
- A diagnosis is usually made.
- When a specific focal diagnosis cannot be made, electrophysiologic studies and diagnostic blockade of suspect structures may be helpful when correlated with the clinical situation.
- Surgical treatment is required for instability (particularly that which threatens neurologic function), radicular compression, or spinal cord compression when neurologic findings are present.
- Intractable pain is another indication for surgery.
- A spectrum of surgical procedures can be employed, and the surgery should be tailored to the patient's individual needs and the abnormalities demonstrated.

REFERENCES

1. **Makela M, Heliovaara M, Sicvers K, et al.** Prevalence, determinants and consequences of chronic neck pain in Finland. *Am J Epidemiol.* 1991;134:1356.
2. **Long DM, BenDebba M, Torgerson WS, et al.** Persistent back pain and sciatica in the United States: Patient characteristics. *J Spinal Disord.* 1996;9:40.
3. **Riley LH 3rd, Long D, Riley LH Jr.** The science of whiplash [commentary on Radanov BP, Sturzenegger M, De Stefano G. Long-term outcome after whiplash injury: A 2-year follow-up considering features of injury mechanism and somatic, radiologic, and psychosocial findings]. *Medicine.* 1995;74:298.
4. **Borghouts J, Koes B, Bouter LM.** The clinical course and prognostic factors of non-specific neck pain: A systematic review. *Pain.* 1998;77:1.
5. **Abel MS.** Occult traumatic lesions of the cervical vertebrae. *Crit Rev Clin Radiol Nucl Med.* 1975;6:469.
6. **Aprill C, Bogduk N.** The prevalence of cervical zygapophyseal joint pain: A first approximation. *Spine.* 1992;17:744.
7. **Gotten N.** Survey of one hundred cases of whiplash injury after settlement of litigation. *JAMA.* 1956;162:865.

8. **Schrader H, Obelieniene D, Bovim G.** Natural evolution of late whiplash syndrome outside the medicolegal context. *Lancet.* 1996;347:1207.

9. **Barnsley L, Lord SM, Bogduk N.** Clinical review; whiplash injury. *Pain.* 1994;58:283.

10. **Rauschning W, McAfee PC, Jonsson H Jr.** Pathoanatomical and surgical findings in cervical spinal injuries. *J Spinal Disord.* 1989;2:213.

11. **Haldeman S.** Diagnostic tests for the evaluation of back and neck pain. *Neurol Clin.* 1996;14:103.

12. **Barnsley L, Bogduk N.** Medial branch blocks are specific for the diagnosis of cervical zygapophysial joint pain. *Region Anesth.* 1993;18:343.

13. **Barnsley L, Lord SM, Bogduk N.** Comparative local anaesthetic blocks in the diagnosis of cervical zygapophysial joint pain. *Pain.* 1993;55:99.

14. **Lord SM, Barnsley L, Bogduk N.** The utility of comparative local anaesthetic blocks versus placebo-controlled blocks for the diagnosis of cervical zygapophysial joint pain. *Clin J Pain* 1995;11:208.

15. **Bogduk N, Aprill C.** On the nature of neck pain, discography, and cervical zygapophysial joint blocks. *Pain.* 1993;54:213.

16. **Lord SM, Barnsley L, Wallis BJ, et al.** A randomized, double-blind, controlled trial of percutaneous radiofrequency neurotomy for the treatment of chronic cervical zygapophysial joint pain. *N Engl J Med.* 1996;335:1721.

17. **Lozano AM, Vanderlinden G, Bachoo R, et al.** Microsurgical C-2 ganglionectomy for chronic intractable occipital pain. *J Neurosurg.* 1998;89:359.

28 OROFACIAL PAIN

Bradley A. Eli, DMD, MS

INTRODUCTION

- It is estimated that more than 90% of all facial pain is the result of dental pathology. Dentists are often the specialists involved in diagnosis and treatment of these conditions.[1,2]
- Patients whose facial pain is unrelated to dental pathology often exhibit multiple signs and symptoms resulting in dental treatment. Misdiagnosis and mismanagement often follow and chronicity can occur.

DIAGNOSTIC GROUPING

- Because of the complexity associated with regional pain of the orofacial structures, many authors have suggested classification or grouping of tissue systems. The clinical characteristics allow the clinician to specify between extracranial, intracranial, musculoskeletal, vascular, neurologic, and psychologic.[1–4]

EXTRACRANIAL PAIN

- Head and neck structures involved with disease and pain include eyes, ears, nose, throat, sinuses, tongue, teeth, and glands. The quality of pain within this region and involving such a broad range of structures can range from mild aching to excruciating. As previously mentioned, the most common cause of pain in the orofacial region is dental pathology. One should consider this diagnosis early in the differential.
- The maxillary sinus is the most commonly affected region to involve disease. The typical descriptor of sinus disease includes constant, aching, pressure and fullness, and often includes the teeth or ear. Fever, congestion, and/or discharge may also be present. Head position or movement can often exacerbate this symptomatology.[1,2]
- Pain of the pulpal tissues or periodontium is often of high intensity and is often localized easily on examination or by patient report. Affected teeth are often painful to palpation or percussion and use of percussion testing is often extremely helpful in the diagnostic process.[1,2]

INTRACRANIAL PAIN

- Although uncommon, neoplasm, hematoma, hemorrhage, edema, aneurysm, and infection of the central nervous system can result in facial pain. Space-occupying lesions are often associated with progressive pain complaints and associated neurologic deficit or signs. Patient descriptors, including the "worst or first," have been identified as specifically pathognomonic of more serious conditions.[1–4]

MUSCULOSKELETAL PAIN

- Musculoskeletal oral facial pain may be the result of temporomandibular joint disorder, myofascial disorders, or systemic rheumatologic, collagen, or cervical spine disease.
- Temporomandibular joint disturbance refers to pain and dysfunction specific to the temporomandibular joint. This is often associated with dysfunctional mandibular movements or function. Palpation of the

region is often associated with exacerbations of pain and trauma is thought to be the main cause of dysfunction within the region. Microtrauma or macrotrauma has been discussed in much of the literature as the etiology of such disorders.[1–5]

- The temporomandibular joint is made up of three bony structures which include the condyle, disc, and skull. Coordinated movements within this structure require maintenance of the disc between the condyle and skull. This position is further complicated by the complex movements within the temporomandibular joint, which include both rotational and translational movements. Rapid displacement can result in pressures that often disrupt the disc–condyle relationship, resulting in incoordination. Mechanical disturbance of this joint is often associated with inflammatory events.[1,3,4]

FACIAL MUSCLE PAIN

- The most common muscle pain disorder of the orofacial region is myofascial pain. Muscle splinting, muscle spasm, and myositis are the most common acute conditions and, based on duration, may precede myofascial pain in etiology.[5]
- Factors associated with aggravation of muscle pain include prolonged muscle tension, poor posture, parafunction, trauma, sleep disturbance, viral infection, metabolic disturbance, and specific joint pathology.[5]

CERVICAL SPINE PAIN

- Disruption in position, structure, and movement can often refer pain into the orofacial region. Careful assessment, history, and clinical examination, including the cervical spine, are paramount to correct identification of etiology and exclusion of referred pain phenomena.[2,4,5]

VASCULAR PAIN

- Discussion regarding vascular etiology of pain refers specifically to the discussion of headache syndromes.
- Because headache is reviewed in a separate chapter (Chapter 25), it should be noted that migraine, as well as tension-type and cluster headaches, may occur anywhere within the trigeminal nerve supply.
- Carotodynia and temporal arteritis are localized to their specific anatomic locations.[1–4]

NEUROLOGIC PAIN

- Neurologic or neuropathic pain is the result of abnormality within nociceptors. Both peripheral and central locations and mechanisms may be involved.
- Decreased inhibition and or increased peripheral activity result in two basic types of pain: paroxysmal and continuous neuralgias.[1,6,7]

PAROXYSMAL NEURALGIAS

- Paroxysmal neuralgias are described as intense, sharp, stabbing, electric-like pains, usually of unilateral presentation involving the specific nerve.
- The intensity of the pain is described as "the worst pain known to man." This can occur in short or extended-duration volleys of pain.[6,7]

TRIGEMINAL NEURALGIA

- Trigeminal neuralgia affects the fifth cranial nerve. It is usually unilateral and is more common in women over the age of 50. Etiology includes idiopathic, demyelination, or vascular malformations.[1,2]
- Additional theory includes pathologic (bone) cavities at the site of previous tooth extraction, periodontal lesions, and previous endodontic therapy.[2]
- The majority of patients describe the classic high-intensity, triggerable pain in association with such activities as eating and talking. Even simple things, such as a cold breeze, can trigger a pain episode.[6,7]
- In addition to the paroxysmal nature of classic trigeminal neuralgia, a pretrigeminal neuralgia has also been described by Fromm. This is of note due to its more constant, dull aching characteristics and is often described by patients as "like a toothache."

GLOSSOPHARYNGEAL NEURALGIA

- Glossopharyngeal neuralgia is more rare than trigeminal neuralgia and involves branches of the glossopharyngeal and vagus nerves.[6,7]
- Symptoms of pain often include the ear, throat, tonsillar pillar, and submandibular regions.
- Triggering mechanisms, including chewing, talking, and swallowing, are often the hallmark.
- Aggressive imaging of the region is recommended because of the high suspicion of regional lesion or pathology associated with this disorder.[2]

DEAFFERENTATION SYNDROMES

- Partial or total loss of nerve supply to a region can result in a painful condition. This can be a direct result of traumatic injury, surgery, or a breakdown of the neural structures.

- Deafferentation-type pain is thought to involve the sympathetic nervous system, as blockade of this system may often eliminate or reduce the complaints of the patient. Characteristic descriptors used with this type of pain seem most commonly to include the words "burning," "stinging," "itching," and "crawling." It is not always present immediately at the time of injury or trauma and may be the result of a breakdown of the central inhibition.

ATYPICAL ODONTALGIA

- This condition has been proposed to describe a painful condition within the oral cavity.
- Additional terms synonymous with atypical odontalgia include phantom tooth pain, atypical facial neuralgia, and idiopathic toothache.
- Four common characteristics have been identified in association with this disturbance:
  ○ Duration longer than 4 months
  ○ Normal radiographic examination
  ○ No clinical observable cause
  ○ Description as a toothache or tooth site pain
- Dental procedures, testing, and diagnostic block of the somatic system are rarely conclusive. Confirmation is associated with positive sympathetic nerve block.[1,2,4]

NEUROMAS AND NEURITIS

- Neuromas and neuritis involve constant regional or localized pain.
- Neuromas are often associated with trauma or direct section of nerve tissue. Stimulation of the region is consistent for diagnostic purposes; however, treatment can be elusive due to recurrence.
- Neuritis as a systemic inflammatory response is often associated with herpes zoster viral infection. Aggressive and early identification and treatment can often decrease or eliminate the constant sequelae of a zoster episode.[6,7]

PSYCHOLOGICAL PAIN

- Psychological illness with reported pain complaints is common. Psychological illness requires the inclusionary criteria present for any other disease.

- Once identified, treatment plans should be developed and presented as clearly and succinctly as those of the other pain etiologies discussed.
- It is important to remember that many of the currently described pain disorders were at one time considered to be a psychological illness. Therefore, care should be exercised when allowing this diagnosis to be made by exclusion.[1,2]

TREATMENT

- Over the past two decades, significant progress has been made in understanding the pathophysiology of painful conditions.[8]
- Treatment of painful conditions of the orofacial region comprises identification of the specific illness and correction of the disorder present. For disorders for which no current curative understanding exists, a management strategy is employed.
- Management of painful conditions attempts to join the most efficient medications and treatment with little or no negative experience, side effect, or misuse potential. This goal can be quite elusive and is the subject of another chapter in this book.

REFERENCES

1. **Okeson JP, ed.** *Orofacial Pain: Guidelines for Assessment, Classification, and Management.* Carol Stream, IL: Quintessence; 1996.
2. **Bell WE.** *Orofacial Pains: Classification, Diagnosis, Management.* 4th ed. Chicago: Year Book; 1989.
3. **Pertes RA, Heir GM.** Temporomandibular disorders and orofacial pain. *Dent Clin North Am.* 1991;35:123–140.
4. **Pertes RA, Gross SG, eds.** *Clinical Management of Temporomandibular Disorders and Orofacial Pain.* Carol Stream, IL: Quintessence; 1995.
5. **Travell JG, Simon DG.** *Myofascial Pain and Dysfunction: The Trigger Point Manual.* Baltimore: Williams & Wilkins; 1999.
6. **Long D.** *Contemporary Diagnosis and Management of Pain.* 2nd ed. Newtown, PA: Handbooks in Health Care; 2001.
7. **Chapman CR, Syrjala KL.** Measurement of pain. In: Bonica JJ, ed. *The Management of Pain. Vol 1.* 2nd ed. Philadelphia: Lea & Febiger; 1990:580–594.
8. *American Pain Society Quality Assurance Standards for Relief of Acute Pain and Cancer Pain.* Proceedings of the 6th World Congress on Pain. New York: Elsevier; 1991.

29 PELVIC PAIN

Ricardo Plancarte, MD
Francisco Mayer, MD
Jorge Guajardo Rosas, MD
Alfred Homsy, MD
Gloria Llamosa, MD

INTRODUCTION

- Pelvic pain in any form, acute or chronic (lasting more than 4–6 months), localized or referred, is common in all age groups.[1]
- Pelvic pain is often accompanied by voiding problems and/or sexual dysfunction.[2,3]
- In one-third to one-half of cases, chronic pelvic pain (CPP) exists without evident pathology,[4] and even if a pathologic condition is visualized, it may not correlate with the pain.[5]
- The pelvis is a very complex neurophysiologic area, with intermingled contributions from the somatic, sympathetic, and parasympathetic nervous systems. Thus, pelvic pain may have mixed nociceptive and/or sympathetic characteristics of somatic, visceral, and/or neurogenic origin.
- Before intervening, a comprehensive, multidisciplinary, diagnostic workup is necessary. This multidisciplinary approach involves coordinating the opinions of the primary care physician as well as those of a selection of specialists in urology, gynecology, obstetrics, gastroenterology, physiotherapy or rehabilitation, pain management, sex therapy, and psychology.
- CPP may occur in 50% or more of patients with a history of physical and/or sexual abuse.[6] If such patients exhibit psychological distress and/or somatization, interventional techniques should be contraindicated or at least delayed.[7]
- Two approaches to the treatment of CPP are advocated: (1) removing the pelvic organs thought to be the pain generators, and (2) treating visible disease without removing pelvic organs.

- Pharmaceutical efficacy in controlling CPP may be achieved at the expense of dysfunction relating to libido, erection, ejaculation, and orgasm (Table 29–1). Carbamazepine, for example, can block testosterone production and result in testicular atrophy as well as gynecomastia and galactorrhea.[8]

NEUROANATOMY OF THE PELVIC AREA

- The pelvic viscera receive neurons from the sympathetic (thoracolumbar) and parasympathetic (craniosacral) systems.
- Most of the input to the pelvic, digestive, and urogenital structures (descending and sigmoid colon, rectum, vaginal fundus, bladder, prostate, prostatic urethra, testes, seminal vesicles, uterus, and ovaries) comes through the superior hypogastric plexus (SHP).
- In females, the corpus, cervix, and proximal fallopian tubes transmit pain through sympathetic fibers that arise from T10 through L1. These fibers include neurons that are part of the uterosacral ligaments and eventually coalesce into the SHP (presacral nerve). The presacral nerve does not receive fibers from the ovaries and lateral pelvic structures, which is why a presacral neurectomy is applicable only to midline pain.
- The lateral pelvis transmits pain via parasympathetic neurons (nervi erigentes) arising from S2 through S4. The presacral nerve divides into the hypogastric nerves that eventually form the inferior hypogastric plexus (IHP), and this plexus subdivides into vesical, middle rectal, and uterovaginal (Frankenhauser's) plexuses. Frankenhauser's plexus lies just lateral to the uterosacral ligaments and medial to the uterine arteries and receives pain sensations only from the corpus and vagina. Unlike presacral neurectomy, which can affect bladder and rectal function, transection of Frankenhauser's plexus during a laparoscopic uterosacral nerve division should not result in constipation or bladder dysfunction.[9]
- Thoracolumbar preganglionic nerves also synapse on postganglionic nerves in sympathetic chain ganglia

TABLE 29–1 Influence of Drugs on Sexual Function

DRUG	LIBIDO	ERECTION	EJACULATION	ORGASM
Antidepressants*		↓	↓↘	↘
Carbamazepine (see text)	↘	±	Failure	
Opioids—tramadol	↘	↘	↘	↘

Note: head-down arrows indicate that function is reduced; inclined arrows indicate that function may or may not be reduced.

*Lane RM. A critical review of selective serotonin reuptake inhibitor-related sexual dysfunction: Incidence, possible etiology and implications for management. *J Psychopharmacol.* 1997;11:72.

that mingle with autonomic sacral parasympathetic projections as well as with the pelvic somatic neuronal pathways.

- The IHP is the major neuronal coordinating center that supplies visceral structures of the pelvis and the pelvic floor. It has a posterolateral retroperitoneal component adjacent to each lateral aspect of the rectum, with interconnections between the right and the left side, and an anterior component associated with the distal extent of the hypogastric plexus, which is referred to as the "hypogastric ganglia" in males and the "paracervical ganglia" in females.
- Efferents from the IHP spread out to innervate the prostate, seminal vesicles, vas deferens, epididymis, penis, and penile corpuscavernosa in the male and the corpora of the clitoris, vagina, and urethra in the female.
- Sensations arising from the pelvic floor are conveyed mainly via the pelvic splanchnic nerve (PSN) to the sacral afferents (S2–4) of the parasympathetic system. Sensations from the testis and epididymis, however, may involve predominantly thoracolumbar (T10–L1) afferents.
- The following pathways may be interrupted by nerve blockade:
  - Spermatic cord (afferents from the testis)
  - SHP (see above)
  - Dorsal root ganglia
  - Sympathetic ganglia (in particular, the ganglion of Walter)
  - Peripheral nerves
  - Pudendal nerve (external anal sphincter, perineal cutaneous, and muscle branches, posterior part of the scrotum and penis [the anterior part is innervated by branches of the ilioinguinal and genitofemoral nerves that arise from L1–2 roots], clitoris, and labia majora)
  - Genitofemoral nerve (cremasteric muscles, spermatic cord, and parietal and visceral structures of the tunica vaginalis)

TABLE 29–2   Causes of Nonmalignant Buttock Pain

Infectious causes
    Furuncle
    Anorectal abscess
    Sacroiliitis
    Epidural abscess

Orthopedic causes
    Trauma
    Facet syndrome (posterior joint syndrome)
    Spondylolisthesis
    Ischial bursitis
    Myofascial syndromes
    Trochanteric bursitis
    Nonspecific low back pain

Neurologic causes
    Degenerative disc disruption
    Epidural process (hematoma, hemorrhage)
    Infarct of the conus medullaris
    Sacral neuropathy (neuritis, neuralgia)

TABLE 29–3   Causes of Nonmalignant Anorectal and Perineal Pain

Vascular causes
    Thrombosed hemorrhoid

Trauma
    Anal fissure
    Related to sexual activity
    Foreign body
    Urethral trauma

Infectious disease
    Herpes simplex
    Syphilis
    Abscess
    Proctitis
    Prostatitis
    Urethritis

Neurologic causes
    Cauda equina tumors
    Neuropathy

Other causes
    Dermatitis
    Muscular pain

CAUSES OF PELVIC PAIN

NONMALIGNANT CAUSES

- Pelvic pain has many causes, some clear and some obscure. (Tables 29–2 to 29–4 summarize the causes of nonmalignant pelvic pain. This chapter does not cover the common causes of CPP in gynecology, urology, or gastroenterology, such as endometriosis, digestive inflammatory diseases, and primary and secondary dysmenorrhea.)
- When the causes are obscure, the temptation to diagnose psychosomatic pain should be overcome, and screening should be conducted in an attempt to uncover organic causes.
- The history and physical examination must include an in-depth assessment of movement arches, sexual activity and performance, parturition, postural habits, and the minor changes that could help reveal the etiology of the pain.
- When a comprehensive evaluation excludes any underlying pathology or when the cause of pain is known but other treatments have failed, a trial of neural blockade may be undertaken to assess the pain's central sympathetic or somatic origin.[10] The institution of a

TABLE 29–4   Causes of Nonmalignant Lower Abdominal Pain

Intestinal causes
  Colitis
  Duodenal ulcer
  Sigmoid or cecal volvulus
  Fecal impaction
  Toxic megacolon
  Ischemic colitis
  Occlusion
  Diverticulosis

Infections
  Colitis
  Peritonitis
  Urinary infection
  Diverticulitis

Vascular
  Aneurysm
  Thrombosis

Urinary tract
  Lithiasis
  Nonspecific cystitis

Other causes
  Poisoning
  Pharmacologic undesirable effects
  Food allergy
  Metabolic disturbances
  Porphyria
  Addisonian crisis
  Ingestion of toxins (cocaine, arsenic, mercury)

differential spinal or epidural block and/or the sequential administration of more specific procedures aimed at the discrete and specific interruption of sympathetic versus somatic nerve impulses could be most helpful.

- CPP, especially urogenital pain, poses the greatest diagnostic challenge.[11,12]
- CPP may be caused by:
  ○ Dysfunctional, high-pressure voiding
  ○ Intraprostatic ductal reflux
  ○ Microorganisms, such as gram-positive uropathogens (*Enterococcus* and *Staphylococcus aureus*) and gram-positive organisms (coagulase-negative *Staphylococcus*, *Chlamydia*, and *Ureaplasma*).[13]
  ○ Cryptic, nonculturable organisms, such as biofilm bacteria, viruses, and cell wall–deficient bacteria
  ○ Autoimmune disorder
  ○ Chemical-urinary metabolites of pyrimidines and purines
  ○ Neuromuscular disorder
  ○ Interstitial cystitis
- The diagnostic protocol consists of assessing symptoms and physical findings and conducting laboratory studies when the patient is not taking antibiotics, α blockers, nonsteroidal anti-inflammatory agents, narcotics, or analgesics.

NONMALIGNANT CAUSES SPECIFIC TO MALES

- CPP syndrome is a common urologic diagnosis in men younger than 50 years, accounts for 173 visits per urologist per year, and poses diagnostic and treatment dilemmas (see Table 29–5).
- In the United States, "chronic prostatitis," with a prevalence rate of 5–8.8%, leads to an estimated 2 million office visits per year and causes a negative impact on quality of life similar to that in patients with unstable angina, recent myocardial infarct, or active Crohn's disease.
- "Chronic prostatitis" is a misnomer; there is no proven prostate disease, and it is unlikely that the syndrome has association with the gland. The anatomic distribution of "chronic prostatitis" includes the prostate, bladder, penis, urethra, testis, epididymis, rectum, and pelvic floor.
- The medical histories of these patients tend to be remarkably similar and include a symptomatic genitourinary constellation of complaints, often coincident with a meaningful psychosocial event. In most cases, the disorder has been diagnosed as prostatitis and treated empirically with potent oral antibiotics despite a lack of microbiologic culture. A urinalysis is generally normal. Because patients often respond dramatically to antibiotic treatment, most urologists prescribe such agents.
- Myofascial trigger points on the pelvic floor and/or abdominal wall are a common cause of "chronic prostatitis."
- Pelvic floor tension myalgia is characterized by continuous habitual contraction of the muscles of the pelvic floor (levator ani and short external rotators of the hip) and may be secondary to a local, painful inflammation. The pain is exacerbated by sitting in cars and is accompanied by suprapubic pressure, genital pain, and variable urinary symptoms. As the pain increases, the tension and contraction of the pelvic muscles also increase, creating a vicious cycle. The prostate is not usually tender, but movement of parapsoriatic fascia by palpation elicits pain.
- Treatment of trigger points and associated referred pain seeks to interrupt these reflexes with such interventions as:
  ○ Pelvic massage therapy, which involves rubbing the muscle fibers along their lengths from origin to insertion with a stripping motion. The urologist should apply as much pressure as the patient can tolerate with moderate pain. The prostate gland and surrounding endopelvic fascia should remain the primary focus of therapy.

TABLE 29–5   Clinical Aspects of Pelvic and Urogenital Pain in Males

	ORCHIALGIA	PROSTATITIS	PROSTADYNIA	PENILE PAIN
Age (years)	30–40		20–60	15–60
Prevalence (%)		25		
Symptoms, radiation	• Abdomen • Back • Legs • Perineum	• Prostadynia (30%)	• Urinary urgency • Dysuria • Pain, discomfort	• Dysesthesia • Hyperesthesia • Hypoesthesia
Sexual dysfunction	• Usually none • Painful ejaculation	• Often • Painful ejaculation for several days	• Usually none • Painful ejaculation	• Possible erectile dysfunction
Main causes	Referred from: • Hip • Nerve entrapment: (ilioinguinal, genitofemoral) • Arterial aneurysms: compression	• Bacterial (acute and chronic) • Nonbacterial	Referred from: • Colon • Rectum • Osteitis pubis	• Paraphimosis • Priapism • Herpes simplex • Trauma • Peyronie disease
Other neuropathic causes	• Epilepsy • Diabetic • Postvasectomy • Discal protrusion • Hydrocele • Varicocele • Spermatocele: often coincidental		• Increased sympathetic activity • Myofascial • Dg of exclusion	• Intracavernous drug injection • Penile prothesis • Pudendal injury
Evaluation	• Clinical • Urologic • Neurologic • Herniography • Physiosexual • Psychosexual • Lumbar sympathetic block	• Bacterial culture, microwave hyperthermia	• Urodynamic • Obstruction • Neurologic • Physiosexual • Psychosexual	• Previous acute history of pain • Neurologic • Physiosexual • Psychosexual

- ○ Ischemic compression, in which specific trigger points are pressed continuously for 60 to 90 seconds.
  - ○ Stretching, anesthetic injections, electrical neuromodulation, and mind–body interactions, such as progressive relaxation exercises and anorectal biofeedback.
- Well-trained physiotherapists who understand myofascial trigger points and soft tissue mobilization are needed for this labor-intensive therapy.
- It is not unusual for a patient to require several months of weekly therapy.

NONMALIGNANT CAUSES SPECIFIC TO FEMALES

- Nononcologic CPP accounts for 10–19% of hysterectomies (a controversial procedure for this indication) and 40% of laparoscopies[14] (see Tables 29–6 and 29–7).
- Pain may arise from the uterus, cervix, or ovaries and be caused by a variety of conditions, including pelvic adhesions, endometriosis, and pelvic congestion. Many of these conditions can be distinguished from levator ani syndrome and coccygodynia by history, physical examination, and, occasionally, laparoscopy.[15]

- The annual prevalence of chronic pelvic pain in the primary care setting among women aged 15 to 73 (38/1000) is comparable to the prevalence of asthma (37/1000) and of back pain (41/1000).[16]
- In the premenstrual period, adnexal tenderness is often reported during a bimanual examination, and the uterus is often retroverted, boggy, and symmetrically enlarged. The patient's level of psychological distress is often high. Dysmenorrhea is a frequent complaint. Uterine pain is felt most characteristically in the hypogastrium and suprapubic regions.
- Endometriosis, when symptomatic, is often only associated with dysmenorrhea, but chronic pain may develop and become severe and constant. The identification of nonpigmented endometriosis in 1986 has increased laparoscopic recognition of this disorder. The severity of pain correlates poorly with the extent of observed disease. Hysterectomy and bilateral salpingo-oophorectomy may relieve pain in more than 90% of cases; preservation of one or both ovaries results in a small but significant recurrence rate.[17]
- Pelvic congestion (overfilling of the pelvic venous system) may be a cause of unexplained, chronic, dull, aching pain secondary to venous stasis or ovarian varices[18] and may be relieved by hormonal treatment.[19]

TABLE 29–6   Clinical Aspects of Pelvic and Urogenital Pain in Females

	VULVODYNIA OR VULVAR HYPERESTHESIA	CLITORAL PAIN
Age	18–59 *Max*: • 18–29 Caucasian • Perimenopausal: dysesthetic essential vulvodynia	Young
Incidence/prevalence (%)	?/? Obstetric: 16–47% dyspareunia 1–5y postepisiotomy	Among African ethnicity
Symptoms, radiation	• Chronic discomfort • Burning, stinging, after acute onset • Irradiation to perineum or pudendal area • Often no other findings except for local signs of dermatoses	• Burning, stinging sensation of the area, exacerbated by contact
Sexual dysfunction	16–20% • Entry dyspareunia (tampon) • Next-day sexual pain • Luteal phase • *Candida* hypersensitivity ±HPV ±Lichen ±Pain	
Main causes	• Dermatosis (cortisone) • Vestibulitis (increased intraepithelial nociceptive nerve free endings?) • Cyclic • Vulvovaginitis • Papillomatosis	Female genital mutilation
Other causes	*Multifactorial*: • Genetic predisposition? • Local therapy: steroid, cream, CO_2 laser, surgery • Pattern of sexual activity • Sexual trauma • Differential diagnosis: pudendal neuralgia? if perimenopausal, vulvodynia	
Evaluation	• Swab test • Routine evaluation of infections • Oxalate critalluria? • Biopsy for: Dermatitis Lichen Herpes LED Behçet's disease • Physiosexual • Psychosexual	

Typically, this pain increases at the end of the day, after prolonged standing, in the premenstrual period, or after nonorgasmic coitus and often is unilateral.

• Dense and vascularized pelvic adhesions may cause CPP, which may be relieved by adhesiolysis.[20]

• Myofascial trigger points with attendant sustained muscular tension and/or painful spasms may be related to stress and autonomic hyperactivity,[21] prolonged sitting,[22] and/or trauma from parturition, sexual activity, or surgery.[23]

• Women with significant central dysmenorrhea may be candidates for laparoscopic uterosacral nerve ablation (LUNA). LUNA should be performed only if the uterosacral ligaments are clearly visualized. It can be achieved using laser or bipolar electrodesiccation and transection/resection with scissors.[24]

• Women with central dysmenorrhea, especially those who have failed LUNA, may benefit from laparoscopic presacral neurectomy (LPSN). Complete familiarization with retroperitoneal anatomy is essential for any surgeon performing LPSN. The superior portion of the presacral nerve runs from the bifurcation of the aorta to the junction of L5–S1 vertebral bodies. The boundaries for LPSN are (1) superiorly, the bifurcation of the aorta; (2) on the right, the right internal iliac artery and right ureter; (3) on the left,

TABLE 29–7 Clinical Aspects of Pelvic and Urogenital Pain in Males and Females

	URETHRAL SYNDROME (US)	PERINEAL PAIN	MYOFASCIAL PAIN
Age	• 15–40 women • Men • Children	18–65	
Symptoms, radiation	• Urinary urgency, frequency, and dysuria (urinary hesitance and pain) • Suprapubic and back pain	• See prostadynia (Table 29–5) for males • See vulvodynia (Table 29–6) for females	*Trigger points*: • Abdominal wall • Pelvic floor: bimanual examination
Sexual dysfunction	None	±	±
Causes	*Increased external urethral sphincter tone*: differential diagnosis—systemic diseases: • Diabetes • Multiple sclerosis • Collagen diseases	Many—extensive differential diagnoses: • Pudendal nerve entrapment • Meningeal cysts • Treat with neuroleptics (catecholamine depletors relieve pain)	• Stress • Autonomic hyperactivity • Prolonged sitting • Parturition • Sexual activity • Surgery • Clinical

Evaluation	• Exclude:
	    Infections
	    Tumors
	    Stones
	• Urodynamic
	• Neurology
	• Psychology
		• Gastroenterologic
		• Proctologic
		• Gynecologic
		• Urologic
		• Neurologic
		• Physiosexual
		• Psychosexual
		• Pudendal block as a diagnostic tool	

the inferior mesenteric and superior hemorrhoidal arteries; (4) inferiorly, just below the division of the right and left inferior hypogastric plexus; and (5) deep, the periosteum of the vertebral bodies.[4]

ANORECTAL PAIN

• Anorectal pain occurs in association with a variety of organic conditions, but the most common functional disorders are levator ani syndrome and proctalgia fugax.

LEVATOR ANI SYNDROME

• This syndrome, also known as puborectalis syndrome, chronic proctalgia, and pelvic tension myalgia,[25] is characterized by a dull, aching, or pressurelike discomfort in the rectum that lasts several hours. Prolonged sitting and defecation precipitate the pain, and some patients experience difficult defecation or a sense of incomplete evacuation.[26] An important clinical finding is palpable tenderness of overly contracted levator ani muscles as the examining finger moves from the coccyx posteriorly to the pubis anteriorly. Often the tenderness is asymmetric and occurs on the left side more frequently than on the right.

• The diagnostic criteria are chronic or recurrent episodes of rectal pain or aching that last 20 minutes or longer and have occurred for at least 3 months in the absence of other causes such as ischemia, inflamma-

tory bowel disease, cryptitis, intersphincteric abscess, anal fissure, hemorrhoids, or coccygodynia.[27]

• The role of anorectal manometry in the evaluation of such patients is not established, but increased anal channel pressures and increased electromyographic activities are often present.[28]

• Treatment includes digital massage to tolerance three or four times per week, the use of muscle relaxants, such as diazepam and methocarbamol, and sitz baths.[3]

PROCTALGIA FUGAX

• Proctalgia fugax is characterized by sudden, severe, aching, gnawing, cramping, or stabbing rectal pain lasting several seconds or minutes before disappearing completely, leaving the patient asymptomatic until the next episode.[29,30]

• Women are more likely than men to experience proctalgia fugax; however, no relationship exists between proctalgia fugax and irritable bowel syndrome.

• The diagnosis depends on the absence of anorectal disease that could produce rectal pain. Although the pain occasionally may last 30 minutes, only 10% of patients report pain lasting longer than 5 minutes; occasionally, pain may awaken the patient from sleep.[31] Reports of associated anal sphincter spasm or contractions of the puborectalis and external anal sphincter muscles have not been substantiated.

• Proctalgia fugax has been treated with clonidine, inhaled salbutamol, nitrates, diltiazem, and caudal epidural blocks.[32]

PELVIC JOINT DYSFUNCTIONS

- A variety of dysfunctions exist within the pelvic joints, including the symphysis pubis joint. Often, symphysis pubis dysfunctions are accompanied by dysfunctions within the sacroiliac (SI) joints. These combined dysfunctions usually manifest as a rotation (anterior or posterior) or a shear (superior or inferior) of the entire bony hemipelvis (innominate).[33]

DYSFUNCTIONAL SYMPHYSIS PUBIS

- With dysfunctional symphysis pubis, pain may be referred to the testicle or the vagina, or down the medial thigh toward the knee on the affected side. If the symphysis alone is dysfunctional, testicle pain occurs after heavy lifting. When the SI joints are involved, low back pain (LBP) occurs with somatic characteristics.
- The diagnosis is made primarily by history and physical examination but may be confirmed with plain radiographs using special stress views and with bone scans. A pelvic MRI may detect an edema within the symphysis pubis.[34,35]
- Patients presenting with pelvic joint dysfunctions do not fit the standard medical paradigms for LBP or groin pain and, thus, present a diagnostic dilemma to physicians not trained in manual medicine techniques. Misdiagnosis is common. The pain does not follow a radicular pattern, and radiculopathy can be excluded with a thorough neurologic evaluation. Further complicating the presentation, secondary trigger points within the gluteus medius, piriformis, and other pelvic muscles may exist as a consequence of the joint imbalances. These trigger points refer symptoms down the leg in the nonradicular patterns of classic myofascial pain.[36]
- Treatment: try to relocate the bone into place with external manipulation. If unsuccessful, surgery is indicated.[33]

SACROILIAC SYNDROME

- Sacroiliac (SI) joint pain may result from spondyloarthropathy, pyogenic or crystal arthropathy, fracture of the sacrum and pelvis, or diastasis.[37]
- The phenomenon of pain emanating from the SI joint in the absence of a demonstrable lesion is termed "SI syndrome" or "SI joint dysfunction" and is presumed to be a mechanical disorder.
- While definitive epidemiologic studies are lacking, SI syndrome appears to occur predominantly in women.[38]
- Diagnostic criteria for SI syndrome[39] include (1) pain in the region of the SI joint with possible radiation to the groin, medial buttocks, and posterior thigh; (2) reproduction of pain by physical examination techniques that stress the joint; (3) elimination of pain with intraarticular injection of local anesthetic; and (4) an ostensibly morphologically normal joint without demonstrable pathognomonic radiographic abnormalities.
- Treatment has included mild oral analgesics and anti-inflammatory agents, diagnostic/therapeutic SI joint injections with an anesthetic and corticosteroid in conjunction with or after a course of physical therapy, muscle balancing and pelvic stabilization exercises, and orthoses.

ISCHIAL SPINE AND PUDENDAL NERVE ENTRAPMENT

- Pudendal nerve entrapment (PNE) causes neuropathic pain.
- In men with PNE, aberrant development and subsequent malpositioning of the ischial spine appear to be associated with athletic activities during their youth. The changes occur during the period of development and ossification of the spinous process of the ischium.
- PNE can cause chronic perineal pain. Patients with PNE typically present with pain in the penis, scrotum, labia, perineum, or anorectal region that is exacerbated by sitting, relieved by standing, and absent when recumbent or when sitting on a toilet seat.
- In PNE, the pudendal nerve is trapped between the sacrotuberous (ST) and sacrospinous (SSp) ligaments and may engage the falciform process of the ST ligament.[40,41]
- Stretching of the pudendal nerve from chronic constipation causes neuropathy.
- Normal vaginal delivery causes measurable neuropathy that lasts approximately 3 months.[42]
- The striking common feature in all patients is that flexion activities of the hip (sitting, climbing, squatting, cycling, and exercising) induce or exacerbate urogenital pain, CPP, or prostatitis-like pain.[43]
- Attention must be paid to (1) the transverse diameter of the ST and SP ligaments that compress the pudendal nerve; (2) the dimensions of the greater sciatic notch (diameter and depth) correlated with age, weight, and body habitus; (3) the cross-sectional area of the greater sciatic notch and the piriformis muscle; and (4) sequential pelvic x-rays in youthful and maturing athletes to measure changes in position and appearance of the ischial spine.
- The primary hypothesis about the etiology is that hypertrophy of the muscles of the pelvic floor during years of youthful athleticism causes elongation and posterior remodeling of the ischial spine. The SSp ligament then rotates, causing the ST and SSp ligaments to overlap. The ligaments act like a lobster claw,

crushing the pudendal nerve as it traverses the interligamentous space. In addition, in this position the pudendal nerve travels a longer course because it is posterior or dorsal to the SSp ligament. In this course it may stretch over the SSp ligament or the ischial spine during squatting, sitting, or rising from a seated position. We surmise that the gluteus muscle, which is intimately attached to the ST ligament, exerts a shearing effect as it extends the hip while the pelvic floor is forced inferiorly during the Valsalva maneuver.

- Pudendal canal decompression leads to pain relief in 70–86% of patients and to improved associated urinary and fecal incontinence in 65–82%.[44]

DIFFERENTIAL DIAGNOSES

- Gynecologic disease, including endometriosis, adhesions (chronic pelvic inflammatory disease), leiomyoma, pelvic congestion syndrome, and adenomyosis
- Gastrointestinal disease, including constipation, irritable bowel syndrome, diverticulitis, diverticulosis, chronic appendicitis, and Meckel's diverticulum
- Genitourinary disease, including interstitial cystitis, abnormal bladder function (bladder dyssynergia), and chronic urethritis
- Myofascial disease, including fasciitis, nerve entrapment syndrome, and hernias (inguinal, femoral, spigelian, umbilical, and incisional)
- Skeletal disease, including scoliosis, L1 through L2 disc disorders, spondylolisthesis, and osteitis pubis
- Psychological disorders, including somatization, psychosexual dysfunction, and depression

MALIGNANT CAUSES

- Pain is not usually an early sign of pelvic neoplasm but is associated with advanced pelvic cancer in about 75% of cases.
- Pelvic pain from malignant causes is usually visceral and occurs when an expanding tumor invades adjacent neural structures, giving rise to a neuropathic component or to somatic pain when the pelvic wall is involved. Visceral or neuropathic pain is commonly referred to the rectum, may be experienced in the lower back, hypogastrium, and perineum, and can be especially troublesome when associated with destruction of the sacrum.
- Visceral pain is the result of smooth muscle spasms of the hollow viscus, distortion of the capsule of solid organs, inflammation, traction or twisting of the mesentery, ischemia, or necrosis.[45,46]

- Neuropathic pain is encountered in 60% of patients with malignant disease of soft tissues invading the nerve trunk and with sacral invasion from carcinoma of the cervix, uterus, vagina, colon, and rectum in women and from penile, prostate, and colorectal carcinoma and sarcoma in men. The infiltration of the perineal nerves results in lumbosacral plexopathies producing symptoms of sensory loss, causalgia, and deafferention. Lumbosacral plexopathy frequently accompanies genitourinary tumors in the pelvis and occasionally develops after radiation to the area. Pain is likely to be neuropathic and is felt in the buttocks, radiating down the leg in the dermatomal distribution of the lumbar nerve roots and, perhaps, extending into the feet.
- Tumor involvement in the epidural space may resemble this pain syndrome but is more likely to be bilateral. Pain may be the initial symptom, but as the disease progresses, sensory and motor deficits may develop.
- Coccygeal plexopathy caused by tumors low in the pelvis may also mimic lumbosacral plexopathy but is more likely to be accompanied by sphincter dysfunction and perineal sensory loss.
- Somatic pain in these patients is due to stimulation of nociceptors in the integument and supporting structures (striated muscles, joints, periosteum, bones, and nerve trunks) by direct extension through fascial planes and lymphatic supplies.
- Primary treatment involves surgery, chemotherapy, and/or radiation therapy to debulk the tumor. When further antitumor therapy is not feasible, pharmacotherapy with NSAIDs, opioids, and adjuvant analgesics is instituted. Invasive approaches are considered if dose-limiting side effects cannot be reversed.[47] Early neurolytic blockade can be appropriate in the context of poor compliance with oral medication for economical or cognitive reasons. Also, infiltrating the plexus before it is rendered inaccessible by invasion of the tumor and/or the surrounding ganglions may increase the success rate.

INTERVENTIONAL TECHNIQUES

GENERAL GUIDELINES

- Lytic or local anesthetic blocks of the autonomic system need to be assessed clinically and with appropriate tests to allow proper evaluation and follow-up.
- Whether done with lytic or local anesthetic solutions, these blocks should be thoroughly explained to the patient and carried on with total consent.

- Routine coagulation tests should be conducted and inquiries made about any previous transfusion or hemorrhagic problems.
- Use of lactate Ringer's preblock infusion is mandatory to prevent hypotension.
- The help of an assistant for regular vital sign checking and proper sedation is necessary.
- Radiologic guidance (fluoroscopy or CT scan) should be used to avoid major neurologic complications.
- One must proceed gently, controlling each step with an aspiration test in each quadrant, and/or test doses, and/or dye injection before injecting a lytic solution.
- Injecting variable quantities (12–20 mL) of air may facilitate the double-contrast image visualization of the space available for the lytic or local anesthetic solution to spread, without diluting it.
- During injection, all of the patient's complaints must be respected and assessed.
- Patients should be carefully observed for 24 hours postprocedure, with an emphasis on neurologic examinations.
- A proper neurosurgical environment must be available in case of a progressive neurologic complication.

INDICATIONS AND TECHNIQUES FOR DIFFERENT INTERVENTIONAL BLOCKS

LUMBAR SYMPATHETIC BLOCK
- Performed at the level of L1–2, the well-known technique of bilateral lumbar sympathetic block may be an effective management tool for some patients with CPP.
- The lumbar sympathetic chain does not innervate pelvic structures directly, but a large amount of injected solution likely diffuses caudally.
- No controlled studies attest to the efficacy of these blocks in testicular pain, although neurophysiologic reasons may explain the role of the lumbar sympathetic chain in conveying testicular pain: some of the testicular afferents enter the spine through thoracolumbar levels.[48]

SUPERIOR HYPOGASTRIC PLEXUS BLOCK
- The SHP, or presacral plexus, lies immediately anterior to the sacral promontory at the level of the L5–S1 interspace, in proximity to the bifurcation of the common iliac vessels. The SHP carries nerve fibers from the pelvic viscera (see above). It is retroperitoneal and bilateral, and contains parasympathetic nerve fibers (S2–4).
- Injection of the SHP requires radiologic guidance, with fluoroscopy or, more efficiently, CT scanning.

- The SHP block is efficacious and safe in patients with advanced cancer.[50,51] Poor results should be expected in patients with extensive retroperitoneal disease overlying the plexus because of inadequate spread of the neurolytic agent.
- SHP block can serve as a less invasive diagnostic, prognostic, and therapeutic tool than such techniques as presacral neurectomy for painful pelvic conditions of nononcologic origin (ie, dysmenorrhea).
- SHP block can be used as a diagnostic tool for referred LBP (viscerosomatic convergence) from the abdomen or pelvis. One of the differential diagnoses of LBP is pain of visceral origin in the pelvis, which is sensed by the patient as LBP. In women who present with CPP *and* LBP, when the pelvic pain resolves with SHP block, we have observed that the LBP does also, indicating that the LBP was a secondary phenomenon referred from the pelvis and did not require primary treatment.
- When the SHP blockade is used for diagnostic/prognostic purposes, we inject 6–8 mL of 0.25% bupivacaine through each needle.
- For therapeutic (neurolytic) blocks, we use a total of 6–8 mL of 10% aqueous phenol through each needle. During manufacture, a small amount of glycerin is added to keep the phenol in solution.[52]
- Hysterectomy is one of the most common gynecologic procedures performed to relieve CPP, but the result is not always positive. It is possible that an SHP block may predict the success of hysterectomy for CPP and, if so, prevent unnecessary hysterectomy. In a prospective clinical trial of 15 women scheduled for hysterectomy who received an SHP block, 11 had 100% relief with the SHP blockade and complete relief after hysterectomy, 2 experienced 90% pain relief with both procedures, 1 patient had 70% improvement and refused surgery, and 1 patient did not improve after SHP blockade and did not have surgery.

Technique
- The SHP can be accessed via a posterior paravertebral, transdiscal, transvascular, or transvaginal approach. We have performed more than 800 SHP blocks using the posterior paravertebral approach, with no complications and minimal side effects.
- An SHP block may be preceded by a single-shot, L4–5 epidural injection of 5–10 mL 1% lidocaine to enhance patient cooperation by reducing reflex muscle spasm, ameliorating the discomfort associated with contact of needles with periosteum, and reducing movement. Alternatively, these goals can be achieved with local infiltration of the intervening muscle planes.

- The patient assumes the prone position with padding placed beneath the pelvis to flatten the lumbar lordosis.
- The lumbosacral region is cleansed aseptically.
- The location of the L4–5 interspace is approximated by palpation of the iliac crests and spinous processes, and then is verified by fluoroscopy.
- Skin wheals are raised 5–7 cm bilateral to the midline at the level of the L4–5 interspace.
- A 7-inch, 22-gauge, short-beveled needle with a depth marker placed 5–7 cm along the shaft is inserted through one of the skin wheals, with the needle bevel directed toward the midline.
- From a position perpendicular in all planes to the skin, the needle is oriented about 30° caudad and 45° mesiad so that its tip is directed toward the anterolateral aspect of the bottom of the L5 vertebral body.
- The iliac crest and the transverse process of L5, which sometimes is enlarged, are potential barriers to needle passage and necessitate the use of the cephalolateral entrance site and oblique trajectory described.
- If the transverse process of L5 is encountered during advancement of the needle, the needle is withdrawn to the subcutaneous tissue and redirected slightly caudad or cephalad. The needle is again advanced until the body of the L5 vertebra is encountered or until its tip is observed fluoroscopically to lie at its anterolateral aspect.
- If the vertebral body is encountered, gentle effort may be made to advance the needle further. If this is unsuccessful, the needle is withdrawn and, without altering its cephalocaudal orientation, is redirected in a slightly less mesiad plane so that its tip is "walked off" the vertebral body. The needle tip is advanced approximately 1 cm past the depth at which contact with the vertebral body occurred, at which point a loss of resistance or "pop" may be felt, indicating that the needle tip has traversed the anterior fascial boundary of the ipsilateral psoas muscle and lies in the retroperitoneal space. At this point the depth marker should, depending on the patient's body habitus, lie close to the level of the skin.
- The contralateral needle is inserted in a similar manner, using the trajectory and the depth of the first needle as a rough guide.
- Biplanar fluoroscopy is used during needle passage to verify needle placement. Anteroposterior views should demonstrate the needle tip's locations at the level of the junction of the L5 and S1 vertebral bodies, and lateral views should confirm placement of the needle tip just beyond the vertebral body's anterolateral margin.
- Injection of 3–4 mL of water-soluble contrast medium through each needle is recommended to further verify accuracy of placement.

- In the anteroposterior view, the spread of the contrast medium should be confined to the paramedian region. In the lateral view, a smooth posterior contour corresponding to the anterior psoas fascia indicates that needle depth is appropriate.
- Alternatively, computerized axial tomography may be used, permitting visualization of the vascular structures.
- Additional precautions include careful aspiration before injection and the use of "test" doses of local anesthetic. Vascular puncture with a risk of subsequent hemorrhage and hematoma formation is possible due to the close proximity of the bifurcation of the common iliac vessels. Intramuscular or intraperitoneal injection may result from an improper estimate of needle depth. These and less likely complications (subarachnoid and epidural injection, somatic nerve injury, renal or ureteral puncture) usually can be avoided by careful observation of technique.

Ganglion Impar Blockade (Ganglion of Walther)

- The ganglion impar is a solitary retroperitoneal structure located at the level of the sacrococcygeal junction that marks the termination of the paired paravertebral sympathetic chains.
- Although the anatomic interconnections of the ganglion impar are poorly understood, its sympathetic component likely predominates.
- Blocking the ganglion impar (ganglion of Walther) can relieve intractable neoplastic perineal pain of sympathetic origin.[53,54]
- The first report of interruption of the ganglion impar for relief of cancer perineal pain appeared in 1990. All 16 patients (13 women, 3 men, ranging in age from 24 to 87 years, median=48 years) had advanced cancer (9 cervix, 2 colon, 2 bladder, 2 rectum, 2 endometrium), and pain had persisted in all cases despite surgery and/or chemotherapy and radiation, analgesics, and psychological support. Each patient had localized perineal pain characterized as burning and urgent (in 8) or of a mixed character (in 8). Pain was referred to the rectum (7), perineum (6), or vagina (3). After preliminary local anesthetic blockade and subsequent neurolytic block, 8 patients experienced complete (100%) relief of pain, and the remainder experienced significant reductions in pain (90% for one, 80% for two, 70% for one, and 60% for four) as determined with a visual analogue scale. Repeated blocks in two patients led to further improvement. Follow-up depended on survival and was carried out for 14–120 days.[55]
- In patients with incomplete relief of pain, residual somatic symptoms may be treated with either epidural injections of steroid or sacral nerve blocks.

Technique

- The stylet is removed from a standard 22-gauge, 3.5-inch spinal needle, which is then manually bent about 1 inch from its hub to form a 25–30° angle. This maneuver facilitates positioning of the needle tip anterior to the concavity of the sacrum and coccyx.
- The needle is inserted through the skin wheal with its concavity oriented posteriorly, and, under fluoroscopic guidance, is directed anterior to the coccyx, closely approximating the anterior surface of the bone, until its tip is observed to have reached the sacrococcygeal junction.
- Retroperitoneal location of the needle is verified by observation of the spread of 2 mL of water-soluble contrast medium, which typically assumes a smooth margined configuration resembling an apostrophe.
- Four milliliters of 1% lidocaine or 0.25% bupivacaine is injected for diagnostic and prognostic purposes, or,

alternatively, 4–6 mL 10% phenol is injected for therapeutic neurolytic blockade.

PERIMEDULLAR BLOCK AND INTRASPINAL OPIOID THERAPY

- Subarachnoid phenol saddle block is appropriate treatment for intractable perineal pain in the presence of urinary diversion and colostomy. It is performed with a spinal needle at the L5–S1 level with the patient seated and inclined backward.
- When the above conditions are not met, the subarachnoid route for neurolysis may be preferred because the spread of the lytic substance in this case is more predictable.
- Because motor paresis can be a complication, perimedullary (spinal or epidural) opioid therapy,[56] with or without dilute concentrations of local anesthetic,[57] is a preferable option.

TABLE 29–8   Current Treatments in Urogenital Pain*

CLINICAL ENTITY	TREATMENT	
	NONINTERVENTIONAL	INTERVENTIONAL
Orchialgia	NSAIDs+antibiotics ±ATD, anticonvulsivants ±Opiates[a] TENS[d]	**Lumbar sympathetic block with LA or phentolamine/lido infusions for sympathetically maintained pain**[b] **SHP blockade**[c]
Prostatitis (nonbacterial)	Antibiotics?[e] Relaxation techniques[f]	Microwave hyperthermia
Prostadynia	Alpha blocking agents[g]	**? Hypogastric block (?)**
Penile pain	Treat underlying diseases	**? Hypogastric block (?) if pudendal nerve injury**
Vulvodynia or vulvar hyperesthesia	Antibiotics, antimycotics Creams: lido, estrogen Low-oxalate diet and Ca citrate to decrease oxalate crystalluria[j] Biofeedback[k]	Perineoplasty: excision of the vulvar vestibule[h,i]; good results (?)
Clitoral pain	?	?
Urethral syndrome (US)	**Electrostimulation** and biofeedback techniques[l]	Various resection, fulguration, and instillation procedures[m]
Perineal pain	And primary disorders And neuroleptic drug exposure (cathecolamine depletors) And Parkinson's disease (anti-Parkinson's therapy)	**Pudendal nerve block** Surgical neurolysis of pudendal nerve[n] or resection of meningeal cysts

*Proposed interventional techniques, apart from surgery, are in boldface. LA, local anesthetics; ATD, antidepressant; TENS, transcutaneous electric nerve stimulation; SHP, superior hypogastric plexus.

[a]Costabile RA HM, Mc Leod DGL: Chronic orchialgia in the pain prone patient: The clinical perspective. *J Urol.* 1991;146:1571.

[b]Wesselmann U. Treatment of neuropathic testicular pain. *Neurology.* 1996;46(Suppl):206.

[c]Baranowski AP, Johnson NS. A review of urogenital pain. *Pain Rev.* 1999;6:53.

[d]Holland JM, Gilbert HC. Phantom orchialgia. *J Urol.* 1994;152:2291.

[e]De la Rosette JJMC, Karhaus HFM. *Eur J Urol.* 1992;22:14.

[f]Moul JW. Prostatitis: Sorting out the different causes. *Postgrad Med.* 1993;94:191.

[g]Barbalias GA, Liastikos GN. Alpha blockers for the treatment of chronic prostatitis in combination with antibiotics. *J Urol.* 1998;159:883.

[h]Woodruff JD, Poliakoff S. Treatment of dyspareunia and vaginal outlet distortions by perineoplasty. *Obstet Gynecol.* 1981;57:750.

[i]Goetsh MF. Simplified surgical revision of the vulvar vestibule for vulvar vestibulitis. *Am J Obstet Gynecol.* 1996;174:1701.

[j]Baggish MS, Johnson Rl. Urinary oxalate excretion and its role in vulvar pain syndrome. *Am J Obstet Gynecol.* 1997;177:507.

[k]Glaser HI. Treatment of vulvar vestibulitis syndrome with EMG biofeedback of pelvic floor musculature. *J. Reprod Med.* 1995;40:283.

[l]Zufall R. Ineffectiveness of the treatment of urethral syndrome in women. *Urology.* 12:1978;337.

[m]Messinger EM. *Campbell's Urology.* Philadelphia: Saunders; 1992.

[n]Robert R BC, Faure A, Lehur PA, et al. La chirurgie du nerf pudendal lors de certaines algies perineales: Evolution et résultats. *Chirurgie.* 1993;119:535.

- Chronic spinal infusion could be carried out through a variety of drug delivery systems ranging from a temporary, percutaneous, tunnelized, epidural catheter to a totally implanted system.[58] Nevertheless, the limited availability and high cost of these implantable devices, as well as development of tolerance, are potential limiting factors.

PERIPHERAL NERVE BLOCK

- Blockade of paravertebral nerves may be considered when pain is referred from the bony pelvis.
- Peripheral neurolysis for the management of cancer pain is well described[59] but seldom used, as most of the pain emanating from the pelvic structures is of sympathetic origin.

PUDENDAL NERVE BLOCK

- The pudendal nerve (PN) lies close to the internal pudendal artery and posterior to the sacrospinous ligament.[60]
- Successful block of the PN bilaterally provides analgesia to the lower third of the vagina and to the posterior two-thirds of the vulva.
- A PN block can be performed:
  ○ Transvaginally, by puncturing the wall of the vagina at the juncture of the ischial spine and the sacrospinous ligament to avoid unintentional needle placement into the rectum, bladder, bowel, or uterine artery.
  ○ Transgluteally, where the nerve is blocked medially to the ischiatic spine slightly below the ischiosacral ligament through a skin wheal and a 3.5-inch, 22-gauge needle.
  ○ Through the buttock, puncturing the PN proximally before its passage through Alcock's canal at the intersection of a vertical line descending from the posterosuperior ischiatic spine and a transversal one (horizontal) crossing the sacrococcygeal joint.[61] A neurostimulator attached to a shielded needle permits precise localization of the PN by reproducing dysesthesia in its distribution area.
- PN block with electromyographic studies of the pelvic floor can help differentiate neuralgia caused by nerve entrapment from other causes of perineal pain.[62,63]

OTHER PERIPHERAL BLOCKS

- Coccygeal, ileoinguinal, and genitofemoral nerve blocks can relieve somatic or neuropathic pelvic pain following trauma of the coccyx or abdominal surgery.

CONCLUSION

- In the yet obscure world of pelvic pain, interventional techniques are helpful when properly designed in a comprehensive evaluation of the patient's psychological, physiologic, and sexual status.

- In the setting of nononcologic pain, these procedures have diagnostic, prognostic, and therapeutic value.
- The use of sympathetic blocks (either the hypogastric or the ganglion impar) seems promising in the setting of chronic pelvic pain, including pain caused by non-bacterial prostatitis and vulvar or clitoral pain.
- In the world of cancer pain, sympathetic blocks may also be used for diagnostic purposes and for predicting the efficacy of neurolytic techniques (Table 29–8).

REFERENCES

1. **Wesselmann U.** Pain of pelvic origin: An updated review [Refresher course syllabus]. IASP; 1999:47.
2. **Wesselmann U, Heinberg LJ.** The urogenital and rectal pain syndromes. *Pain.* 1997;73:269.
3. **Huffman JW.** Dyspareunia of vulvo-vaginal origin: Causes and management. *Postgrad Med.* 1983;73:287.
4. **Reiter RC.** Nongynecologic somatic pathology in women with chronic pelvic pain and negative laparoscopy. *J Reprod Med.* 1991;36:253.
5. **Stout AL.** Relationship of laparoscopic findings to self report of pelvic pain. *Am J Obstet Gynecol.* 1991;164:73.
6. **Toomey TC.** Relationship of physical or sexual abuse to pain and psychological assessment variables in chronic pelvic pain patients. *Pain.* 1993;53:105.
7. **Walker EA.** Medical and psychiatric symptoms in women with childhood sexual abuse. *Psychosom Med.* 1992;54:658.
8. **Nezhat C.** A simplified method of laparoscopic presacral neurectomy for the treatment of central pelvic pain due to endometriosis. *Br J Obstet Gynecol.* 1992;99:659.
9. **Elbaya TA, El-Halwagy HE.** Focus on primary care: Chronic pelvic pain in women. *Obstet Gynecol Surv.* 2001; 56:757.
10. **Raj PP.** *Cancer Pain, Local Anesthetic Blockade.* Philadelphia: Lippincott; 1993.
11. **Baranowski AP, Johnson NS.** A review of urogenital pain. *Pain Rev.* 1999;6:53.
12. **Patt RB.** Pelvic pain. In: *Pain Medicine—A Comprehensive Review.* Mosby; 1996:440–448.
13. **Anderson RU.** Management of chronic prostatitis— Chronic pelvic pain syndrome. *Urol Clin North Am.* 2002;29:235.
14. **Peterson HB, Philips JM.** American Association of Gynecologic Laparoscopists' 1988 survey membership on operative laparoscopy. *J Reprod Med.* 1990;35:587.
15. **Wald A.** Functional anorectal and pelvic pain. *Gastroenterol Clin North Am.* 2001;30:243.
16. **Zondervan KT, Yudkin PL, Vessey MP, et al.** Prevalence and incidence in primary care of chronic pelvic pain in women: Evidence from a national general practice database. *Br J Obstet Gynaecol.* 1999;106:1149.
17. **Stovall TG, Ling FW, Crawford DA.** Hysterectomy for chronic pelvic pain of presumed uterine etiology. *Obstet Gynecol.* 1990;75:676.

18. **Edwards RD, et al.** Pelvic pain syndrome: Successful treatment of a case by ovarian vein embolization [Case Report]. *Clin Radiol*. 1993;47:429.

19. **Reginald PW, et al.** Medroxyprogesterone acetate in the treatment of pelvic pain due to venous congestion. *Br J Obstet Gynecol*. 1989;96:1148.

20. **Peters AA, et al.** A randomized clinical trial on the benefits of adhesiolysis in patients with pelvic adhesions and chronic pelvic pain. *Br J Obstet Gynaecol*. 1992;99:59.

21. **Duncan CH.** A psychosomatic study of pelvic congestion. *Am J Obstet Gynecol*. 1952;64:1–12.

22. **McGiveney JQ.** The levator syndrome and its treatment. *South Med J*. 1965;58:505.

23. **Drossman DA.** Sexual and physical abuse in women with functional or organic gastrointestinal disorders. *Ann Intern Med*. 1990;113:828.

24. **Morales AJ, Murphy AA.** Endoscopic treatment for endometriosis. *Obstet Gynecol Clin*. 1999;26:121.

25. **Sinaki M, Merritt JL, Stilwell GK.** Tension myalgia of the pelvic floor. *Mayo Clin Proc*. 1977;52:717.

26. **Grant SR, Salvati EP, Rubin RJ.** Levator syndrome: An analysis of 316 cases. *Dis Colon Rectum*. 1975;18:161.

27. **Whitehead WE, Wald A, Diamant NE, et al.** Functional disorders of the anus and rectum. *Gut*. 1999;45 (Suppl 2):1155.

28. **Grimaud JC, Bouvier M, Naudy B, et al.** Manometric and radiologic investigations and biofeedback treatment of chronic idiophatic anal pain. *Dis Colon Rectum*. 1991;34:690.

29. **Thompson WG.** Proctalgia fugax. *Dig Dis Sci*. 1981;26:1121.

30. **Khan A, Ahmed M, Talati J.** Seminal vesicle cystic dilatation masquerading as proctalgia fugax. *Br J Urol*. 1989;64:428.

31. **Kamm MA, Hoyle CHV, Burleigh DE, et al.** Hereditary intestinal anal sphincter myopathy causing proctalgia fugax and constipation. *Gastroenterology*. 1991;100:809.

32. **Amaranath I, Wexner SD.** Caudal epidural block in the management of proctalgia fugax. *Am J Pain Manage*. 1994;4:153.

33. **Greenman PE.** Principles of diagnosis and treatment of pelvic girdle dysfunctions. In: Greenman PE, ed. *Principles of Manual Medicine*. Baltimore: Williams & Wilkins; 1991:225.

34. **Chamberlain WE.** The symphysis pubis in the roentgen examination of the sacroiliac joint. *Am J Roentgenol Radium Ther*. 1930;24:621.

35. **Death AB, Kirby RL, MacMillan CL.** Pelvic ring mobility: Assessment by stress radiography. *Arch Phys Med Rehabil*. 1982;63:204.

36. **Travell JG, Simons DG.** *Myofascial Pain and Dysfunction: The Trigger Point Manual*, Vol 2: *The Lower Extremities*. Baltimore: Williams & Wilkins; 1992.

37. **Bellamy N, Park W, Rooney PJ.** What do we know about the sacroiliac joint? *Semin Arthritis Rheum*. 1983;12:282.

38. **Schwarzer AC, Aprill CN, Bogduk N.** The sacroiliac joint in chronic low back pain. *Spine*. 1995;20:31.

39. **Fortin JD, Dwyer AP, West S, et al.** Sacroiliac joint: Pain referral maps upon applying a new injection/arthrography technique. Part I: Asymptomatic volunteers. *Spine*. 1994;19:1475.

40. **Robert R, Prat-Pradal D, Labat JJ, et al.** Anatomic basis of chronic perineal pain: Role of the pudendal nerve. *Surg Radiol Anat*. 1998;20:93.

41. **Shafik A.** Pudendal canal syndrome: A new etiological factor in prostatodynia and its treatment by pudendal canal compression. *Pain Digest*. 1998;8:32.

42. **Tetzschner T, Sorensen M, Lose G, et al.** Pudendal nerve function during pregnancy and after delivery. *Int Urogynecol J Pelvic Floor Dysfunct*. 1997;8:66.

43. **Amarenco G, Lanoe Y, Perrigot M, et al.** A new canal syndrome: Compression of the pudendal nerve in Alcock's canal or perineal paralysis of cyclists [French]. *Presse Med*. 1987;16:399.

44. **Shafik A.** Pudendal canal syndrome: A cause of chronic pelvic pain. *Urology*. 2002;60:199.

45. **Rigor BM Sr.** Pelvic cancer pain. *J Surg Oncol*. 2000;75:280.

46. **Bonica JJ.** Cancer pain. In: Bonica JJ, ed. *Management of Pain*. Philadelphia: Lea & Febiger; 1990.

47. **Patt RB.** Therapeutic decision making for invasive procedures. In: Patt RB, ed. *Cancer Pain*. Philadelphia: Lippincott; 1993.

48. **Plancarte R, Aldrete JA.** Hypogastric plexus block: Retroperitoneal approach. *Anesthesiology*. 1989;71:A739.

49. **Plancarte R, Amescua C, Py HRB, Aldrete JA.** Superior hypogastric plexus block for pelvic cancer pain. *Anesthesiology*. 1990;73(2):236–239.

50. **Plancarte R.** Superior hypogastric plexus block: A very effective and underutilized diagnostic and therapeutic procedure. Paper presented at: Worldwide Pain Conference 2000; San Francisco, California; July 19, 2000.

51. **Kent E, Lema M.** Neurolytic superior hypogastric block for cancer related pelvic pain. *Reg Anesth*. 1992;17(Suppl):19.

52. **Plancarte R, de Leon-Casasola OA, El-Helaly M, Allende S, Lema MJ.** Neurolytic superior hypogastric plexus block for chronic pelvic pain associated with cancer. *Reg Anesth*. 1997;22(6):562–568.

53. **Plancarte R, Patt RB, et al.** Presacral blockade of the ganglion of Walther (ganglion impar). *Anesthesiology*. 1990;73:A751.

54. **Patt R, Plancarte R.** Superior hypogastric plexus and ganglion impar. In Hahn MB, McQuillan PM, Sheplock GJ, eds. *Regional Anesthesia: An Atlas of Anatomy and Techniques*. St. Louis: Mosby; 1996.

55. **Patt RB, Plancarte R.** Superior hypogastric plexus block: A new therapeutic approach for pelvic pain. In Waldman SD, Winnie A, eds. *Interventional Pain Management*. Philadelphia: Saunders; 1996:387–391.

56. **Wang JK.** Intrathecal morphine for intractable pain secondary to pelvic cancer of pelvic organs. *Pain*. 1985;21:99.

57. **Du Pen S, et al.** Chronic epidural bupivacaine–opioid infusion in intractable cancer pain. *Pain*. 1992;49:293.

58. **Waldmann SD, et al.** Intraspinal opioid therapy. In: Patt RB, ed. *Cancer Pain*. Philadelphia: Lippincott; 1993.

59. **Patt RB.** Peripheral neurolysis and the management of cancer pain. *Pain Digest*. 1992;2:30.

60. **Kayser Enneking F.** Gynecology and urology. In: Brown D, ed. *Regional Anesthesia and Analgesia*. Philadelphia: Saunders; 1996.

61. **Baude C.** Les douleurs pelvi-perinéales chroniques, in douleurs pelviennes et anopérineales chroniques-Une prise en charge multidisciplinaire. Lyon: Formation S; 2000:1–77.
62. **Bensignor MF LJ, Robert R, Ducrot P**. Diagnostic and therapeutic pudendal nerve block for patients with perineal non-malignant pain. In: *8th World Congress on Pain*. Paris: IASP;1996:56.
63. **Robert R BC, Faure A, Lehur PA, et al.** La chirurgie du nerf pudendal lors de certaines algies perineales: Evolution et résultats. *Chirurgie*. 1993;119:535.

30 THORACIC PAIN

P. Prithvi Raj, MD

INTRODUCTION

- Pain of the thoracic region is a frequently encountered complaint for specialists in pain management.
- Thoracic pain is often generated from disorders of the viscera contained within the thoracic cavity.
- Diagnosis of these syndromes is difficult because of the vague quality of the visceral pain and from the referred pain that frequently coexists.
- The diagnostic dilemma is further complicated by the fact that efferent somatosensory and efferent visceral impulses of both the somatosensory and autonomic nervous systems impinge on the spinal cord at the same place, approximately within the levels of T1 to T7.
- Acute angina (heart T1 to T4) may, therefore, be experienced as epigastric discomfort, left shoulder or arm pain, left chest pain, or right-sided chest and arm pain.
- Although many acute thoracic pain syndromes exist, only the more chronic syndromes that are likely to be encountered in a pain center are discussed in this chapter.
- Table 30–1 lists some of the common acute pain states encountered in the thoracic region.
- Thoracic pain can be categorized as visceral, musculoskeletal, myofascial, neurogenic, and other.

VISCERAL PAIN

LUNGS AND TRACHEA

- Visceral afferent fibers from the trachea and bronchi are carried to the central nervous system (CNS) through afferent fibers of the vagus and upper thoracic sympathetic nerves (T2 to T7).
- Pain associated with the trachea and bronchi radiates to the sternum.
- The lung parenchyma and the visceral pleura are insensate and, thus, do not produce pain following surgery or trauma.
- The parietal pleura transmits pain along somatic nerves, including the brachial plexus (C8, T1), intercostal nerves (T1 to T12), and phrenic nerves (C3 to C5).
- Pain from the parietal pleura (eg, arising from carcinoma, pneumonia, or pleurisy) is often sharp, piercing, and knifelike and is worsened by effort or deep respiration.
- Parietal pleural pain radiates to the supraclavicular region, the shoulder area, and the area supplied by the intercostal nerve.[1]

TABLE 30–1 Thoracic Pain

VISCERAL	MUSCULOSKELETAL	NEUROGENIC	MISCELLANEOUS
Thorax	Bony origin	Herpes zoster	Vascular
	Rib/sternum	Acute	Angina
		Postherpetic neuralgia	Pulmonary infarct
			Aortic
Lung/trachea	Costochondritis (Tietze's syndrome)		
Pneumonia	Vertebrae		
Pleurisy	Disk disease		
Carcinoma (Pancoast)	Facet syndrome		
	Compression fracture: osteoporosis (steroids)		
	Degenerative joint disease		
	Bone metastases		
Heart	Soft tissue	Causalgia (CRPS)	Infectious disease
Myocarditis	Muscle ligaments	Posttrauma	
Mediastinitis	Breast	Postsurgery	
Angina			
Esophagus	Posttrauma	Myelopathies	Metastatic disease
Carcinoma	Postsurgery	Demyelination	
Esophagitis		Spinal cord injury	

- Although this pain may initially be confused with angina, angina is not exacerbated by coughing or deep respiration.

PAIN MANAGEMENT

- Intrapleural catheters may be placed for intermittent or continuous infusion of local anesthetic or narcotic agents to block the affected intercostal nerves.[1]
- Intermittent or continuous epidural blocks using local anesthetics and steroids alone or in combination may be used to block pain mediated by spinal nerve roots and autonomic visceral components.
- The use of transcutaneous electrical neural stimulation (TENS) and myofascial trigger point injections in spastic paraspinal muscle may help breathing and improve the patient's clinical condition.
- Pain associated with the trachea and bronchi because of carcinoma may improve after vagotomy.[2]
- Pain associated with cancerous involvement of the visceral pleura and surrounding tissues should be treated with an aggressive multidisciplinary approach, including tricyclic antidepressants, narcotic analgesics, nerve blocking techniques, psychological counseling, and a strong emotional support system.[3]

HEART

- The visceral afferent fibers of the heart are transmitted through the vagus, the cervical ganglia (middle and inferior cervical nerves), and the upper five thoracic ganglia (thoracic cardiac nerves), and enter the central nervous system at T1 to T5 (see Figure 30–1).
- Most cardiogenic pain is secondary to ischemia.
- Whether ischemia is due to coronary artery vasospasm, coronary atherosclerosis, or acute coronary arterial insufficiency, the symptoms may be similar: substernal, crushing, or epigastric pain—a feeling of tightness, constriction, and heaviness that may become progressively more severe or intense.
- The pain frequently radiates to the left sternal border, left shoulder, arm, and neck, and there may be an accompanying feeling of impending doom.
- Acute infectious processes, such as endocarditis and myocarditis, produce symptoms of pleuritic substernal or epigastric pain that may be lancinating or paroxysmal or that may become continuous and more severe.

PAIN MANAGEMENT

- Acute treatment includes administration of oxygen, reduction of myocardial work through rest, and administration of coronary artery dilating agents, such as

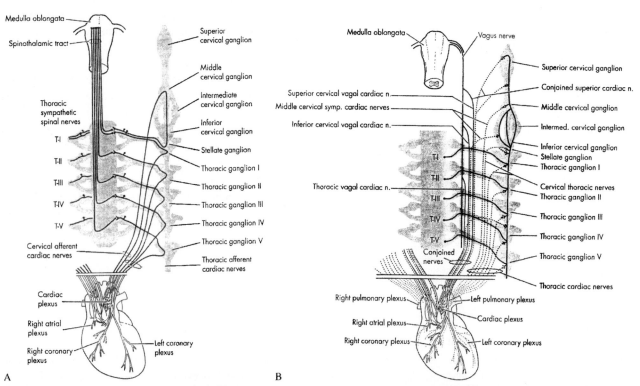

FIGURE 30–1 Autonomic nerve supply to the heart. (A) Efferent nerve supply. (B) Afferent nerve supply. Redrawn from Bonica JJ, ed. *Sympathetic Nerve Blocks for Pain Diagnosis and Therapy.* Vol 1. New York: Winthrop Breon; 1984.

β-blockers, calcium channel-blocking drugs, nitrites, sedatives, antibiotics, and antiviral agents, as indicated.
- Coronary artery revascularization or balloon angioplasty may be indicated.
- The pain produced by these acute processes may be relieved by potent narcotic analgesics, continuous epidural blockade, or stellate ganglion block.[2]
- Acute treatment is rarely given in the pain clinic setting, but it is imperative that myocardial ischemia be excluded as an etiology of chest pain before initiating any treatment involving chest pain.
- Chronic chest pain or referred sympathetic pain (shoulder–hand syndrome) may be treated by stellate ganglion block or by interruption of preganglionic sympathetic nerves T2 to T5.
- The possibility of cardiac causalgia following the onset of angina pectoris has been suggested.
- Cardiac causalgia is characterized by constant burning and chronic substernal chest discomfort.
- Hyperesthesia of the sternum and the chest wall over the painful area may be present.
- Although nitroglycerin and rest do not relieve the pain of cardiac causalgia, calcium channel-blocking drugs may be effective.
- The role of sympathetic nervous system blockade with respect to cardiac causalgia has not been evaluated.

ESOPHAGUS

- Visceral afferent fibers from the esophagus are carried through inferior cervical sympathetic nerves and the vagus (upper esophagus T2 to T5) and through thoracic cardiac sympathetic nerves and the stellate ganglion (lower esophagus T5 to T8) to the CNS.
- Pain from the upper esophagus radiates to the midsubsternal area, lower neck, lateral chest, and arms, whereas lower esophageal pain (esophagitis, spasm of the gastroesophageal junction) radiates to the area over the heart or epigastrium.
- Esophageal pain is paroxysmal, occurring with swallowing and radiating to the back at the level of the lesion.
- Pain associated with inflammation, acidic conditions, chemical irritation, mechanical irritation or dilation, and/or autonomic dysfunction may be relieved with antacids, histamine H_2-blocking drugs, misoprostol (Cytotec), metoclopramide hydrochloride (Reglan), or antiflatulents.
- Pain from esophageal cancer described as substernal, epigastric, and exacerbated by swallowing may be relieved by blocking spinal nerve roots T2 to T5 for upper esophageal lesions in combination with vagotomy or by blocking T5 to T8 for lower esophageal lesions.

MUSCULOSKELETAL PAIN

- Thoracic musculoskeletal pain is a frequent complaint and may be related to trauma, postsurgical changes, infectious processes, degenerative changes, overuse phenomenon, or inflammatory processes.
- The site of the pain may involve the vertebrae, the bony thorax, and the soft tissue or musculoligamentous structures.

COSTOCHONDRITIS (TIETZE'S SYNDROME)

- Pain of the costochondral junctions along the anterior chest wall may follow blunt chest trauma; persistent coughing, as with chronic obstructive pulmonary disease or acute respiratory infection; overuse of the upper extremity (from activities such as washing windows and painting); or chest surgery.
- True Tietze's syndrome is most frequently unilateral, involving the second and third costal cartilages (see Figure 30–2).[4]
- This pain is described as mild to moderate over the anterior chest wall.
- If the pain is severe enough, the patient may confuse it with a myocardial infarction.
- Differential diagnosis includes underlying malignancy and sepsis.
- Tietze's syndrome, which is often a diagnosis of exclusion, occurs in all age groups (including children) but is most frequently observed in persons younger than 40 years of age.
- Bulbous swellings that may persist for several months and point tenderness over the costochondral junctions are characteristic of Tietze's syndrome.
- Exacerbations and remissions of the pain can remain localized or radiate to the arm and shoulder.

PAIN MANAGEMENT
- Treatment may include local heat, nonsteroidal anti-inflammatory drugs (NSAIDs), local infiltration with a local anesthetic solution/steroid combination, intercostal nerve blocks, or electroacupuncture therapy.
- TENS may be useful until the irritative process or inflammatory reaction subsides.[1,3]

COSTOCHONDRITIS

- Costochondritis presents as inflammation of multiple costochondral or costosternal articulations.
- It may radiate widely and mimic intrathoracic and intraabdominal disease.

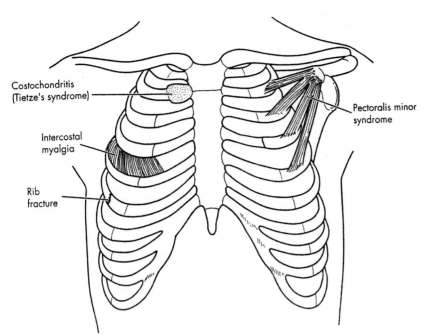

FIGURE 30–2 Costochondritis (Tietze's syndrome).

- Because multiple articulations are usually involved, local tenderness is elicited with palpation, which may reproduce the symptoms of the radiating pain.
- Costochondritis most frequently occurs in adults 40 years of age and older.[5]
- Additional costochondral pain problems include trauma to the sternum and ribs, with subsequent fractures, dislocations, and separation of the ribs, cartilage, and sternum.

PAIN MANAGEMENT

- Treatment is similar to that of Tietze's syndrome once the diagnosis is made and other underlying causes of cardiac, gastrointestinal, and arthritic processes and myofascial strain have been ruled out.
- Costochondral arthritis, osteoporosis, infection, and trauma or delayed healing following thoracic surgery can be a challenge to therapeutic interventions.
- TENS can be very helpful when the electrical signal is used in a crossed fashion over the area of pain.
- Electroacupuncture therapy is a useful adjunct.
- Periodic intercostal nerve blocks and thoracic epidural or intrapleural catheter techniques have been described.
- If permissible, local infiltration near the site of pain may be beneficial.

VERTEBRAL DISORDERS

- Painful disorders of the thoracic vertebrae may involve osteoporosis, compression fractures, thoracic facet syndrome, ankylosing spondylitis, postural abnormalities (scoliosis), or injuries involving forced or violent flexion or extension movement of the spine.
- Pain associated with fractures, infections, degenerative arthritic processes, metabolic bone disease, or primary or metastatic malignancies is also commonly encountered.
- Compression fractures of the thoracic vertebrae that are due to trauma, osteoporosis secondary to aging or corticosteroid use, and degenerative changes are common.
- Patients complain of encircling pain along the intercostal nerves, aggravated by twisting motions, coughing, or postural changes.
- In the acute setting, fractured vertebrae and ribs produce severe, constricting pain of the thorax, which may inhibit respiration.
- The pain is generally accompanied by severe muscle spasms of the intercostal and paraspinous muscles, inhibiting the patient from obtaining adequate sleep or movement.

PAIN MANAGEMENT

- Treatment consists of local heat or ice, TENS, NSAIDs, and nonopioid and opioid analgesics.
- Nerve-blocking techniques, such as single-shot and continuous epidural blocks, single-level or multiple-level intercostal blocks, paravertebral somatic nerve blocks, and intrapleural catheter techniques, can also be used.

MYOFASCIAL PAIN

- The paravertebral muscles (eg, the longissimus thoracis and iliocostalis muscles) are a common source of thoracic pain.
- Pain can be reproduced by pressure on the trigger area and is often relieved by massage, vapo-coolant spray, or the injection of a local anesthetic/steroid mixture.

POSTTHORACOTOMY PAIN

- Chronic pain after thoracotomy can be due to various etiologic mechanisms.
- Some authors suggest that surgical excision of intercostal nerves, designed to relieve pain, may result in late postoperative pain caused by neuroma formation. This technique has been condemned.
- Complications of chemically induced intercostal neuritis with the use of absolute alcohol resulted in a recommendation against the use of such agents.[6,7]
- Many of the common causes of postthoracotomy pain are amenable to therapeutic interventions.

ENTRAPMENT OF NERVE FIBERS IN SCAR TISSUE

- In the thoracic region, one may encounter noxious input from cutaneous receptors of a mild to severe degree secondary to scar tissue formation or nerve entrapment in scar tissue.
- When nerve fibers are trapped in scar tissue, a light touch on the scar produces intense radiating pain, sometimes accompanied by burning pain from associated reflex sympathetic dystrophy.
- The pain can be described as dull and aching, with frequent bouts of sharp, shooting pain associated with particular movement.
- Localized pain can be aggravated by direct pressure on the scar itself, and one might find referred pain to areas more closely associated with the scar tissue or more remote.
- Patients complain of exquisite tenderness over areas of the scar, hyperalgesia, and incapacitation.
- Injection of the scar with a local anesthetic agent is diagnostic.

PAIN MANAGEMENT
- Repeated injection of a local anesthetic mixed with a steroid is likely to provide long-term relief.
- Cryoablation, chemical neurolysis, excision of intercostal nerves, or thoracic dorsal root entry zone lesions (DREZ) of the spinal cord may give rise to more "permanent," prolonged effects.
- Ablation of irregular bundles of nerve element, such as neuromas, may prove beneficial but neuroablative procedures may result in either less intense or more intense pain.
- It is suggested that neuromas found in scar tissue may give rise to the "viscerosensory reflex."
- It is thought that the internal viscera are connected embryologically to cutaneous manifestations throughout the entire body. By pressing on or moving the various connective tissue elements of the somatosensory areas served by the same neurologic tissue, one can produce visceral or autonomic symptoms.
- Thus, injection of a painful cutaneous scar may alleviate abdominal or thoracic visceral pain that may appear to be remote from the site itself.
- Several clinicians recommend cryoanalgesia of involved intercostal nerves at the time of surgery to prevent postthoracotomy pain and pulmonary complications[7,8]; however, cryoanalgesia is not without possible complications, because secondary neuralgia may occur.
- Others have suggested the use of TENS for treatment of postthoracotomy pain.[6,9]
- For acute postthoracotomy pain management, epidural narcotic infusions may be more effective than cryoanalgesic measures or TENS.[10]

NEUROMA

- A palpable neuroma in the scar, loss of pinprick sensation over the skin, and elicitation of pain on palpation are diagnostic.
- Repeated injections of a local anesthetic/steroid mixture may relieve the pain.
- Persistent pain from a localized neuroma may respond well to neurolytic injection of phenol or to cryolysis.

SYMPATHETIC DYSTROPHY

- Burning pain associated with hyperpathia, decreased skin temperature over the area, and increased sweating characterize this syndrome.
- Pain is relieved by paravertebral sympathetic block, nerve root block, or epidural block of sympathetic fibers.
- This pain may also respond to the use of calcium channel-blocking drugs, blockers, antidepressants, anti-inflammatory medications, and neural stabilizing agents, such as fluphenazine.

MYOFASCIAL TRIGGER POINTS

- Tender trigger points located in the pectoral and anterior serratus muscles and accompanied by spasm in those muscles are a common source of anterior chest pain (see Figure 30–2).
- Pain is reproduced by pressure on the trigger point and relieved by local anesthetic injection or vapocoolant spray technique.
- The pain is not relieved by intercostal block because the pectoral muscles are innervated by the branches of the brachial plexus.
- TENS and physical therapy involving stretching exercises, deep massage, and passive then active range-of-motion techniques are helpful in preventing recurrence.[3,11]
- Myofascial trigger points can also be the source of postthoracotomy pain.
- They can be located by careful palpation of the paravertebral tissues.
- Local injections, TENS, and epidural blocks as well as local heat and ice, physical therapy, and anti-inflammatory agents may be helpful.

NEUROGENIC PAIN

- It is important to mention pain syndromes of the thorax, acute herpes zoster, and chronic postherpetic neuralgia.
- Additional pain syndromes in the thoracic region involving nerve tissue or damage to nerve tissue include causalgia and intercostal neuropathies following trauma, surgical intervention, or intraneural injection.
- Irritation of the intercostal nerves can also occur following osteoarthritis of the joint space and destruction or tumor invasion of the intercostal nerve, with resultant mechanical compression.
- Hematoma or infiltration neuritis and postinjection neuritis can affect the intercostal nerves.
- Lesions of the spinal cord, including myelopathies, demyelination, and spinal cord traumatic injuries, may also contribute to thoracic pain.
- Causalgia involving any of the thoracic somatic nerves, thoracic intercostal nerves, or the spinal cord itself may be present.

OTHER CAUSES OF PAIN

SURGICAL SCARS

- Painful scars can occur after thoracic surgery.
- They cause a characteristic pain syndrome that usually persists for at least 2 months after the procedure.

- A continuous aching or burning sensation often extends beyond the scar.
- In addition, there is sensory loss and absence or sweating along the scar.
- Temperature, touch, pressure, and emotional factors can exacerbate the pain.
- The appearance of the scar is not significant. Smooth scars can be painful, and indurated scars can be painless.
- Histologic examination shows a chaotic formation of neural elements; neuromas may be present.
- The pain has been attributed to imperfect nerve regeneration.

PAIN MANAGEMENT
- TENS, analgesics, antidepressants, anticonvulsants, local infiltration of anesthetics and corticosteroids, and nerve blocks have been used with varying degrees of success.
- Many patients have undergone scar resection with no pain relief.
- Delayed chest pain also may occur as a result of sternal wire sutures.[11,12]

PAIN AFTER BREAST SURGERY

- Chest pain may be felt after extensive breast surgery, such as radical mastectomy.
- Patients usually have a burning pain in the axilla and upper chest; this may radiate to the medial part of the arm.
- The pain probably is secondary to transection of the intercostobrachial nerve.
- Postmastectomy surgical pain rarely lasts longer than 3 months after surgery.
- Some patients may have chronic pain after mastectomy. This pain frequently is in a nonanatomic area on the anterior chest wall and is extremely sensitive to touch.

PSYCHIATRIC CAUSES

- Panic disorder, depression, and other psychiatric maladies also may be manifested as chest pain.[13–15]

REFERENCES

1. **Fineman SP.** Long-term post-thoracotomy cancer pain management with interpleural bupivacaine. *Anesth Analg.* 1989;68:694.

2. **Ramamurthy S.** Pain in thoracic region. In: Raj PP, ed. *Practical Management of Pain.* Chicago: Year Book Medical; 1986:464.

3. **Levy MH.** Integration of pain management into comprehensive cancer care. *Cancer.* 1989;63:2329.

4. **Fam AG, Smythe HA.** Musculoskeletal chest wall pain. *Can Med Assoc J.* 1985;133:379.

5. **Calabro JJ, Jeghers H, Miller KA, et al.** Classification of anterior chest wall syndrome (C). *JAMA.* 1980;243:1420.

6. **Rooney SM, Subhash J, Melormack P.** A comparison of pulmonary function tests for postthoracotomy pain using cryoanalgesia and transcutaneous nerve stimulation. *Ann Thorac Surg.* 1986;41:204.

7. **Maiwand O, Makey AR.** Cryoanalgesia for relief of pain after thoracotomy. *Br Med J.* 1981;282:49.

8. **Glynn CJ, Lloyd JW, Bernard JDW.** Cryoanalgesia in the management of pain after thoracotomy. *Thorax.* 1980; 35:325.

9. **Stubbing JF, Jellicoe JA.** Transcutaneous electrical nerve stimulation after thoracotomy. *Anesthesia.* 1988;43:296.

10. **Gough JD, Williams AB, Vaughan RS, et al.** The control of post-thoracotomy pain: A comparative evaluation of thoracic epidural fentanyl infusions and cryoanalgesia. *Anaesthesia.* 1988;43:780.

11. **Richter JE.** Practical approach to the diagnosis of unexplained chest pain. *Med Clin North Am.* 1991;75:1203.

12. **Roll M, Kollind M, Theorell T.** Clinical symptoms in young adults with atypical chest pain attending the emergency department. *J Intern Med.* 1991;230:271.

13. **Brand DL, Beck JG, Wielgosz AT.** Unexplained chest pain: Future directions for research. *Med Clin North Am.* 1991; 75:1209.

14. **Bradley LA, Scarinci IC, Richter JE.** Pain threshold levels and coping strategies among patients who have chest pain and normal coronary arteries. *Med Clin North Am.* 1991; 75:1189.

15. **Eagle KA.** Medical decision making in patient with chest pain. *N Engl J Med.* 1991;324:1282.

31 AIDS-RELATED PAIN SYNDROMES

Benjamin W. Johnson, Jr., MD, MBA, DAPBM

INTRODUCTION

- Improved treatment and rehabilitation modalities for patients with acquired immunodeficiency syndrome (AIDS), such as highly active antiretroviral therapy (HAART), have resulted not only in prolonged survival but also in the manifestation of an increasing number of AIDS-related pain syndromes.
- The tendency to consider AIDS-related pain as a correlate of cancer pain is being challenged due to the emerging chronicity of the disease process. A more appropriate paradigm for AIDS-related pain treatment would be the multidisciplinary chronic pain management model.
- The incidence of pain in ambulatory HIV-infected patients ranges from 40 to 60% and increases with disease progression.
- In a 2-year longitudinal study, 69% of AIDS patients had moderate-to-severe pain that interfered with their daily living.[1]
- Pain was reported in 30% of patients with AIDS admitted to the hospital, and pain treatment was required in 50% of hospitalized patients with AIDS.[2]
- In a hospice, 53% of patients with advanced AIDS reported pain.[3]

THE MULTIDISCIPLINARY/ MULTIMODAL APPROACH TO THE PATIENT WITH AIDS-RELATED PAIN

- Undertreatment of AIDS-related pain is common. In 1996, only 8% of patients with severe AIDS-related pain were receiving opioids for relief, and only 10% were receiving adjunct pain medications. The reasons underlying the undertreatment of patients with AIDS-related pain are multifactorial.
- The complexity of AIDS-related pain, combined with the complexity of the AIDS patient, requires a multidisciplinary/multimodal approach to evaluation and management. The services required for the evaluation and management of these patients include:
  - Medical management: antiviral agents, antibiotics, antituberculosis agents, and so on
  - Palliative care: management of medications for relief of pain
  - Behavioral management: cognitive-behavioral intervention, biofeedback, guided imagery, mood-altering agents, and so on
  - Social services: financial assistance, vocational testing, housing issues, and so on
  - Rehabilitation services: physical therapy, occupational therapy, and so on
  - Interventional care: procedural interventions for relief of pain

COMMON AIDS-RELATED PAIN SYNDROMES

- Patients with AIDS often experience several types of pain simultaneously.

- The most common pain symptoms are headaches, peripheral neuropathy, and arthralgias.[4]
- The most common locations for pain are the extremities, head, and upper and lower gastrointestinal tract.
- AIDS-related pain can also develop from the pharmacologic treatment for the disease process and its complications. These pharmacologic agents include: chemotherapeutic agents, antiviral agents, antitubercular drugs, and colony-stimulating factors.

NEUROPATHIC PAIN

HEADACHES
- Headache is the most common of AIDS-related pain syndromes.

Causes
- Cerebral toxoplasmosis
- Meningitis
- Complications of dural puncture
- Chemotherapeutic agents
- Interferon-α2a + vinblastine
- Azidothymidine (AZT)
- Tumor necrosis factor (TNF)

Treatment Strategies
- Pharmacologic therapy:
  ○ Nonsteroidal anti-inflammatory drug (NSAID) therapy
  ○ Neuropathic pain medications, such as gabapentin
  ○ Opioid therapy
  ○ Epidural blood patch (for postdural puncture headache)
- Nonpharmacologic therapy:
  ○ Biofeedback training
  ○ Transcutaneous electrical nerve stimulation (TENS)
  ○ Muscle relaxation therapy

PAINFUL DISTAL SENSORY PERIPHERAL NEUROPATHY

Incidence
- Nearly 30% of patients with AIDS are affected by peripheral neuropathy.[5]

Signs and Symptoms
- Mechanical allodynia and hyperalgesia

Proposed Mechanisms
- *Axonal atrophy*: Decreased intraepidermal nerve fiber density is associated with increased neuropathic pain, low CD4 counts, and high plasma HIV RNA levels.[6]

- *Mitochondrial toxicity*[7]: DNA polymerase γ-inhibition causes abnormal mitochondrial DNA synthesis. Depletion of the nerve fiber's mitochondrial DNA causes axonal degeneration. The following antiviral agents have been implicated[8]:
  ○ 2′3′-Dideoxycytidine (ddC)
  ○ Didanosine (ddI)
  ○ Lamuvidine (3TC)
  ○ Stavudine (d4T)
  ○ Fialuridine (FIAU)
- *Vacuolar myelopathy*: Immune-mediated myelin and oligodendrocyte injury and impairment of neural repair mechanisms are associated with S-adenosyl-L-methionone (SAM) deficiency.
- *Necrotizing vasculitis*: Inflammatory destruction of the vasa nervorum causes ischemic neuronal injury and neuropathic pain.

PROGRESSIVE POLYRADICULOPATHY
- Progressive polyradiculopathy[9] is often associated with cytomegalovirus infection.
- Signs and symptoms:
  ○ Flaccid paralysis
  ○ Pain and paresthesias
  ○ Areflexia
  ○ Urogenital sphincter dysfunction

DIFFUSE INFILTRATIVE LYMPHOCYTOSIS SYNDROME
- This condition causes a painful peripheral neuropathy due to persistent lymphocytosis, which improves with corticosteroids and zidovudine.

TREATMENT STRATEGIES

Neuropathic Pain Medications
- Anticonvulsants: gabapentin
- Antidepressants
- Calcium channel/NMDA antagonists[10]
- Opioid analgesics (Although less effective for neuropathic pain, these analgesics remain the "gold standard" for pain relief.)

Neuroaugmentation
- TENS, spinal cord stimulation, and peripheral stimulation are reversible modalities to consider for long-term pain relief.
- The depressed immune status of HIV patients, however, suggests that caution be exercised before considering invasive therapeutic modalities, due to potential infectious complications.

Interventional Pain Therapy
- Caution must be exercised in the use of corticosteroids in this population, as corticosteroids have been

implicated in the extracutaneous spread of Kaposi's sarcoma.[11]

MUSCULOSKELETAL PAIN

CAUSES OF MUSCULAR PAIN
- Pyomyositis, which produces inflammatory mediators that lower the threshold for noxious stimulation, thereby causing muscular pain with benign stimulation
- Rhabdomyolysis, associated with simvastatin use
- Muscular infiltration by Kaposi's sarcoma[12]

CAUSES OF BONE PAIN
- Avascular necrosis due to corticosteroid usage
- Osteoporosis due to reduced activity and/or poor nutrition
- Invasion by Kaposi's sarcoma[13]
- Tuberculous arthritis and/or bone invasion

TREATMENT STRATEGIES
- NSAIDs (COX-2 agents are preferable if patient is also using corticosteroids, to reduce adverse gastrointestinal and platelet effects.)
- Opioid analgesics
- Physical therapy
- Nutritional counseling and intervention
- Medical/surgical intervention as indicated for disease management

VISCERAL PAIN

ABDOMINAL PAIN
- Etiology: infection, typically *Cryptosporidium, Microsporidium*, cytomegalovirus

ORAL PAIN: APHTHOUS STOMATITIS
- Esophagitis: herpes simplex, *Candida*
- Hepatobiliary: hepatitis, AIDS cholangiopathy
- Pancreatitis
- Cytomegalovirus-induced enterocolitis and/or small bowel perforation
- Urolithiasis

ANORECTAL ABSCESSES
- Cancer: Kaposi's sarcoma, oropharyngeal lesions

OTHER CAUSES
- Urolithiasis (Indinavir is associated with renal colic.)
- Anorectal pain: fissures, ulcerations

TREATMENT STRATEGIES
- Medical treatment of disease process
- Opioid analgesics

- Interventional pain therapy
  - Celiac plexus/splanchnic nerve blocks for upper abdominal pain
  - Superior hypogastric plexus blocks for pelvic pain
  - Ganglion impar blockade for perineal pain

BARRIERS TO EFFECTIVE TREATMENT OF AIDS-RELATED PAIN

COMPLICATING FACTOR

- The population of patients with AIDS is a special needs group[14] requiring intensive multidisciplinary treatment modalities.

MEDICAL/SURGICAL INTERVENTION

- The incidence of infectious complications due to surgical procedures in HIV patients is difficult to determine accurately because of the presence of confounding variables.[15] Most reports in the literature suggest that interventions can be performed safely if strict aseptic technique is observed.

REHABILITATIVE INTERVENTION

- These modalities can be difficult to execute due to such issues as:
  - Anal sphincter dysfunction in patients with polyradiculitis
  - Sedation or dysphoria in patients taking opioid analgesics
  - Allodynia due to painful peripheral neuropathies

BEHAVIORAL INTERVENTION

- These modalities may require working with the following confounding factors:
  - Nontraditional family dynamics: gay lovers, estranged spouses, estranged parents, extended families
  - Substance abuse history
  - Psychiatric disorders

PHARMACOLOGIC INTERVENTION

OPIOID THERAPY
- Opioid therapy must be prescribed with caution and monitoring due to:
  - Possible history of substance abuse

○ Possible worsening of psychiatric disorders (AIDS dementia complex)
○ Interference with behavioral modification therapy: dysphoria, sedation, hallucinations
• Parenteral routes may be more beneficial in patients with AIDS-related gastrointestinal disturbances.
• Transdermal formulations.

NONOPIOID THERAPY
• The use of adjunctive medications (anticonvulsants, antidepressants, antianxiety agents) is strongly advised, when indicated, to minimize the use of opioids.

INTERVENTIONAL THERAPIES

NEUROBLOCKADE TECHNIQUES: VISCERAL OR SYMPATHETIC BLOCKS
• Celiac plexus blocks for abdominal pain
• Stellate ganglion and lumbar sympathetic blocks for sympathetically mediated pain and vascular insufficiency
• Presacral plexus blocks for pelvic pain
• Ganglion impar blocks for rectal pain
• Peripheral nerve blocks
  ○ Nerve root blocks
  ○ Peripheral nerve blocks (ilioinguinal, intercostal blocks)
  ○ Botulinum toxin for myofascial pain
• Central nerve blocks
  ○ Epidural nerve blocks
  ○ Intrathecal blocks

NEUROBLOCKADE AGENTS
• Temporary: local anesthetics, steroids
• Neurodestructive: phenol, alcohol, heat, cryo (see Chapter 49)

ALTERNATIVE AND COMPLEMENTARY INTERVENTIONS

• Acupuncture, acupressure, Feldenkrais, and other such modalities are a highly desirable adjunct because of their noninvasive nature.

CONCLUSION

• The multidisciplinary evaluation and management of the patient with AIDS-related pain permits timely comprehensive care of the highest quality.
• The use of multimodality treatment facilitates delivery of the most beneficial care with the least adverse effects, when compared with unimodal treatment models.

REFERENCES

1. **Frich LM, Borgbjerg FM.** Pain and pain treatment in AIDS patients: A longitudinal study. *J Pain Symptom Manage.* 2000;19:339.
2. **Young DF.** Neurological complications of cancer chemotherapy. In: Silverstein A, ed. *Neurological Complications of Therapy: Selected Topics.* New York: Futura; 1982:57.
3. **Schofferman J, Brody R.** Pain in far advanced AIDS. In: Foley KM, ed. *Advances in Pain Research and Therapy.* Vol 16. New York: Raven; 1990:379.
4. **Singer IF, Zorilla C, Fahy-Chandon B, et al.** Painful symptoms reported by ambulatory HIV-infected men in a longitudinal study. *Pain.* 1993;54:15.
5. **Parr GJ.** Peripheral neuropathies associated with human immunodeficiency virus infection. *Ann Neurol.* 1988;23 (Suppl):349 .
6. **Polydefkis M, Yannoutsos CT, Cohen BA, et al.** Reduced intraepidermal nerve fiber density in HIV-associated sensory neuropathy. *Neurology.* 2002;58:115.
7. **Dalakas MC, Semino-Mora C, Leon-Monzon M.** Mitochondrial alterations with mitochondrial DNA depletion in the nerves of AIDS patients with peripheral neuropathy induced by 2'3'dideoxycytidine (ddC). *Lab Invest.* 2001; 81:1537.
8. **Dalakas MC.** Peripheral neuropathy and antiretroviral drugs. *J Peripher Nerv Syst.* 2001;6:14.
9. **Fuller GN.** Cytomegalovirus and the peripheral nervous system in AIDS. *J Acquir Immune Defic Syndr* 1992;5(Suppl 1): S33.
10. **Lipton SA.** HIV-related neuronal injury: Potential therapeutic intervention with calcium channel antagonists and NMDA antagonists. *Mol Neurobiol.* 1994;8:181.
11. **Trattner A, Hodak E, David M, et al.** Kaposi's sarcoma with visceral involvement after intraarticular and epidural injections of corticosteroids. *J Am Acad Dermatol.* 1993; 29(5, Pt 2):890.
12. **Haddow LJ, Davies S, Buckingham S, et al.** Kaposi's sarcoma infiltrating skeletal muscle. *Sex Transm Infect.* 2002;78:464.
13. **Ritz-Quillac L, Machet L, Machet MC, et al.** Bone involvement in a case of Kaposi's sarcoma. *Dermatology.* 1999;198:73.
14. **Breitbart WS, Panye DK, Passik AD.** Psychiatric and psychological aspects of cancer pain. In: Parris WCV, ed. *Cancer Pain Management: Principles and Practice.* Boston: Butterworth-Heineman; 1997:253.
15. **Jones S, Schechter CB, Smith C, et al.** Is HIV infection a risk factor for complications of surgery? *Mt Sinai J Med.* 2002;69:329.

32 ARTHRITIS

Zuhre Tutuncu, MD
Arthur Kavanaugh, MD

INRODUCTION

- Pain, one of the cardinal features of arthritis, is the result of the action of numerous inflammatory mediators and inflammatory cell-derived products on local nerves.
- Although pain is a subjective feeling, it is one of the criteria that are used in clinical practice to assess patients' overall functioning, disease activity, and response to therapy.
- Musculoskeletal disorders affect 20 to 45% of the population.
- Pain, soreness, aches, stiffness, swelling, weakness, and fatigue account for more than 95% of all initial muscloskeletal presentations.
- Chronic disability from muscloskeletal disorders affects 6.1 to 10% of the population.
- The most common inflammatory and noninflammatory conditions in men and women, by age in approximate order of prevalence, are listed in Table 32–1.
- Arthritis is a general term that describes more than 100 conditions. Specific management of pain in arthritic conditions requires differentiation of the type of arthritis. The primary goals of the patient's evaluation are to discern if the complaint is:
  - Inflammatory or noninflammatory
  - Articular or periarticular in origin
  - Acute or chronic
  - Mono/oligoarticular or polyarticular
- Muscloskeletal conditions are often classified as having inflammatory or noninflammatory symptoms or signs that reflect the nature of the underlying pathologic process. Specific features that are useful in distinguishing inflammatory versus noninflammatory conditions are noted in Table 32–2.[1]

EVALUATION

- While evaluating the patient, the physician should determine whether the complaint originates from articular or periarticular structures.
- Periarticular structures include tendon, bursa, ligament, muscle, bone, fascia, nerve, or overlying skin. Periarticular joint pain is usually focal and pain is experienced on active motion in a few, specific planes.
- Pain in arthritic conditions is present on both active and passive motion of the joint in all planes and it is diffuse and produces deep tenderness.
- On presentation, the clinician should also determine if the arthritis is acute or chronic, based on whether the

TABLE 32–1   Common Rheumatologic Conditions*

	MEN		WOMEN	
AGE	NONINFLAMMATORY	INFLAMMATORY	NONINFLAMMATORY	INFLAMMATORY
18–34	Injury/overuse[†] Low back pain	Spondyloarthropathies Gonoccocal arthritis Gout	Injury/overuse Low back pain	Gonoccocal arthritis RA SLE
35–65	Low back pain Injury/overuse OA Entrapment syndromes[‡]	Bursitis Gout Spondyloarthropathies USP	Osteoporosis Low back pain Injury/overuse Fibromyalgia Entrapment syndromes OA Raynaud's phenomenon	Bursitis RA USP
>65	OA Low back pain Osteoporosis Fracture	Bursitis Gout USP RA Pseudogout Polymyalgia rheumatica Septic arthritis	Osteoporosis OA Fibromyalgia Low back pain Fracture	Bursitis USP RA Gout Pseudogout Polymyalgia rheumatica Septic arthritis

*Conditions are listed in approximate order of prevalence.
[†]Injury/overuse includes fracture, soft tissue injuries, tendonitis, and nonarticular rheumatism.
[‡]Entrapment syndrome includes carpal tunnel and tarsal tunnel syndromes; spondyloarthropathies include ankylosing spondylitis, psoriatic arthritis, and Reiter's syndrome.
RA, rheumatoid arthritis; SLE, systemic lupus erythematosus; OA, osteoarthritis; USP, undifferentiated seronegative polyarthritis.

TABLE 32–2 Specific Features That Are Useful in Distinguishing Inflammatory From Noninflammatory Conditions

	CHARACTERISTICS OF CONDITION	
FEATURE	INFLAMMATORY	NONINFLAMMATORY
Joint pain	Yes (with activity and rest)	Yes (with activity)
Joint swelling	Soft tissue	Bony (if present)
Local erythema	Sometimes	Absent
Local warmth	Sometimes	Absent
Morning stiffness	Prolonged (>60 min)	Variable (<60 min)
Systemic symptoms	Common	Rare
ESR, CRP	Increased	Normal for age
Hemoglobin	Normal or low	Normal
Serum albumin	Normal or Low	Normal
Synovial fluid, WBCs/mm^3	≥2000	<2000
Synovial fluid %PMNs	≥75%	<75%

complaint has been present 6 weeks or less (acute) or longer than 6 weeks (chronic).

- The extent of articular involvement is defined as monoarticular (one joint), oligoarticular or pauciarticular (two to four joints), or polyarticular (more than four joints). These approaches can help the physician categorize the complaint as:
  ○ Acute inflammatory mono/oligoarthritis (eg, septic arthritis, gout, pseudogout, viral arthritis, Reiter's syndrome, Lyme disease, acute rheumatic fever, hemarthrosis, palindromic rheumatism)
  ○ Chronic inflammatory mono/oligoarthritis (eg, tuberculous arthritis, fungal arthritis, psoriatic arthritis, spondyloarthropathy, pseudogout, sarcoidosis, juvenile chronic arthritis)
  ○ Acute noninflammatory mono/oligoarthritis (eg, mechanical derangement, trauma)
  ○ Chronic noninflammatory mono/oligoarthritis (eg, osteoathritis, osteonecrosis, neuropathic arthritis, hemarthrosis, pigmented villonodular synovitis, foreign body synovitis)
  ○ Acute inflammatory polyarthritis (eg, viral arthritis, septic arthritis, acute rheumatic fever, Reiter's syndrome)
  ○ Chronic inflammatory polyarthritis (eg, rheumatoid arthritis, psoriatic arthritis, enteropathic arthritis, crystal-induced arthritis, juvenile arthritis, Lyme disease, systemic lupus erythematosus (SLE), scleroderma, mixed connective tissue disease, polymyalgia rheumatica, polymyositis)
  ○ Chronic noninflammatory polyarthritis (eg, osteoarthritis, hemochromatosis, etc)[2]

OSTEOARTHRITIS

GENERAL

- Osteoarthritis (OA) is the most common noninflammatory arthritic condition.
- It typically affects the joints of the hand, spine, and weight-bearing joints (hips, knees).
- OA generally involves more than one joint but can also occur as monoarthritis.
- Approximately 12% of the adult population has symptomatic OA, characterized by joint pain, crepitus, stiffness after immobility, and limitation of motion. A greater percentage will have radiologic changes.
- The clinical joint symptoms are associated with defects in the articular cartilage that lead to changes in the underlying bone.
- OA is either primary/idiopathic or secondary.

EVALUATION

- Secondary causes of OA include trauma, obesity, congenital disorders, metabolic disorders, neuropathic disorders, and hemophilia.
- Laboratory tests tend to be normal for age. Synovial fluid is usually amber, clear, and noninflammatory with normal viscosity.
- Typical radiographic changes include loss of joint space, subchondral sclerosis, bony cysts, and reactive osteophyes.
- Articular erosions and osteoporosis are rare.
- It is important to note that radiographic findings do not necessarily correlate with clinical symptoms.
- When possible, synovial fluid aspiration should be done to evaluate all patients with acute onset of arthritis. Synovial fluid analysis provides unique and valuable information.
- The primary goal of synovial fluid analysis is to discern whether a synovial effusion is noninflammatory, inflammatory, septic, or hemorrhagic. There are a few disorders for which the synovial fluid analysis is diagnostic, for example, infectious and crystal-induced arthritis.
- Arthrocentesis may be therapeutic as well as diagnostic. For tense effusions, in which intra-articular pressure is high, removing fluid relieves symptoms and may decrease joint damage.
- Importantly, if present, septic arthritis should be diagnosed immediately and it should be treated with appropriate intravenous antibiotics and intensive follow-up.

TREATMENT

- The goals of therapy in OA are to relieve pain, maintain function, protect articular structures, and educate the patient.
- As there is no medication that has been shown to stop or reverse the disease process underlying OA, education about the disease and the rationale for therapy helps patients adhere to therapy.
- Pharmacologic therapy in pain management includes nonnarcotic analgesics, topical agents (eg, capsaicin), nonacetylated salicylates, nonsterodial anti-inflammatory drugs (NSAIDs) (initially analgesic dose), and intra-articular corticosteroids.
- Intra-articular corticosteroid injection may provide temporary or sustained relief of pain.
- Chronic use of strong narcotics and oral corticosteroids should be discouraged.
- Modification of activities, exercise (biking, walking, swimming), weight loss, splinting, joint protection, ambulatory assistive devices, physical therapy, hydrotherapy, heat/cold application, and self-help programs are nonpharmacologic measures that can play a crucial role in improving range of motion and stability and in decreasing pain.
- For those with advanced disease joint replacement surgery may dramatically improve the quality of life. Surgery should be considered for patients who experience intractable/refractory pain, loss of function or mobility, and radiographic evidence of advanced degenerative disease in the joint.
- A survey of 440 practicing rheumatologists revealed the following preferences for initial treatment of OA of the knee: nonnarcotic analgesic: 37%; low-dose NSAIDs: 35%; high-dose NSAIDs: 13%; physical therapy: 10%; and intra-articular corticosteroids: 6%. If the initial treatment failed to curtail symptoms, the preferred second therapy was intra-articular corticosteroid: 33%; high-dose NSAIDs: 30%; low-dose NSAIDs: 23%; physical therapy: 8%; and nonnarcotic analgesics: 5%.

CHRONIC INFLAMMATORY ARTHRITIS

- Chronic inflammatory arthritis is an inflammatory articular condition that has persisted more than 6 weeks.
- If fewer than three joints are involved, the patient has chronic mono/oligoarthritis. Synovial fluid analysis should be considered in such conditions.
- If chronic tuberculosis or fungal arthritis is suspected, synovial biopsy may be indicated. Gout and pseudogout are the other conditions that might be considered with mono/oligoarthritis.
- Patients who present with chronic oligo- or polyarthritis should be evaluated for other chronic inflammatory conditions including connective tissue diseases.
- Table 32–3 describes joint and extra-articular manifestations and laboratory findings, which, if present, may assist in the diagnosis of a specific chronic inflammatory arthritis.

RHEUMATOID ARTHRITIS

GENERAL

- Because rheumatoid arthritis (RA) is the most common type of chronic inflammatory arthritis, RA should be a major consideration in patients with symmetric arthritis of more than 6 weeks in duration and morning stiffness.

TABLE 32–3 Chronic Inflammatory Polyarthritis: Diagnosis

DIAGNOSIS	JOINT MANIFESTATIONS	EXTRA-ARTICULAR MANIFESTATIONS	LABORATORY FINDINGS
RA	Symmetric polyarthritis involving typical joints	Rheumatoid nodules, vasculitis, ocular, pulmonary lesions	Elevated RF* in ≥80% of patients
Spondyloarthropathy	Asymmetric oligoarthritis Inflammatory back pain Sacroiliitis	Typical skin rash Ocular involvement Genitourinary tract inflammation Bowel inflammation	Radiographic findings of sacroiliitis HLA-B27
Psoriatic arthritis	Asymmetric oligoarthritis Erosive peripheral arthritis (DIP and/or PIP joints) Spondylitis	Psoriatic skin lesions Nail changes	Negative RF in 80% of patients
Gout	Episodic mono/oligoarthritis	Tophi	Intra-articular MSU crystals in synovial fluid Elevetad serum urate levels
Systemic lupus erythematosus	Nondeforming inflammatory arthritis	Malar rash, photosensitivity, alopecia, oral/genital sores, digital ulcers	ANA, other autoantibodies Hematologic abnormalities

*RF, rheumatoid factor; MSU, monosodium urate; ANA, antinuclear antibody; DIP, distal interphalangeal; PIP, proximal interphalangeal.

TABLE 32–4   Revised Criteria for the Classification of Rheumatoid Arthritis

1. Stiffness in and around the joints lasting 1 h before maximal movement
2. Arthritis of three or more joint areas, simultaneously, observed by a physician
3. Arthritis of the proximal interphalangeal, metacarpophalangeal, or wrist joints
4. Symmetric arthritis
5. Rheumatoid nodules
6. Positive test for serum rheumatoid factor
7. X-ray changes characteristic of RA (erosions and/or periarticular osteopenia in hand and/or wrist joints

A person can be classified as having RA if four or more criteria are present at any time.
   Criteria 1 through 4 must be present for at least 6 wk.
   Criteria 2 through 5 must be observed by a physician.

- RA is a chronic, systemic, inflammatory disorder of unknown etiology.
- Its primary site of pathology is the synovium of the joints. The synovial tisues become inflamed and proliferate, forming pannus, which invades bone, cartilage, and ligament and leads to damage and deformities.
- RA affects approximately 1% of the population.
- Women are affected about three times more often than men.
- The peak onset is between 35 and 50 years of age.
- Diagnostic criteria for the classification of RA are summarized in Table 32–4.

EVALUATION

- No laboratory or diagnostic test by itself is diagnostic in RA.
- Rheumatoid factor (RF) is the test that is most closely associated with RA. It is present in 75 to 85% of the patients with established RA.
- Other laboratory tests that can be helpful in supporting the diagnosis of RA include synovial fluid analysis, measurement of acute phase reactants (erythrocyte sedimentation rate [ESR], C-reactive protein [CRP]), and complete blood count (CBC).
- Elevations in ESR and/or CRP levels provide a surrogate measure of inflammation and may be useful in establishing the diagnosis and gauging the response to therapy.
- In RA, synovial fluid analysis is expected to be non-inflammatory (Table 32–2).
- Early in the disease course plain radiographs may show only soft tissue swelling or joint effusion.
- Nearly 70% of patients develop bony erosions within the first 2 years of disease.

- Erosions may be seen in virtually any joint but are most common in the metacarpophalangeal (MCP), metatarsophalangeal (MTP), and wrist joints.

TREATMENT

- Although OA and RA are different arthritic conditions, pain management principles are similar.
- Goals of therapy in rheumatoid arthritis are to educate the patient, relieve pain, reduce inflammation, protect articular structures, control systemic involvement, and maintain function.
- The approach to treatment of RA has changed dramatically over the past decade.
- It is now recognized that the long-term prognosis for RA patients is poor and warrants the institution of aggressive therapy within the first few months of onset of RA.
- Most if not all RA patients should initially receive symptomatic treatment with NSAIDs.
- Low-dose corticosteroids (≤10 mg) may also be introduced at the beginning of therapy in selected patients.
- RA patients, especially those with aggressive disease, should receive disease-modifying drugs (DMARDs) very early in the disease course.
- Methotrexate (with concomitant folate) is the most commonly used DMARD. Other DMARDs include hydroxychloroquine, sulfasalazine, leflunomide, tumor necrosis factor (TNF) inhibitors (infliximab, etanercept, adalimumab), cyclosporin, cyclophosphamide, azathioprine, and minocycline.
- Altering the disease progression with DMARDs has great impact on pain management.
- Some RA patients may require intraarticular corticosteroid injections when they have one or two joint flareups.
- Pain management is not limited to NSAIDs. Some physicians prescribe antidepressants or narcotic analgesics in patients who are recalcitrant to therapy.
- Ambulatory/assistive devices, orthotics/splints, physical/occupational therapy, exercise, rest, and self-help programs are nonpharmacologic agents that are helpful in treatment of pain and maintenance of functional status.

REFERENCES

1. **Ruddy S, Harris E, Sledge CB, eds.** *Kelley's Textbook of Rheumatology.* Philadelphia: WB Saunders; 2001.
2. **Cush JJ, Kavanaugh AF, eds.** *Rheumatology Diagnosis and Therapeutics.* Philadelphia: Lippincott Williams & Wilkins; 2000.

33 CANCER PAIN

Bradley W. Wargo, DO
Allen W. Burton, MD

EPIDEMIOLOGY

- The World Health Organization (WHO) estimates that by 2021, there will be 15 million new cases of cancer worldwide. As new treatments increase survival rates, cancer patients will live longer with pain from the disease and its treatment.[1]
- Cancer pain and its undertreatment are epidemic.[2] Up to 50% of patients undergoing treatment for cancer and up to 90% of patients with advanced cancer have pain.[3] Most (an estimated 70%) cancer pain is due to tumor involvement with soft tissue, viscera, nerves, or bone and to structural changes in the body secondary to the tumor (eg, muscle spasm or imbalance).
- Up to 25% of cancer pain is due to therapy, including chemotherapy, radiotherapy, immunotherapy, and/or surgery.
- Cancer pain can be categorized as: (1) pain caused by the cancer itself, (2) pain related to treatment, and (3) other pain, including osteoarthritis, degenerative disc disease, and diabetic neuropathy.[4]
- The impact of cancer pain is multiplied by the interaction of pain and its treatments with other common cancer symptoms: fatigue, dyspnea, weakness, nausea, constipation, and impaired cognition.
- Nearly all cancer-related pain is associated with and magnified by psychologic and spiritual distress.

ASSESSMENT

- The patient with cancer requires a careful and detailed history and physical examination to elicit the true nature of the pain. In addition, if there are multiple pain complaints, then each pain issue needs to be considered separately.
- When compiling a pain history in a patient with cancer, the history must include the standard pain questions:
  - Location
  - Intensity
  - Quality
  - Duration/temporal pattern
  - Initiating factors
  - Radiating components
  - Previous therapy or treatments (pharmacologic and nonpharmacologic)
  - Associated psychologic components
  - Associated social/family components
  - Other chronic pain diagnoses and treatments
- Questions must also be asked about the cancer diagnosis, progression, and treatments because cancer treatments and metastasis can cause pain (eg, chemotherapy and radiotherapy can induce neuropathies; thoracotomy and mastectomy can lead to postoperative pain syndromes).
- Any new pain in a patient with cancer is assumed to be disease progression until proven otherwise.
- The physical examination should also be detailed, as specific sensory or motor exam findings may indicate tumor location (primary or metastatic).
- After the physical examination, imaging can confirm the diagnosis:
  - Plain films: fractures, visceral pathology
  - Bone scans: increased bone growth or destruction
  - Magnetic resonance imaging: evaluation of soft tissue pathology, especially spinal neoplastic disease
  - Computed tomography: bone pathology
  - Electromyography/nerve conduction studies

MANAGEMENT

TREATMENT GUIDELINES

- The most effective form of treatment of any cancer-related pain is treatment of the cancer itself, which in the majority of cases reduces or eliminates the pain. Early intervention is the key to preventing the development of posttherapy neuralgias as well as to helping the patient tolerate potentially difficult oncologic treatment protocols. Appropriately dosed opioids are the cornerstone of effective cancer pain management. Management of opioid-related side effects and the appropriate use of adjuvants and procedures complete the treatment armamentarium.
- The control of pain involves modifying the source of the pain, altering the central perception of pain, and blocking the transmission of the pain to the central nervous system. An individual care plan must be designed and implemented, and reassessed at regular intervals to ensure that both the quality and the quantity of a patient's life are optimized.[5]
- Cancer pain can be treated effectively in 85–95% of patients with an integrated program of systemic, pharmacologic, and anticancer therapy.[5] The remaining patients can be appropriately treated with invasive procedures.
- Several algorithms exist for the treatment of cancer-related pain. The first was WHO's analgesic ladder (Figure 33–1). A more detailed treatment guideline was later published by the National Cancer Care Network (NCCN).[6] Use of a cancer pain treatment

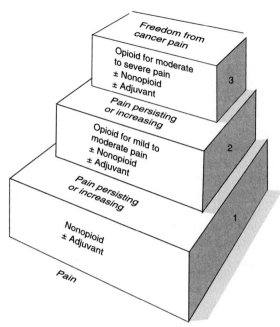

FIGURE 33–1 WHO analgesic ladder for the treatment of cancer pain.

algorithm by oncologists improves cancer patients' symptom control.[7]

- Although oversimplified, the basic tenets of the WHO analgesic ladder remain helpful in the treatment of cancer pain: begin with a nonopioid analgesic (aspirin, acetaminophen, nonsteroidal anti-inflammatory drugs [NSAIDs]) and increase to intermediate or stronger opioids and/or adjuvant medications as needed.

- Our group within the University of Texas M. D. Anderson Cancer Center has published a modified and condensed version of the NCCN guideline that fits on a pocket card (Figure 33–2).[8] Our recommendation is to prescribe stronger opioids and adjuvants sooner and to reassess treatment frequently to deal with increased pain levels. One need not start on the bottom rung of the ladder. In cases of severe pain, it is sometimes appropriate to initiate strong opioids and or adjuvant analgesics.

- The specifics of which opioid, starting dose, and adjuvants to use rest largely in the realm of the art of medicine; little comparative evidence exists that would permit us to recommend specific analgesic combinations and doses.

- In general, treatment intensity may be based on pain reported on a written or verbal numeric or facial expression pain intensity scale and on the patient's degree of opioid tolerance. On the analog/numeric pain scale, where 0 is no pain and 10 is the worst pain imaginable, pain scaled 1 to 3 corresponds to mild

pain, 4 to 6 refers to moderate pain, and 7 to 10 signifies severe pain.

- Mild-to-moderate opioids include propoxyphene, codeine, and hydrocodone, and strong opioids include morphine, oxycodone, fentanyl, and methadone. Common nonopioid and opioid analgesics are described in Table 33–1.

SELECTING THE APPROPRIATE ANALGESIC DOSE

- The appropriate analgesic dose depends on the pain scale result and history of opioid therapy. The efficacy of the therapy should be periodically reassessed, with dosing adjusted as necessary.

NONOPIOID ANALGESICS

- The nonopioid analgesics (WHO Step 1) are characterized by a ceiling effect, above which there is no additive affect. NSAIDs achieve analgesia mainly by decreasing circulating levels of inflammatory mediators released at the site of tissue injury—specifically by inhibiting the enzyme cyclooxygenase. Cyclooxygenase (COX) catalyzes the conversion of arachidonic acid to prostaglandins and leukotrienes, which sensitizes nerves to painful stimuli.[4] The new class of COX-2-specific NSAIDs produce analgesia and anti-inflammation activity equivalent to those of nonselective NSAIDs, without the COX-1 side effects of gastrointestinal toxicity and inhibition of platelet aggregation.[1]

WEAK TO MODERATE OPIOIDS

- The so-called weak to moderate potency opioids (WHO Step 2) are frequently combined with an NSAID or acetaminophen to create a synergistic effect. The limitation of this combination therapy is that there is an analgesic ceiling associated with NSAIDs as well as a dose-dependent toxicity. It is at this step that we employ the analgesic adjuvants listed in Table 33–2. Such adjuvants treat concurrent symptoms that exacerbate pain, produce independent analgesia for specific types of pain, and increase the analgesic efficacy of opioids.[5]

- Note that the following weak to moderate opioids are listed on the Drug Enforcement Agency's Schedule 3; thus, prescriptions may be phoned in, written for multiple refills, and written on standard prescription pads.
  - Hydrocodone, the most commonly prescribed opioid analgesic in the United States, is available only in combination with acetaminophen in oral formulation.

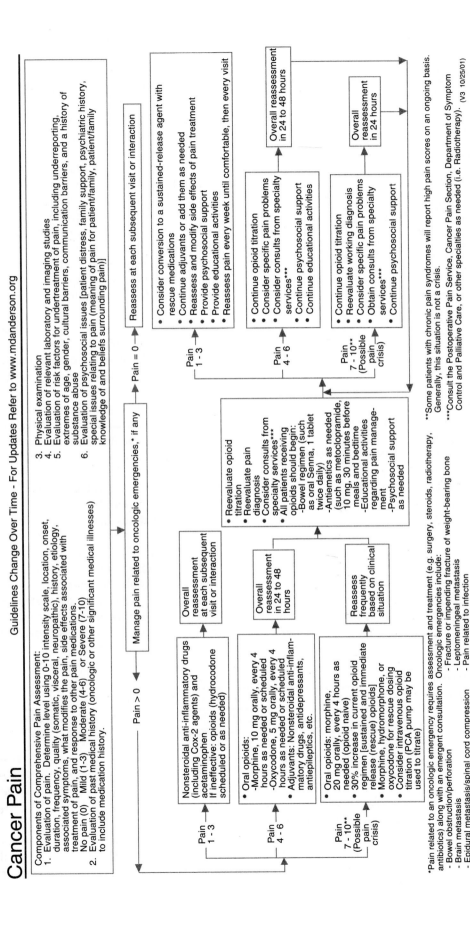

FIGURE 33–2 M. D. Anderson cancer pain treatment guideline. From Bruera et al.[8]

TABLE 33–1   Common Nonopioid and Opioid Analgesics

MEDICATION CLASS	MEDICATION	ADULT STARTING DOSE
Nonopioids	Acetaminophen	325–650 mg PO q4–6h
	Tramadol	50–100 mg PO q6h
NSAIDs	Ibuprofen	400–800 mg PO q6–8h
	Salicylate	500–750 mg PO q8–12h
	Naproxen	250–500 mg PO q8–12h
	Ketorolac	15–30 mg IV q6–8h
COX-2-specific NSAIDs	Celecoxib	100–200 mg PO q12–24h
	Rofecoxib	12.5–25 mg PO q24h
	Valdecoxib	10–20 mg PO q24h
Short-acting opioids	Hydrocodone	5–10 mg PO q4h prn
	Morphine	10–30 mg PO q3–4h prn
	Oxycodone	5–10 mg PO q3–4h prn
	Hydromorphone	1–3 mg PO q3–4h prn
	Transmucosal fentanyl (Actiq)	200–400 µg TM q3–8h
Long-acting opioids	Morphine controlled-release	15 mg PO q12h
	Oxycodone controlled-release	10 mg PO q12h
	Transdermal fentanyl (Duragesic)	25 µg/h, replaced q72h
	Methadone	2.5–10 mg PO q8–12h

- Propoxyphene is most commonly combined with acetaminophen or aspirin.
- Acetaminophen with codeine is another commonly prescribed weak opioid.
- Tramadol is a weak mu agonist available as a sole agent or in combination with acetaminophen.

"STRONG" OPIOIDS

- The pure opioid agonists (WHO Step 3) do not have a ceiling effect and are dose-limited only by dose-dependent side effects. Opioid analgesics bind to the μ receptor. Investigators have identified multiple μ_1 receptors, and this genetic polymorphism may result in varying expression of these receptors in different patients, which would explain why some patients respond better to one opioid class than to another.[1]
  - ○ Morphine, the gold standard of opioid analgesics, forms the basis by which all other classes of opioids are compared. Morphine is converted to morphine-3-glucoronide (M3G) and morphine-6-glucoronide (M6G) via glucoronyl transferase in the liver. M3G has low affinity for the opioid receptor but may be responsible for the neuroexcitatory toxic effects of morphine.[9] M6G has potent opioid activity but is converted in a smaller quantity than other metabolites. Because these metabolites are renally excreted, they should be used cautiously in patients with renal impairment. Morphine is available in immediate-release and controlled-release formulations. Morphine is also available in parenteral and preservative-free formulations (suitable for neuraxial use).
  - ○ Oxycodone, which is potent when used as a sole agent, is also combined with acetaminophen or an NSAID, which limits the dose. Oxycodone is currently available in immediate- and sustained-release oral preparations.
  - ○ Hydromorphone is available in oral and parenteral formulations (including preservative-free formulations suitable for neuraxial use). The controlled-release formulation available in other countries will soon be sold in the United States.
  - ○ Fentanyl is a semisynthetic opioid available in transdermal, parenteral, neuraxial, and transmucosal formulations that is useful in the management of severe cancer pain in the opioid-tolerant patient (Table 33–3). Transdermal and oral transmucosal fentanyl citrate (Actiq) are difficult to titrate and should be reserved for patients with chronic pain who have exhausted oral opioid options. The suggested equivalency ratio is 100:1 (oral morphine:fentanyl transdermal patch in mil-

TABLE 33–2   Adjuvant Analgesics

MEDICATION CLASS	MEDICATION	ADULT STARTING DOSE
Anticonvulsants	Gabapentin (Neurontin)	100–300 mg PO qhs, with dose escalations to 3600 mg/d divided tid
	Tiagabine (Gabitril)	2–4 mg PO q24 h, with dose escalations to 56 mg/d divided bid to qid
Tricyclic antidepressants	Amitriptyline (Elavil)	10–25 mg PO every night
	Nortriptyline (Pamelor)	10–25 mg PO every morning
	Desipramine (Norpramin)	10–25 mg PO every morning
Selective serotonin reuptake inhibitors	Sertraline (Zoloft)	25–50 mg PO qd
	Paroxetine (Paxil)	10–20 mg PO qd
Psychostimulants	Dextroamphetamine (Dexedrine)	5–10 mg PO every morning and noon
	Methylphenidate (Ritalin)	5–10 mg PO every morning and noon
Bisphosphonates	Etidronate (Didronel)	5–10 mg/kg/d PO*, †
	Pamidronate (Aredia)	90 mg IV every month*, †

*Diener KM. Bisphosphonates for controlling pain from metastatic bone disease. *Am J Health-Syst Pharm.* 1996;53:1917–1927.
†LaCivita CL. Pain management for bone metastases. *Am J Health-System Pharm.* 1996;53:1907.

TABLE 33–3 Transdermal Fentanyl Equivalency Ratio*

IV/SC MORPHINE	ORAL MORPHINE	TRANSDERMAL FENTANYL
20 mg	60 mg	25 µg/h
40 mg	120 mg	50 µg/h
60 mg	180 mg	75 µg/h
80 mg	240 mg	100 µg/h

*From Bruera et al.[8]

ligrams per 24 hours). It is important to prescribe breakthrough doses of another opioid with initiation of the patch. The patch dose should not be increased more frequently than every 3 days, and the increase should be based on the additional amount of breakthrough opioid required during a 3-day period. When rotating a patient off the fentanyl patch, a new opioid should be started 12 hours after removal of the patch. Breakthrough medication should be available during and after this critical period.

○ Methadone, a long-acting opioid available parenterally and orally, has the added benefit of creating an *N*-methyl D-aspartate (NMDA) receptor antagonizing effect for cancer pain patients with neuropathic pain. Methadone has great utility when used cautiously in low doses and titrated upward carefully.

ROUTES OF ADMINISTRATION

- In patients not responding to oral medications (or unable to use their gastrointestinal tract), the other routes of administration are:
  ○ Sublingual/transmucosal
  ○ Rectal
  ○ Intramuscular
  ○ Subcutaneous
  ○ Transdermal
  ○ Transmucosal
  ○ Parenteral
  ○ Intracerebroventricular
  ○ Epidural/subarachnoid[10]

BREAKTHROUGH PAIN

- The appropriate interval for dosing depends on the opioid used and the route of administration, and dosing of short- or long-acting opioids should be scheduled at intervals that prevent breakthrough pain.[11]
- Each breakthrough dose should be approximately 10% of the total daily opioid dose.

- Long-acting dosage forms of morphine sulfate (Oramorph) and oxycodone (OxyContin) are given every 8 to 12 hours. Breakthrough doses of immediate-release products should always be prescribed in conjunction with these long-acting pharmaceuticals.

OPIOID SIDE EFFECTS

- The most common opioid side effects include nausea and vomiting, constipation, cognitive impairment, myoclonus, sedation, and respiratory depression. These side effects are generally self-limiting, except for constipation, which can be managed with a consistent regimen of bowel stimulants and laxatives.
- When starting a patient on opioids, we prophylactically administer metoclopramide for nausea and Senekot S for constipation.
- Sedation can be managed by decreasing the dose of the opioid, rotating opioids, or adding a psychostimulant.

OPIOID ROTATION

- The long-term use of opioid analgesics may lead to opioid tolerance, but tolerance to a specific opioid does not predict tolerance to equianalgesic doses of other opioids—a finding referred to as "incomplete cross-tolerance." Table 33–4 presents the equianalgesic doses for opioid conversion. Due to incomplete cross-tolerance it is important to decrease the daily dose of a new opioid by 30–50%.
- At our institution, we convert all opioid analgesics to a morphine equivalent daily dose (MEDD), to better assess opioid usage and requirements.
- Methadone is unique in its nonlinear conversion ratios; at low morphine doses methadone is close to a 1:1 conversion, whereas at high doses (>300 mg/d morphine) methadone is much more potent and the conversion ratio may be 20:1. When converting to methadone in patients on high-dose opioids, therefore, a 90% reduction in dosing is appropriate.[12,13] Because of its long half-life, methadone must be titrated upward slowly and carefully, using a short-acting opioid liberally until the methadone therapeutic dose is attained.

ANALGESIC ADJUVANTS: NEUROPATHIC PAIN

- Neuropathic pain can be caused by the direct invasion of tumor into nervous structures, by

TABLE 33–4 Conversion Table for Opioids*

OPIOID	IV/SC OPIOID TO IV/SC MORPHINE	IV/SC MORPHINE TO IV/SC OPIOID	ORAL OPIOID TO ORAL MORPHINE	ORAL MORPHINE TO ORAL OPIOID
Hydromorphone	5	0.2	5	0.2
Meperidine	0.13	8	0.1	10
Levorphanol	5	2	5	0.2
Oxycodone	—	—	1.5	0.7
Hydrocodone	—	—	0.5	2

Oral morphine to IV/SC morphine: *divide by 3*; IV/SC morphine to oral morphine: *multiply by 3*
Example
To convert from hydromorphone 4 mg PO every 4 h plus two extra 2-mg doses of hydromorphone per day (4 mg) to oral morphine immediate-release (IR):
   1. Total opioid amount: oral hydromorphone equals 28 mg/d.
   2. 28 mg×5=oral morphine 140 mg/d; 30% decrease=oral morphine 98 mg/d.
   3. New regimen: oral morphine IR 100 mg divided by 6 doses=oral morphine IR 15 mg every 4 h around the clock plus 7.5 mg every 2 h prn for breakthrough pain.

*From Bruera et al.[8]

antineoplastic therapy, or by other cancer-related causes including[14]:
   ○ Chemotherapy-induced peripheral neuropathies (ie, cisplatin, paclitaxel, and vincristine)
   ○ Radiotherapy-induced plexopathies (brachial, lumbar, and sacral)
   ○ Postherpetic neuralgia
- A third of cancer patients suffer from neuropathic pain.[12] Many symptoms of neuropathic pain (ie, burning, lancing, electric shock-like allodynia and hyperalgesia) can be managed with adjuvant medications, including:
   ○ Antiepileptic drugs (AEDs)
   ○ Heterocyclic antidepressants
   ○ Topical anesthetics (ie, lidocaine—the Lidoderm Patch)
   ○ NMDA receptor antagonists (ie, dextromethorphan, methadone, and ketamine)

ANALGESIC ADJUVANTS: OTHER

- The COX-2-specific NSAIDs produce analgesia and anti-inflammation activity equivalent to those of the nonselective NSAIDs, without the COX-1 side effects of gastrointestinal toxicity and inhibition of platelet aggregation.[1]
- Any of the serotonin-specific reuptake inhibitors are useful in patients with situational depression.
- Low-dose benzodiazepines or butyrophenones (ie, haloperidol) are useful in treating anxiety.
- Low-dose heterocyclic antidepressants or the sedative-hypnotics (eg, zolpidem [Ambien] and zaleplon [Sonata]) are used to treat insomnia.
- For nausea, we optimize the bowel regimen and use metoclopramide scheduled and as needed.

- For appetite stimulation, we use low-dose dronabinol (Marinol 2.5–5 mg twice daily).

INTERVENTIONAL PAIN MANAGEMENT

- When other analgesic measures have failed to provide adequate pain control or cause intolerable side effects, or when the risk:benefit ratio is highly favorable for a certain procedure, we use the following interventional techniques. The timing of the use of such modalities is controversial; one study found significantly fewer side effects in cancer pain patients with intrathecal therapy versus oral medical management.[10]
   ○ Neurolytic blocks (eg, celiac plexus block for pancreatic pain)
   ○ Neuraxial analgesia in the form of epidural port-a-caths or tunneled catheters, intrathecal tunneled catheters, intraventricular catheters, or implanted intrathecal catheter/pump systems
   ○ Vertebroplasty (for painful compression fractures or painful metastasis)
- We generally go to neuraxial techniques when the patient has poor analgesia or intolerable opioid side effects despite opioid rotation.
- Patients using neuraxial pain control methods must receive adequate follow-up to have their pumps refilled and/or dosage adjusted as needed. Frequently, drug combinations including local anesthetics and clonidine are useful in neuropathic pain states.[15]
- Finally, in desperate situations where the pain is difficult to control, it may be appropriate to perform neurosurgical destructive procedures such as:
   ○ Anterolateral cordotomy (spinothalamic tractotomy)
   ○ Stereotactic mesencephalotomy
   ○ Midline myelotomy

○ Hypophysectomy
○ Dorsal root entry zone lesions

PALLIATIVE CARE

- Palliative care is the active, total care of patients whose disease is not responsive to curative treatments. Control of symptoms (including pain) and provision of psychological, social, and spiritual support are paramount.[16] The goal of palliative care is to achieve the best possible quality of life for patients and their families. This growing area of medicine is often practiced in inpatient units, with a transitional approach that involves sending some patients home with home hospice care. This is a very patient-centered, multidisciplinary method of caring for a dying patient.

CONCLUSION

- As in other areas of pain management, the tenets of good cancer pain management are similar to those of any sound medical practice.
- Examine the patient carefully, set realistic treatment goals, and then administer medications and interventional treatments in concord with the patient and the oncologist.
- Remember to enlist the help of consultants with difficult cases (including specialists in physical medicine, hospice, and palliative care).

REFERENCES

1. **Lucas LK, Lipman AG.** Recent advances in pharmacotherapy for cancer pain management. *Cancer Pract.* 2002; 10(Suppl 1):S14–S20.
2. **Hewitt DJ.** The management of pain in the oncology patient. *Obstet Gynecol Clin.* 2001;28(4).
3. **Cleeland CS, Gonin R, Hatfield AK, et al.** Pain and its treatment in outpatients with metastatic cancer. *N Engl J Med.* 1994;330:592–596.
4. **Chang HM.** Cancer pain management. *Med Clin North Am.* 1999;83(3).
5. **Levy MH.** Drug therapy: Pharmacologic treatment of cancer pain. *N Engl J Med.* 1996;335:1124–1132.
6. **Benedetti C, Brock C, Cleeland C, et al.** NCCN practice guidelines for cancer pain. *Oncology.* 2000;11:135–150.
7. **DuPen SL, Du Pen AR, Polissar N, et al.** Implementing guidelines for cancer pain management: Results of a randomized controlled clinical trial. *J Clin Oncol.* 1999; 17:361–370.
8. **Bruera E, Burton A, Cleeland C.** *Cancer Pain Guidelines.* Houston: Univ of Texas M. D. Anderson Cancer Center; 2001.
9. **Reddy SK, Shanti BF.** Cancer pain: Assessment and management. *Primary Care Cancer.* 2000;20: 44–52.
10. **Smith TJ, Staats PS, Deer T, et al.** Randomized clinical trial of an implantable drug delivery system compared with comprehensive medical management for refractory cancer pain: Impact on pain, drug-related toxicity, and survival. *J Clin Oncol.* 2002;20:4040–4049.
11. **Portenoy RK, Payne D, Jacobsen P.** Breakthrough pain: Characteristics and impact in patients with cancer pain. *Pain.* 1999;81:129–134.
12. **Grond S, Radbruch L, Meuser T, et al.** Assessment and treatment of neuropathic cancer pain following WHO guidelines. *Pain.* 1999;79:15–20.
13. **Mancini I, Lossignol DA, Body JJ.** Opioid switch to oral methadone in cancer pain. *Curr Opin Oncol.* 2000; 12:308–313.
14. **Norton JA, Edwards AD.** Pain in adults with cancer. In: *The Massachusetts General Hospital Handbook of Pain Management.* Lippincott Williams & Wilkins; 2002; 453–469.
15. **Walker SM, Goudas LM, Cousins MJ, et al.** Combination spinal analgesic chemotherapy: A systemic review. *Anesth Analg.* 2002;95:674–715.
16. **Patrick DL, Engelberg RA, Curtis JR.** Evaluating the quality of dying and death. *J Pain Symptom Manage.* 2001; 22:717–726.

34 CENTRAL PAIN

Michael G. Byas-Smith, MD

BRAIN: ISCHEMIC INJURY

DESCRIPTION OF PROBLEM

- Most cases of central poststroke pain (CPSP) occur after a thalamic stroke, but injury to other regions of the brain can give rise to chronic pain including injury to the cortex (see Figures 34–1 and 34–2.)
- The diagnosis of CPSP is made after identifying a definable lesion of the brain in concert with characteristic painful symptoms that do not result from peripheral disease.[1]
- The painful region may encompass a small area of body but typically is large, ignoring sclerotomal, dermatomal, and myotomal distributions.
- CPSP is often of an intractable nature and effective treatment options are limited.
- No pain quality is pathognomonic for central pain, but constant burning and aching are common descriptions mixed with recurring acute sharp/shooting sensations (see Table 34–1).

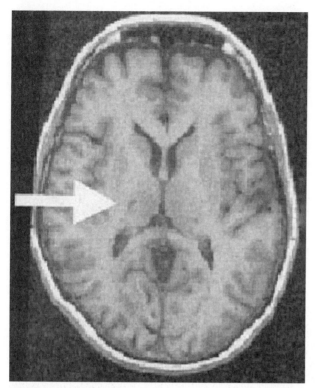

FIGURE 34–1 Magnetic resonance image of brain. Arrow points to infarction region on this T2-weighted image in a patient with a thalamic infarct.

- The intensity of the pain is typically not extreme but considerably irritating and distracting.

PATHOPHYSIOLOGY OF PAIN
- Most investigators agree that central CPSP is caused by perturbations of the somatosensory systems.[2]
- Central pain is independent of abnormalities in muscle function, coordination, vision, hearing, vestibular functions, and higher cortical functions.
- Nonsensory symptoms are not necessary for the development of central pain.
- The two most widely discussed mechanisms for these sensory changes are the ectopic activity hypothesis and the neuroplastic change, synaptic reorganization hypothesis.[3]
  ○ The mechanism for ectopic activity involves the spontaneous or evoked discharge of neurons linked to the processing of somatosensory information. As a consequence of an imbalance in sensory neuronal input and altered synaptic connections, the patient perceives discomfort.
  ○ The neuroplastic changes and hypersensitivity states that occur during and after nerve injury to the somatosensory system result from the activation of *N*-methyl-D-aspartate (NMDA) receptors by excitatory amino acids.

MULTIPLE SCLEROSIS

DESCRIPTION OF PROBLEM
- The body region involved in the ongoing pain virtually always displays thermal sensory abnormalities often with cold or tactile allodynia.
- Chronic pain in multiple sclerosis patients is a common finding and is believed to have a central nervous system origin. It is estimated that at least 25% of all patients with multiple sclerosis suffer from central pain.[4]
- Like other central pain syndromes, patients complain of a variety of different symptoms and body locations.
  ○ The qualities of pain include: aching, burning, cutting, cramplike sensations, prickling, and others.
  ○ The symptoms can be reported as being deep, superficial, or a combination of the two. The symptoms can be intermittent but the more severe cases involve constant nagging pain.
  ○ The location of the pain can vary, but very commonly patients report symptoms in the lower extremities and will have pain involving multiple

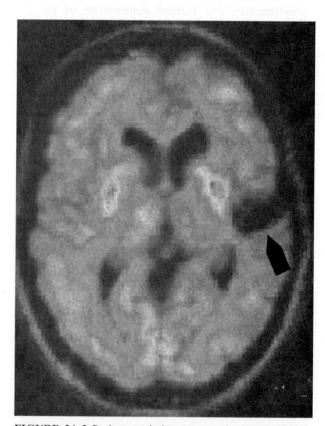

FIGURE 34–2 Positron emission tomography image of brain. Arrow identifies an infarction region in the right hemisphere (SII somatosensory cortex). This patient experienced pain over the entire left side of her body.

TABLE 34–1 Mechanism-Directed Treatment Approach to Central Pain

SYMPTOM/SIGN	POSSIBLE MECHANISM	MODULATING TREATMENT
Spontaneous pain (paroxysms)	Ectopic activity	Anticonvulsants (gabapentin, lamotrigine, topiramate, carbamazepine, oxcarbazepine)
		Antiarrythmics (lidocaine, mexiletine)
Spontaneous pain (burning, aching)	Sensitized nociceptors?	Tricyclic antidepressants (desipramine, amytriptyline)
		α_2-Receptor agonists (clonidine)
		Opioids (morphine, methadone)
		Dorsal column stimulation
Sympathetically maintained pain (burning, aching)	Pathologic activity in sympathetic nervous system	α Receptor antagonists (phentolamine, prazosin)
		α_2 Receptor agonists (zanaflex, clonidine)
		Ganglionic blockade
Spatial and temporal summation	Progressive discharges in spinal neurons	NMDA receptor antagonists (ketamine, dextromethorphan, amantadine, memantine, methadone)
Thermal allodynia	Central neuroplastic changes due to unmasking of cold-sensitive cells	Tricyclic antidepressants (desipramine, amytriptyline)
		Anticonvulsants (lamotrigine)
Dynamic mechanical allodynia	Neuroplastic changes, synaptic reorganization	NMDA receptor antagonists (ketamine, dextromethorphan, amantadine, memantine, methadone)
		Anticonvulsant (gabapentin)
Static mechanical allodynia	Sensitization of C nociceptors	Mexiletine, lamotrigine, carbamazepine, opioids
Punctate mechanical allodynia	Neuroplastic changes via Aδ fibers	Antiarrythmics (lidocaine, mexiletine)
		Anticonvulsants (gabapentin, lamotrigine, topiramate, carbamazepine, oxcarbazepine)

areas of the body upper extremities and lower extremities and truncal distribution of painful symptoms.
- A trigeminal neuralgia is also a common feature in patients with multiple sclerosis.

PATHOPHYSIOLOGY OF PAIN

- The diagnosis of central pain in multiple sclerosis is based partly on exclusion and partly on specific criteria (as defined by Boivie).[3]
  - Nontrigemimal central pain and duration of pain longer than 6 months and no other known causes or suspected causes of peripheral generators of pain.
  - This in combination with the diagnostic criteria for multiple sclerosis such as radiologic exams demonstrating lesions and showing demyelination in the central nervous system (see Figure 34–3).
- Patients can present with a range of neurologic disabilities but there has not been any evidence to suggest that severity of the neuromuscular symptoms correlates with the intensity and incidence of pain.
- The demyelinating plaques that characterize multiple sclerosis can occur throughout the central nervous system and are frequently found in the spinal cord.
- The central pain from multiple sclerosis is thought to be secondary to disruptions in the spinal thalamic track pathways.

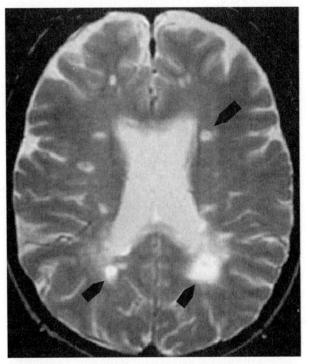

FIGURE 34–3 Magnetic resonance image of brain. Arrows identify plaques throughout the brain tissue in this patient diagnosed with multiple sclerosis.

- The lesions found in multiple sclerosis patients are thought to be the source of the ongoing pain, creating an imbalance and neuronal modulation of sensory information, particularly in regions involving pain and/or the involvement of abnormal discharges from sensory fibers and pathways native to the central nervous system.

SPINAL CORD

TRAUMATIC ISCHEMIC INJURY

DESCRIPTION OF PROBLEM
- Painful sensations are a common and troublesome sequela of paraplegia and quadriplegia following a spinal cord injury.
- The incidence of pain in this population has been reported to be as high as 96%.[5]
- Severe debilitating pain is present in a smaller percentage of patients but is typically resistant to a variety of therapeutic interventions.
- A number of classification schemes for the different types of painful syndromes have been devised over the years. In general, this schema divides the syndromes into categories related to symptoms occurring at the level of the injury below the chord injury and secondary to pathologic changes that occur as a consequence of the trauma.[6]
- Of these syndromes, central dysesthetic pain is by far the most difficult to manage.
- Dysesthetic pain syndrome has been defined as the presence of pain caudad to the site of injury for any period at least 4 weeks postinjury with the initial presentation of pain typically within the first year. The prevalence of dysesthetic pain is greatest in patients with incomplete quadriplegia, with pain sensations commonly referred to the lower extremities and posterior trunk below the zone of injury.[7]
- Using the McGill pain questionnaire the most commonly used descriptors of the sensations include: cutting, burning, piercing, radiating, cruel, and nagging.

PATHOPHYSIOLOGY OF PAIN
- The physiologic hypothesis concerning this altered neurologic state has not varied considerably over the past 50 years.[8]
- These mechanisms include:
  ○ Loss of balance between different sensory channels
  ○ Loss of spinal inhibitory mechanisms
  ○ Presence of pattern generators within the injured cord
- The bottom line is that a variety of abnormal electrophysiologic and neurochemical abnormalities are potentially in play in any given patient.[9,10]
- A variety of abnormal sensations are possible, some of which may be responsive to specific of therapies, but many others resist that treatment (see Table 34–1).

CORD LESIONS/SYRINGOMYELIA

DESCRIPTION OF PROBLEM
- Syringomyelia is one of several cord lesions that commonly give rise to central pain.
- Its hallmark is the development of an expanding post-traumatic cyst with ascension of the motor and sensory levels, increasing motor disability, and development of new pain.
- Claimed incidences for syringomyelia vary between 1 and 3.2% using clinical criteria in the pre-MRI era and up to 59% using MRI.[11]
- This disorder may take months to years to fully develop and as such is characteristically a late complication of cord injury.
- Patients with this problem usually complain of aching and burning pain at the level of the lesion, sometimes extending above and below the level of the lesion.
- Assessment of sensory and motor functions coupled with MRI helps determine the diagnosis.
- Continuous escalation in pain intensity is the natural course of pain associated with syringomyelia.
- Surgical intervention to decompress the cyst may not bring the pain under control.

PATHOPHYSIOLOGY OF PAIN
- Despite many hypotheses, the pathophysiology of syringomyelia is still not well understood.
- The advent of MRI techniques has greatly facilitated diagnosis of the condition (see Figure 34–4).
- The associated pain is presumably related to disturbances in the somatosensory apparatus of the cord and all the neurophysiologic derangements are potentially involved (see Table 34–1).

APPROACHES TO TREATMENT OF CENTRAL PAIN SYNDROMES

ANTICONVULSANT THERAPY

- The anticonvulsant medications have taken center stage in the management of neuropathic pain syndromes in general.
- With the exception of gabapentin, most anticonvulsant drugs presumably relieve neuropathic pain symptoms via sodium channel blockade.[1]
- The newer seizure medications have a much better side effect profile compared with older-generation medications and provide similar levels of analgesia.
- Consequently patients tolerate the higher doses of drug generally needed to achieve pain relief.
- Drugs like gabapentin, lamotrogine, and topiramate are examples of drugs that have led the way to greater use of anticonvulsants for nerve injury pain.

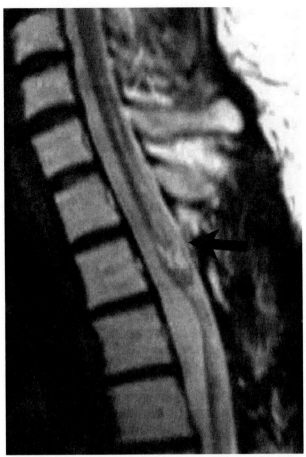

FIGURE 34–4 Magnetic resonance image of spine. Arrow identifies a cystic lesion in the spinal cord of a patient who was diagnosed as having syringomyelia.

- Older-generation drugs such as carbamazepine, phenytoin, and valproic acid are still used, but usually as second- and third-line alternatives.
- Unfortunately there are no control studies on the use of many of these medications after spinal cord injury and in other central pain syndromes, but the evidence is strong that nerve injury pain is responsive to this therapy.
- There is no clear rationale for choosing one medication over another as the initial treatment, but gabapentin has become the front-line anticonvulsant of choice in many practices throughout the world.

ANTIDEPRESSANT DRUGS

- Prior to the advent of second-generation anticonvulsant drugs, tricyclic antidepressant drugs were the front-line, nonopioid treatment for control of central pain.
- Rarely are patients with central pain syndromes or neuropathic pain symptoms of peripheral origin managed with a single agent.

- Polypharmacy is the method of the day and antidepressant medications should be included in the regimen.
- Parallel to anticonvulsants, newer antidepressants with fewer side effects have been brought to the market, but reports of better or equal analgesic potency in comparison to the older drugs have been slow to come.
- Consequently, amitriptyline, nortriptiline, and desiprimine continue to be commonly prescribed for control of central pain.
- These agents are thought to modulate the somatosensory pathways by enhancing the descending inhibitory system.
- Some patients may also benefit from the positive mood-altering effects observed in the higher dose range.

ANTIARRHYTHMIC DRUGS

- The oral anesthetic antiarrhythmic agents have been shown to be effective in management of neuropathic pain lesions in controlled studies, but these drugs, for example, mexiletine, are not well tolerated and can be proarrhythmic in certain populations.
- Mexiletine should be the third or fourth choice when developing a treatment strategy.

OPIOIDS

- There has been considerable controversy over the use of opioid analgesics for chronic management of neuropathic pain syndromes.
- Central pain syndromes tend to be refractory and require higher dosages to realize relief, and the opioids are no exception.
- A number of studies have shown the opioids to be effective in treating neuropathic pain syndromes, but very few systematic studies exist.
- Opioid medications in comparison to other therapies, including nonpharmacologic approaches, are rated highest in patient satisfaction among multiple sclerosis patients.[4]
- Opioids have several potential analgesic sites of operation at the spinal cord and brain level of the central nervous system.
- Treatment decisions regarding the use of opioids are, for the most part, based on case reports and clinical experiences, but the consensus among pain management specialists is that it is appropriate to use this class of medications chronically to control central pain.
- It is important to remember that patients with central pain syndromes typically show greater resistance to analgesic therapy when compared with patients with peripheral neuropathies.

- Opioids are the most commonly used medications in multiple sclerosis patients.

ELECTRICAL STIMULATION

TRANSCUTANEOUS ELECTRICAL NERVE STIMULATION

- Nerve stimulation treatments have been studied for patients with pain from spinal cord injury.
- The so-called TENS unit, or transcutaneous electrical nerve stimulation, has been shown to be effective in patients who experience pain at the level of injury.
- The technique is less effective below the site of injury. These conclusions are based on anecdotal reports in small case series, but the therapy is fairly inexpensive and is not associated with any significant risk to the patient at trial.

DORSAL COLUMN STIMULATION

- Implanted spinal cord stimulators have been used as well.
- The published data would suggest that this approach may not be indicated in that the results at this point have been disappointing. Additional study is needed.

INTRATHECAL ANALGESIC THERAPY

- Continuous infusion of intrathecal medications is used in select cases, particularly for spinal cord injury-induced central pain. Additional investigation is needed to validate any benefit.
- There are published studies showing acute relief of symptoms following administration of morphine and clonidine.
- Clonidine is most beneficial when spasms accompany the painful symptoms.

NMDA RECEPTOR ANTAGONISTS

- Blockade of these receptors and secondary messenger systems can prevent and reverse these hypersensitivity states in animal preparations.
- While not as successful as the anticonvulsants, agents that possess NMDA receptor-blocking effects have been used clinically with a modicum of success.

DORSAL ROOT ENTRY ZONE LESIONING

- Surgical treatments for spine cord lesions have been used for many years.

- The dorsal root entry zone (DREZ) lesioning technique is the most common.
- To date, the procedure has not been proven effective and should not be considered until all other approaches have been exhausted.

GAMMA KNIFE RADIAL SURGERY

- For severe cases, some institutions are using gamma knife radial surgery (GKS) for treatment of multiple sclerosis-associated trigeminal neuralgia.[12] If successful, the technique will probably be expanded to other central pain disorders.

OTHER ALTERNATIVE APPROACHES TO THERAPY

- A variety of so-called alternative treatments have been studied for these patients including acupuncture, massage, relaxation, and chiropractic techniques.
- Because the traditional therapies have not proven to be effective for most patients with severe central pain disorders, a significant number of patients seek alternative approaches to controlling their symptoms.
- Cannabinoids are among a growing list of agents that are being tested for use in battling this difficult and debilitating disease. Further research is needed to elucidate the benefit of these therapies.

REFERENCES

1. **Jensen TS.** Anticonvulsants in neuropathic pain: Rationale and clinical evidence. *Eur J Pain.* 2002;6(Suppl A):61–68.
2. **Dworkin RH.** An overview of neuropathic pain: Syndromes, symptoms, signs, and several mechanisms. *Clin J Pain.* 2002;18:343–349.
3. **Boivie J.** Central pain. In: Wall P, Melzack R, eds. *Textbook of Pain.* 4th ed. Edinburgh: Churchill Livingstone; 1999: 879–914.
4. **Kalman S, Osterberg A, Sorensen J, Boivie J, Bertler A.** Morphine responsiveness in a group of well-defined multiple sclerosis patients: A study with i.v. morphine. *Eur J Pain.* 2002;6:69–80.
5. **Warms CA, Turner JA, Marshall HM, Cardenas DD.** Treatments for chronic pain associated with spinal cord injuries: Many are tried, few are helpful. *Clin J Pain.* 2002;18:154–163.
6. **Cardenas DD, Turner JA, Warms CA, Marshall HM.** Classification of chronic pain associated with spinal cord injuries. *Arch Phys Med Rehabil.* 2002;83:1708–1714.

7. **Davidoff G, Roth E, Guarracini M, Sliwa J, Yarkony G.** Function-limiting dysesthetic pain syndrome among traumatic spinal cord injury patients: A cross-sectional study. *Pain.* 1987;29:39–48.
8. **Beric A.** Central pain and dysesthesia syndrome. *Neurol Clin.* 1998;16:899–918.
9. **Loeser JD, Melzack R.** Pain: An overview. *Lancet.* 1999;353:1607–1609.
10. **Wiesenfeld-Hallin Z, Aldskogius H, Grant G, Hao JX, Hokfelt T, Xu XJ.** Central inhibitory dysfunctions: Mechanisms and clinical implications. *Behav Brain Sci.* 1997;20:420–425.
11. **Bodley R.** Imaging in chronic spinal cord injury: Indications and benefits. *Eur J Radiol.* 2002;42:135–153.
12. **Rogers CL, Shetter AG, Ponce FA, Fiedler JA, Smith KA, Speiser BL.** Gamma knife radiosurgery for trigeminal neuralgia associated with multiple sclerosis. *J Neurosurg.* 2002;97:529–532.

35 COMPLEX REGIONAL PAIN SYNDROME

Paul J. Christo, MD
Srinivasa N. Raja, MD

HISTORY

- In 1864, Dr. Silas Mitchell and colleagues described a chronic pain syndrome with severe burning pain that followed injury to peripheral nerves from gunshot wounds sustained in the Civil War.
- Mitchell called what we now know as chronic regional pain syndrome (CRPS) Type II, "causalgia or burning pain." Rene Leriche, a French surgeon, later connected the sympathetic nervous system to causalgia by noting that sympathectomy provided pain relief in many of his patients.
- The term "reflex sympathetic dystrophy," or CRPS Type I, is used for a syndrome similar to causalgia that lacks a specific nerve lesion.
- "Reflex sympathetic dystrophy" (RSD), however, is a misnomer as it implies a reflex mechanism associated with a hyperactive sympathetic nervous system (SNS), and animal models suggest that altered neuromodulation, nerve hyperexcitability, and central sensitization may also contribute to CRPS.[1] To incorporate new pathophysiologic evidence and establish uniform terminology and diagnostic criteria, the International Association for the Study of Pain (IASP) proposed taxonomy that grouped the disorders under the term "complex regional pain syndromes." Type I CRPS corresponds to RSD and occurs without

an identifiable nerve lesion. Type II (previously "causalgia") results from a specific nerve injury.
- Diagnostic criteria for CRPS Types I and II include:
  - Regional, spontaneous pain, allodynia, or hyperalgesia not limited to the territory of a single peripheral nerve and disproportionate to a known inciting event.
  - Evidence of edema, changes in skin blood flow, or abnormal sudomotor activity in the region of the pain.
  - Presence of a noxious event or cause of immobilization (absent in 5–10% of patients).
  - No other condition that can otherwise account for the degree of pain and dysfunction.
  - Ability to differentiate CRPS from other neuropathic pain states by the presence of edema, vasomotor, and sudomotor dysfunction.
- The fact that the somatosensory symptoms of CRPS Type II extend beyond the course of the affected peripheral nerve distinguishes this syndrome from an isolated peripheral mononeuropathy.[2]

EPIDEMIOLOGY

- CRPS may be triggered by a variety of insults, such as trauma, surgery, inflammation, stroke, nerve injury, and immobilization.
- The syndrome occurs frequently in young adults and more frequently in women than in men.
- No correlation exists between the severity of injury and the resulting painful syndrome.[3]
- Patients with certain neoplasms of the lung, breast, central nervous system, and ovary, and patients suffering from stroke or myocardial infarction, may exhibit signs and symptoms of CRPS.[3]
- Even psychologic stressors and poor coping skills can influence the natural history and severity of CRPS.[4]

PATHOPHYSIOLOGIC MECHANISMS

- Although several pathophysiologic mechanisms have been postulated for CRPS, the disease is still poorly understood.
- Many believe that dysfunction of the sympathetic nervous system and/or an upregulation of adrenoceptors may play an important role in this syndrome.
- Animal models show that peripheral nerve injury induces the sprouting of sympathetic nerve fibers around sensory neurons in the dorsal root ganglion.
- In some models of nerve injury, mechanical allodynia and thermal hyperalgesia are alleviated by surgical or chemical sympathectomy.

- Abnormal nerve sprouting and C-fiber excitation by the sympathetic nervous system may explain the abnormal discharges observed in peripheral nerves following nerve damage.[5]
- Human studies implicate the SNS less clearly. In fact, variations in response to sympathetic blockade and high rates of relapse raise questions about the role of the sympathetics in the pathophysiology of CRPS.[1]
- Investigators postulate that concurrent central changes in the dorsal horn of the spinal cord participate in maintaining the hyperexcitable state of CRPS. The generation of central sensitization and consequent activation of *N*-methyl-D-aspartate (NMDA) receptors may sustain this neuronal hyperexcitability following nerve injury. Further, NMDA antagonists can attenuate the neurochemical cascade that leads to central sensitization. NMDA-induced hyperalgesia and loss of spinal inhibitory control may explain the phenomenon of neuropathic pain.

CLINICAL MANIFESTATIONS

- Great heterogeneity of symptoms exists in patients suffering from CRPS.
- The signs and symptoms of CRPS reflect changes in the sensory, autonomic, and motor systems.
- Patients frequently describe burning and stinging pain. Many report hyperesthesia to ordinary cutaneous stimuli such as contact with clothing or cool breezes. Moreover, patients often relate pain from nonpainful stimuli (allodynia) or exaggerated responses to painful stimuli (hyperalgesia).
- Temperature changes in the environment may exacerbate the pain.
- Other common pain descriptors include "aching, shooting, squeezing, and throbbing."
- Certain patients may even guard the affected region from cutaneous or thermal stimulation by wearing a glove or sock or exhibiting protective postures.
- Vasomotor disturbances in CRPS include temperature asymmetry and/or skin color changes.[6]
- Patients may complain that an extremity feels warm and appears red or feels cool and looks dusky or gray.
- Sudomotor changes are seen as an asymmetry of either hyperhidrosis or dryness in the painful region.
- Patients may present with evidence of edema in the affected limb that appears shiny or smooth.
- Motor dysfunction may manifest as dystonia, muscle spasms, tremor, or weakness of the painful muscle groups. More severe cases, or CRPS, can cause muscle atrophy and contractures. Occasionally, patients report myoclonic movements or complain of myofascial pain in the affected region. Trophic disturbances

in the affected limb may present as alteration in skin, nails, or hair pattern.
- If selective sympathetic blockade in the absence of somatic blockade relieves pain and/or allodynia, the patient is regarded as having a sympathetically maintained pain (SMP) component.
- If sympathetic blockade fails to alleviate the pain associated with CRPS, the syndrome is viewed as sympathetically independent pain. The results of sympathetic blockade need to be interpreted with caution, however, due to the potential for false positive and negative results.[3,7]
- A triad of stages (acute, dystrophic, and trophic) based on progressive signs and symptoms in CRPS has been proposed[8]; however, a prospective study of more than 800 patients with a diagnosis of RSD/causalgia could not substantiate a sequential progression of the syndrome. In a study of 113 patients, cluster analysis revealed three subgroups based on homogeneity of signs, symptoms, and duration of CRPS.[9] Interestingly, these subgroups did not differ in duration of CRPS, which argues against a chronologic progression of the disease. For instance, the subgroup presenting with severe CRPS features (stage III) experienced the shortest disease duration of the three groups.
- Most investigators believe that emotional and behavioral changes accompany CRPS. Many patients experience depression, anxiety, and fear. No well-designed studies have connected these psychologic symptoms to the cause or the result of the syndrome, however, and the psychologic distress of CRPS is generally considered a normal result of sustained pain and disability.

DIAGNOSIS

- The IASP criteria for diagnosis of CRPS do not list the number of signs and symptoms needed to make a diagnosis. An investigation of the internal and external validity of the IASP criteria led to a proposal of enhancing the criteria to require that a patient display at least one sensory (hyperesthesia), vasomotor (temperature or skin color changes), sudomotor/edema (sweating or edema asymmetry in the affected limb), or motor/trophic (trophic changes or motor dysfunction) symptom and at least one objective sign in two or more of the following categories: sensory (hyperalgesia or allodynia), vasomotor (temperature or skin color asymmetry), sudomotor/edema (edema or sweating abnormalities), or motor/trophic (weakness, tremor, dystonia; hair, nail, skin changes).[6,10]
- The diagnosis of CRPS remains clinical, though tests can aid in confirmation.

- Patients with CRPS can exhibit a wide spectrum of dysfunction including SMP or independent pain, autonomic changes, and neuropathy.
- Testing can clarify the existence of SMP and autonomic dysfunction or can rule out conditions that mimic CRPS. For instance, vascular studies can rule out deep vein thrombosis or vascular insufficiency, EMG/NCT can rule out peripheral neuropathy, radiographs and MRI can rule out bone, disc, or soft tissue pathology, and blood testing can rule out infection, cellulitis, or rheumatologic disease.
- Other tests can reinforce the diagnosis of CRPS by detecting abnormalities in sympathetic activity or blood flow in affected limbs. Note that outcome research has not supported the prognostic or therapeutic value of any of these tests.[3] Common tests are described below.

THERMOGRAPHY

- Uses an infrared thermometer to detect cutaneous thermal changes in two extremities.
- A difference of 1.0°C is considered significant.

QUANTITATIVE SENSORY TESTS

- Measure the intensity of stimuli needed to produce sensations such as touch, vibration, warmth, coolness, and heat and cold pain thresholds.
- These tests are used to help detect sensory abnormalities related to hyperesthesia, hyperalgesia, allodynia, and temperature changes associated with neuropathic pain.

PLAIN RADIOGRAPHS

- Display a patchy osteopenia as soon as 2 to 3 weeks after the onset of CRPS.
- As the syndrome progresses, a ground-glass appearance to the bony anatomy reflects generalized osteopenia and cortical erosions.

THREE-PHASE BONE SCINTIGRAPHY

- Intravenous administration of technetium-(^{99m}Tc)-labeled diphosphonate or polyphosphate detects osseous abnormalities in the affected limb sooner than do plain films.
- The test is divided into three phases (angiographic images, regional blood pooling, and bony uptake of ^{99m}Tc).

- In CRPS patients, the third phase reveals an abnormally diffuse increased joint uptake affecting the painful extremity only.

SUDOMOTOR TESTING

- The resting sweat output test measures the sweat output of nonstimulated skin in both the painful and nonpainful limbs.
- The quantitative sudomotor axon reflex test measures the sweat output provoked by an electric current and then by cutaneous application of methacholine or acetylcholine.
- In CRPS patients, the latency after electric current stimulation and prolonged sweating is shorter in the affected extremity.

SYMPATHETIC BLOCKS

- Local anesthetic blockade of the sympathetic chain (stellate ganglion block for the upper extremity and lumbar sympathetic block for the lower extremity) is an important diagnostic tool, especially if the block produces pain relief.
- A positive response (pain relief) is not necessary to diagnose CRPS, however.
- Patients with CRPS and SMP who experience symptomatic improvement following local anesthestic sympathetic blocks may benefit from having a series of blocks incorporated into their treatment regimen.
- Due to the risk of false positive and false negative tests associated with these procedures, a pharmacologic sympathetic block with phentolamine can be used to diagnose a sympathetically maintained component of CRPS. Phentolamine is a nonspecific α-adrenergic receptor antagonist that is infused intravenously at 1 mg/kg over 10 minutes. A positive response (pain reduction) implies involvement of adrenergic mechanisms in the pain state.[3]

TREATMENT

- Successful treatment of CRPS relies on an aggressive multidisciplinary approach that focuses on pain relief, physical rehabilitation, and control of psychologic dysfunction.

PHYSICAL THERAPY

- Physical therapy is integral to the treatment of CRPS. Yet, no randomized controlled trials report a favorable impact on the natural history of CRPS.[11]

- The treatment consists of progressive desensitization following adequate analgesia. This usually includes the use of heat, cold, vibration, massage, and contrast baths.
- Once the patient tolerates these interventions, isometric strengthening exercises are introduced.
- Finally, more aggressive treatment modalities that facilitate mobilization and resumption of activity in the affected limb are instituted: range of motion exercises, isotonic strengthening, and aerobic conditioning.
- Patients may require months to complete this process and also may experience a transient increase in their pain and swelling at the beginning of physiotherapy.

PHARMACOTHERAPEUTIC AGENTS

- Few placebo-controlled trials have been performed to assess treatment efficacy in patients with CRPS.
- Several medications, however, have been studied in controlled trials for the treatment of pain associated with postherpetic neuralgia and diabetic neuropathy.[11]

CORTICOSTEROIDS
- Studies have reported effective treatment of CRPS with corticosteroids.[11]
- Steroids may suppress CRPS-induced ectopic neural discharges and reduce the inflammatory component of the syndrome.
- Chronic use of steroids, however, is not recommended due to an unfavorable risk:benefit ratio.

TRICYCLIC ANTIDEPRESSANTS
- This class of medication can reduce pain, alleviate depression, and facilitate sleep in patients with CRPS.
- Randomized, controlled trials provide evidence that antidepressants treat neuropathic pain[12] in patients with postherpetic neuralgia and diabetic neuropathy.
- The mechanism of action may relate to reuptake inhibition of norepinephrine and serotonin in the central nervous system. These neurotransmitters may promote the effects of the descending, antinociceptive pathways in the CNS.
- Selective serotonin reuptake inhibitors are less effective in treating neuropathic pain.[13]
- Tricyclic antidepressants can produce conduction abnormalities, anticholinergic side effects, orthostatic hypotension, and sedation.

ANTICONVULSANTS
- Anticonvulsants (especially phenytoin and carbamazepine) are effective in treating neuropathic pain associated with trigeminal neuralgia and diabetic neuropathy.[12]
- FDA has recently approved gabapentin as an agent for the treatment of postherpetic neuralgia.
- Studies have found gabapentin to be effective in treating pain from postherpetic neuralgia[14] and diabetic neuropathic pain.
- Only case series and clinical observation suggest that gabapentin may be useful in treating CRPS.

OPIOIDS
- Neuropathic pain responds less favorably to opioid treatment; therefore, opioids are added only when CRPS-related pain responds poorly to other drug therapies.
- Because NMDA receptor antagonists effectively treat neuropathic pain, methadone is an appropriate first-line opioid for CRPS because of its NMDA receptor-blocking properties, followed by other long-acting opioid preparations of morphine, oxycodone, or fentanyl.
- Opioids can permit more complete participation in physical therapy and rehabilitation in patients with intractable CRPS-related pain.

TOPICAL AGENTS
- Lidocaine patches are useful in treating the allodynic component of CRPS in focal areas of pain.
- Capsaicin can produce analgesia in CRPS and peripheral neuropathy through its release and reuptake inhibition of substance P.[11] Unfortunately, patients are unable to tolerate the burning sensation associated with capsaicin treatment.

OTHER DRUG THERAPIES
- Randomized, controlled trials have not confirmed the efficacy of calcium channel blockers, bisphosphonates, oral α-adrenergic agents (prazosin, phenoxybenzamine), calcitonin, ketamine, clonidine, or muscle relaxants.
- Intrathecal baclofen, however, may be useful in treating the dystonia or nociceptive flexor reflexes associated with CRPS.[15]

SYMPATHETIC BLOCKS

- Sympathetic blockade with local anesthetics for diagnostic or therapeutic reasons has been used for many years as an integral component of the treatment plan for CRPS. The anecdotal literature suggests efficacy, but a systematic review (meta-analysis) revealed weak evidence for sympathetic blockade as a therapeutic modality[1] because fewer than one-third of patients obtained complete pain relief. Moreover, none of these studies permitted estimation of the duration of pain relief among those patients who responded to initial sympathetic blockade.

- Despite this finding, patients who derive meaningful relief from diagnostic sympathetic block (SMP) merit a series of frequent sympathetic ganglion blocks with local anesthetic for several weeks.
- Cervical or lumbar sympathetic blocks are performed intermittently or in series. Such blocks should spare both sensory and motor function, thus permitting patients to participate in physical therapy and rehabilitation.
- Physical therapy is often initiated subsequent to the blocks to maximize the analgesic effects of the blockade.
- If relapses occur or if repetitive blocks produce temporary pain relief, surgical sympathectomy, radiofrequency lesioning, or chemical neurolysis can be considered.
- In patients who fail to respond to sympathetic blocks, epidural or somatic blocks (brachial or lumbar plexus) can facilitate the transition to physical therapy.

REGIONAL AND NEURAXIAL BLOCKADE

- Lumbar, brachial, or epidural local anesthetic injections also block the corresponding sympathetic nerves.
- Similar to sympathetic blocks, somatic blocks can be performed in series or intermittently.
- Great care must be taken to ensure proper range of motion during physical therapy given that affected limbs are anesthetized during regional or neuraxial anesthesia.

NEUROMODULATION

- The mechanism of action of spinal cord stimulation (SCS) is incompletely understood but may involve inhibition of sympathetic function and changes in spinal or supraspinal GABA-mediated neurochemistry.[3]
- The use of SCS for the treatment of CRPS is controversial.
- A randomized, controlled trial of 36 patients with CRPS unresponsive to treatment demonstrated a statistically significant decrease in pain intensity with SCS.[16] Patients receiving SCS noted a significant decrease in their painful symptomatology but no improvement in functional status.
- In carefully screened patients with CRPS and in the context of multidisciplinary treatment, SCS can improve health-related quality of life.

- Epidural or intrathecal clonidine administered to CRPS patients reduces associated pain.[11]

CONCLUSION

- Most experts agree that only pieces of the CRPS puzzle have been discovered.
- Many authors wonder whether animal models for SMP can accurately depict the complexity of pain manifested in humans.[1]
- The clinical criteria for CRPS must be refined to improve the sensitivity and specificity of diagnosis.
- CRPS treatments are diverse, but no single treatment is uniformly effective.
- A multidisciplinary approach to the alleviation of pain and restoration of function that includes one or more modalities such as medications, sympathetic/somatic blockade, physical therapy, psychologic intervention, neuromodulation, and neuraxial analgesia is recommended.

REFERENCES

1. **Cepeda MS, Lau J, Carr DB.** Defining the therapeutic role of local anesthetic sympathetic blockade in CRPS: A narrative and systematic review. *Clin J Pain.* 2002;18:216.
2. **Rho RH, Brewer RP, Lamer TJ, et al.** Complex regional pain syndrome [concise review for clinicians]. *Mayo Clinic Proc.* 2002;77:174.
3. **Raja SN, Grabow TS.** Complex regional pain syndrome I (reflex sympathetic dystrophy). *Anesthesiology.* 2002; 96:1254.
4. **Lynch ME.** Psychological aspects of regional sympathetic dystrophy: A review of the adult and paediatric literature. *Pain.* 1992;49:337.
5. **McLachlan EM, Janig W, Devor M, et al.** Peripheral nerve injury triggers noradrenergic sprouting within dorsal root ganglia. *Nature.* 1993;363:543.
6. **Harden RN.** Complex regional pain syndrome. *Br J Anaesth.* 2001;87:99.
7. **Hogan QH, Abrams SE.** Neural blockade for diagnosis and prognosis. *Anesthesiology.* 1997;86(1):216–241.
8. **Galer BS, Schwartz L, Allen RJ.** Complex regional pain syndromes—type I: Reflex sympathetic dystrophy, and type II: Causalgia. In: Loeser JD, ed. *Bonica's Management of Pain.* 3rd ed. Philadelphia: Lippincott Williams & Wilkins; 2001:388.
9. **Bruehl S, Harden RN, Galer BS, et al.** Complex regional pain syndrome: Are there distinct subtypes and sequential stages of the syndrome? *Pain.* 2002;95:119.
10. **Harden RN, Bruehl S, Galer BS, et al.** Complex regional pain syndrome: Are the IASP diagnostic criteria valid and sufficiently comprehensive? *Pain.* 1999;83:211.

11. **Kingery WS.** A critical review of controlled clinical trials for peripheral neuropathic pain and complex regional pain syndrome. *Pain*. 1997;73:123.
12. **McQuay HJ, Tramer M, Nye BA, et al.** A systematic review of antidepressants in neuropathic pain. *Pain*. 1996;68:217.
13. **Watson CP.** The treatment of neuropathic pain: Antidepressants and opioids. *Clin J Pain*. 2000;16(2, Suppl):S49.
14. **Rice ASC, Maton S, et al.** Gabapentin in postherpetic neuralgia: A randomized, double blind, placebo controlled study. *Pain*. 2001;94:215.
15. **van Hilten BJ, van de Beek WJ, Hoff JI, et al.** Intrathecal baclofen for the treatment of dystonia in patients with reflex sympathetic dystrophy. *N Engl J Med*. 2000;343:625.
16. **Kemler MA, Barendse GA, van Kleef M, et al.** Spinal cord stimulation in patients with chronic reflex sympathetic dystrophy. *N Engl J Med*. 2000;343:618.

36 GERIATRIC PAIN

F. Michael Gloth III, MD, FACP, AGSF

THE SCOPE OF THE PROBLEM

- In no segment of our population is pain more prevalent than in our seniors.
- Studies indicate that as many as half of community-dwelling seniors suffer from pain that interferes with their ability to function normally. The prevalence of pain in nursing homes is an estimated 80%, with analgesics used in 40–50% of residents.[1]
- One of the greatest risk factors for having inadequately treated pain is simply being over 70 years of age.[2]

REASONS FOR THE VULNERABILITY OF SENIORS TO PAIN

- Reasons for poor pain management include lack of physician training, inadequate pain assessment, and the reluctance of physicians to prescribe opioids.[3]
- As most elderly patients take multiple medications for comorbid conditions, prescribing for the older adult in pain can be daunting.[4]
- Pain has not been studied thoroughly in elderly subjects, and most studies have focused on threshold levels of mechanical, electrical, or thermal stimuli.[5,6]
- With age, pain tolerance decreases, and pain complaints increase in frequency.
- Aging changes the dispersal of medications throughout the body, as well as blood flow to organs, protein binding, and body composition.

- Most analgesics are metabolized primarily by the liver and/or kidneys, and renal function typically declines with age, although routine indicators of renal function (eg, serum creatinine) may show little change.
- Factors that impede pain control include depression,[7] secondary gain, anxiety, and mentally focusing on the pain.

ASSESSMENT

- A formal pain assessment, a prerequisite to adequate pain control, is a challenge in seniors.[1–3]
- The 2002 version of the American Geriatrics Society's *Guidelines for Management of Persistent Pain in Older Adults* promotes use of pain scales that lack optimal standardization in seniors and cannot be applied in the presence of common disabilities, such as visual impairment.[4]
- The Functional Pain Scale (see Figure 36–1), which has been standardized in an older population for reliability, validity, and responsiveness,[5] has three levels of assessment:
  ○ First, the patient rates pain as "tolerable" or "intolerable." (Intolerable pain should be considered an urgent matter requiring immediate further evaluation and intervention with frequent follow-up to ensure improvement into the "tolerable" range as rapidly as possible.)
  ○ Second, a functional component adjusts the score depending on whether a person can respond verbally.
  ○ Finally, the 0–5 scale allows rapid comparison with prior pain levels (responsiveness). Ideally all patients should reach a 0–2 level, preferably 0–1.
- It may be difficult to determine the etiology of pain in seniors because their symptoms can differ from those of younger patients. For example, certain types

0 = No Pain

1 = Tolerable (and doesn't prevent any activities)

2 = Tolerable (but prevents some activities)

3 = Intolerable (but can use telephone, watch TV, or read)

4 = Intolerable (and can't use telephone, watch TV, or read)

5 = Intolerable (and unable to talk because of pain)

FIGURE 36–1 The Functional Pain Scale. Responsiveness and validity data have been collected in a frail, elderly population. From Gloth et al.[5]

of visceral pain may be less intense in seniors[6]; thus, a "surgical abdomen" may present without leukocytosis or marked pain. In older patients, myocardial infarctions may be "silent," but a common complaint, like headache, may be due to a serious cause, like temporal arteritis, cervical osteoarthritis, depression, congestive heart failure, subdural hematoma, or electrolyte disturbance.[7]

- After analysis of a patient's pain history and physical examination for obvious or subtle manifestations of a serious disease, an aggressive treatment plan should be initiated.

TREATMENT

- Curing the source of pain is ideal at any age, but aggressive palliation is appropriate in cases that lack a cure or while waiting for a cure to take effect.

NONPHARMACOLOGIC INTERVENTIONS

- In an older population with a high risk of adverse events, nonpharmacologic options should be considered first.
- At the outset nociception can be suppressed by chilling the area to reduce release of prostaglandins and other mediators that may sensitize C fibers, chilling or warming the area to encourage the release of endogenous opioids,[8] and modifying the noxious response either centrally or peripherally.
- Transcutaneous electrical nerve stimulation, percutaneous electrical nerve stimulation, and acupuncture release endogenous opioids.
- Nerve blocks and tumor site radiation may be useful.
- Alternative or complementary medical interventions, such as relaxation techniques, biofeedback (particularly with vascular headaches), and hypnosis, are options. Because chronic pain patients may be using these therapies without oversight, it is useful to obtain a good history on *all* therapies being used.
- Physical therapy and occupational therapy offer a variety of modalities that improve pain relief.[9]

PHARMACOLOGIC INTERVENTIONS

- When considering pharmacologic interventions in older adults, it may be necessary to emphasize safety before efficacy.
- Cost is another priority consideration.
- When, on hospitalization, pharmacologically noncompliant patients receive medications as prescribed, overmedication may occur and cause adverse events.

- Because of the potential for drug interactions, elimination of unnecessary medications is advisable.
- Doses may require adjustment to account for the altered pharmacokinetics and bioavailability in the elderly.
- More research is needed to determine if, in this population, it is safer or more effective to prescribe low doses of multiple analgesics with different mechanisms of action or to maximize doses of individual medications.

NONOPIOIDS

- Nonopioids, such as acetaminophen, are generally the first line of therapy for mild to moderate pain. Acetaminophen is usually well tolerated in the elderly but may be contraindicated in patients taking drugs metabolized through the liver or with hepatic disease.
- Cyclooxygenase 2 (COX-2) inhibitors have the best gastrointestinal (GI) safety profile of nonsteroidal anti-inflammatory drugs (NSAIDs). Because of its availability as a liquid, relatively rapid onset of action, lack of association with sulfa allergies, and long duration of effect that permits once-a-day dosing, the COX-2 inhibitor rofecoxib is particularly useful in seniors. COX-2 inhibitors, however, do not provide an antiplatelet cardioprotective benefit.
- Some NSAIDs, for example, ibuprofen, inhibit the antiplatelet activity of aspirin, and it is not known if low-dose aspirin therapy obviates the GI safety of COX-2 agents.
- Many older patients, especially those who are homebound, take antiepileptic agents, or have fat malabsorption syndromes, are deficient in vitamin D. This deficiency is a potential cause of deep musculoskeletal pain or superficial light pressure pain. Vitamin D and calcium supplementation decrease rates of fracture and the attendant pain.
- Tricyclic antidepressants, some antiepileptic agents (eg, clonazepam, carbamazepine, gabapentin, and phenytoin), and mexiletine are recommended for neuropathic pain. As most of these agents are approved for other indications, selection may be predicated on using a single agent to combat multiple problems. Effective doses for pain are usually below those needed for the treatment of depression or seizures.
- Amitriptyline and anxiolytics, such as hydroxyzine, that are associated with anticholinergic effects should be avoided in seniors.

OPIOIDS

- Although addiction risk is low with opioids used for acute pain in patients who are not substance abusers (<0.1%), elderly patients may associate opioids with addiction, and this may be an issue even in the final days of life.

- To counteract constipation with opioid use, patients should consume adequate hydration and bulk fiber (so long as hydration is maintained) and should be as mobile as possible. A senna product is often helpful, and when chronic cathartics must be used, an agent such as sorbitol usually provides relief within days. Sorbitol is well tolerated, lacks long-term GI effects, and is relatively inexpensive. Patients may request reimbursable prescription lactulose, which carries a caution label for use in diabetics.
- Some adverse events, such as pruritus, may be associated with receptor binding and may be remedied by using a more potent opioid.
- In the elderly, a short-acting opioid should be administered first, appropriate dosing established, and then a switch made to a controlled-release formulation.
- Regular dosing provides better pain relief with fewer narcotics than does intermittent dosing, which should be avoided.
- Inpatients should be told they may refuse a scheduled medication if they do not need it or are developing side effects, but nurses should inform the attending physicians immediately should this occur.
- Patients require close attention (for change in cognition, physical findings, and pain) during the first 24 hours after an opioid adjustment.
- Patient-controlled analgesia, with oral or parenteral agents, can lead to the best pain control with the least amount of opioid.
- Opioids may be started at doses too low for the elderly under the "start low and go slow" principle; thus, medication should be increased by 50–100% when pain relief is inadequate. If patients metabolize opioids quickly and experience breakthrough pain after 8 hours of adequate pain relief, the dosing frequency should be increased to every 8 hours instead of increasing the dosage.
- A controlled-release morphine or oxycodone should never be prescribed more frequently than every 8 hours. If breakthrough pain occurs after 3 to 4 hours of relief, the amount of medication should be increased without changing the dosing schedule.
- Older patients who metabolize medication slowly may get relief with less frequent dosing at surprisingly small quantities of opioids, such as 15–30 mg of controlled-release morphine every 24 hours.
- Greater amounts of analgesic may be necessary to bring pain under control than to maintain control once the anxiety associated with inadequate pain control is eliminated.
- It would be catastrophic to crush long-acting, controlled-release agents for older patients who have difficulty swallowing pills.

- Use of short-acting opioids may facilitate tolerance and lead to higher opioid dosage requirements for adequate pain control.
- Meperidine has been associated with a host of adverse events in seniors and should be avoided either alone or in combination with a product such as hydroxyzine, which is anticholinergic and can be associated with orthostatic hypotension and confusion.
- Opioids that are antagonistic to the μ-receptor are less desirable, given the high prevalence of unrecognized and untreated depression in seniors who can benefit from the euphoric component that occurs with binding of the μ-receptor.
- There is no role in seniors for agonist–antagonist agents.
- The transdermal fentanyl patch may be useful when oral medication cannot be administered and subcutaneous or intraspinal routes are too cumbersome. In the older patient, however, these patches should be avoided as a first-line agent because age-related changes in body temperature and subcutaneous fat and water may cause fluctuation in absorption. Deaths have occurred in opioid-naive seniors using one 50-μg patch per hour. Thus, older patients should never be started on doses higher than 25 μg/h. Peak serum levels occur in 8–12 hours, and removal leaves a subcutaneous reservoir of active drug with a half-life of approximately 18 hours.
- In elderly patients, the route of administration is an important consideration because of age-related changes in skin integrity and GI absorption and motility.
- Terminally ill patients may present with symptoms resembling opioid toxicity that are really manifestations of the dying process. Great care must be taken before ordering an opioid antagonist, such as naloxone, which can cause an agonizing withdrawal in patients who have used opioids for a prolonged period.

ADVERSE EVENTS
- Adverse drug reactions occur in elderly patients more than twice as often as in younger subjects and increase with the number of medications. Thus, an elderly patient taking six medications is 14 times more likely to have an adverse reaction than a younger one.
- Patients taking opioids, particularly older males with enlarged prostates, should be queried about urinary retention.
- Suspected adverse events should be evaluated thoroughly. Often, reactions may be misinterpreted as side effects from medication. For example, the exhausted sleep of a patient whose longstanding pain has finally been relieved may be mistaken as a side effect of morphine.

- Dementia occurs in approximately 5% of the population 65 years and older and in more than 20% after age 85. Disorientation often increases when a patient is moved to a different environment, such as a hospital. Previously undetected dementia may become manifest following an overnight hospitalization, even in the absence of infection or use of centrally acting medication.
- An older patient who demonstrates a mental status change while in the hospital must be carefully evaluated. Infections, such as pneumonia or those occurring in the urinary tract, may present solely as a change in mental status and improve rapidly with appropriate antibiotic therapy.

ADJUVANT ANALGESICS

- For refractory nonmalignant pain in the frail elderly, nonopioids can often be used to reduce the dosage in an opioid regimen.
- Analgesic adjuvants, such as NSAIDs and amphetamines, may improve opioid tolerance and pain resolution.
- The adjuvant use of agents such as nortriptyline, clonazepam, carbamazepine, phenytoin, gabapentin, tramadol, and mexiletine is beneficial for neuropathic pain.[10,11]
- Antiepileptic medications also are used to manage certain painful conditions, including trigeminal neuralgia (or glossopharyngeal neuralgia), which may occur frequently in elderly patients. Gabapentin is indicated for postherpetic neuralgia and may be effective when administered initially at 100 mg orally one to three times daily and increased by 300 mg/d as needed. Clonazepam, carbamazepine, or phenytoin may serve as an alternative. The greatest concern with antiepileptic agents is their propensity to disrupt balance and to interfere with vitamin D metabolism.[12]

OTHER ISSUES AFFECTING SUCCESSFUL PAIN CONTROL

- The staff of multispecialty pain clinics or colleagues in other disciplines should be consulted whenever pain control is not achieved.
- The role of spirituality in pain control has not received adequate attention and may be important in seniors.
- Many of our frail, older patients do or will live in a nursing home or assisted living facility where the prevalence of inadequately controlled pain is high. Thus, quality assurance measures for these institutions should include evaluation and protocols for good pain management.[13–18]

REFERENCES

1. **Ferrell BA, Ferrell BR, Osterweil D.** Pain in the nursing home. *J Am Geriatr Soc.* 1990;38:409.
2. **Cleeland CS, Gonin R, Hatfield AK, et al.** Pain and its treatment in outpatients with metastatic cancer. *N Engl J Med.* 1994;330:592.
3. **Von Roenn JH, Cleeland CS, Gonin R, et al.** Physician attitudes and practice in cancer pain management: A survey from the Eastern Cooperative Oncology Group. *Ann Intern Med.* 1993;119:121.
4. **AGS Panel on Persistent Pain in Older Persons.** The management of persistent pain in older persons. *J Am Geriatr Soc.* 2002;50(6, Suppl):S205.
5. **Gloth FM III, Scheve AA, Stober CV, Chow S, Prosser J.** The Functional Pain Scale (FPS): Reliability, validity, and responsiveness in a senior population. *J Am Med Dir Assoc.* 2001;2(3):110.
6. **Marco CA, Schoenfeld CN, Keyl PM, et al.** Abdominal pain in geriatric emergency patients: Variables associated with adverse outcomes. *Acad Emerg Med.* 1998;5:1163.
7. **Gordon RS.** Pain in the elderly. *JAMA.* 1979;241:2491.
8. **Hyman SE, Cassem NH.** Pain. In: Rubenstein E, Federman DD, eds. *Scientific American Medicine.* Vol 11: *Neurology.* New York: Scientific American; 1994:12.
9. **Hölmich P, Uhrskou P, Ulnits L, et al.** Effectiveness of active physical training as treatment for longstanding adductor-related groin pain in athletes: Randomised trial. *Lancet.* 1999;353:439.
10. **Harati Y, Gooch C, Swenson M, et al.** Double-blind randomized trial of tramadol for the treatment of the pain of diabetic neuropathy. *Neurology.* 1998;50:1842.
11. **Morellow CM, Leckband SG, Stoner CP, et al.** Randomized double-blind study comparing the efficacy of gabapentin with amitriptyline on diabetic peripheral neuropathy pain. *Arch Intern Med.* 1999;159:1931.
12. **Gloth FM III, Gundberg CM, Hollis BW, et al.** The prevalence of vitamin D deficiency in a cohort of homebound elderly subjects compared to a normative matched population in the United States. *JAMA.* 1995;274:1683.
13. **Schumacher GA, Goodell H, Hardy JD, et al.** Uniformity of the pain threshold in man. *Science.* 1940;92:110.
14. **Sherman DE, Robillard E.** Sensitivity to pain in the elderly. *Can Med Assoc J.* 1960;83:944.
15. **Parmelee PA, Katz IR, Lawton MP.** The relation of pain to depression among institutionalized aged. *J Gerontol.* 1991;46:P15.
16. **Pitkala KH, Strandberg TE, Reijo ST.** Management of nonmalignant pain in home-dwelling older people: A population-based survey. *J Am Geriatr Soc.* 2002;50:1861.
17. **Gloth FM III.** Pain management in older adults: Prevention and treatment. *J Am Geriatr Soc.* 2001;49:188.
18. **Gloth FM III.** Geriatric pain: Factors that limit pain relief and increase complications. *Geriatrics.* 2000;55(10):46.

37 MYOFASCIAL PAIN AND FIBROMYALGIA

Robert D. Gerwin, MD

INTRODUCTION

- Muscular pain may be one of the most common reasons for visits to physicians when one includes complaints associated with low back pain, neck and shoulder pain, arthritis, and tension headache in addition to primary myalgias.
- The prevalence of localized muscle pain is reported to be 20%, and that of widespread muscle pain, as high as 10%.[1]

MYOFASCIAL PAIN SYNDROME

- Myofascial pain syndrome (MPS) may be acute or chronic, regional or widespread, but, in every case, it is associated with tenderness or pain localized to a linear or nodular hardening in a muscle that is called a "myofascial trigger point."[2]

CLINICAL FEATURES

- Motor:
  - Taut (hardened) band of muscle that runs the length of the muscle
  - Twitch or local contraction of muscle band on mechanical stimulation
  - Restricted range of motion
  - Weakness
- Sensory:
  - Tenderness (allodynia, hypersensitivity) of the taut band (known as the myofascial trigger point or zone)
  - Referred pain
- Autonomic:
  - Skin temperature changes
  - Lacrimation
  - Piloerection (goose bumps)
- Viscerosomatic syndromes:
  - Cardiac
  - Esophageal–gastrointestinal–hepatic
  - Genitourinary
- MPS results from acute (eg, whiplash) or chronic (eg, repetitive strain syndromes) muscle overload.
- Muscle that is fatigued and/or eccentrically loaded is susceptible to injury.[3]

- An abnormal motor end-plate mechanism is thought to cause taut bands that extend between myotendinous junctions.[2]
- Injured or inflamed muscle rapidly leads to central sensitization, lowering the threshold to nociceptive and nonnociceptive stimulation and producing hypersensitivity, allodynia (the phenomenon of nonpainful stimulation being perceived as painful), and referred pain.[4]
- MPS can persist long after the initial injury has resolved.
- Myofascial trigger zones may develop in the referred pain zone as well as in muscles that are agonists or antagonists of the muscle(s) that was initially injured.

CLINICAL PRESENTATION

- Pain generally occurs with activity but, in more severe cases, can be present at rest and interfere with sleep.
- Taut (hardened) bands shorten affected muscles and increase their diameter or cross-sectional bulk, which can result in nerve entrapment syndromes, such as the piriformis syndrome of the sciatic nerve, brachial plexus compressions in the interscalene compartment and the thoracic outlet, and the hyperabduction syndrome of the pectoralis minor muscle. In these syndromes of intermittent compression, electromyogram and nerve conduction study results are usually normal.
- Range of motion may be limited because of taut muscle bands or pain, and weakness may occur in affected muscles; the mechanism, thus, may involve central fatigue from persistently contracted taut bands within the muscle.[5]
- Referred pain, a spinal cord and thalamic phenomenon, often occurs with or without pain in the primary trigger zone.
- Referred pain syndromes can be mistaken for other conditions (radiculopathy or viscerosomatic pain syndromes).
- Some typical myofascial pain syndromes are:
  - Piriformis syndrome (entrapment of the sciatic nerve)
  - Interscalene compartment syndrome (entrapment of the brachial plexus)
  - Thoracic outlet-like syndrome (entrapment of the brachial plexus between the clavicle and first rib)
  - Hyperabduction syndrome
  - Viscerosomatic syndromes (cardiac, gastrointestinal, hepatic, genitourinary)
  - Headaches (chronic tension type, with or without migraine)
  - Temporomandibular joint syndrome

○ Frozen shoulder
• Mechanical stimulation of the primary trigger zone reproduces the pain, including referred pain.

DIAGNOSIS

• Identification of the primary trigger zone that reproduces the patient's pain is made by physical examination and reproduction of pain on palpation.
• A taut band of muscle is palpable and tender.
• Limited range of motion is a frequent and helpful sign, but motion may appear normal in hypermobile people.
• Referred pain may be elicited after 4–5 seconds.
• In the case of deep muscles like the multifidi, needling the muscle may be necessary to elicit the symptoms.
• Laboratory tests may identify coexisting, aggravating, or perpetuating conditions but do not support the clinical diagnosis of MPS.

TREATMENT

• Treatment is specific (treating the trigger point directly), general (treating pain and sleeplessness), and corrective (identifying and correcting the predisposing and perpetuating factors that may lead to and aggravate MPS) (Tables 37–1, 37–2, and 37–3).
• First, the clinician must inactivate the myofascial trigger point to relieve pain and restore normal function.
• Second, conditions that create and maintain trigger points, such as significant foot pronation, leg length inequality, and ergonomic stresses, must be corrected or eliminated.

TABLE 37–1   Treatment of MPS: Physical Modalities

Primary
  Local trigger point compression
  Local trigger point stretch
  Myofascial release
  Muscle play
  Therapeutic stretch
  Self-stretch
  Muscle reeducation
Adjunctive
  Intermittent cold
  Postisometric relaxation
  Strain–counterstrain
  Dry needling or injection (local anesthetic or botulinum toxin)
  Massage
  Ultrasound
  Electrical stimulation
  Acupuncture

TABLE 37–2   Needling or Injection of the Trigger Point

Purpose
  Diagnostic
  Rapid relief of pain
  Facilitation of manual (physical) therapy
Medications
  Short-acting local anesthetics without epinephrine
  "Dry needling" with no drug (mechanical stimulation of the trigger point alone)
  Botulinum toxin

• Inactivation of the trigger point is achieved manually or by needling the trigger point (Table 37–1). Most techniques compress and stretch the trigger point, followed by muscle reeducation and restoration of normal muscle sequencing during movement. Postisometric relaxation, reciprocal inhibition, and contract–relax techniques are all useful in stretching muscle.
• In hypermobile patients, therapeutic and self-stretching are relatively contraindicated, and treatment is directed locally to the trigger point.
• Ultrasound aids in the inactivation of trigger points, though no controlled study has confirmed this.
• Electrical stimulation reduces pain and allows manual treatment to proceed more comfortably.
• Strengthening to maintain improvement is reserved until muscle pain has been significantly reduced.

TRIGGER POINT NEEDLING
• Trigger point needling or injection of a local anesthetic relieves pain but has not been compared with placebo in a controlled trial.
• Needling or injection confirms a diagnosis if the pain is relieved rapidly.
• This therapy is precise; the needle should enter the trigger zone and elicit a twitch response for best results. Outcome does not vary whatever the material injected or if only dry needling (no material injected) is done.[6]
• The effect of needling or injection is often temporary, lasting days, and should be combined with manual (physical) therapy (Table 37–2).

TABLE 37–3   Pharmacologic Treatment of MPS

Over-the-counter drugs
Nonsteroidal anti-inflammatory drugs
Antidepressant drugs (those that inhibit reuptake of serotonin and norepinephrine, like the tricyclic antidepressants and venlafaxine)
Muscle relaxants
Antispasticity drugs (tizanidine)
Anticonvulsants
Opioid analgesics (preferably long-acting, slow-release)
Botulinum toxin

- Procaine 0.5% is recommended for injection because it is the least myotoxic of the local anesthetics, and it is extremely short-acting, an advantage should a nerve be blocked.
- Lidocaine 1% is more commonly used, however, because of its wide availability, and 0.1 or 0.2 cc will inactivate a trigger point.
- Injection of 25 units of botulinum toxin type A or 1250 units of botulinum toxin type B into the trigger zone (except in head and neck muscles, where 5–10 units of botulinum toxin type A are injected) produces longer-lasting pain relief than does dry needling or the injection of local anesthetics. Open-label studies have shown promise in treating MPS with botulinum toxin, but one small, randomized, double-blind, placebo-controlled trial showed only a trend toward improvement of those injected a second time 6 weeks after the initial injection. A randomized, controlled study of the use of botulinum toxin type A in low back pain, however, showed significantly greater efficacy of the toxin compared with saline.[7] Myofascial trigger points were definitely injected in that study.

PHARMACOLOGIC TREATMENT

- Pharmacologic treatment (Table 37–3) is directed toward pain relief and sleep improvement.
- Acetaminophen and aspirin provide short-term pain relief in mild pain states.
- Nonsteroidal anti-inflammatory drugs (NSAIDs) are not used for any anti-inflammatory purpose in muscle but for their analgesic activity, including that against postinjection pain. If NSAIDs are used for a long period, the selective COX-2 inhibitors should be used.
- Some anticonvulsant drugs (carbamazepine, gabapentin, and pregabalin) are effective in the treatment of neuropathic pain. Other of the newer anticonvulsants (topiramate, lamotrigine) have had mixed results in trials of treatment of neuropathic pain. Nevertheless, anticonvulsant medications may reduce muscle pain and can be given a trial in patients with MPS.
- Tizanidine, an α_2-adrenergic agonist, is efficacious in the treatment of MPS. The major adverse effects are daytime drowsiness, dry mouth, and the possibility of an initial drop in blood pressure. The drug is started at a low dose of 1–2 mg at night and then titrated upward to effectiveness on a twice or three times daily schedule.
- Cyclobenzaprine, related to the tricyclic antidepressants, has garnered mixed reports about its efficacy in treating MPS and is not recommended except as adjunctive treatment.
- Carisoprodol is to be avoided because it is highly addictive.

- In one study, the benzodiazepine derivative clonazepam (start with 0.5 mg every night and titrate upward) was effective in treating MPS.
- Sleep disruption can be treated with melatonin (3 mg every night), drugs such as zolpidem (5–10 mg every night), or antidepressants such as trazodone (50–150 mg every night).
- Opioids are used strictly for pain relief. They can be liberating for someone who is disabled by pain, but they can cause physical dependence and, rarely, addiction; create constipation; and impair cognitive function. If considered for long-term use, only long-acting, slow-release forms should be used, such as controlled-release forms of morphine sulfate, oxycodone, methadone, and fentanyl. These drugs should be used only by physicians experienced in their management.
- Tramadol alone at 50–100 mg every 4–6 hours or with acetaminophen up to 800 mg/d can be used for pain of moderate intensity. *Caution*: Tramadol in combination with certain antidepressant drugs can lower the seizure threshold.

OTHER TREATMENT OPTIONS

- Acupuncture is useful for pain relief. In a form of acupuncture called superficial dry needling, the needle is placed 2–3 mm under the skin over the trigger point.[8] Relaxation of the trigger point can be seen. The usual manual treatment protocol follows (Table 37–1).
- When the clinician identifies depression or other emotional stress that might underlie and aggravate the MPS, screening by a social worker, psychologist, or psychiatrist for psychologic treatment is in order.
- Psychologic treatment options for MPS include education, cognitive behavioral therapy, and antidepressants or antianxiolytics when indicated.
- Activation of the limbic system can reinforce neck and shoulder trigger points. This is an outgrowth of cognitive-behavioral therapy.

SUMMARY

- MPS patients are treated with manual inactivation of the trigger point (physical therapy, including trigger point compression, massage, local and therapeutic stretching, and self-stretching). *Warning*: Stretching should be done cautiously or not at all in hypermobile MPS individuals.
- Trigger points that do not release manually are needled or injected with local anesthetic. Botulinum toxin is used as a long-lasting trigger point injection in cases where needling or local anesthetic combined with physical therapy does not give long-term relief.

- Postural, ergonomic, mechanical (structural), hormonal, nutritional, and other medical precipitating and perpetuating factors are identified and corrected.
- Strengthening, including lumbar stabilization, is performed when pain levels are reduced enough to allow the patient to perform resistive and stabilizing exercises without an undue increase in pain.
- Counseling and cognitive-behavioral therapies are employed where warranted.
- Medications are used when necessary to treat symptoms:
  - Sleep disturbance: melatonin 3 mg every night, trazodone 50–150 mg every night, amitriptyline 25–50 mg every night, or zolpidem 5–10 mg every night.
  - Antispasticity drugs: tizanidine starting at 1–2 mg every night and titrating to effectiveness two or three times daily up to 8 mg three times daily can significantly reduce pain.
  - Muscle relaxants: cyclobenzaprine 10 mg three times daily or methylcarbamoyl 500–750 mg three times daily, for short-term use. Carisoprodol should be avoided.
- Analgesics are for short-term use, the type depending on the severity of the pain. For acute, severe pain, rapid-onset, short-duration opioids like oxycodone/APAP 5/325 and hydrocodone/APAP 5/500, every 4 hours as needed, are used. For pain that is subacute or for chronic severe pain, slow-release, long-acting opiates like controlled-release morphine sulfate and oxycodone, methadone, or fentanyl patch are used, starting at low doses and titrating upward to efficacy. For lesser pain tramadol starting at 50 mg two to four times daily and titrating to effectiveness (50–100 mg every 4–6 h/d, maximum dose of 800 mg/d) or NSAIDs are used. For mild pain, over-the-counter preparations are satisfactory.

FIBROMYALGIA SYNDROME

- Fibromyalgia syndrome (FMS) is a chronic, widespread muscular pain syndrome that is the second most common disorder seen by rheumatologists.
- FMS is not a disease *per se* but rather is a syndrome that can have multiple etiologies.

CLINICAL FEATURES

- Pain appears to be related to neuroplastic changes of the central nervous system that result in general hypersensitivity to all types of stimuli through the unmasking of dormant synapses and reduction of central inhibition.[9]

- FMS patients have decreased serum serotonin levels and impaired central serotonin metabolism as well as elevated levels of cerebrospinal fluid substance P.[8,10] They have low levels of insulin-like growth factor 1[11] and decreased function of the hypothalamic–pituitary–adrenal axis with low serum androgen levels that correlate with poor physical functioning and with pain.[12]
- The hallmark of FMS is widespread muscular pain in three or four quadrants of the body (ie, upper and lower and right and left sides) of 3 or more months' duration.
- Pain is often accompanied by unusual fatigue and disturbed sleep.
- FMS occurs in about 3.5% of women and 0.5% of men and is more common with advancing age. It occurs in children as well as adults.
- FMS is comorbid with many other conditions, such as rheumatoid arthritis, systemic lupus erythematosus, Lyme disease, hepatitis, Sjögren's syndrome, and myofascial pain syndrome.

CLINICAL PRESENTATION

- Patients with FMS complain of widespread muscle pain that interferes with activity, fatigue out of proportion to any sleep disorder, and impaired sleep (they usually awaken feeling tired).
- FMS patients often have associated problems of depression, headache, joint pain, morning stiffness, Raynaud's phenomenon, bladder irritability, irritable bowel syndrome, and painful intercourse.
- Many of these associated conditions are the result of myofascial trigger point syndromes that coexist with FMS (eg, muscular headaches, morning stiffness, and pelvic floor or viscerosomatic pain syndromes).
- FMS patients complain of difficulty concentrating and of short-term memory impairment.
- Symptoms can be so severe they cause many to seek disability retirement.

DIAGNOSIS

- The diagnosis is based on the history of chronic, widespread pain and the presence of bilateral muscle tenderness (tender points) that affects the upper and lower halves of the body.
- The American College of Rheumatology (ACR) established criteria for the diagnosis of FMS to aid in the development of clinical studies, and these criteria have been adopted for clinical use.[13] The presence of tenderness at 11 or more of 18 preselected sites has a

**TABLE 37–4   Tender Point Sites for
Fibromyalgia Examination**

Suboccipital
Lower anterior cervical
Upper trapezius
Supraspinatus
Parasternal at second rib
Lateral epicondylar region
Anterior gluteal fold
Greater trochanter of the hip
Medial fat pad above the knee (vastus medialis)

diagnostic sensitivity of 88% and a specificity of 81%. Nine sites are examined bilaterally (Table 37–4). There need not be 11 or more tender points at any given examination in clinical practice, but, over time, muscle tenderness must be widespread, which the criteria ensure.

- The tender point examination is conducted by palpating muscle with a force sufficient to blanche the fingernail, approximately 4 kg pressure.
- In clinical practice, tenderness is not confined to the sites designated in the ACR criteria but must be present in a widespread distribution. Care should be taken when examining for tenderness to distinguish tender, taut muscle bands of myofascial trigger points so as not to confuse FMS with MPS.
- The associated problems of joint stiffness, Raynaud's phenomenon, interstitial cystitis, and so on need not be present to diagnosis FMS.
- Other causes of widespread, chronic muscle pain should be excluded (Table 37–5).
- Orthostatic hypotension is seen in many patients with FMS; blood pressure and pulse should be taken supine, immediately after standing, and 2 minutes after standing.[14]
- Numerical rating scales for pain (0=no pain, 10=worst possible pain) are useful for assessing the degree of pain a patient is experiencing.
- The Fibromyalgia Impact Questionnaire assesses the impact of pain on a patient's life.[15]
- A polysomnogram or sleep disorder consultation may be necessary to diagnose treatable sleep disturbances.

TREATMENT

PHARMACOLOGIC TREATMENT
- As with MPS, over-the-counter analgesics may be used to treat pain when necessary.
- Nonsteroidal, anti-inflammatory drugs.
- Muscle relaxants and antispasticity drugs (cyclobenzaprine 10 mg three times daily).

- Tricyclic antidepressants that inhibit the reuptake of serotonin and norepinephrine provide short-term improvement. Amitriptyline, at doses of 25–50 mg every night, has been the most thoroughly studied and has led to improvement for as long as 6 months. Tramadol may cause seizures when used with a variety of antidepressant drugs and, therefore, should either be avoided or be used with caution in association with amitriptyline. Fluoxetine at 20 mg daily and sertraline at 50 mg daily are also effective. Antidepressants improve sleep, fatigue, and pain but not the tender point count.
- Anticonvulsants reduce neuropathic pain and can be used nonspecifically in FMS. In one study, pregabelin was effective in treating FMS, but this drug is not yet available.
- Antispasticity drugs (tizanidine starting at 1–2 mg every night, slowly titrating upward).
- Opiates.
- Nutritional supplements (S-adenosyl-L-methionine).
- Hormone therapy:
  ○ Growth hormone titrated to an insulin-like growth factor 1 (IGF-1) level of 250 mg/mL improves FMS after about 6 months of treatment at a cost of approximately $1000/mo. Symptoms recur after treatment is stopped. Growth hormone is not recommended for routine management.
  ○ When hypothyroidism coexists with FMS, thyroid supplementation may resolve FMS symptoms. No data support the use of other kinds of hormonal therapy.
- Some studies have found that S-adenosyl-L-methionine at 200 mg/d improves pain, fatigue, mood, and morning stiffness.

PHYSICAL TREATMENT

- Graded aerobic exercise is the most effective form of physical therapy, in the short and long term (up to 4 years).[16] Moderately intense aerobic exercise two or

TABLE 37–5   Differential Diagnoses for Fibromyalgia

Myofascial pain syndrome
Drug-induced: statin cholesterol-lowering drugs
Hypothyroidism
Iron deficiency
Vitamin B_{12} deficiency
Infections
    Candidiasis
    Parasitic
    Bacterial (*Mycoplasma*)
Sleep apnea, restless leg syndrome
Myoadenylate deaminase deficiency

three times per week, with minimal eccentric muscle activity, improves physical functioning, cardiovascular fitness, and self-efficacy, but pain levels, tender point counts, mood and depression, and sleep and fatigue may not improve.[17]

- Physical therapy otherwise is useful primarily to identify and treat coexistent problems, such as MPS, postural dysfunctions, and ergonomic stresses.
- Electrical stimulation.
- Acupuncture is an effective complementary therapy.

PSYCHOLOGIC TREATMENT

- Education.
- Teaching coping skills and relaxation training constitutes cognitive-behavioral therapy (educational content varied considerably among studies).
- Biofeedback, especially combined with exercise, improves function and reduces tender points.
- Hypnosis and meditation-based stress reduction each improve pain ratings and function and can reduce the number of tender points.
- Psychotherapy.

OTHER TREATMENT

- A multidisciplinary treatment program combining behavioral modification, education, and physical training is effective.[18]
- Treatment of sleep disturbance is important and should include attention to sleep hygiene (darkened room, using the bed only for sleep and sexual intercourse) and medications to promote sleep, such as melatonin 3 mg before bedtime, trazodone 50–150 mg at bedtime, or a pharmaceutical such as zolpidem 5–10 mg at bedtime. Amitriptyline improves sleep.
- There is no evidence to support the use of magnesium or magnesium-malic supplements, DHEA, guaifenesin, corticosteroids, sex hormones, and herbal supplements.
- The associative disorders of headache, interstitial cystitis, irritable bowel syndrome, irritable bladder syndrome, dysmenorrhea, and dyspareunia should be treated symptomatically, but muscular (myofascial) causes of these conditions that can be treated specifically should be assessed.
- Trigger point injections are used to treat coexistent MPS, but injection of tender points with local anesthetics or with corticosteroids has no proven benefit in FMS.

SUMMARY

- Diagnosis is positive in identifying widespread muscle tenderness in a person with a history of chronic, widespread pain, and negative in excluding other causes of widespread myalgia.
- An antidepressant drug that inhibits uptake of both serotonin and norepinephrine, such as amitriptyline 25–50 mg every night or venlafaxine SR at 150–300 mg/d, is used to relieve pain and improve sleep.
- Sleep is improved with trazodone 50–150 mg nightly, melanotonin 3 mg nightly, or a drug such as zolpidem 5–10 mg nightly. A sleep consultation should be sought if the patient suffers a serious sleep disorder or significant daytime hypersomnia. Caffeine and other drugs that interfere with sleep, such as opiates, and sympathomimetic drugs such as nasal decongestants should be avoided.
- A moderately intensive aerobic exercise program that avoids excessive eccentric resistive exercise should be instituted.
- Pain is treated with a suitable analgesic if necessary.
- A multidisciplinary approach combining graded aerobic exercise, cognitive-behavioral therapy, and patient education should be used.
- Coexistent conditions (such as hypothyroidism, iron deficiency, and vitamin B_{12} deficiency) and comorbid MPS, ergonomic and postural stressors, and psychologic disorders are treated.
- Comorbid MPS is treated with trigger point injections or needling.
- Complementary/alternative methods of treatment, such as supplementation with S-adenosyl-L-methionine, use of acupuncture, and biofeedback, should be considered.

REFERENCES

1. **Kissel JT, Miller R.** Muscle pain and fatigue. In: Schapira AHV, Griggs RC, eds. *Muscle Diseases.* Woburn, Mass: Butterworth–Heinemann; 1999:33.
2. **Simons DG, Travell JG, Simons LS.** *Myofascial Pain and Dysfunction: The Trigger Point Manual.* Vol 1. Baltimore: Williams & Wilkins; 1999:19, 69.
3. **Newham DJ, McPhail G, Mills KR, et al.** Ultrastructural changes after concentric and eccentric contractions of human muscle. *J Neurol Sci.* 1983;61:109.
4. **Mense S, Simons D.** *Muscle Pain: Understanding Its Nature, Diagnosis, and Treatment.* Philadelphia: Lippincott Williams & Wilkins; 2001:158.
5. **Loscher WN, Nordlund MM.** Central fatigue and motor cortical excitability during repeated shortening and lengthening actions. *Muscle Nerve.* 2002;25:864.

6. **Cummings TM, White AR.** Needling therapies in the management of myofascial trigger point pain: A systematic review. *Arch Phys Med Rehabil.* 2001;82:986.

7. **Foster L, Clapp L, Erickson M, et al.** Botulinum toxin A and chronic low back pain: A randomized, double blind study. *Neurology.* 2001;56:1290.

8. **Pillemer SR, Bradley LA, Crofford LJ.** The neuroscience and endocrinology of fibromyalgia. *Arthritis Rheum.* 1997;40:1928.

9. **Coderre TJ, Katz J, Vaccarino AL.** Contribution of central neuroplasticity to pathological pain: Review of clinical and experimental evidence. *Pain.* 1993;52:259.

10. **Russell IF.** Neurochemical pathogenesis of fibromyalgia syndrome. *J Musculoskel Pain.* 1996;4:61.

11. **Bennet RM, Cook DM, Clark SR.** Hypothalamic–pituitary–insulin-like growth factor axis dysfunction in patients with fibromyalgia. *J Rheumatol.* 1997;24:1384.

12. **Dessein PH, Shipton EA, Joffe BI.** Hyposecretion of adrenal androgens and the relation of serum adrenal steroids, serotonin and insulin-like growth factor-1 to clinical features in women with fibromyalgia. *Pain.* 1999;83:313.

13. **Wolfe F, Smythe HA, Yunus MB, et al.** The American College of Rheumatology 1990 criteria for the classification of fibromyalgia: Report of the multicenter criteria committee. *Arthritis Rheum.* 1990;33:160.

14. **Rowe PC, et al.** Neurally mediated hypotension and chronic fatigue syndrome. *Am J Med.* 1998;105(3A):15S.

15. **Burckhardt CS, Clark SR, et al.** The fibromyalgia impact questionnaire: Development and validation. *J Rheumatol.* 1991;18:728.

16. **Gowans SE, deHueck A, Voss S, et al.** A randomized, controlled trial of exercise and education for individuals with fibromyalgia. *Arthritis Care Res.* 1999;12:120.

17. **Clark SR, Jones KD, Burckhardt CS, Bennett RM.** Exercise for patients with fibromyalgia: Risks versus benefits. *Curr Rheumatol Rep.* 2001;3:135.

18. **Burckhardt CS, Mannerkorpi K, Hedenberg L, et al.** A randomized, controlled clinical trial of education and physical training for women with fibromyalgia. *J Rheumatol.* 1994;21:714.

38   PEDIATRIC PAIN

Robert S. Greenberg, MD

CHILDREN HAVE PAIN, TOO

- As it has in adults, pain has long been undertreated in children, but this neglect is no longer acceptable, and clinicians now realize the necessity of considering and treating pain and painful procedures in children.

REASONS FOR THE UNDERTREATMENT OF PAIN IN CHILDREN

- Despite increasing awareness of the importance of treating pain as a disease, pain is still inadequately managed, even in adults. This problem may be more acute in children who lack the ability to demand relief from pain.

- Small children, especially preverbal infants, cry in reaction to discomfort (hunger, heat or cold, wet clothing, boredom, tiredness, frustration, presence of strangers) as well as to pain; therefore, it is easy to discount or misinterpret crying caused by pain. Astute caregivers, however, learn to distinguish the wails of prelanguage babies (he's sleepy, she's hungry) and either meet their needs or distract them from their discomfort.

- Fear/anxiety exacerbates pain; yet adults may fail to appreciate the level of fear/anxiety felt by a young child about to undergo even a minimally painful experience. This is especially true if the child does not understand what is happening or why it is happening—only that it hurts.

- If the caregiver who usually takes away his or her pain (or pangs) is involved in the painful procedure, the young child may experience anxiety-increasing confusion.

- Some adults have a cavalier attitude about children's pain. If the adult knows the child's pain will soon subside, the adult may believe it is not worth treating.

- Some adults believe that it is an important life lesson and part of "growing up" for a child to learn to bear pain.

- Adults generally shed tears only in response to emotional distress, while children shed tears readily for a host of reasons. Some adults believe that children, especially boys, should be taught never to cry.

- Sometimes adults think that a child's complaint of pain is merely a ruse. If a child says her or his stomach hurts on a school day, for example, the adult may think the child simply wants to stay home from school.

- These attitudes join with the limited ability of children to provide clinically relevant information about their pain and the persistence of misinformation about pain to hinder appropriate pain management in children.

- Thus, the "coming of age" of the recognition, definition, and management of pain in children is very recent.

NEED FOR A MULTIDISCIPLINARY APPROACH

- The multidisciplinary approach needed to achieve adequate pain management in adults with chronic pain may be even more important in children, and this multidisciplinary approach should involve parents or guardians whenever possible.

- In fact, achieving adequate pain management in children requires that the child/patient, patient's family, and medical professionals establish good lines of communication so they can educate each other about the problem and potential solutions.
- A multidisciplinary approach allows all involved to achieve clarity about the purpose of pain management and to set realistic goals.

FACTORS THAT MODULATE PEDIATRIC PAIN

CHILD-SPECIFIC FACTORS

- Age
- Sex
- Temperament
- Previous pain experience
- Family environment
- Cognitive/developmental level
  - How well the child can interpret information about the cause and prognosis of pain

TABLE 38–1 The CHEOPS Scale

PARAMETER	FINDING	POINTS
Cry	None	1
	Moaning	2
	Crying	2
	Screaming	3
Facial expression	Smiling	0
	Composed	1
	Grimace	2
Child verbal	Positive	0
	None	1
	Complaints other than pain	1
	Pain complaints	2
	Pain and nonpain complaints	2
Torso	Neutral	1
	Shifting	2
	Tense	2
	Shivering	2
	Upright	2
	Restrained	2
Touch	Not touching	1
	Reach	2
	Touch	2
	Grab	2
	Restrained	2
Legs	Neutral	1
	Squirming, kicking	2
	Drawn up, tensed	2
	Standing	2
	Restrained	2

- Ability to identify pain triggers
- Expectations about treatment efficacy
- Knowledge and ability to execute practical drug and nondrug therapy
- Ability to recognize stress and knowledge about how to deal with it

BEHAVIORAL FACTORS

- Repertoire of distress responses
- Ability to accommodate drug and nondrug therapy
- Management and resolution of stressful situations
- Ability to participate in routine activities (home, school, sports, social)

EMOTIONAL FACTORS

- Anticipatory anxiety, which may heighten distress and accelerate/escalate the effect of the initiating factor
- Fear regarding an undiagnosed condition and/or continuing pain
- Situation-specific stress (home, school, sports, social)
- Frustration regarding disruption to activities that serve as positive reinforcers of life
- Underlying/inherent anxiety or depression

PAIN ASSESSMENT IN CHILDREN

OBJECTIVE/OBSERVATIONAL/BEHAVIORAL

- Enables the clinician to translate objective/observed aspects of the patient's condition into an interpretation of pain. This method is used for children who cannot perform a self-assessment.
- Special scales may be used for children with special problems (obtunded, mental retardation, physical disabilities, etc).
- CHEOPS (see Table 38–1):
  - This scale is suggested for children 1–5 years of age.
  - Sum of all six parameters: minimum score = 4; maximum score = 13.
- Self-report:
  - Enables the patient to translate his or her own sense of pain into an objective scale for others to record and follow.
  - The FACES method for providing self-reports of pain was developed for use in children (see Figure 38–1).
  - A visual analogue scale or numeric scale can also be used (see Figure 38–2).

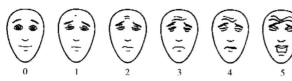

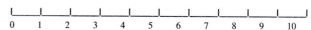

FIGURE 38–1 When using the FACES scale, explain to the child that each face is for a person who feels happy because he has no pain (hurt) or sad because he has some or a lot of pain. Face 0 doesn't hurt at all.[1]

FIGURE 38–2 When using a numeric scale, explain to the child that at one end of the line is a 0, which means that a person feels no pain (hurt). At the other end is a 10, which means the person feels the worst pain imaginable. The numbers 1 to 9 range from a very little pain to a whole lot. Ask the child to choose the number that best describes how well he or she is feeling. On this scale, a 10 is equivalent to a 5 on the FACES scale in Figure 38–1.[2]

PAIN TREATMENT IN CHILDREN

NSAIDs

- Mode of action: inhibition of cyclo-oxygenase
- Used in the initial/basic treatment of most pediatric pain
- Can cause decreased platelet effect (especially aspirin) and bone reformation (ibuprofen, ketorolac, naproxen), so avoid if there is a history of gastrointestinal bleeding, airway or intracranial surgery, or bone fracture ("osteotomies" and spine)

- Should be used (if not contraindicated) for most pain as an adjunct to severe pain, for example, treatment with opioids to decrease overall opioid use (see Table 38–2)

OPIOIDS

- Receptors μ, κ, δ, σ
- Physiologic effects
  - Analgesia
  - Sedation

TABLE 38–2 NSAIDs Used to Treat Pediatric Pain*

DRUG	AVAILABILITY	DOSING REGIMEN	CAVEATS
Acetaminophen Feverall Liquiprin Panadol Tempra Tylenol APAP Paracetamol	Drops: 100 mg/mL Elixir: 80, 120, 160, 325 mg/5 mL Tablets: 120, 325, 500 mg Chewable tabs: 80, 120, 160 mg Caplets: 160, 325, 500 mg Rectal suppository: 80, 120, 325, 650 mg	15 mg/kg/dose PO q4h 30 mg/kg/first dose PR Max dose: 75 mg/kg/d or 4 g/day	Excellent analgesic base if given around the clock Caution in renal and/or hepatic failure Caution in G6PD deficiency
Aspirin Anacin Bayer Buffered Empirin ASA	Tablets: 81, 325, 650 mg Chewable tablets: 81 mg Caplets: 80, 165, 625, 500, 650 mg Rectal suppository: 60, 120, 200, 325, 650 mg	10–15 mg/kg PO q4h Max dose: 4 g/d	Generally not used for pain, except for arthritic/chronic conditions Caution: Reye's syndrome association, eg, contraindicated during viral syndrome
Choline magnesium trisalicylate Trilisate	Solution: 500 mg/mL Tablets (scored): 500, 750, 1000 mg	7.5–15 mg/kg PO q6h	Does not have much effect on platelets Can be split bid
Ibuprofen Advil Motrin Medipren Nuprin	Suspension: 100 mg/mL Tablets: 200, 400, 600, 800 mg	4–10 mg/kg PO q6h	Excellent base analgesic if given around the clock, especially for musculoskeletal pain May affect bone reformation
Ketorolac Toradol	Injection: 15, 30 mg/mL Tablets: 10 mg	0.5 mg/kg IV (IM) or PO q6h Max total dose: 120 mg/kg/d 5-day maximum duration of therapy	Keep well hydrated Caution if renal impaired or history of GI bleeding May affect bone reformation
Naproxen Aleve Naprosyn	Suspension: 125 mg/mL Tablets: 200, 250, 375, 500 mg	5 mg/kg PO q8–12h Max total dose: 30 mg/kg/d	May affect bone reformation
Propacetamol Pro-Dalfalgan (not available in United States)	Injection: reconstituted from powder, usually 10 mg/mL	30 mg/kg IV (over 20 min) q6h Max adult dose: 8 g /day 2-day maximum duration of therapy	Excellent postoperative analgesic base if given around the clock Caution in renal and/or hepatic failure Caution in G6PD deficiency

*Paraphrased from Yaster et al.[2]

- ○ Dysphoria and euphoria
- ○ Nausea and vomiting
- ○ Miosis
- ○ Seizures
- ○ Psychotomimetic behaviors, excitation
- ○ Antitussive
- ○ Respiratory depression (decreased minute ventilation)
- ○ Bronchospasm
- Drugs
  - ○ Fentanyl
  - ○ Hydromorphone
  - ○ Morphine
  - ○ Methadone
  - ○ Codeine
  - ○ Oxycodone
  - ○ Nalbuphine
  - ○ Butorphanol
  - ○ Tramadol
  - ○ Naloxone (antagonist)
- Routes of administration
  - ○ Intravenous (IV), intramuscular (IM), subcutaneous (SC)
  - ○ Epidural, intrathecal
  - ○ Nasal
  - ○ Oral/enteral
  - ○ Transmucosal
  - ○ Sublingual
  - ○ Oral
  - ○ Transdermal
- Standard doses
- Equipotencies
- Specific receptor effects?

ADJUVANT AGENTS

- These drugs, while most commonly associated with treatment of depression, have become recognized as effective adjuvants in many acute (and chronic) pain scenarios.
- Some of the most likely to be useful in acute pain management are listed in Table 38–3.

TABLE 38–3 Adjuvant Agents Used to Treat Pediatric Pain

CLASS	DRUG (TRADE NAME)	DOSING REGIMEN	NOTES
Amphetamines (can be added as a means to counter the sedative and potentiate the analgesic effects of high-dose opiates)	Methylphenidate (Concerta, Ritalin, Ritalin-SR)	0.3 mg/kg/dose (2.5–5 mg/dose) PO with breakfast and lunch. May increase in 5-mg intervals weekly unless side effects appear	Caution in hypertension, glaucoma, Tourette's syndrome
	Dextroamphetamine (Dexedrine)	5 mg PO q. May increase in 5-mg intervals weekly unless side effects appear	
Antinarcoleptics	Modafinil (Provigil)	3–5 mg/kg PO qam (usually 100–200 mg/d)	Especially helpful when opioids cause severe sedation yet are still not completely analgesic, eg, sickle cell crises
Anticonvulsants	Gabapentin (Neurontin)	5 mg/kg or 300 mg PO qhs. May increase to 300 qmg PO tid	A good option for neuropathies/chronic pain. Take time to work (2–3 weeks). May cause somnolence, dizziness, nystagmus
Alpha agonists	Clonidine (Catapress)		Will also cause some sedation and lower blood pressure
	Tizanidine (Zanaflex)	Approx 50 μg/kg/dose PO q6–8h	Good to ameliorate the muscle spasm associated with orthopedic manipulation. Less sedation and hypotension than with clonidine
Benzodiazepines	Diazepam (Valium)	0.1–0.2 mg/kg IV q2–6h (depending on needs). 0.2–0.3 mg/kg PO q4–6h	Used especially for muscle spasm/spasticity which can cause severe pain postorthopedic/genitourinary procedures. Can cause burning on IV injection. Long half-life in neonates
	Lorazepam (Ativan)	0.05–0.1 mg/kg IV q4–8h. 0.05–0.2 mg/kg PO q6–8h	Sometimes tolerated better than diazepam: less hypotension and sedation. See precautions for diazepam

LOCAL ANESTHETICS

PHARMACOLOGY

- See Table 38–4.
- Amides (bupivacaine, lidocaine, etidocaine, ropivacaine, mepivacaine, prilocaine).
- Esters (chloroprocaine, procaine, tetracaine, cocaine).
- pK_a=pH at which half of the drug is in ionized form.
- Generally, weak bases that exist in aqueous solutions in nonionized and ionized forms. Only the nonionized form can cross the nerve membrane to block the sodium channel.
- Protein binding:
  - Bind to plasma proteins.
  - α_1-acid glycoproteins are the predominant protein-binding local anesthetics.
    - Increased in inflammatory disease and cancer (less risk)
    - Decreased in children <6 months of age (greater risk of free agent causing toxicity)
  - Lipid solubility: Highly lipid-soluble agents cross nerve membranes readily and may ascend along the nerve membrane.

FACTORS AFFECTING NEURAL BLOCKADE

- Na^+ channel blockers
- Minimum effective blocking concentration
  - Fiber size/myelinization
  - pK_a
  - Acid–base
  - Local calcium concentration
  - Nerve stimulation rate
  - Local concentration effects
  - Temperature

TOXICITY

- Peak absorption is site-dependent: intercostal, intratracheal > caudal/epidural > brachial plexus > distal peripheral > subcutaneous
- Total drug dose
- Clinical signs of toxicity:
  - Central nervous system: visual disturbance, tinnitus, anxiety, twitching, convulsions, cardiorespiratory depression, coma, death
  - Cardiovascular system: vasodilation, hypotension, ventricular dysrhythmias, myocardial depression, cardiovascular collapse
  - Respiratory system: respiratory arrest, hypoxia
  - Allergy: uncommon with amides, more likely vasovagal reaction; ester allergy more common, especially with patients allergic to *para*-aminobenzoic acid
  - Methemoglobinemia: associated with prilocaine, especially in newborns, eg, EMLA

TREATMENT REGIMEN

- Start with ABCs.
- Prolonged CPR (especially with bupivacaine) may be required.

COMMON APPLICATIONS

Axial Blocks

- Caudal/lumbar/thoracic epidural
- Intrathecal/spinal anesthesia

Regional Blocks

- Penile
- Ilioinguinal/iliohypogastric
- Femoral/3-in-1
- Axillary
- Bier/intravenous
- Transdermal

INTRAVENOUS PATIENT-CONTROLLED ANALGESIA

- As pain, especially acute, postoperative pain, is not of constant intensity, and the person who best knows the pain is the patient, patient-controlled analgesia systems have been well-accepted, even in the pediatric population.
- In the situation where a child is too young or too sick (ie, debilitated) to provide his or her own initiation of drug dosing (pushing a button), a properly trained nurse or parent/guardian can intervene and provide the necessary dose of medication.

PRINCIPLES OF PCA

- Patient/parent/nurse-controlled analgesia systems all have similar elements.
  - Drug in a reservoir
  - Mechanized/computerized management of drug delivery
  - Means to deliver drug (intravenous line, subcutaneous access)
  - Programmed regimen to deliver drug
    - Basal infusion=a continuous delivery of medication.
    - Bolus infusion=dose of medication to be delivered on demand of the patient/parent/nurse.
    - Lockout doses=maximum number of doses that can be delivered to a patient in a certain period (eg, doses/hour).
    - Lockout time=minimum number of minutes that must transpire between doses.
- Drugs commonly used for PCA in the pediatric population are listed in Table 38–5.

TABLE 38-4 Common Drugs Used in Pediatric Nerve Blocks

DRUG/TYPE OF BLOCK	pK$_a$	PROTEIN BINDING (%)	EQUI-EFFECTIVE CONCENTRATION	POTENCY	CONCENTRATION (%)	ONSET	DURATION (min)	MAXIMAL DOSES WITHOUT EPINEPHRINE (mg/kg)	MAXIMAL DOSES WITH EPINEPHRINE (mg/kg)
Chloroprocaine	8.7	—	2	4				8	10
Infiltration					1–2	Rapid	30–45		
Epidural					2–3	Rapid	30–60		
Procaine	8.9	6	2	1				7	8.5
Tetracaine	8.5	76	0.25	16					
Spinal					1	Slow	60–150		
Bupivacaine	8.1	96	0.25	16				2	3
Infiltration					0.25–0.5	Slow	90–360		
Peripheral					0.25–0.5	Slow	120–360		
Epidural					0.125–0.5	Slow	120–360		
Lidocaine	7.9	64	1	4				5	7
Infiltration					0.5–1.0	Rapid	30–60		
Topical					2–10	Rapid	30–60		
Peripheral					1.0–2.0	Rapid	30–90		
Epidural					0.3–2.0	Rapid	30–90		
Spinal					5.0	Rapid	30–90		
Mepivacaine	7.6	78	1	2				5	6
Infiltration					1.0	Slow	60–90		
Peripheral					1–1.5	Slow	60–120		
Epidural					1.5–2.0	Slow	60–120		
Prilocaine	7.9	55	1	3				5	7
Ropivacaine	8.1	94	0.2	14					
Epidural					0.2–0.5	Slow	60–240		

TABLE 38–5 Common Drugs/Starting Regimens for PCA

DRUG	CONCENTRATION	BASAL (μg/kg/h)	BOLUS (μg/kg/dose)	LOCKOUT min	LOCKOUT doses/h	COMMENTS
Fentanyl	10 μg/mL	0.5	0.5	15	3	Commonly used for infants. May have facial pruritus/blanching
Nalbuphine	1 mg/mL	20	20	8	5	May have a ceiling effect and fewer side effects
Morphine	1 mg/mL	20	20	8	5	May also be sedating
Hydromorphone	0.2 mg/mL	4	4	8	5	May have fewer side effects and be less sedating

SYSTEMATIZING MANAGEMENT
- Protocol development
- Systemwide education
  - Parent/nurse/physician education
  - Observation/assessment
  - Management of side effects
  - Management of operational failures

EPIDURAL ANALGESIA

PRINCIPLES OF REGIONAL ANALGESIA
- Anatomy/placement
  - The epidural potential space can be injected with a variety of medications from several access points along the patient's back: cervical, thoracic, lumbar, and caudal. Furthermore, in smaller children (<5 years of age), it is not difficult to enter the epidural space from the caudal site and then thread a catheter within the space to a higher level.
  - In larger children and adults, the lumbar or thoracic epidural space is entered from a puncture in the lower or upper back, respectively.
  - Nearly all epidural placements in children occur at the time of the surgical procedure, with the child asleep.

DIAMOND THEORY
- Sympathetic, sensory, motor blockade:
  - Local anesthetics are the mainstay of axial analgesia in children (see above discussion of local anesthetics).

- The three basic effects of local anesthetics placed in the epidural space are sympathetic blockade, diminution (or ablation) of the afferent pain signals to the brain, and blockade of outgoing, efferent, motor signals.
  - The height (or cephalocaudal dimension) of the block depends on the volume of the agents injected relative to the point of injection. In contrast to intrathecal injections, the baricity of the agent and the position of the patient have little, if any, effect.
- Anesthesia versus analgesia: The density of the block, or the differential effect of the agents on sympathetic (always), sensory (usually), or motor (sometimes) pathways, depends on the amount of agent injected (concentration).
- Adjuvants: Pathways that contribute to postoperative pain can be affected by epidural injection of agents before, during, and/or after the operative procedure. In addition to local anesthetics, opiate agonists and α agonists improve and augment effects while reducing the overall side effect profile.
  - Opiates (fentanyl, hydromorphone, morphine)
  - Clonidine

COMMON DRUG REGIMENS

Single-Shot Caudal
- With a 22-gauge needle (or angiocatheter), a single injection can be given for intra- and postoperative pain relief.
- This can be performed for common outpatient procedures such as herniorrphy and circumcision.

TABLE 38–6 Local Anesthetics Used for Epidural Anesthesia in the Pediatric Population

LOCAL ANESTHETIC	BASAL (mL/kg)	BOLUS (mL/kg)	LOCKOUT min	LOCKOUT doses/h	MAXIMUM DELIVERED (mg/kg/h)
Infant: lidocaine (2 mg/mL)	0.5	0	N/A	N/A	1
Child: lidocaine (3 mg/mL)	0.2	0.1	15	3	1.5
Bupivacaine (0.8 mg/mL)	0.2	0.1	15	2	0.32
Bupivacaine (1 mg/mL)	0.2	0.1	15	2	0.4
Ropivacaine (1.5 mg/mL)	0.2	0.1	15	2	0.6
Ropivacaine (2 mg/mL)	0.2	0.1	15	2	0.8

TABLE 38–7 Additives (Opiate and/or Clonidine) Used to Improve the Analgesic Effect of Epidural Analgesia (and May Permit Using a Lower Concentration)

DRUG GROUP	DRUG	CONCENTRATION	COMMENTS
Opiate	Fentanyl	1–2 µg/mL	Tends to stay in area of deposition
	Hydromorphone	10–20 µg/mL	May ascend up the spinal cord somewhat
	Morphine	10–20 µg/mL	Tends to ascend cephalad and is more likely to be associated with respiratory depression

Local anesthetic	Lidocaine
	  Max dose: 1.5 mg/kg/h
		Infants: 1 mg/mL
		  Children: 3 mg/mL
		Older children: 5 mg/mL
			Serum levels may be monitored (keep ≤4 mcg/mL) to reduce risk of toxicity

	Bupivacaine Max dose: 0.4 mg/kg/h	0.0625–0.125%	Gives a good differential block for postoperative analgesia at lower concentrations
	Ropivacaine Max dose: 0.8 mg/kg/h	0.1–0.2%	Less cardiac toxicity at equianalgesic concentrations
α-agonist	Clonidine	0.5–1 mg/mL	Potentiates both local anesthetic and opiate May be associated with some hypotension and sedation

Epidural PCA
- Continuous epidural analgesia (with or without bolus, depending on the patient's ability to participate) can be provided via the caudal, lumbar, or even thoracic route.
- Doses are calculated based on the total dose allowed of local anesthetic using mg programming in the pump.
- Local anesthetics and additives used for epidural PCA are described in Tables 38–6 and 38–7.

MANAGEMENT OF SIDE EFFECTS
- Nausea/vomiting: ondansetron, diphenhydramine, droperidol, metoclopramide
- Itching: diphenhydramine, hydroxyzine, butorphanol, naloxone infusion
- Constipation: Senokot
- Urinary retention: urinary catheter

TRANSITION TO HOME
- Basal analgesia is converted to oral analgesia.
- Once the patient can tolerate eating some food, oral analgesics (eg, oral opioids, see Table 38–8) are given, the basal infusion is discontinued (leaving the bolus only for awhile as a rescue), and then PCA is discontinued.

PRESCRIPTION FILLING

- It is best not to assume that every drug is available in every neighborhood pharmacy, especially the liquid forms of opiates.

TABLE 38–8 Common Oral Opiates Used to Treat Pediatric Pain

DRUG	WITH ACETAMINOPHEN	AVAILABILITY	DOSE
Codeine		Solution: 15 mg/5 mL Syrup: 10, 60 mg/5mL	0.5–1.2 mg/kg q4h
	120 mg	Solution: 12 mg/5 mL Tablet	Based on codeine
Tylenol #1	300 mg	7.5 mg	
Tylenol #2	300 mg	15 mg	
Tylenol #3	300 mg	30 mg	
Tylenol #4	300 mg	60 mg	
Hydrocodone	120 mg	Solution: 2.5 mg/5 mL	Based on hydrocodone 0.1 mg/kg q4h
Vicodin	500 mg	Tablet: 2.5 or 5 mg	
Hydromorphone		Tablet: 2, 4 mg	0.2 mg/kg q4h
Dilaudid		Rectal suppository: 3 mg	0.2 mg/kg q6h
Methadone		Solution: 5, 10 mg/5 mL	0.1 mg/kg q4h
Morphine		Solution: 10, 20, 100 mg/5 mL	0.3–0.5 mg/kg q4h
MS-Contin		Tablets: 10, 15, 30 mg Extended release: 15, 30, 60, 100 mg	0.3–0.5 mg/kg q4h
Oxycodone		Solution: 1 mg/mL	0.1 mg/kg q4h
		Tablet: 5 mg	0.1 mg/kg q4h
Percoset	25 mg	5 mg	Based on acetaminophen
Tylox	500 mg	5 mg	
Oxycontin		Extended release: 10, 20, 40 mg	

FOLLOW-UP

- It is easy to neglect to follow up once patients have gone home. A simple call may reveal problems that can be solved by an experienced clinician.

REFERENCES

1. **Schechter, Berde, and Yaster.** *Pain in Infants, Children, and Adolescents.* Baltimore: Lippincott Williams & Wilkins; 2003.
2. **Yaster et al.** *Pediatric Pain Management and Sedation Handbook.* Baltimore: Mosby, 1997.

39 PERIPHERAL NEUROPATHY

Mitchell J. M. Cohen, MD

EPIDEMIOLOGY

- The peripheral neuropathies are a large class of disorders with multiple presentations and etiologies.
- The epidemiology of this heterogeneous group of disorders is difficult to study, and their prevalence varies with clinical, regional, and socioeconomic contexts.
- Diabetic neuropathy is most often seen in general medical practice, postherpetic neuralgia in geriatric medicine, traumatic neuropathy in the urban emergency room, and neuropathy secondary to niacin deficiency (pellagra) in low-income populations.
- According to the best available data, the population prevalence of peripheral neuropathies in North America and Europe is 2–3%. Up to 10% of the geriatric population may be affected.[1]

PATHOPHYSIOLOGY

DEFINITIONS OF CLASSES OF PERIPHERAL NEUROPATHY

- Peripheral neuropathy is a general term referring to a group of disorders that may involve a single nerve or nerve root (mononeuropathies), multiple individual identified nerves (mononeuropathy multiplex), and/or small-fiber syndromes that do not conform to specific dermatomes (peripheral polyneuropathies).
- The peripheral polyneuropathies represent systemic disease of the peripheral nerves, commonly present with stocking–glove distribution, and often first affect the toes because the longest nerve fibers are most

vulnerable. As it progresses, the disease affects the next longest fibers in the calves, proximal legs, fingers, hands, and then chest.
- Polyneuropathies tend to be symmetric. Mononeuropathies tend to be asymmetric.
- Acute-onset neuropathies of either type must be aggressively evaluated, since acute symmetric polyneuropathy can be associated with fatal illness (eg, Guillain–Barré syndrome) and acute mononeuropathy with preventable permanent neurologic damage (eg, limiting neuropathy associated with vasculitis through steroid therapy).

COMMON NEUROPHYSIOLOGIC ELEMENTS IN PERIPHERAL NEUROPATHIES

- Various etiologic events and conditions lead to peripheral nerve damage, including diabetes, uremia, amyloidosis, alcoholism, autoimmune diseases, thyroid disease, vasculitis, radiation and antineoplastic drug treatments, HIV and acute herpes zoster infections, nutritional deficiencies, compression and entrapment from anatomic changes or scar tissue, and trauma. Some of these conditions lead to axonal degeneration of the neuron; others lead to loss of the myelin sheath.
- One-third of cases develop in the context of diabetes mellitus. Alcoholism is the second most common cause. A large number of peripheral neuropathies are idiopathic.
- The various peripheral neuropathies have some pathophysiologic changes in common. These changes are driven by excitatory inflammatory products and extravasated neuronal content, such as hydrogen ions, potassium ions, nerve growth factor, catecholamines, serotonin, prostaglandins, cytokines, and bradykinin.
- In response to this excitation, the neuronal cell membranes become unstable, and increased sodium channels are expressed on the neuronal surface. Neuronal firing thresholds to chemical, mechanical, and thermal stimuli decrease. Spontaneous firing and ectopic impulses also occur in the damaged neurons.
- The central nervous system receives increasing input from these altered primary peripheral pain afferents (nociceptors) and develops central sensitization or "windup."
- In central sensitization, spinal cord transmission cells develop functional changes that parallel those in the peripheral nerves: transmission cells develop lower firing thresholds, spontaneously fire, and show broadened receptive fields. The fact that these cells can fire in response to a wider-than-normal range of inputs provides one explanation for allodynia, the

experience of pain in response to a nonnoxious stimulus (eg, light touch). Activation of *N*-methyl-D-aspartate (NMDA)-type glutamate receptors and the related increased influx of calcium to transmission cells appear to be important components of the windup process.

- Wide-dynamic-range cells in the dorsal horn are among the transmission cells most frequently implicated in the central sensitization process.
- Glutamate and aspartate continually provoke increased firing in sensitized spinal cord cells, which can lead to cell exhaustion and death. Since the preponderance of spinal cord cells is inhibitory, the net effect is further acceleration of pain transmission.[2]

CLINICAL FEATURES

- Peripheral neuropathies involve (1) baseline, spontaneous pain and (2) evoked, stimulus-dependent pain.
- The baseline pain can have a burning and/or pins-and-needles sensation, either steady in quality or episodic, which can be lightning-like, lancinating, or crampy.
- Evoked pain can be intense, with a crescendo after stimulation of the symptomatic area, and can amplify any of the baseline pain qualities. Patients often describe evoked pain as more fearsome than their baseline pain.
- Evoked pains all involve abnormal responses to stimulation. Hyperalgesia involves a lowered nociceptor firing threshold; hyperpathia involves a raised threshold with a delayed but explosive response to stimulation; and allodynia involves conscious pain experience from nonnoxious stimuli.
- In peripheral polyneuropathies, walking short distances may provoke increased burning and cramping sensations in the feet.
- In postherpetic neuralgia affecting the T7 dermatome, tight clothing, a seatbelt harness, or a blanket's touch can provoke paroxysms of cramping, stabbing pain.
- In small-fiber polyneuropathies, such as occur in diabetes, as symptoms progress proximally from the toes, additional neurologic findings and impairments develop, including loss of deep tendon reflexes, motor weakness, and muscle atrophy. Foot drop, gait disturbance, and severe functional losses accrue over time.
- Fear of evoked pain can also significantly restrict activities, especially those involving crowds and an increased likelihood that the affected area may be bumped. Patients may be forced to abandon swimming, dancing, and other activities associated with evoked pain.
- Peripheral neuropathies become complicated by a variety of comorbid neuropsychiatric conditions, including sleep disturbance, decreased concentration due to distraction by pain, major depression, and anxiety disorders.[3]

DIAGNOSIS

- When possible, any medical diagnosis underlying the neuropathy (eg, diabetes, hypothyroidism, multiple myeloma, and uremia) must first be established and managed.
- Complete history, physical, and laboratory examinations are essential, as so many conditions can give rise to peripheral neuropathies. When history and physical do not provide an underlying diagnosis, laboratory assessment becomes important.
- If serum electrolytes, electrolytes, creatinine, and urea nitrogen are normal, a standard rheumatologic screen, thyroid function tests, and chest x-ray should be obtained. If these are normal, patient history determines the next studies, based on assessment of individual risk factors and physical findings.
- The next level of studies can include HIV antibody testing, Lyme titers, serum protein electrophoresis (to rule out multiple myeloma and paraproteinemias), skeletal survey (to rule out tumor and multiple myeloma), B_{12} and folate levels, lumbar puncture (to rule out Guillain–Barré and multiple sclerosis), and nerve biopsy.
- Electrodiagnostic studies document mononeuropathies and mononeuropathy multiplex but often fail to reveal small-fiber polyneuropathies. Electromyography may distinguish demyelinating diseases from axonal damage.
- Quantitative sensory testing (QST) is emerging as a more sensitive method of demonstrating small-fiber neuropathies, but is not yet widely used or available.
- A significant number of peripheral neuropathies end up classified as idiopathic.

MANAGEMENT

- In established peripheral neuropathies, the treatment goals are symptomatic pain control, reduced impairments (eg, improved sleep and concentration), and enhanced function (eg, greater walking endurance, socialization). Pain elimination and cure are not realistic treatment goals.
- Pain control involves rational polypharmacy with drugs that exert antineuropathic effects by different presumed mechanisms.
- Sodium channel agents act, in part, by blocking the increased sodium channels expressed on affected

peripheral nerves. Established agents in this class include carbamazepine, oxcarbazepine, tricyclic antidepressants, and topical lidocaine.

- Calcium channel agents act, in part, by blocking the influx of calcium that occurs as part of central sensitization. Established agents in this class include gabapentin and oxcarbazepine.[4,5]
- Drugs that enhance the descending inhibition of pain act at levels from the cortex down to the dorsal horn of the spinal cord. Established agents in this class include opioids, tramadol, and tricyclic antidepressants.[6]
- Many other agents used to treat peripheral neuropathies are associated with inadequate evidence of efficacy, including topical capsaicin, levodopa, ketamine, dextromethorphan, and selective serotonin reuptake inhibitors (SSRIs).
- Many patients require combined therapy with agents from different classes as well as standard antineuropathic analgesia plus rescue medication. A sample regimen could include daily application of a topical lidocaine patch plus gabapentin plus short-acting oxycodone as needed for rescue analgesia during severe pain flares.
- Sleep disorders, major depression, and anxiety disorders must be aggressively treated. Tricyclic antidepressants tend to normalize sleep, have antineuropathic analgesic effects, and reduce mood and anxiety symptoms.
- When tolerability and safety are problems with tricyclics, and formal sleep disorders such as apnea are ruled out, zolpidem or low-dose treatment with trazadone or quetiapine may improve sleep.
- SSRIs are very effective in controlling depression and anxiety, although they have little effect on pain in nondepressed patients.
- Pain coping can be enhanced with relaxation training, biofeedback, supportive psychotherapy, regular exercise, and increased social function.

REFERENCES

1. **Martyn C, Hughes R.** Epidemiology of peripheral neuropathy. *J Neurol Neurosurg Psychiatry.* 1997;62:310.
2. **Devor M.** Neuropathic pain and injured nerve: Peripheral mechanisms. *Br Med Bull.* 1991;47:619.
3. **Hughes RA.** Peripheral neuropathy. *BMJ.* 2002;324:466.
4. **Backonja M, Beydoun A, Edwards KR, et al.** Gabapentin for the symptomatic treatment of painful neuropathy in patients with diabetes mellitus: A randomized controlled trial. *JAMA.* 1998;280:1831.
5. **Rowbotham M, Hardon N, Stacey B, et al.** Gabapentin for the treatment of postherpetic neuralgia: A randomized controlled trial. *JAMA.* 1998;280:1837.
6. **Watson C, Babul N.** Efficacy of oxycodone in neuropathic pain: A randomized trial in postherpetic neuralgia. *Neurology.* 1998;50:1837.

40 POSTSURGICAL PAIN SYNDROMES

Amar B. Setty, MD
Christopher L. Wu, MD

INTRODUCTION

- The extent of the problem of postoperative chronic pain is illustrated by the fact that, in a survey conducted in pain clinics in Scotland and Northern England, 20% of patients believed their operation was a cause of their chronic pain and half of these attributed their pain entirely to the surgical procedure.[1]
- Neuropathic pain develops after tissue trauma from surgical procedures.
- After peripheral nerve injury, changes such as sprouting, spontaneous activity in nerve endings, and peripheral sensitization occur.
- Combined with the loss of somatosensory input from distal nerves, the increased activity from damaged nerves leads to the central sensitization that, in turn, leads to spontaneous pain and hyperalgesia.[2] This basic mechanism underlies postoperative pain syndromes.
- Recent studies have increased our knowledge of the subject. Nevertheless, significant variations in results exist because of the lack of randomized controlled trials and the varying methodology and definitions for chronic pain.[1,3] For instance, is the time scale 3, 6, or 12 months? Does postoperative pain refer only to new-onset symptoms or can it be a progression of preoperative symptoms?
- A useful set of criteria define postoperative chronic pain syndrome as[1]:
  - Pain that develops after a surgical procedure
  - Pain of at least 2 months' duration
  - Exclusion of other causes of the pain
  - Exclusion of preexisting pain

POSTAMPUTATION PAIN SYNDROME

- Pain after limb amputation is the best studied postoperative syndrome. This pain is broadly categorized as residual limb pain (stump pain) or phantom limb pain.

CHARACTERISTICS

- Residual limb pain is characterized by paresthesias and hyperalgesia in the stump[1] and is caused by neuroma formation at the site followed by spinal cord modulation.
- Phantom limb sensation and pain are central phenomena often explained by Melzack's neuromatrix theory, which holds that a matrix exists for each body part and this matrix persists in the absence of the body part.[3] Even after loss of the limb, therefore, the "pain memory" may continue.
- In these patients, modulation takes place at the somatosensory cortex,[4,5] subcortex, and thalamus. These changes may occur prior to amputation in patients with extensive loss of limb function.[4]
- Peripheral and spinal cord neuroplastic changes may also contribute to amputation pain.[4]
- Almost all patients experience phantom sensations, and the phantom limb may seem to resemble the amputated limb in shape and function.
- Eventually, phantom limb sensations may fade.
- Telescoping occurs when the distal phantom limb sensation approaches the stump and eventually is perceived within the stump.[5]
- Both stump and phantom limb pain may be episodic.[1,3]
- Some reports describe the pain intensity as mild. Others describe it as severe in as many as 40% of patients.[1]
- The duration of phantom pain episodes ranges from more than 15 hours a day in approximately 25% of patients to less than 1 hour in 20%.
- Approximately 25% of patients report 20 or more days of phantom pain per month, but half may have pain 5 days or less a month.[1]
- Phantom pain can occur after removal of body parts other than limbs, including the rectum, breast, tongue, teeth, and genitals.[1]

INCIDENCE

- The incidence of postamputation pain ranges from 30 to 83%[1,3] (see Table 40–1). Lower estimates tend to come from older studies that relied on patients' request for pain medicine to determine incidence.[5]
- Phantom limb pain occurs less often in children and in those missing a limb as a result of congenital limb deficiency.[5]
- The incidence of stump pain ranges from 5 to 62%.[1,3]

TABLE 40–1 Incidence of Postamputation Pain

STUDY	STUMP PAIN INCIDENCE (%)	PHANTOM PAIN INCIDENCE (%)
Finch et al[a]	18	30
Sherman et al[b]	—	78
Jensen et al[c]	—	59–65
Pohjolainen [d]	5	53
Krane and Heller[e]	—	83
Nikolajsen et al[f]	—	55–81
Wartan et al[g]	57	55
Fisher and Hanspal[h]	—	31
Nikolajsen et al[i]	—	59–79
Kooijman et al[j]	49	51
Fraser et al[k]	—	69
Gallagher et al[l]	48	69

[a]Finch DR, Macdougal M, Tibbs DJ, et al. Amputation for vascular disease: The experience of a peripheral vascular unit. *Br J Surg.* 1980; 67:233.
[b]Sherman RA, Sherman CJ, Parker L. Chronic phantom and stump pain among American veterans: Results of a survey. *Pain.* 1984;18:83.
[c]Jensen TS, Krebs B, Nielsen J, et al. Immediate and long-term phantom limb pain in amputees: Incidence, clinical characteristics and relationship to pre-amputation limb pain. *Pain.* 1985;21:267.
[d]Pohjolainen T. A clinical evaluation of stumps in lower limb amputees. *Prosthet Orthot Int.* 1991;15:178.
[e]Krane EJ, Heller LB. The prevalence of phantom limb sensation and pain in pediatric amputees. *J Pain Symptom Manage.* 1995;10:21.
[f]Nikolajsen L, Ilkjaer S, Christensen JH, et al. Randomised trial of epidural bupivacaine and morphine in prevention of stump and phantom pain in lower-limb amputation. *Lancet.* 1997;350:1353.
[g]Wartan SW, Hamann W, Wedley JR, et al. Phantom pain and sensation among British veteran amputees. *Br J Anaesth.* 1997;78:652.
[h]Fisher K, Hanspal RS. Phantom pain, anxiety, depression, and their relation in consecutive patients with amputated limbs: Case reports. *BMJ.* 1998;316:903.
[i]Nikolajsen L, Ilkjaer S, Jensen TS. Effect of preoperative extradural bupivacaine and morphine on stump sensation in lower limb amputees. *Br J Anaesth.* 1998;81:348.
[j]Kooijman CM, Dijkstra PU, Geertzen JH, et al. Phantom pain and phantom sensations in upper limb amputees: An epidemiological study. *Pain.* 2000;87:33.
[k]Fraser CM, Halligan PW, Robertson IH, et al. Characteristics of phantom limb phenomena in upper limb amputees. *Prosthet Orthot Int.* 2001;25:235.
[l]Gallagher P, Allen D, Maclachlan M. Phantom limb pain and residual limb pain following lower limb amputation: A descriptive analysis. *Disabil Rehabil.* 2001;23:522.

- Stump pain persists in 5 to 10% of patients.[5]
- Phantom pain occurs in 30 to 83% of patients.
- Phantom limb pain begins usually within 3 weeks of amputation.[1]
- The frequency of painful episodes decreases in the first year but prevalence does not change.[1,3]
- Half of individuals with phantom limb pain report no change in the intensity of their pain over time.[3]
- Stump pain exists in 66% of patients with phantom limb pain and in half of those without phantom pain.[3]
- The pain is often perceived to exist in the same location as the now-phantom limb.[5]

RISK FACTORS

- Increased pain preoperatively increases the probability of postoperative phantom limb pain at 3-month follow-up by 33–72%.[3,5]
- Postoperative stump pain is associated with phantom pain.
- Nonpainful phantom paresthesias also correlate with the presence of phantom pain.[1,3]
- Pain may be more common after amputation for cancer than for trauma.[3]
- No known associations exist with age, sex, site of amputation, ethnicity, or educational level.[1,5]
- The effect of intraoperative anesthetic or surgical technique on postamputation pain is unknown.[3]
- Other factors that may influence this pain include genetic predisposition, anxiety, attention/distraction, urination/defecation, weather changes, and stump manipulation.[5]

PREVENTION AND TREATMENT

- Prolonged preoperative and postoperative treatment of pain with regional anesthesia may decrease the risk of phantom and stump pain, but the data are equivocal.[3]
- This pain is not alleviated by stump procedures (further amputation, neuroma excisions, etc).[1]
- Opioids may provide pain relief,[5] perhaps because of cortical reorganization.[6]
- Pain treatment may include calcitonin (100–200 IU up to five times a day), antidepressant drugs, anticonvulsant drugs, nonsteroidal anti-inflammatory drugs, tramadol, transcutaneous electrical nerve stimulation, acupuncture, hypnosis, or biofeedback.[5,7] Case reports describe the use of continuous peripheral blockade for treatment of this pain.[7]
- Ketamine may reduce spinal sensitization via N-methyl D-aspartate receptor antagonism.[5]
- Some investigators suggest that if pain treatment starts early, the success rate will be higher (80–90%) than if it is started later (30%).[7]
- Dorsal root entry zone lesions, cordotomy, thalamotomy, and sympathectomy provide short-term relief.[5]
- Functional prostheses and rehabilitation may help.[1,5]

POSTTHORACOTOMY PAIN SYNDROME

CHARACTERISTICS

- Postthoracotomy pain syndrome (PTPS) manifests as an aching or burning pain along the thoracotomy scar that may persist months after surgery.[8]
- This pain is usually related to intercostal nerve injury from either rib resection or retraction.[1]
- PTPS occurs in the first weeks after surgery.
- If the occurrence of pain is delayed in patients with cancer, tumor recurrence must be excluded.[1]
- Intensity varies: 80% rate pain as 4 or less on the 11-point numeric rating scale.[1]
- Although pain is often severe at 1 month, it usually subsides by 1 year.[8]
- The pain is severe in 3–5% at 1 year.[9]

INCIDENCE

- The incidence of PTPS may exceed 50%[3] (see Table 40–2).
- Prevalence varies between 5 and 67%.[1,3]
- Incidence, prevalence, and intensity decrease with time.[1,3]

TABLE 40–2   Incidence of Postthoracotomy Pain

STUDY	CHRONIC PAIN INCIDENCE (%)
Dajczman et al[a]	54
Kalso et al[b]	44
Landreneau et al[c]	22–44
Bertrand et al[d]	61–63
Perttunen et al[e]	61
Obata et al[f]	33–67
Hu et al[g]	41
Senturk et al[h]	62
Ochroch et al[i]	21

[a]Dajczman E, Gordon A, Kreisman H, et al. Long-term postthoracotomy pain. *Chest.* 1991;99:270.
[b]Kalso E, Perttunen K, Kaasinen S. Pain after thoracic surgery. *Acta Anaesthesiol Scand.* 1992;36:96.
[c]Landreneau RJ, Mack MJ, Hazelrigg SR, et al. Prevalence of chronic pain after pulmonary resection by thoracotomy or video-assisted thoracic surgery. *J Thorac Cardiovasc Surg.* 1994;107:1079.
[d]Bertrand PC, Regnard JF, Spaggiari L, et al. Immediate and long-term results after surgical treatment of primary spontaneous pneumothorax by VATS. *Ann Thorac Surg.* 1996;61:1641–1645.
[e]Perttunen K, Tasmuth T, Kalso E. Chronic pain after thoracic surgery: A follow-up study. *Acta Anaesthesiol Scand.* 1999;43:563.
[f]Obata H, Saito S, Fujita N, et al. Epidural block with mepivacaine before surgery reduces long-term post-thoracotomy pain. *Can J Anaesth.* 1999;46:1127.
[g]Hu JS, Lui PW, Wang H, et al. Thoracic epidural analgesia with morphine does not prevent postthoracotomy pain syndrome: A survey of 159 patients. *Acta Anaesthesiol Sin.* 2000;38:195.
[h]Senturk M, Ozcan PE, Talu GK, et al. The effects of three different analgesia techniques on long-term postthoracotomy pain. *Anesth Analg.* 2002;94:11.
[i]Ochroch EA, Gottschalk A, Augostides J, et al. Long-term pain and activity during recovery from major thoracotomy using thoracic epidural analgesia. *Anesthesiology.* 2002;97:1234.

RISK FACTORS

- Pain in the immediate postoperative period predicts the development of PTPS.
- The severity of postoperative pain is a significant predictor of PTPS (36% of patients with minor postoperative pain develop PTPS vs 56% of patients with moderate-to-severe acute postoperative pain).[3,9]
- Pain in the immediate postoperative period may be the only factor that predicts PTPS.[10]
- PTPS may be related to the patient's preoperative pain state.[1,3]
- The incidence at 1 month and 1 year is increased in females versus males.[8]
- Malignancy is not associated with increased incidence.[9]
- PTPS may be associated with nerve dysfunction (loss of superficial abdominal reflex).[3]
- The incidence of PTPS does not appear to be decreased by video assistance during thoracoscopic procedures.[1,3]

PREVENTION AND TREATMENT

- Intraoperative and postoperative use of epidural analgesia with local anesthetics decreases PTPS significantly compared with postoperative use of intravenous opiates.[11]
- No significant difference in PTPS occurs with use of postoperative patient-controlled epidural analgesia versus postoperative intravenous analgesia.[12]
- Intercostal nerve cryoablation may decrease PTPS.[3]

POSTMASTECTOMY PAIN SYNDROME

CHARACTERISTICS

- Postmastectomy pain syndrome (PMPS) can involve chest wall, breast, scar, and arm/shoulder pain as well as phantom breast sensations or pain.[1,3]
- The mechanism is probably nerve damage from surgery, radiation, chemotherapy, or tumor recurrence.[1,3]
- Onset is within the first weeks following a surgical procedure. Pain from recurrent cancer or radiation usually takes 5 years to develop.[1]
- Women with PMPS are often misdiagnosed and undertreated, and have poor pain control.[1]

INCIDENCE

- The incidence of PMPS is up to 50% after surgery for cancer but varies by type of pain.[3]

- Breast or chest wall pain incidence at 3 weeks is 35% and decreases to 23% at 1 year. In the same period, hyperesthesia decreases from 38 to 13%.[3]
- The prevalence stays at 30% over a 6-year period.[1]
- Arm pain incidence is stable between 3 and 15 months (55% vs 51%).[3]
- The incidence of phantom breast pain is approximately 13% at 3 weeks and 17% at 6 years.[1]

RISK FACTORS

- Preoperative breast pain may be a risk factor for postoperative phantom breast pain, although this suggestion is controversial.[3]
- Preoperative depression and anxiety are associated but not statistically significant.[3]
- Mastectomy with reconstruction (incidence 49%) is more likely than mastectomy alone (31%) or elective breast reduction (22%) to lead to PMPS.
- Reconstruction with prosthesis implantation has the highest risk of chronic pain (53%).[13]
- A large retrospective trial found that chronic pain is more common after breast-conserving surgery compared with radical surgery, but this finding was not replicated in small, prospective trials.[3]
- Axillary dissection increases the risk of chronic arm pain.[3]
- The severity of acute postoperative pain and level of analgesic requirements predict chronic pain in the breast and ipsilateral arm.[3]
- Postoperative radiation therapy is a risk factor for chronic pain and possibly for phantom sensations.[3]
- Altered sensation in the intercostobrachial nerve is associated with neuralgia.[3]

TREATMENT

- One randomized study found pain relief with topical capsaicin.[14]

POSTCHOLECYSTECTOMY CHRONIC PAIN

CHARACTERISTICS

- Postcholecystectomy chronic pain syndrome involves poorly characterized and multifactoral abdominal pain.[3]
- Symptoms include:
  - Indigestion[1,3]
  - Noncolicky pain[1]

- ○ Dull or mild abdominal pain[1,3]
- ○ Severe abdominal pain[1,3]
- ○ Scar pain[1,3]

INCIDENCE

- Varies from 3 to 56%[3]

MECHANISMS[3]

- Sphincter of Oddi dysfunction
- Bile duct stones
- Ulcer
- Colonic dysfunction
- Scar pain

RISK FACTORS

- Risk factors[1,3] include psychologic vulnerability, being female, and long-standing preoperative pain.
- Risk is decreased with classic "gallbladder attack symptoms."
- Surgical approach (laparoscopic vs open) is not a factor.
- Pain at 6 weeks predicts pain at 1 year.
- It is unknown if neuraxial or regional anesthesia can decrease the risk.

POSTINGUINAL HERNIA CHRONIC PAIN

CHARACTERISTICS

- Pulling, tearing, or sharp pain of moderate to severe intensity adjacent to a scar from inguinal hernia repair[15]
- May be neuropathic or somatic[15]
- May lead to difficulty in walking or to sexual dysfunction[16]

INCIDENCE

- The incidence varies from "rare" to more than 30%.[3,15]
- One large study found an incidence of 28.7% for pain at 1 year and functional impairment in half of the patients.[17]
- Technique affects incidence: Open repair was associated with a 63% incidence of pain at 12 months versus a 15% incidence after 9 months with laparoscopic repair.[1]

MECHANISMS

- Ischemic: secondary to tension in the operative site or tight closure of the deep or superficial inguinal ring with edema formation.[18]
- Nerve trauma during dissection with neuroma formation and secondary neuropathy.[18]

RISK FACTORS

- Risk factors include ambulatory surgery,[15] age less than 40 years,[15] preoperative pain,[15] pain in the immediate postoperative period,[15] and mesh repair.[16,18]
- Increased pain at 1 and 4 weeks postoperatively correlates with higher rates of moderate to severe pain at 12 months.[16]
- Recurrent hernia repair has a fourfold higher incidence of moderate-to-severe pain.[16]
- It is unclear if risk is lower with laparoscopic than with open procedures.[3,16]
- Lower incidences are reported for procedures performed at dedicated hernia centers.[18]
- It is unknown if neuraxial or regional anesthesia can decrease the risk.

OTHER POSTOPERATIVE PAIN SYNDROMES

POSTSTERNOTOMY

- Chronic pain incidence is 27% after thymectomy (mostly women) and 28% after coronary artery bypass grafting (mostly men).
- Pain is due to bone fracture, incomplete healing, osteomyelitis, sternocostal chondritis, costal fracture, brachial plexus injury, or nerve entrapment caused by sternal wires.
- Risk factors include younger age, increased New York Heart Association class, and pain in the immediate postoperative period.[19]
- Saphenous vein grafts may lead to chronic leg pain.[1]
- Some studies implicate internal mammary artery harvest.[19]

POSTSYMPATHECTOMY

- This syndrome is characterized by burning thigh pain.
- Incidence is 12–35% for open and phenol techniques.[1]

POSTVASECTOMY

- Vasectomy may lead to chronic testicular pain for 5–33% of patients.
- Adequate local anesthesia may prevent this pain.[1]

POSTRECTAL AMPUTATION

- Perineal pain may develop in 12% after abdominoperitoneal resection for rectal cancer.[1]

CONCLUSION

- Preoperative pain increases the risk for postoperative pain. This may be related to modulation of the peripheral and central nervous system.
- Structural changes or alterations of inhibitory and facilitatory mechanisms[20] maintain the pain state.
- Peripheral factors include neuroma formation in surgically cut nerves with spontaneous and abnormally induced activity. A neuroma can lead to hyperalgesia, allodynia, and chronic pain.[5]
- Acute postoperative pain is another contributor.
- The trauma of surgery may lead to sensitization and subsequent peripheral/central changes that cause chronic pain.
- Psychological vulnerability and genetic predisposition are implicated but need further study.
- Treatment options have been inadequately studied.
- Traditional treatments, such as opiates, anti-inflammatory drugs, anticonvulsants, and other nonopiate analgesics, are the primary therapies.

REFERENCES

1. **Macrae WA.** Chronic pain after surgery. *Br J Anaesth.* 2001; 87:88.
2. **Gottrup H, Andersen J, Arendt-Nielsen L, et al.** Psychophysical examination in patients with post-mastectomy pain. *Pain.* 2000;87:275.
3. **Perkins F, Kehlet H.** Chronic pain as an outcome of surgery. *Anesthesiology* 2000;93:1123.
4. **Grusser SM, Winter C, Schaefer M, et al.** Perceptual phenomena after unilateral arm amputation: A pre–post-surgical comparison. *Neurosci Lett.* 2001;302:13.
5. **Nikolajsen L, Jensen TS.** Phantom limb pain. *Br J Anaesth.* 2001;87:107.
6. **Huse E, Larbig W, Flor H, et al.** The effect of opioids on phantom limb pain and cortical reorganization. *Pain.* 2001;90:47.
7. **Lierz P, Schroegendorfer K, Choi S, et al.** Continuous blockade of brachial plexus with ropivicaine in phantom pain: A case report. *Pain.* 1998;78:135.
8. **Gotoda Y, Kambara N, Sakai T, et al.** The morbidity, time course and predictive factors for persistent post-thoracotomy pain. *Eur J Pain.* 2001;5:89.
9. **Pertunen K, Tasmuth T, Kalso E.** Chronic pain after thoracic surgery: A follow-up study. *Acta Anaesthesiol Scand.* 1999;43:563.
10. **Katz J, Jackson M, Kavanagh B, et al.** Acute pain after thoracic surgery predicts long term post-thoracotomy pain. *Clin J Pain.* 1996;12:50.
11. **Obata H, Saito S, Fujita N, et al.** Epidural block with mepivicaine before surgery reduces long term post-thoracotomy pain. *Can J Anaesth.* 1999;46:1127.
12. **Senturk M, Ozcan PE, Talu GK, et al.** The effects of three different analgesia techniques on long-term postthoracotomy pain. *Anesth Analg.* 2002;94:11.
13. **Wallace MS, Wallace AM, Lee J, et al.** Pain after breast surgery: A survey of 282 women. *Pain.* 1996;66:195.
14. **Dini D, Bertelli G, Gozza A, et al.** Treatment of the post mastectomy syndrome with topical capsaicin. *Pain.* 1993; 54:223.
15. **Poobalan AS, Bruce J, King PM, et al.** Chronic pain and quality of life following open inguinal hernia repair. *Br J Surg.* 2001;88:1122.
16. **Callesen T, Bech K, Kehlet H.** Prospective study of chronic pain after groin hernia repair. *Br J Surg.* 1999;86:1528.
17. **Bay-Nielsen M, Perkins FM, Kehlet H.** Pain and functional impairment 1 year after inguinal herniorrhaphy: A nationwide questionnaire study. *Ann Surg.* 2001;233:1.
18. **Condon RE.** Groin pain after hernia repair. *Ann Surg.* 2001;233:8.
19. **Kalso E, Mennander, Tasmuth T, et al.** Chronic post sternotomy pain. *Acta Anaesthesiol Scand.* 2001;45:935.
20. **Oliver HG, Smith W, Tassonyi E, et al.** Preoperative back pain is associated with diverse manifestations of central neuroplasticity. *Pain.* 2002;97:189.

41 PREGNANCY AND CHRONIC PAIN

James P. Rathmell, MD
Christopher M. Viscomi, MD
Ira M. Bernstein, MD

INTRODUCTION

- Pain occurs during pregnancy in nearly all women.
- Even during the course of an otherwise uncomplicated pregnancy, common musculoskeletal conditions can cause severe pain.
- Patients with longstanding painful disorders who enter pregnancy present management challenges.

USE OF MEDICATIONS DURING PREGNANCY

- Medical management of the pregnant patient should begin with attempts to minimize the use of all medications and use nonpharmacologic therapies whenever possible.
- When opting for drug therapy, the clinician must consider any potential for harm to the mother, the fetus, and the course of pregnancy.
- With the exception of large polar molecules (such as heparin and insulin), nearly all medications reach the fetus to some degree.
- The most critical period for minimizing maternal drug exposure is during early development — from conception through the tenth menstrual week of pregnancy (the tenth week following start of the last menstrual cycle). Drug exposure prior to organogenesis (prior to the fourth menstrual week) usually has an all-or-none effect: the embryo either does not survive or develops without abnormalities. Drug effects later in pregnancy typically lead to single- or multiple-organ involvement, developmental syndromes, or intrauterine growth retardation.
- The US Food and Drug Administration (FDA) has developed a five-category labeling system for all approved drugs in the United States (Table 41–1).

This labeling system rates the potential risk for teratogenic or embryotoxic effects based on available scientific and clinical evidence.

USE OF MEDICATIONS IN THE BREASTFEEDING MOTHER

- High lipid solubility, low molecular weight, minimal protein binding, and the deionized state all facilitate excretion of medications into breast milk. The neonatal dose of most medications obtained through breastfeeding is 1 to 2% of the maternal dose.
- Only small amounts of colostrum are excreted during the first few postpartum days; thus, early breastfeeding poses little risk to the infant whose mother received medications during the delivery period.
- The majority of breast milk is synthesized and excreted during and immediately following breastfeeding. Taking medications after breastfeeding or during times when the infant has the longest interval between feedings and avoiding long-acting medications minimize drug transfer via breast milk.
- The American Academy of Pediatrics Committee on Drugs has categorized medications in relation to the safety of maternal ingestion by breastfeeding mothers (Table 41–2).

TABLE 41–1   FDA Pregnancy Risk Classification Categories for Medications Used in Pain Management*

FDA CLASSIFICATION	DEFINITION	EXAMPLE
Category A	Controlled human studies indicate no apparent risk to the fetus. The possibility of harm to the fetus seems remote.	Multivitamins
Category B	Animal studies do not indicate a fetal risk or animal studies do indicate a teratogenic risk, but well-controlled human studies have failed to demonstrate a risk.	Acetaminophen Butorphanol, nalbuphine[†] Caffeine Fentanyl, hydrocodone, methadone, meperidine, morphine, oxycodone, oxymorphone[†] Ibuprofen, naproxen, indomethacin Metoprolol Paroxetine, fluoxetine Prednisolone, prednisone
Category C	Studies indicate teratogenic or embryocidal risk in animals, but no controlled studies have been done in women or there are no controlled studies in animals or humans.	Aspirin, ketorolac Codeine, propoxyphene[†] Gabapentin Lidocaine, mexiletene Nifedipine Propranolol Sumatriptan
Category D	There is positive evidence of human fetal risk, but in certain circumstances, the benefits of the drug may outweigh the risks involved.	Amitriptyline, imipramine Diazepam Phenobarbital Phenytoin Valproic acid
Category X	There is positive evidence of significant fetal risk, and the risk clearly outweighs any possible benefit.	Ergotamine

*Adapted from *Fed. Regist.* 1980;44:37434–37467.
[†]All opioid analgesics are FDA Risk Category D if used for prolonged periods or in large doses near term.

TABLE 41–2   Classification of Maternal Medication Use During Pregnancy*

CLASSIFICATION	DEFINITION	EXAMPLE
Category 1	Medications should not be consumed during lactation. Strong evidence exists that serious adverse effects on the infant are likely with maternal ingestion of these medications during lactation.	Ergotamine
Category 2	Effects on human infants are unknown, but caution is urged.	Amitriptyline, desipramine, doxepin, fluoxetine, imipramine, trazadone Diazepam, lorazepam, midazolam
Category 3	Medications are compatible with breastfeeding.	Carbamazepine, phenytoin, valproate Atenolol, propranolol, diltiazem Codeine, fentanyl, methadone, morphine, propoxyphene Butorphanol Lidocaine, mexiletene Acetaminophen Ibuprofen, indomethacin, ketorolac, naproxen Caffeine

*Adapted with permission from American Academy of Pediatrics Committee on Drugs.[1]

MEDICATIONS COMMONLY USED IN PAIN MANAGEMENT

NONSTEROIDAL ANTI-INFLAMMATORY DRUGS

- Aspirin remains the prototypical nonsteroidal anti-inflammatory drug (NSAID) and is the most thoroughly studied of this class of medications. First-trimester exposure to aspirin does not pose appreciable teratogenic risk. Prostaglandins appear to trigger labor and the aspirin-induced inhibition of prostaglandin synthesis may result in prolonged gestation and protracted labor.
- Aspirin has well known platelet-inhibiting properties and, theoretically, may increase the risk of peripartum hemorrhage.
- Neonatal platelet function is inhibited for up to 5 days after delivery in aspirin-treated mothers. Although low-dose aspirin therapy (60–80 mg/d) has not been associated with maternal or neonatal complications, higher doses appear to increase the risk of intracranial hemorrhage in neonates born prior to 35 weeks of gestation.[2]
- Circulating prostaglandins modulate the patency of the fetal ductus arteriosus. NSAIDs have been used therapeutically in neonates with persistent fetal circulation to induce closure of the ductus arteriosus via inhibition of prostaglandin synthesis. In utero, patency of the ductus arteriosus is essential for normal fetal circulation.
- Indomethacin has shown promise for the treatment of premature labor, but its use has been linked to antenatal narrowing and closure of the fetal ductus arteriosus.[3]
- Neither ibuprofen nor naproxen has been linked to congenital defects. Use of ibuprofen and naproxen during pregnancy may result in reversible oligohydramnios (reflecting diminished fetal urine output), mild constriction of the fetal ductus arteriosus, and an increased incidence of persistent pulmonary hypertension in the newborn.
- In a large series of NSAID use during pregnancy, naproxen and ibuprofen were most frequently used during the first and second trimesters because many patients stopped therapy once pregnancy was recognized and many of the rheumatic conditions remitted later in pregnancy. Under these conditions, there was no significant difference in pregnancy outcome (duration of pregnancy and labor, vaginal delivery rate, maternal bleeding requiring transfusion, or incidence of congenital anomalies) or the health status of offspring at long-term follow-up (ranging from 6 months to 14 years).
- In breastfeeding women, salicylate transport into breast milk is limited by its highly ionized state and high degree of protein binding. Caution should still be exercised if more than occasional or short-term aspirin use is contemplated during lactation as neonates have very slow elimination of salicylates. Both ibuprofen and naproxen are also minimally transported into breast milk, and are considered compatible with breastfeeding; these agents are generally better tolerated than indomethacin.
- Acetaminophen provides similar analgesia without the anti-inflammatory effects seen with NSAIDs. Acetaminophen has no known teratogenic properties, does not inhibit prostaglandin synthesis or platelet function, and is hepatotoxic only in extreme overdosage. If persistent pain demands use of a mild analgesic during pregnancy, acetaminophen appears to be a safe and effective first-choice agent.
- Acetaminophen does enter breast milk, although maximal neonatal ingestion would be less than 2% of

a maternal dose and it is considered compatible with breastfeeding.

OPIOID ANALGESICS

- Much of our present knowledge about the effects of chronic opioid exposure during pregnancy comes from studies of opioid-abusing patients. Pregnancy outcomes in studies of drug-abusing mothers must be interpreted with caution when attempting to establish the risks of a prescribed narcotic regimen in the pregnant patient with pain.
- Most studies suggest that methadone maintenance is associated with longer gestation and increased birth weight when compared with outcomes of untreated opioid abusers. However, both methadone-maintained and untreated opioid-abusing pregnant women deliver infants with lower birth weights and smaller head circumference than do drug-free controls. No increase in congenital defects has been observed in offspring of methadone-consuming patients.
- Neonatal abstinence syndrome occurs in between 30 and 90% of infants exposed to either heroin or methadone in utero. Neonatal withdrawal symptoms may be more frequent if the maternal daily methadone dose exceeds 20 mg. The majority of infants who will have symptomatic narcotic withdrawal are symptomatic by 48 hours postpartum, but there are reports of withdrawal symptoms beginning 7–14 days postpartum.
- Methadone levels in breast milk appear sufficient to prevent opioid withdrawal symptoms in the breastfed infant. The American Academy of Pediatrics considers methadone doses of up to 20 mg/d to be compatible with breastfeeding.
- Recognition of infants at risk for neonatal abstinence syndrome and institution of appropriate supportive and medical therapy typically result in little short-term consequence to the infant.
- There is no evidence to suggest a relationship between exposure to any of the opioid agonists or agonist–antagonists during pregnancy and large categories of major or minor malformations.
- The most extensive data are available for codeine and propoxyphene. No evidence was found for either agent to suggest a relationship to large categories of major or minor malformations.
- There are substantial data demonstrating no congenital anomalies associated with hydrocodone, meperidine, methadone, morphine, or oxycodone use during pregnancy.
- There are few reported exposures to other opioids, but there have been no reports linking the use of fentanyl, hydromorphone, oxymorphone, butorphanol, or nalbuphine with congenital defects.
- Postoperative analgesia for most pregnant women undergoing nonobstetric surgery can be readily provided using narcotic analgesics. Fentanyl, morphine, and hydromorphone are all safe and effective alternatives when a potent opioid is needed for parenteral administration. There are a range of safe and effective oral analgesics: For mild pain, acetaminophen alone or in combination with hydrocodone is a good alternative; for moderate pain, oxycodone alone or in combination with acetaminophen is effective; more severe pain may require morphine or hydromorphone, both of which are available for oral administration.
- Opioids are excreted into breast milk. Pharmacokinetic analysis has demonstrated that breast milk concentrations of codeine and morphine are equal to or somewhat greater than maternal plasma concentrations. The American Academy of Pediatrics considers use of many opioid analgesics including codeine, fentanyl, methadone, morphine, and propoxyphene to be compatible with breastfeeding.

LOCAL ANESTHETICS

- Few studies have focused on the potential teratogenicity of local anesthetics. Lidocaine and bupivacaine do not appear to pose significant developmental risk to the fetus. Only mepivacaine has any suggestion of teratogenicity; however, the number of patient exposures is inadequate to draw conclusions.
- Neither lidocaine nor bupivacaine appears in measurable quantities in the breast milk after epidural local anesthetic administration during labor. Intravenous infusion of high doses (2–4 mg/min) of lidocaine for suppression of cardiac arrhythmias led to minimal levels in breast milk. Based on these observations, continuous epidural infusion of dilute local anesthetic solutions for postoperative analgesia should result in only small quantities of drug actually reaching the fetus. The American Academy of Pediatrics considers local anesthetics to be safe for use in the nursing mother.

STEROIDS

- Most corticosteroids cross the placenta, although prednisone and prednisolone are inactivated by the placenta. Fetal serum concentrations of prednisone are less than 10% of maternal levels. No increase in malformations has been seen among patients exposed to corticosteroids during their first trimester of pregnancy. The use of corticosteroids during a limited trial of epidural steroid therapy in the pregnant patient probably poses minimal fetal risk.

- In the mother who is breastfeeding, less than 1% of a maternal prednisone dose appears in the nursing infant over the next 3 days. This amount of steroid exposure is unlikely to impact infant endogenous cortisol secretion.

BENZODIAZEPINES

- First-trimester exposure to benzodiazepines may be associated with an increased risk of congenital malformations. Diazepam may be associated with cleft lip/palate as well as congenital inguinal hernia. Benzodiazepine use immediately before delivery also risks fetal hypothermia, hyperbilirubinemia, and respiratory depression.
- In the breastfeeding mother, diazepam and its metabolite desmethyldiazepam can be detected in infant serum for up to 10 days after a single maternal dose. This is due to the slower metabolism in neonates compared with adults. Infants who are nursing from mothers receiving diazepam may show sedation and poor feeding. It appears most prudent to avoid any use of benzodiazepines during organogenesis, near the time of delivery, and during lactation.

ANTIDEPRESSANTS

- Antidepressants are often employed in the management of migraine headaches, as well as for analgesic and antidepressant purposes in chronic pain states.
- Although there are case reports of human neonatal limb deformities after maternal amitriptyline and imipramine use, large human population studies have not revealed association with any congenital malformation with the possible exception of cardiovascular defects after maternal imipramine use. There are no reports linking maternal desipramine use with congenital defects. Withdrawal syndromes have been reported in neonates born to mothers using nortriptyline, imipramine, and desipramine, with symptoms including irritability, colic, tachypnea, and urinary retention.
- Amitriptyline, nortriptyline, and desipramine are all excreted into human milk. Amitriptyline, nortriptyline, desipramine, clomipramine, and sertraline were not found in quantifiable amounts in nurslings and no adverse effects were reported. The American

Academy of Pediatrics considers antidepressants to have unknown risk during lactation.

ANTICONVULSANTS

- Most data regarding the risk of major malformation in fetuses of women taking anticonvulsants are derived from the treatment of epilepsy. Among epileptic women receiving phenytoin, carbamazepine, or valproic acid, the risk of a congenital defect was approximately 5%, or twice that of the general population. Neural tube defects and, to a lesser extent, cardiac abnormalities predominate in the offspring of women taking carbamazepine and valproic acid and can be detected during routine prenatal screening (elevated α-fetoprotein level).
- Fetal hydantoin syndrome has been associated with phenytoin, carbamazapine, and valproate use during pregnancy; the syndrome consists of variable dysmorphic features including microcephaly, mental deficiency, and craniofacial abnormalities. The appearance of this syndrome may be predicted either by fetal genetic screening or by measuring amniocyte levels of the enzyme responsible for phenytoin metabolism.
- While anticonvulsants have teratogenic risk, epilepsy itself may be partially responsible for fetal malformations. Perhaps pregnant women taking anticonvulsants for chronic pain may have a lower risk of fetal malformations than those taking the same medications for seizure control.
- Patients contemplating childbearing who are receiving anticonvulsants should have their pharmacologic therapy critically evaluated. Those taking anticonvulsants for neuropathic pain should strongly consider discontinuation during pregnancy, particularly during the first trimester. Consultation with a perinatologist is recommended if continued use of anticonvulsants during pregnancy is being considered. Frequent monitoring of serum anticonvulsant levels and folate supplementation should be initiated, while maternal α-fetoprotein screening may be considered to detect fetal neural tube defects.
- Gabapentin, a new anticonvulsant, is being used for treatment of neuropathic pain syndromes. Insufficient data exist to counsel patients regarding the fetal risk of gabapentin use during pregnancy.
- The use of anticonvulsants during lactation does not seem to be harmful to infants. Phenytoin, carbamazepine, and valproic acid appear in small amounts in breast milk, but no adverse effects have been noted. No data exist on gabapentin use during lactation.

ERGOT ALKALOIDS

• Ergotamine can have significant therapeutic efficacy in the episodic treatment of migraine headaches. However, even low doses of ergotamine are associated with significant teratogenic risk, while higher doses have caused uterine contractions and abortions.

• During lactation, ergot alkaloids are associated with neonatal convulsions and severe gastrointestinal disturbances.

CAFFEINE

• Caffeine is often used in combination analgesics for the management of vascular headaches. There are no identifiable risks with moderate caffeine ingestion (100 mg/m^2, a dose similar to that found in 2 cups of brewed coffee), while ingestion of more than 300 mg/d is associated with decreased birth weight. Caffeine ingestion combined with tobacco use increases the risk of delivering a low-birth-weight infant.

• Moderate ingestion of caffeine during lactation (up to 2 cups of coffee per day) does not appear to affect the infant. Breast milk usually contains less than 1% of the maternal dose of caffeine, with peak breast milk levels appearing 1 hour after maternal ingestion. Excessive caffeine use may cause increased wakefulness and irritability in the infant.

EVALUATION AND TREATMENT OF PAIN DURING PREGNANCY

• Severe pain during pregnancy most often arises from an extreme form of one of the more common musculoskeletal pain syndromes of pregnancy.

• Back pain and migraine headaches during pregnancy are also common problems that are encountered in practice.

MUSCULOSKELETAL CONSIDERATIONS IN PREGNANCY

ABDOMINAL WALL AND LIGAMENTOUS PAIN

• Pain in the abdomen brings a pregnant woman to the obstetrician early. In most cases, the problem is not serious and the majority of cases can be diagnosed by physical examination alone. One of the most common causes of abdominal pain early in pregnancy is miscarriage and presents with abdominal pain and vaginal bleeding. Unruptured ectopic pregnancy and ovarian torsion may present with vague hypogastric

pain and suprapubic tenderness. Once these conditions requiring the immediate attention of an obstetrician are ruled out, myofascial causes of abdominal pain should be considered.[5]

• The round ligaments stretch as the uterus rises in the abdomen. If the pull is too rapid, small hematomas may develop in the ligaments (Figure 41–1). This usually begins at 16–20 weeks of gestation, with pain and tenderness localized over the round ligament which radiates to the pubic tubercle. Treatment is bed rest and local warmth along with oral analgesics in more severe cases.

• Less common is abdominal pain arising from hematoma formation within the sheath of the rectus abdominis muscle (Figure 41–2). As the uterus expands, the muscles of the abdominal wall become greatly overstretched. Severe pain localized to a single segment of the muscle often follows a bout of sneezing. Diagnosis of rectus hematoma is made when localized pain is exacerbated by tightening the abdominal muscles (raising the head in the supine position). Ultrasonography can be helpful in confirming the diagnosis. Conservative management with bed rest, local heat, and mild analgesics is often all that is needed.

HIP PAIN

• Two relatively rare conditions, osteonecrosis and transient osteoporosis of the hip, occur with somewhat

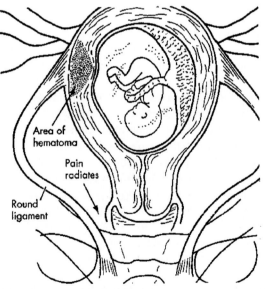

FIGURE 41–1 Abdominal pain arising from stretch and hematoma formation in the round ligament typically presents between 16 and 20 weeks of gestation with pain and tenderness over the round ligament that radiates to the pubic symphysis. Adapted with permission from Chamberlain.[4]

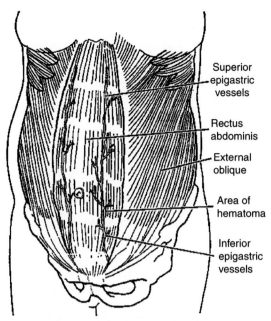

FIGURE 41–2 Stretch of the abdominal wall in pregnancy can lead to tearing of the rectus abdominis muscle or inferior epigastric veins and formation of a painful hematoma within the rectus sheath. Pain is well localized and can be severe, often starting after a bout of coughing or sneezing. Adapted with permission from Chamberlain.[4]

greater frequency during pregnancy. While the exact etiology is not known, high levels of estrogen and progesterone in the maternal circulation and increased interosseous pressure may contribute to the development of osteonecrosis.

- Transient osteoporosis of the hip is a rare disorder characterized by pain and limitation of motion of the hip and osteopenia of the femoral head. Both conditions present with hip pain during the third trimester, which may be either sudden or gradual in onset.
- Osteoporosis is easily identified, with plain radiography demonstrating osteopenia of the femoral head with preservation of the joint space. Osteonecrosis is best evaluated with MRI, which demonstrates changes before they appear on plain radiographs.
- Both conditions are managed symptomatically during pregnancy. Limited weight bearing is essential in transient osteoporosis of the hip to avoid fracture of the femoral neck.

POSTERIOR PELVIC PAIN

- The hormonal changes that occur during pregnancy lead to widening and increased mobility of the sacroiliac synchondroses and the symphysis pubis as early as the 10th to 12th weeks of pregnancy. This type of pain is described by a large group of pregnant

women and is located in the posterior part of the pelvis distal and lateral to the lumbosacral junction.
- Many terms have been used in the literature to describe this type of pain including "sacroiliac dysfunction," "pelvic girdle relaxation," and even "sacroiliac joint pain." The pain radiates to the posterior part of the thigh and may extend below the knee leading to misinterpretation as sciatica. The pain is less specific than sciatica in distribution and does not extend to the ankle or foot. Differentiating between back and posterior pelvic problems is a challenge.

BACK PAIN

- Back pain occurs at some time during pregnancy in about half of women and is so common that it is often looked on as a normal part of pregnancy. The lumbar lordosis becomes markedly accentuated during pregnancy and may contribute to the development of low back pain. Endocrine changes during pregnancy may also play a role in the development of back pain.[5]
- Although radicular symptoms often accompany low back pain during pregnancy, herniated nucleus pulposus (HNP) has an incidence of only 1:10,000. Pregnant women do not have an increased prevalence of lumbar intervertebral disc abnormalities. Direct pressure of the fetus on the lumbosacral nerves has been postulated as the cause of radicular symptoms.
- Back pain during pregnancy assumes one of three common patterns (Figure 41–3): pain localized to the sacroiliac area that increases as pregnancy progresses

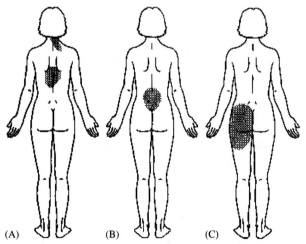

(A) (B) (C)

FIGURE 41–3 Three types of pain were reported by a group of 855 women studied between 12 menstrual weeks of pregnancy and delivery. Forty-nine percent of women reported back pain at some point during pregnancy: (A) high back pain by 10%; (B) low back pain by 40%; (C) sacroiliac pain by 50%. Adapted with permission, from Ostgaard.[6]

(also termed posterior pelvic pain) or pain localized to either the midthoracic area (high back) or the lumbar area (low back) that either decreases or does not change during the course of pregnancy. True sciatica with a dermatomal distribution occurs in only 1% of pregnant women.[6]

• Evaluation begins with a thorough history, which often points the clinician to other causes. Patients with both preterm labor and premature rupture of membranes may present with low back pain accompanied by uterine contractions and changes in the cervical os. Urologic disorders including hydronephrosis, pyelonephritis, and renal calculi may also present with low back discomfort. Major morphologic changes occur in the collecting system of pregnant women including dilation of the calices, renal pelves, and ureters.[7]

• Physical examination should include complete back and neurologic evaluations. Particular attention should be directed toward the pelvis and sacroiliac joints during examination. Posterior pelvic pain (sacroiliac dysfunction) can often be distinguished from other causes of low back pain based on physical examination. Positive straight leg raise (typical low back pain with or without radiation to the ipsilateral lower extremity) during physical examination is consistent with either sacroiliac subluxation or herniated nucleus pulposus. Unilateral loss of knee or ankle reflex or presence of sensory or motor deficit is suggestive of lumbar nerve root compression.

• Pregnancy is not an absolute contraindication to radiographic evaluation. No detectable growth or mental abnormalities have been associated with fetal exposure to less than 10 rad — the dose received during a typical three-view spinal series typically does not exceed 1.5 rad. Plain radiographs contribute vital information primarily when fracture, dislocation, and destructive lesions of the bone are suspected.

• MRI has revolutionized diagnostic imaging during pregnancy, proving effective and reliable in the diagnosis of both infections and neoplasms. Although MRI appears to be safe during pregnancy, there are no long-term studies examining the safety of fetal exposure to intense magnetic fields during gestation. Practical guidelines for use of radiographic studies in the evaluation of pregnant patients are given in Table 41–3.[8]

• Few of the commonly used strategies to prevent low back pain during pregnancy are universally effective. The American College of Obstetricians and Gynecologists recommends specific muscular conditioning exercises to promote good posture and prevent low back pain during pregnancy.

TABLE 41–3 Guidelines for Use of Neurodiagnostic Imaging in the Pregnant Patient*

• Determine the necessity of a radiologic examination and the risks involved.
• If possible, perform the examination only during the first 10 days postmenses or, if the patient is pregnant, delay the examination until the third trimester or preferably postpartum.
• Determine the most efficacious use of radiation for the problem.
• Use MRI if possible.
• Avoid direct exposure to the abdomen and pelvis.
• Avoid contrast agents.
• Do not avoid radiologic testing purely for the sake of pregnancy. Remember, you are responsible for providing the best possible care for the patient. The risk to the pregnant patient of not having an indicated radiologic examination is also an indirect risk to the fetus.
• If significant exposure is incurred by a pregnant patient, have a radiation biologist (usually stationed in the radiology department) review the radiology examination history carefully so that an accurate dose estimate can be ascertained.
• The decision to terminate pregnancy due to excessive radiation exposure is an extremely complex issue. Because any increased risk of malformations is considered to be negligible unless radiation doses exceed 0.1 to 0.15 Gy (10 to 15 rad), the amount of exposure that an embryo or fetus would likely receive from diagnostic procedures is well below the level for which a therapeutic abortion should be considered.
• Consent forms are neither required nor recommended. The patient should be informed verbally that any radiologic examinations ordered during pregnancy are considered necessary for her medical care. She should also be informed that the risks to the fetus from CT/plain films are very low and that there are no known risks to humans of MRI. Having the patient sign a consent increases the perceived risks and adds needlessly to her concerns during and after the examination.

*Adapted, with permission, from Schwartz, 1994.[8]

• Reassurance and simple changes in the patient's activity level often suffice to reduce symptoms to a tolerable level.

• If pain remains poorly controlled, referral to a physical therapist for evaluation and instruction in body mechanics and low back exercises may be beneficial. Aquatic exercise programs can be particularly helpful to the parturient and offer the added benefit of reducing the effects of gravity on the mother's musculoskeletal system. Massage and the surface application of heat or ice may also be useful.

• Mechanical support devices may help reduce symptoms of back pain and sacroiliac dysfunction. Widely available devices include a nonelastic trochanteric belt designed to support the abdomen and the use of a wedge-shaped pillow designed to support the abdomen of a pregnant woman while sleeping on her side.

• While the incidence of herniated nucleus pulposus during pregnancy is low, radicular symptoms are common and often accompany sacroiliac subluxation and myofascial pain syndromes. While the risk to the fetus following a single dose of epidural corticosteroid appears to be low, epidural steroids should be reserved for the parturient with the new onset of signs (unilateral loss of deep tendon reflex, sensory/motor change in a dermatomal distribution) and symptoms consistent with lumbar nerve root compression.

- Acetaminophen is the first analgesic to consider for management of minor back pain. While NSAIDs are the cornerstone of the pharmacologic management of back pain in nonpregnant individuals, their use during pregnancy remains controversial. Severe back pain may require treatment with narcotics and necessitate hospital admission for parenteral administration of opioid analgesics. Progressive ambulation over several days using the assistance and instruction of a skilled physical therapist is usually successful. Short courses of oral or parenteral opioids appear to add little risk to the fetus.

MIGRAINE HEADACHE DURING PREGNANCY

- Nearly 25% of women suffer from migraine headaches, with the peak incidence during childbearing years. Migraines occur more often during menstruation, which has been attributed to a sudden decline in estrogen levels. During pregnancy, a sustained 50- to 100-fold increase in estradiol occurs. Indeed, 70% of women report improvement or remission of migraines during pregnancy.[9]
- Migraine headaches rarely begin during pregnancy. Initial presentation of headaches during pregnancy should initiate a thorough search for potentially serious causes. The literature is replete with reports of intracranial pathology that mimicked migraines during pregnancy including strokes, pseudotumor cerebri, tumors, aneurysms, arteriovenous malformations, and cerebral venous thrombosis. Metabolic causes of headache during pregnancy include drug use, most notably, cocaine, anti-phospholipid antibody syndrome, and choriocarcinoma.
- Patients who present with their first severe headache during pregnancy should receive a complete neurologic examination and should be strongly considered for MRI, toxicology screen, and serum coagulation profiles. In the patient who presents with sudden onset of the "worst headache of my life," subarachnoid hemorrhage should be ruled out. Progressively worsening headaches in the setting of sudden weight gain should suggest preeclampsia or pseudotumor cerebri. The triad of elevated blood pressure, proteinuria, and peripheral edema points toward preeclampsia; hyperreflexia and elevated serum uric acid are also found in patients with preeclampsia.

- For those pregnant women with a history of migraines prior to pregnancy and a normal neurologic examination, the therapeutic challenge is to achieve control of the headaches while minimizing risk to the fetus. Nonpharmacologic techniques, including relaxation, biofeedback, and elimination of certain foods, often suffice for treatment.
- If pharmacologic therapy appears warranted, acetaminophen with or without caffeine is safe and effective. The short-term use of mild opioid analgesics like hydrocodone, alone or in combination with acetaminophen, also appears to carry little risk. When oral analgesics prove ineffective, hospital admission and administration of parenteral opioids may be required.

CONCLUSION

- Many physicians find themselves apprehensive about treating pain in pregnant patients. Evaluation and treatment are limited by the relative contraindication of radiography in the workup and the risks associated with pharmacologic therapy during pregnancy.
- Familiarity with common pain problems as well as the maternal and fetal risks of pain medications can allow the pain practitioner to help women achieve a more comfortable pregnancy.
- A single health care provider should be designated to coordinate specialist evaluations and integrate their suggestions into a single, integrated plan of care.

REFERENCES

1. American Academy of Pediatrics Committee on Drugs. The transfer of drugs and other chemicals into human milk. *Pediatrics.* 1994;93:137–150.
2. **Briggs GG, Freeman RK, Yaffe SJ.** *Drugs in Pregnancy and Lactation.* Baltimore: Williams & Wilkins; 1990.
3. **Niebyl JR.** Nonanesthetic drugs during pregnancy and lactation. In: Chestnut DH, ed. *Obstetric Anesthesia: Principles and Practice.* St. Louis: Mosby; 1994:229–240.
4. **Chamberlain G.** ABC of antenatal care: Abdominal pain in pregnancy. *BMJ.* 1991;302:1390.
5. **MacEvilly M, Buggy D.** Back pain and pregnancy: A review. *Pain* 1996;64:405–414.
6. **Ostgaard HC, Andersson GBJ, Karlsson K.** Prevalence of back pain in pregnancy. *Spine.* 1991;16:549.
7. **Rungee JL.** Low back pain during pregnancy. *Orthopedics.* 1993;16:1339–1344.
8. **Schwartz RB.** Neurodiagnostic imaging of the pregnant patient. In: Devinsky O, Feldmann E, Mainline B, eds. *Neurological Complications of Pregnancy.* New York: Raven Press; 1994:243–248.

9. **Silverstein SD.** Headaches and women: Treatment of the pregnant and lactating migraineur. *Headache.* 1993;33: 533–540.

FURTHER READING

Rathmell JP, Viscomi CM, Ashburn MA. Acute and chronic pain management in the pregnant patient. *Anesth Analg.* 1997;85:1074–1087.

Rathmell JP, Viscomi CM, Bernstein IM. Pain management during pregnancy and lactation. In: Raj PP, ed. *Practical Management of Pain.* 3rd ed. St. Louis: Mosby Year Book; 2000:196–211.

42   SICKLE CELL ANEMIA

Richard Payne, MD

INTRODUCTION

- Sickle cell anemia was identified in the United States in 1910 by Herrick, who observed sickle-shaped red blood cells (RBCs) in an anemic black medical student in Chicago.[1]
- Sickle cell anemia is an inherited autosomal dominant disorder, resulting from a single amino acid substitution in which valine replaces glutamic acid.[2] The sickled morphology occurs when RBCs are placed in an environment of decreased oxygen tension.[3–7]
- Fetal hemoglobin (HbF; the β-globin chain in adult hemoglobin is replaced by a γ chain) persists into the first months of life and inhibits blood from sickling when it constitutes >20% of the total hemoglobin.[8]
- Hydroxyurea, which increases the production of HbF, is reserved for patients with severe disease and, compared with placebo, reduces the number of (1) vaso-occlusive crisis (VOC) episodes (including the time to first and second VOC), (2) acute chest syndromes, and (3) transfusions.[9]

CLINICAL MANIFESTATIONS OF DISEASE

- Pain is a cardinal feature of sickle cell disease; however, the timing, severity, and frequency of painful episodes vary greatly.

- In general, approximately 20% of patients have pain rarely; 60% have one or two episodes each year, and 20% have more than two episodes per month and are considered severely affected.[10]
- The classic VOC is a relatively unpredictable ischemic event that occurs when rigid sickled cells obstruct blood vessels. Table 42–1 lists the factors that influence the frequency of VOCs.
- Pain can be severe and is usually present in the bone, chest, and abdomen.
- Children may experience sickle cell dactylitis, most likely caused when avascular necrosis of the marrow produces swelling in the dorsal surfaces of the hands and feet. Repetitive splenic infarction in children produces recurrent abdominal pain and, eventually, an autosplenectomy.
- Other manifestations of the disease include aplastic and megaloblastic crises, sequestration crises (ie, sudden massive pooling of RBCs, especially in the spleen), hemolytic crises, osteomyelitis (especially *Salmonella typhimurium*), priapism, renal failure, jaundice and hepatomegaly, ischemic leg ulceration, stroke, and a host of other ischemic manifestations in every organ.[11]
- The acute chest syndrome, an important variant of VOC, manifests as chest pain, with or without fever, in association with a pulmonary infiltrate.
- The acute chest syndrome may be caused by lung infarction or rib infarction with associated pleuritis and chest splinting and is associated with a higher mortality than other forms of VOC, particularly in children placed on intravenous opioid infusions who are not carefully monitored.[12,13]
- The most common causes of death for sickle cell patients are listed in Table 42–2.[14]
- Appropriate management of the acute chest syndrome includes the judicious use of opioids and aggressive respiratory treatments, especially the use of incentive spirometry.

TABLE 42–1   Factors Influencing the Frequency of Vaso-occlusive Crises

Increase frequency
• Cold weather
• Young adult males (15–25 years old)
• Pregnancy (especially third trimester)
Decrease frequency
• Presence of α-thalassemia
• Elevated HbF levels (>30% total hemoglobin)
• RBC membrane polymorphisms (inhibit aggregation to vascular endothelium)

TABLE 42–2 Causes of Death in Patients with Sickle Cell Anemia

Causes of death

- Pulmonary fat embolism
- Acute multi-organ system failure
- Acute chest syndrome
- Renal failure
- Seizures

Factors associated with risk of early death

- Persistent leukocytosis
- Depressed HbF levels

"ROUTINE" MANAGEMENT OF VASO-OCCLUSIVE CRISES

- Standard treatment approaches to the management of a VOC episode include intravenous hydration, oxygen inhalation, and parenteral analgesics (opioids and nonopioids).
- Some experts assert that routine intravenous hydration is unnecessary in the absence of clinically apparent dehydration.
- The use of oxygen therapy is even more controversial: in a controlled clinical trial in which patients were randomized to inhalation of 50% oxygen or room air, the duration of severe pain, the consumption of analgesics, and the length of hospitalization did not differ, even though the oxygen-treated group had a reduction in reversibly sickled cells.[15]

GUIDELINES FOR ANALGESIC USE

- Tables 42–3 and 42–4 summarize information on the use of analgesics. The principles of pharmacologic management of acute and chronic sickle cell pain are similar to those for the management of pain in any group of patients with a serious, potentially life-limiting medical disorder.[16,17]
- Bone pain is a particularly prominent feature of VOC and other forms of sickle cell pain; therefore, nonselective and COX-2-selective nonsteroidal anti-inflammatory drugs (NSAIDs) are used commonly as single agents or in combination with other analgesics, especially opioids (Tables 42–3 and 42–4).
- Although widely used, meperidine is associated with signs of central nervous system excitability, including seizures, related to accumulation of the normeperidine metabolite. Given the effects of sickle cell disease on kidney function, these patients are vulnerable to this toxic effect of meperidine, which should not

be a first-line opioid for the treatment of acute or chronic pain.
- Emergency department guidelines for the treatment of sickle cell pain emphasize the need to evaluate patients quickly to assess and treat infections and treat pain aggressively. Some institutions have established day treatment hospitals for sickle cell patients so that pain management can be achieved efficiently by a group of clinicians who know the patient best.

SUBSTANCE ABUSE CONCERNS

- The prevalence of substance abuse disorders in sickle cell patients appears to be grossly exaggerated, especially if one considers iatrogenic substance abuse.[18]
- One study demonstrated that hematologists and emergency department physicians estimated that approximately 25% of adult sickle cell patients are addicted to illegal substances, when the published prevalence of addiction is actually much lower[19]: no addiction found in 600 adults[16]; "addiction" in 3 and "dependence" in 7 of 101 patients[17]; and drug abuse "suspected" in 9 and "definite" in 5 of 114.[18]
- The term *pseudo-addiction* has been used to describe drug-seeking behavior in patients who are provoked by inadequate control of pain.[20] Sickle cell patients are at great risk for displaying "pseudo-addiction" behavior when their pain is inadequately controlled.

TABLE 42–3 Some Nonselective and COX-2-Selective NSAIDs Used to Manage Sickle Cell Pain

DRUG TYPE	NAME/BRAND	TYPICAL STARTING DOSE
Acetaminophen	Tylenol and others	650 mg q4h PO
Aspirin	Multiple	650 mg q4h PO
Ibuprofen	Motrin and others	200–800 mg q6h PO
Choline–magnesium trisalicylate	Trilisate	1000–1500 mg tid PO
Diclofenac sodium	Voltaren	50–75 mg q8-12 PO
Naproxen	Naprosyn	250–750 mg q12h PO
Naproxen sodium	Anaprox	275 mg q12h PO
Meloxicam	Mobic	7.5 mg PO daily
Ketorolac	Toradol	10 mg q4–6h PO (not to exceed 10 d)
Ketorolac		60 mg (initial), then 30 mg q6h IV or IM (not to exceed 5 d)
Celecoxib*	Celebrex	200 mg bid
Rofecoxib*	Vioxx	25 mg daily PO
Valdecoxib*	Bextra	20 mg PO daily

*Selective for COX-2 isoenzyme.

TABLE 42–4   Commonly Used Opioids for Moderate-to-Severe Pain

	USUAL STARTING DOSE	COMMENT
WHO STEP I/II OPIOIDS		
Codeine (with aspirin or acetaminophen)	60 mg q3–4h PO	• Fixed combination with aspirin or acetaminophen=DEA schedule III; single entity=DEA II.
Tylenol #2 (15 mg codeine)		• Usually 250-mg aspirin or acetaminophen/tablet
Tylenol #3 (30 mg codeine)		• Take care not to reach toxic doses of aspirin and acetaminophen
Tylenol #4 (60 mg codeine)		
Hydrocodone (with aspirin or acetaminophen)	10 mg q3–4h PO	• Same as for codeine
		• Vicodin Extra Strength has 750-mg acetaminophen/tablet
Lorcet, Lortab, Vicodin, etc		
Oxycodone	10 mg q3–4h PO	• Available in controlled-release formulation (as single entity)
Roxicodone (single entity)		
Percocet, Percodan, Tylox, etc		
Tramadol	50 mg qid PO	• Although a μ-opioid agonist, it is not scheduled as an opioid
Ultram (single entity)		• Also blocks catecholamine reuptake
Ultracet (tramadol +ibuprofen)		• Nausea common side effect
		• Seizures may occur in doses >400 mg/d
WHO STEP II/III OPIOIDS		
Morphine	30 mg q3–4h PO	• Standard by which all other opioids are compared
Immediate release (MSIR)	10 mg q3–4h IV	• MSIR is preferred rescue analgesic for controlled-release preparations
Sustained release (MS Contin, Oramorph, Kadian, Avinza)	30 mg q12h PO	• Some clinicians do not view MS Contin and Oramorph as therapeutically interchangeable
		• MS Contin available in 15-, 30-, 60-, 100-, and 200-mg tablets.
		• Oramorph available in 15-, 30-, 60-, and 100-mg tablets only
		• Morphine also available as suppository
OxyContin		• Twice as potent as morphine
		• Available in 10-, 20-, and 40-mg tablets; imediate-release oxycodone also considered step II/III opioid and recommended as rescue medicine for OxyContin
Hydromorphone	20 mg q12h PO	• Sustained-release formulation in clinical development
Dilaudid, others	6 mg q12h PO	• Available in 2-, 4-, and 8-mg tablets
		• Available as suppository
Fentanyl	50 μg/h q72h	• Only opioid available for transdermal administration
Duragesic (transdermal)	50 μ/h via continuous infusion	• Potency relative to morphine close to 100:1
Sublimaze, others		• Many patients require oral rescue doses
Methadone	20 mg q6–8h PO	• Very stigmatized because of use to treat heroin addiction
Dolophine, others	10 mg q6–8h IV	
Levorphanol	4 mg q6–8h PO	• Relatively long-acting
Levo-Dromoran opioid		• Incidence of psychotomimetic effects may be higher than with other opioids

REFERENCES

1. **Herrick JB.** Peculiar elongated and sickle-shaped red corpuscles in a case of severe anemia. *Arch Intern Med.* 1910;6:517.

2. **Taliaferro WH, Huck JG.** The inheritance of sickle-cell anemia in man. *Genetics.* 1923;8:594.

3. **Ingram VM.** Gene mutations in human hemoglobin: The chemical difference between normal and sickle cell haemoglobin. *Nature.* 1957;180:326.

4. **Conley CL.** Sickle-cell anemia: The first molecular disease. In: Wintrobe MM, ed. *Blood, Pure and Eloquent.* New York: McGraw-Hill; 1980:319.

5. **Beutler E.** The sickle cell disease and related disorders. In: Beutler E, Lictman MA, Coller BS, Kipps TJ, eds. *Williams' Hematology.* 5th ed. New York: McGraw-Hill; 1995:616.

6. **Embury SH, Dozy AM, Miller J, et al.** Concurrent sickle-cell anemia and alpha-thalassemia: Effect on severity of anemia. *N Engl J Med.* 1982;306:270.

7. **Stevens MCG, Padwick M, Serjeant GR.** Observations on the natural history of dactylitis in homozygous sickle cell disease. *Clin Pediatr.* 1981;20:311.

8. **Noguchi CT, Rodger GP, Serjeant G, et al.** Levels of fetal hemoglobin necessary for treatment of sickle cell disease. *N Engl J Med.* 1988;318:96.

9. **Charache S, Terrin ML, Moore RD, et al.** Effect of hydroxyurea on the frequency of painful crises in sickle cell anemia. *N Engl J Med.* 1995;332:1317.

10. **Ballas SK, Delengowski A.** Pain measurement in hospitalized adults with sickle cell painful episodes. *Ann Clin Lab Sci.* 1993;23:358.

11. **Baum KF, Dunn DT, Maude GH, et al.** The painful crises of homozygous sickle cell disease: A study of risk factors. *Arch Intern Med.* 1987;147:1231.

12. **Rucknagel DL, Kalinyak KA, Gelfand MJ.** Rib infarcts and acute chest syndrome in sickle cell diseases. *Lancet.* 1991;337:831.

13. **Cole TB, Spinkle RK, Smith SJ, et al.** Intravenous narcotic therapy for children with severe sickle cell pain crises. *Am J Child.* 1986;140:1255.

14. **Platt OS, Brambilla DJ, Rosse WF, et al.** Mortality in sickle cell disease: Life expectancy and risk factors for early death. *N Engl J Med.* 1994;330:1639.
15. **Zipursky A, Robieux IC, Brown, EJ, et al.** Oxygen therapy in sickle cell disease. *Am J Pediatr Hematol Oncol.* 1992;14:222.
16. **Brozovic M, Davies SC, Yardumian A, et al.** Pain relief in sickle cell crisis. *Lancet.* 1986;2:624.
17. **Vichinsky EP, Johnson PR, Lubin RB.** Multidisciplinary approach to pain management in sickle cell disease. *Am J Pediatr Hematol Oncol.* 1982;4:328.
18. **Portenoy RK, Payne R.** Acute and chronic pain. In: Lowinson JH, Ruiz P, Millman RB, Langrod JG, eds. *Substance Abuse: A Comprehensive Textbook.* Baltimore: Williams & Wilkins; 1992:691.
19. **Shapiro BS, Benjamin LJ, Payne R, et al.** Sickle cell-related pain: Perceptions of medical practitioners. *J Pain Symptom Manage.* 1997;14:168.
20. **Weissman DE, Haddox JD.** Opioid pseudo-addiction: An iatrogenic syndrome. *Pain.* 1989;36:363.

43 SPASTICITY

R. Samuel Mayer, MD

DEFINITIONS AND DIFFERENTIAL DIAGNOSIS

- Muscle tone is "the sensation felt as one manipulates a joint through a range of motion, with the subject attempting to relax."[1] Abnormalities of muscle tone are often painful. Differentiation of various forms of abnormal muscle tone is critical because the etiology and, therefore, the treatment of each differ.
- Spasticity has been defined as a "motor disorder characterized by a velocity-dependent increase in tonic stretch reflexes (muscle tone) with exaggerated tendon jerks, resulting from the hyperexcitability of the stretch reflex, as one component of the upper motor neuron syndrome."[2] Spasticity is associated with damage to the spinal cord or the corticospinal tracts in the brain.
- Rigidity "has an even or uniform quality throughout the range of motion, like that noted in bending a lead pipe or pulling a strand of toffee. When released, the limb does not assume its original position, as happens in spasticity."[3] Rigidity is associated with lesions of extrapyramidal tracts of the brain, especially in the basal ganglia.
- Muscle cramp occurs when "a random restless stretching movement [induces] a hard contraction of a single muscle which cannot be voluntarily relaxed."[3]
- Tetany, a sustained muscle contraction elicited by minimal stimulation, has a characteristic appearance on electromyography with fast-frequency doublets and triplets. Tetany results from muscle membrane abnormalities such as hypocalcemia.
- States of persistent fasciculation occur in "stiff-man" syndrome and amyotrophic lateral sclerosis.
- Dystonia is a focal, continuous, muscular contracture of the neck (torticollis) or limb muscles (eg, writer's cramp). Its pathophysiology is poorly understood.

EVALUATION

- Evaluation of the patient with spasticity requires an interdisciplinary approach, as mere physical examination provides inadequate information on which to base management.
- Team members often include:
  ○ Physiatrist
  ○ Neurologist
  ○ Physical and occupational therapists
  ○ Orthopedic surgeon
  ○ Neurosurgeon
  ○ Anesthesiologist
  ○ Psychologist
- Increased muscle tone, particularly extensor tone, often helps patients with standing and ambulation.
- The role that tone plays in either impeding or facilitating functional activities must be fully assessed.[4]
- It is critical to observe the patient performing functional activities, such as bed *and* wheelchair transfers.

HISTORY

- Important questions include:
  ○ Do the spasms cause pain?
  ○ Do the spasms inhibit sleep?
  ○ Does the muscle tone interfere with activities of daily living?
  ○ Does the muscle tone aid in standing?
  ○ Do muscle contractures cause poor hygiene or skin breakdown?
  ○ How does muscle tone vary with position?
  ○ Is the spasticity localized or generalized?
  ○ How long has the patient had this condition?

QUANTIFICATION

- Modified Ashworth Scale[5] (Table 43–1)
- Range of motion
- Muscle stretch reflexes and clonus[6]
- Gait analysis
- Electrodiagnostic studies (H-reflex)[7]
- Viscoelastic measurements[8]

TABLE 43–1   Modified Ashworth Scale

1	Minimal increase in tone
1a	Minimal increase in tone with catch
2	Moderate increase in tone
3	Limited range of motion
4	Rigid contracture

TREATMENT PARADIGM

- Management of abnormal muscle tone relies on several factors from the evaluation.
  ○ Etiology (brain vs spinal cord, corticospinal vs extrapyramidal tracts)
  ○ Generalized versus localized involvement
  ○ Duration of symptoms and course of disease process
  ○ Goal of treatment (pain, functional use or restoration of range of motion)

PHYSICAL MODALITIES

- The first line of treatment always involves the use of physical modalities to control tone.
- Range-of-motion exercises prevent contractures but do not increase range of motion.
- Serial casting or dynamic splinting is required to relieve contractures that have already occurred.[9]
- Ultrasound enhances the effectiveness of tendon stretching.
- Ice can relieve acute muscle spasm.[10]
- Positioning can reduce muscle tone.

ORAL MEDICATIONS

- Table 43–2 outlines commonly used medications.
- Side effects often limit the usefulness of oral medications.
- In most cases, the use of oral medications should be reserved to treat generalized disorders.
- The choice of medication depends largely on the etiology of abnormal muscle tone.

INTRATHECAL MEDICATIONS

- Baclofen is the primary intrathecal medication in clinical use for spasticity.
- Baclofen is delivered by a pump implanted in an abdominal pocket, which connects via tubing to the intrathecal space.
- The baclofen enters the central nervous system directly, allowing for much smaller doses and minimizing side effects, such as sedation. The drug effect is, therefore, maximized.[11,12]

INTRATHECAL TRIALS

- Most patients should receive trial dosing of intrathecal baclofen prior to pump placement.
- A bolus trial involves injecting a single dose of baclofen and monitoring the patient's response for the next 6 hours. Dosing generally starts at 50 μg, with a 25-μg increase on subsequent days should the initial dose be ineffective.
- Catheter trials involve the dosing of medication through an externalized pump for several days to monitor effectiveness. Such trials are particularly useful in patients whose response may be less predictable (eg, dystonic cerebral palsy or ambulatory multiple sclerosis patients).

INTRATHECAL BACLOFEN COMPLICATIONS

- Underdosing can cause hypertonicity, pruritus, and/or withdrawal seizures.
- Overdosing can cause somnolence, hypotonia, respiratory depression, and/or seizures.
- Catheter complications (approximately 5% lifetime incidence) include kinks, disconnections, and iatrogenic holes.
- Pump failure is usually due to depleted battery life (approximately 5 years), rarely from mechanical problems. There is an automated low-battery alarm.
- Infection in the abdominal pocket is rare, and meningoencephalitis is very rare.

TABLE 43–2   Oral Medications

DRUG	INDICATION	ACTION	SIDE EFFECTS
Baclofen	Spinal spasticity	GABA agonist	Sedation, weakness, seizure
Dantrolene	Brain or spinal spasticity	Muscle Ca^{2+} channels	Weakness, liver toxicity
Tizanidine	Brain or spinal spasticity	α agonist	Orthostasis, sedation, dry mouth
Diazepam	Brain or spinal spasticity	GABA stimulation	Sedation, tolerance/addiction
Sinemet	Rigidity	Dopaminergic	Orthostasis, hallucinations, dyskinesias
Cyclobenzaprine	Myalgia	Tricyclic antidepressant	Orthostasis, dry mouth, sedation, atrioventricular block
Methocarbamol	Myalgia	Interneuronal blockade	Sedation, tolerance/addiction

INTRATHECAL DOSING

- Intrathecal doses range widely from 50 to 1500 μg/d and are highly individualized, so an experienced clinician should be monitoring.
- Dosing can be single daily bolus, simple continuous, or complex continuous (in which higher doses are given during times of the day when tone is worse).
- The pump is refilled every 1–4 months depending on dosing.

INJECTIONS

- Injections are first-line therapy for localized abnormalities of muscle tone,[13] and are notably effective for focal dystonias.[14]
- Botulinum toxins A and B are commercially available in the United States. The cost is approximately $400 per dose for average size muscles. Botulinum toxins can be injected by anatomic localization into larger superficial muscles but require electrodiagnostic guidance for smaller, deeper muscles.
- Phenol and ethanol are relatively easy to prepare for hospital and custom pharmacies and cost less than $50 per dose. These injections require electrodiagnostic localization to maximize effect and minimize complications (dysesthesia from injecting mixed motor/sensory nerves).

INJECTION TECHNIQUE

- Table 43–3 designates muscle groups, which should be injected for common patterns of spastic deformity.
- There are two methods of electrodiagnostic localization of muscles:
  - Electromyographic localization with a Myoject needle is used for larger superficial muscles with active voluntary movement. Endplate noise or motor unit potentials are identified.[15]
  - Motor point blocks are performed by using minimal electrical stimulation through the needle and observing muscle twitch when the needle is near the neuromuscular junction. This can be used for muscles without voluntary movement or muscles that are small or deep.[16]

ORTHOPEDIC SURGERY

- Tendon releases for intractable contractures require control of spasticity to prevent recurrence.[17]
- Tendon transfers can improve function for certain joint movements (eg, ankle dorsiflexion, wrist extension).

NEUROSURGERY

- Dorsal rhizotomy can be very effective in children with spastic cerebral palsy. It is not commonly performed in adults.[18]
- Surgical treatment of Parkinson's disease and other extrapyramidal disorders is beyond the scope of this chapter.

TABLE 43–3   Muscle Groups Involved in Patterns of Spastic Deformity

DEFORMITY	MUSCLES INVOLVED
Shoulder adduction/internal rotation	Pectoralis major, subscapularis
Elbow flexion/pronation	Brachialis, pronator teres
Clenched fist	Flexor digitorum superficialis/profundus, flexor pollicis longus, flexor carpi radialis
Hip adduction	Adductor magnus/longus
Knee flexion	Semitendinosus, semimembranosus, biceps femoris
Equinovarus	Gastrocnemius, soleus, tibialis posterior

REFERENCES

1. **Lance JW, McLeod JG.** Disordered muscle tone. In: *Physiological Approach to Clinical Neurology.* Boston: Butterworth; 1981.
2. **Lance JW.** Symposium synopsis. In: Feldman RG, Young RR, Koella WP, eds. *Spasticity: Disordered Muscle Control.* Chicago: Year Book Medical; 1980.
3. **Adams RD, Victor M.** *Principles of Neurology.* 5th ed. New York: McGraw-Hill; 1993.
4. **Katz RT, Dewald JPA, Schmitt BD.** Spasticity. In: Braddom RL, et al, eds. *Physical Medicine and Rehabilitation.* 2nd ed. Philadelphia: WB Saunders; 2000.
5. **Bohanon RW, Smith MB.** Interrater reliability on a modified Ashworth scale of muscle spasticity. *Phys Ther.* 1987;67:206.
6. **Ada L, Vattanaslip W, O'Dwyer NJ, et al.** Does spasticity contribute to walking dysfunction after stroke? *J Neurol Neurosurg Psychiatry.* 1998;64:628.
7. **Katz RT.** Electrophysiologic quantification of spastic hypertonia. In: Katz RT, ed. *Spasticity. State of the Art Reviews in Physical Medicine and Rehabilitation.* Vol. 8. Philadelphia: Hanley & Belfus; 1994.
8. **Lehman JF, Price R, deLateur B, et al.** Spasticity: Quantitative measurements as a basis for assessing effectiveness of therapeutic intervention. *Arch Phys Med Rehabil.* 1989;70:6.

9. **Booth BJ, Doyle M, Montgomery J.** Serial casting for the management of spasticity in the head-injured adult. *Phys Ther.* 1983;63:1960.

10. **Price R, Lehman JF, Boswell-Bessette S, et al.** Influence of cryotherapy on spasticity at the human ankle. *Arch Phys Med Rehabil.* 1993;74:300.

11. **Penn RD, Savoy SM, Corcos D, et al.** Intrathecal baclofen for severe spinal spasticity. *N Engl J Med.* 1989;320:1517.

12. **Parke B, Penn RD, Savoy SM, et al.** Functional outcome after delivery of intrathecal baclofen. *Arch Phys Med Rehabil.* 1989;70:30.

13. **Robinson LR, Wang L.** Botulinum toxin injections. *Phys Med Rehabil Clin North Am.* 1995;6:897.

14. **NIH Consensus Development Conference Statement.** Clinical use of botulinum toxin. *Arch Neurol.* 1991;48:1294.

15. **Barbano RL.** EMG guidance for injection of botulinum toxin: Needle EMG guidance is useful. *Muscle Nerve.* 2001;24:1567.

16. **Khalili AA, Betts HB.** Peripheral nerve block with phenol in the management of spasticity: Indications and complications. *JAMA.* 1967;200:1155.

17. **Pinzur MS.** Surgical correction of lower extremity problems in patients with brain injury. *J Head Trauma Rehabil.* 1987;2:34.

18. **McDonald CM.** Selective dorsal rhizotomy: A critical review. *Phys Med Rehabil Clin North Am.* 1991;2:891.

44   SUBSTANCE ABUSE

Steven D. Passik, PhD
Kenneth L. Kirsh, PhD

INTRODUCTION

- Approximately one-third of the US population have used illicit drugs, and an estimated 6–15% have a substance use disorder.[1–3]
- In diverse patient populations with chronic pain issues, a history of drug abuse presents a constellation of stigmatizing physical and psychosocial issues that can complicate the management of the underlying disease and undermine therapies.
- The interface between the therapeutic use of potentially abusable drugs and the abuse of these drugs is complex and must be understood to optimize pain management.
- Additional studies are needed to clarify the epidemiology of substance abuse and addiction in chronic pain patients.
- Chronic pain patients can be adequately and successfully treated only when addiction problems are noted

by staff, and these patients' special needs are addressed.[4]

DEFINITION OF ADDICTION IN CHRONIC PAIN

- Definitions of addiction that include phenomena related to physical dependence or tolerance cannot be the model terminology for medically ill populations who receive potentially abusable drugs for legitimate medical purposes.
- A more appropriate definition of addiction notes that it is a chronic disorder characterized by "the compulsive use of a substance resulting in physical, psychological or social harm to the user and continued use despite that harm."[5]
- Any appropriate definition of addiction must include the concepts of loss of control over drug use, compulsive drug use, and continued use despite harm.
- The concept of "aberrant drug-related behavior" is a useful component of definitions of abuse and addiction and recognizes the broad range of behavior that may be considered problematic by prescribers.
- If drug-taking behavior in a medical patient can be characterized as aberrant, a "differential diagnosis" for this behavior can be explored (see Table 44–1).

PSYCHIATRIC COMPLICATIONS

- Impulsive drug use may indicate the existence of another psychiatric disorder, diagnosis of which may have therapeutic implications.
- Patients with borderline personality disorder can express fear and rage through aberrant drug taking and may behave impulsively and self-destructively during pain therapy. One of the more worrisome aberrant drug-related behaviors, forging a prescription for a controlled substance, can be an impulsive expression of fear of abandonment and may have little to do with true substance abuse in a borderline patient.[6]

TABLE 44–1 Differential Diagnosis of Aberrant Drug-Taking Attitudes and Behavior

Addiction
Pseudoaddiction (inadequate analgesic)
Other psychiatric diagnoses
    Encephalopathy
    Borderline personality disorder
    Depression
    Anxiety
Criminal intent

- Patients who self-medicate for anxiety, panic, depression, or even periodic dysphoria and loneliness can present as aberrant drug takers.
- Careful diagnosis and treatment of psychiatric problems can at times obviate the need for such self-medication with opioids.

DETERMINING ABERRANCY OF BEHAVIOR

- In assessing the differential diagnosis for drug-related behavior, it is useful to consider the degree of aberrancy (see Table 44–2).
- The less aberrant behaviors (such as aggressively complaining about the need for medications) are more likely to reflect untreated distress of some type, rather than addiction-related concerns.
- Highly aberrant behaviors (such as injection of an oral formulation) are more likely to reflect true addiction. Although empirical studies are needed to validate this conceptualization, it may be a useful model when evaluating aberrant behavior.

NEED FOR A TAILORED APPROACH

- The differential between patients with no history of substance abuse and those who are prior addicts, as well as all the gradations between, has created a need for tailoring chronic pain management to the patient.
- To this end, we offer an oversimplified three-level conceptualization of prototypical patients and the amount of follow-up necessary for each (see Table 44–3). These caricatures should be used to create mental prototypes that are useful in the assessment of chronic pain patients.

TABLE 44–2 Examples of Behaviors Indicative of Aberrancy at Both Ends of the Continuum

BEHAVIORS _LESS_ INDICATIVE OF ABERRANCY	BEHAVIORS _MORE_ INDICATIVE OF ABERRANCY
Drug hoarding during periods of reduced symptoms	Prescription forgery
Acquisition of similar drugs from other medical sources	Concurrent abuse of related illicit drugs
Aggressive complaining about the need for higher doses	Recurrent prescription losses
Unapproved use of the drug to treat another symptom	Selling prescription drugs
Unsanctioned dose escalation one or two times	Multiple unsanctioned dose escalations
Reporting psychic effects not intended by the clinician	Stealing or borrowing another patient's drugs
Requesting specific drugs	Obtaining prescription drugs from nonmedical sources

TABLE 44–3 Three-Level Conceptualization of Prototypical Patients and the Corresponding Level of Care and Follow-up Needed for Chronic Pain Management

PROTOTYPE PATIENT	REQUIREMENTS FOR CARE
"Nice little old lady" (uncomplicated patient)	Minimal structure required due to lack of comorbid psychiatric problems and lack of connection to drug subculture
	Routine medical management generally sufficient
	Suggested practice includes 30-day supply of medications with liberal rescue dose policy
	Monthly follow-ups
"The chemical coper"	Behavior resembles that of addicts with a central focus on obtaining drugs
	Needs structure, psychiatric input, and drug treatments that decentralize the pain medication from their coping
	Decentralize meaning: reduce the meaning of medications, undo conditioning, and undo drug-related socialization
	Best accomplished via use of pain-related psychotherapy
"Addicted patient"	Requires the most structure including frequent visits
Active abuser	Give patient a limited supply of medications
Patient in drug-free recovery	Drug choices should be tailored for long-acting opioids with little street value
Patient in methadone maintenance	Rescues offered judiciously
	Implement use of urine toxicology screening and follow-up on results
	Require patient to be in active recovery programs or psychotherapy

ASSESSMENT: THE 4 As APPROACH

- The 4 As (analgesia, activities of daily living, adverse events, and aberrant drug-taking behaviors) are the clinical domains that reflect progress toward pain management and the goal of a full and rewarding life (see Table 44–4).[7]

ANALGESIA
- Analgesia is not necessarily the most important outcome of pain management.
- An alternate view is how much relief it takes for patients to feel that their life is meaningfully changed so they can work toward the attainment of their goals.

ACTIVITIES OF DAILY LIVING
- "Activities of daily living" refers to quality-of-life issues and functionality.
- Patients must understand that they must comply with all of their recommended treatment options so that they are better able to return to work and to avocations and social activities.

TABLE 44–4   The 4 As of Outcome of Pain Management

OUTCOME AREA	EXPLANATION
Analgesia	This refers to the actual amount of relief experienced by the chosen opioid therapy The most obvious A, but it should not be considered the only important part of opioid therapy
Activities of daily living	This refers to whether or not the patient on opioid therapy has become more active as a result of opioid therapy The domains of interest include physical, social, emotional, and family functioning as well as improved sleep
Adverse side effects	This refers to finding out whether or not the opioid therapy chosen has intolerable side effects for the patient Typical adverse effects to screen for include constipation, nausea, sedation, and mental clouding
Aberrant drug-related behaviors	This may be better referred to as "ambiguous noncompliance behaviors" In essence, this refers to whether or not the patient is engaging in socially undesirable behaviors with the opioid therapy that may or may not be indicative of addiction Problem behaviors include self-escalating dose, hoarding medications, seeking out multiple providers for prescriptions, prescription forgery, and stealing prescription drugs

ADVERSE EVENTS

- Patients must also be made aware of the adverse side effects inherent in the treatment of their pain condition with opioids and other medications.
- Side effects must be aggressively managed so that they do not overshadow the potential benefits of drug therapy.
- The most common side effects of opioid analgesics include constipation, sedation, nausea and vomiting, dry mouth, respiratory depression, confusion, urinary retention, and itching.

ABERRANT DRUG-TAKING BEHAVIOR

- Patients must be educated through contracts, or other means, about the parameters of acceptable drug taking.
- Even overall good outcome in every other domain might not constitute satisfactory treatment if the patient is not compliant with the contract in worrisome ways.
- Dispensing pain medicine in a highly structured fashion may become necessary for some patients who are in violation or constantly on the fringes of appropriate drug taking.

OPTIMIZING DRUG THERAPY FOR SUBSTANCE ABUSERS WITH PAIN

- Optimal drug therapy for substance abusers with pain first employs the basic principles of good pain treatment with consideration of the unique pharmacologic needs of addicts and then adds the psychosocial, recovery, and additional structures necessary to attempt to maximize the likelihood of a good outcome (see Figure 44–1).
- Substance abusers are complex patients with two distinct diseases. Treatment of one with the assumption that it is most important and will "take care" of the other is a common mistake that results in additional suffering for the patient from either or both illnesses.
- Good opioid pain treatment in any patient follows two key rules:
  - The clinician must maintain an accepting and thoughtful attitude toward self-reports of pain.
  - The decision to use an opioid must be followed by skill in titration that focuses on balancing analgesia and side effects.

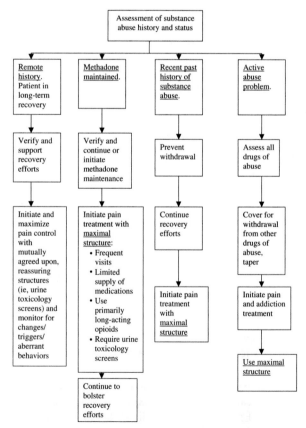

FIGURE 44–1 Flowchart of optimal pain management for chronic pain patients with substance abuse issues.

- Connecting with the patient and forming a therapeutic bond can often improve the reliability of self-report if trust can be maintained by both parties.
- Pain reports should be followed by nonjudgmental, interested, and concerned assessment that both recognizes them as a cry of distress and helps the patient to articulate what she or he most needs help with.
- Drug addicts are often alexithymic (many are unable to describe distress as other than "good" or "bad"), and this trait often leads to global distress in the face of negative emotions associated with pain and chronic illness.[8]
- Drug selection in such patients is often limited to sustained-release delivery to avoid feeding into compulsive pill popping and/or use of opioids in the service of chemical coping.[9]
- Use of a drug with a relatively low street value is recommended for patients who are battling for recovery but maintain unavoidable contact with the addiction subculture.
- Titration should be aimed at and continued until effect or toxicity, bearing in mind that addicts are often highly tolerant and require very large doses of opioids for pain control.

URINE TOXICOLOGY SCREENING

- Urine toxicology screening can be very useful for diagnosing potential abuse and for monitoring patients with a history of abuse.
- Urine toxicology screens, however, are employed infrequently in tertiary care centers.[10]
- When screens are ordered, documentation tends to be inconsistent about the reasons for the order or follow-up recommendations based on the results. In one survey, nearly 40% of the charts listed no reason for obtaining the screen, and the ordering physician could not be identified nearly 30% of the time.[10]

OUTPATIENT MANAGEMENT

- A written contract between the treatment team and the patient helps provide structure for the treatment plan, establishes clear expectations of the roles played by both parties, and outlines the consequences of aberrant drug taking.
- The inclusion of spot urine toxicology screens in the contract can be useful in maximizing treatment compliance. Expectations regarding attendance of clinic visits and management of the supply of medications should also be stated.

- The amount of drug dispensed per prescription should be limited and refills made contingent on clinic attendance.
- Requiring the patient to document attendance at a 12-step program should be considered as a condition for ongoing prescribing.
- Family members and friends should be involved in the treatment to help bolster social support and functioning. Becoming familiar with the family may help the treatment team identify family members who are drug abusers and who may potentially divert the patient's medications.

INPATIENT MANAGEMENT

- Inpatient management of patients with active substance abuse problems includes and expands on the guidelines for outpatient settings.
- First the patient's drug use should be discussed openly and the patient reassured that steps will be taken to avoid adverse events, such as drug withdrawal.
- In certain situations, such as for preoperative patients, patients should be admitted several days in advance when possible for stabilization of the drug regimen.
- It is important to provide the patient with a private room near the nurses' station to aid in monitoring the patient and to discourage attempts to leave the hospital for the purchase of illicit drugs.
- Visitors should be required to check in with nursing staff prior to visitation.
- Daily urine specimens should be collected for random toxicology analysis, and pain and symptom management frequently reassessed.
- Open and honest communication between the clinician and the patient reassures the patient that these guidelines were established in his or her best interest.

PATIENTS IN RECOVERY

- Pain management with patients in recovery presents a unique challenge.
- Due to fear of ostracism from some programs (eg, Alcoholics Anonymous), some patients may be leery of taking opioids. Thus, the first choice should be to explore nonopioid therapies with these patients, which may require referral to a pain center.[11]
- Alternative therapies may include the use of nonopioid or adjuvant analgesics, cognitive therapies, electrical stimulation, neural blockades, or acupuncture.
- If opioids are prescribed, it is necessary to structure opioid use with opioid management contracts, random urine toxicology screens, and occasional pill

counts. If possible, attempts should be made to include the patient's recovery program sponsor to garner his or her cooperation and aid in successful monitoring of the condition.

REFERENCES

1. **Colliver JD, Kopstein AN.** Trends in cocaine abuse reflected in emergency room episodes reported to DAWN. *Public Health Rep.* 1991;106:59.
2. **Groerer J, Brodsky M.** The incidence of illicit drug use in the United States, 1962–1989. *Br J Addiction.* 1992;87:1345.
3. **Regier DA, Farmer ME, Rae DS, et al.** Comorbidity of mental disorders with alcohol and other drug abuse. *JAMA.* 1990;264:2511.
4. **Bruera E, Moyano J, Seifert L, Fainsinger RL, Hanson J, Suarez-Almazor M.** The frequency of alcoholism among patients with pain due to terminal cancer. *J Pain Symptom Manage.* 1995;10:599.
5. **Rinaldi RC, Steindler EM, Wilford BB, Goodwin D.** Clarification and standardization of substance abuse terminology. *JAMA.*1988;259:555.
6. **Hay J, Passik SD.** The cancer patient with borderline personality disorder: Suggestions for symptom-focused management in the medical setting. *Psychooncology.* 2000;9:91.
7. **Passik SD, Weinreb HJ.** Managing chronic nonmalignant pain: Overcoming obstacles to the use of opioids. *Adv Ther.* 2000;17:70.
8. **Handelsman L, Stein JA, Bernstein DP, et al.** A latent variable analysis of coexisting emotional deficits in substance abusers: Alexithymia, hostility, and PTSD. *Addict Behav.* 2000;25:423.
9. **Bruera E, Moyano J, Seifert L, et al.** The frequency of alcoholism among patients with pain due to terminal cancer. *J Pain Symptom Manage.* 1995;10:599.
10. **Passik S, Schreiber J, Kirsh KL, et al.** A chart review of the ordering and documentation of urine toxicology screens in a cancer center: Do they influence patient management? *J Pain Symptom Manage.* 2000;19:40.
11. **Parrino M.** State Methadone Treatment Guidelines. Washington, DC. TIPS 1 DHHS publication (SMA) 93-1991.

45   BIOPSYCHOSOCIAL FACTORS IN PAIN MEDICINE

Rollin M. Gallagher, MD, MPH
Sunil Verma, MBBS

INTRODUCTION

- Chronic, uncontrolled pain is likely the most expensive health care problem in the United States. It is the most frequent symptom for which patients seek medical care, is associated with substantial economic and psychosocial cost, and is often undertreated or mistreated.
- Because persistent pain has an emotional component and is frequently accompanied by depression and/or anxiety, patients benefit from a comprehensive assessment and multidisciplinary treatment.[1,2]
- Psychological factors play a significant role in chronic pain and in the transition of acute to chronic pain, and neuroscientific and clinical evidence has exposed the close relationship between pain and mood states.[3]
- Fishbain[4] used the Diagnostic and Statistical Manual of Mental Disorders (DSM-IV) to categorize psychiatric comorbidities with pain disorders as:
  - Axis I comorbidity, for example, a major psychiatric disorder, such as depression (the most common) or substance abuse, somatoform disorders, anxiety disorders, and a miscellaneous group comprising psychotic disorders, schizophrenia, delusional disorders, and bipolar affective disorders.
  - Axis I and Axis II (personality disorders) comorbidity, for example depression (Axis I) *and* antisocial disorder (Axis II).
  - Axis I psychoactive substance abuse disorder and other psychiatric disorders, for example, alcohol dependence *and* depression.
  - Comorbidity within psychoactive substance abuse disorders, for example, cocaine *and* alcohol dependence.
  - Comorbidity of an Axis I disorder with an Axis III medical condition, for example, depression *and* diabetic neuropathy.

PAIN AND DEPRESSION

- Many studies and reviews have documented the high degree of comorbidity between depression and chronic pain, and there is evidence that the incidence of depression among patients with chronic pain is higher than for other chronic medical illnesses, even in patients without apparent risk of depression.
- A risk model for depression following chronic pain (depicted in Figure 45–1) was derived from a study comparing women with temporomandibular pain and dysfunction syndrome with community controls matched for socioeconomic status and with first-degree relatives of patients and controls.[5]
- Phenomenologically, depression plays an important role in the experience of chronic pain. Thus, depressed patients report higher levels of pain, greater disability, and greater interference due to pain; tend to be less active; and display more pain behavior than do nondepressed patients with pain.
- A systematic review of prospective, cohort studies implicated distress, depressed mood, and somatiza-

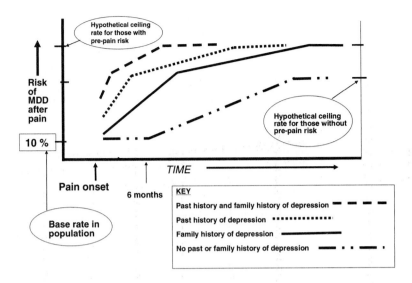

FIGURE 45–1 Hypothetical risk model for depressive illness in persons who develop chronic pain.

tion as factors in the transition of acute to chronic low back pain.[6]

- Depression can augment pain-related impairment and cause it to persist even in populations with access to excellent health care.
- A 24-month prospective study involving 228 well-insured, elderly residents of a retirement community who underwent semiannual evaluations of pain, depression, physical impairment, and health care utilization revealed that[7]:
  - Pain and depression were commonly comorbid.
  - Increasing depression was associated with increasing pain-related impairment.
  - This comorbidity was usually sustained longitudinally.[8]
  - Even mild, subclinical depression can increase health care utilization.[9]
- The presence of any physical symptom increased the likelihood of a diagnosis of a mood or anxiety disorder in a sample of primary care patients by as much as threefold.[10] Relatively high rates of mood disorder (34–46%) occurred with the following regional pain complaints:
  - 34% of patients with joint or limb pain
  - 38% of patients with back pain
  - 40% of patients with headache
  - 46% of patients with chest pain
  - 43% of patients with abdominal pain

MANAGING DEPRESSION IN PAIN PATIENTS

SCREENING FOR DEPRESSION

- The successful management of depression begins with a thorough initial assessment to establish a diag-

nosis and investigate potential biopsychosocial risks and strengths. Simple screening instruments or strategies include:
  - The Beck Depression Inventory
  - During the review of systems (to reduce bias), determining if the patient has depressed mood, loss of interest or enjoyment, and/or multiple sites of pain
- Because (1) a significant false negative rate for identifying depression may accompany an initial evaluation of chronic pain[11] and (2) the risk of developing depression is high during the course of chronic pain, clinicians should periodically screen for depression during treatment, particularly when pain symptoms, impairment, or disability change or an additional life stressor occurs.

DIAGNOSING A MOOD DISORDER

- The history-gathering should solicit information on:
  - Current illness and symptoms
  - Previous psychiatric disorders, including mania
  - Treatment, including treatment response
  - General medical condition
  - Substance abuse
  - Familial psychiatric illness
  - Psychological development, coping skills, and response to previous life events
  - Mental status
  - Selective physical and laboratory examination as indicated
  - Whether the patient has major depression, minor depression, dysthymia, bipolar illness, or substance or medically induced mood disturbance
  - Whether the patient has marital problems (because marital satisfaction and a negative spousal response to pain are related to depressive symptoms)[12]

EVALUATING PATIENT SAFETY

- Because chronic pain is associated with suicide[4] and violence,[13] careful assessment of these risks will indicate if a patient is best treated on an inpatient or outpatient basis.
- All suicidal patients should be evaluated by a properly trained professional to assess risk and arrange appropriate management.
- The assessment of suicide risk should consider the presence of suicidal ideation, plans made by the patient, the availability of means/methods, and the lethality of contemplated methods.
- Pain clinicians should be aware that depression increases the risk for anger attacks, that persons with chronic pain who are in treatment have higher rates of violent ideation than do samples of community controls, and that the presence of depression increases risk.[13]
- Other factors increasing risk include job dissatisfaction, unemployment, workers' compensation, work rehabilitation programs, litigation, and when physicians diagnose malingering.[14]
- An antagonistic relationship among workers' compensation insurer, employer, and injured worker may threaten the well-being of a patient's family.
- At initial evaluation and when there is a treatment setback, the physician should ask patients if they are experiencing angry outbursts or angry thoughts and, if so, whether they can control these events.

ESTABLISHING AND MAINTAINING A THERAPEUTIC ALLIANCE

- Developing a trusting and positive working relationship with the patient and, if possible, with the patient's family or significant others is important to ensure safe and effective treatment.
- Successfully titrating medications to their analgesic and antidepressant potential requires that the clinician and patient communicate effectively about potential side effects, toxicity, drug interactions, and therapeutic targets.
- An effective working relationship starts with patient education about the painful condition, the goals of treatment, the rationale for treatment choices, and the clinician's expectations of the patient's responsibilities for record-keeping, adherence, and follow-up.
- Trust in this relationship is critical when dealing with matters of safety, such as toxicity, suicide, and violence.

EDUCATING THE PATIENT AND THE PATIENT'S FAMILY

- All patients and, when possible, appropriate family members should receive education about depression, pain, and the relationship between pain and depression.
- Uninformed family members may discourage patients from taking psychotropic medication because they fear side effects or addiction.
- It is appropriate to educate groups of patients in 7–10 sessions that cover various aspects of pain, mood, stress, anxiety, relationships, activities, and other pain-related issues, including the rational use of medications. Spouses may also benefit from these sessions.
- Longitudinal, open-ended support groups help patients maintain treatment gains.

TREATMENT ADHERENCE

- Successful treatment of depression requires close adherence to treatment plans for long or indefinite durations to ensure full remission and prevent relapse or recurrence.
- To enhance adherence to treatment, side effects must be carefully explained.
- In the early stages of treatment, clinicians must base interventions to enhance treatment adherence on the understanding that patients with pain and depression may be poorly motivated and unduly pessimistic about their chance of recovery.

PHARMACOLOGIC MANAGEMENT OF DEPRESSION

- The 22 compounds approved by the US Food and Drug Administration (FDA) as antidepressants are classified in Table 45–1.
- Although no single drug is most effective in depression, dual-action antidepressants with noradrenergic and serotonergic reuptake inhibition may provide the most effective treatment.[15]
- More than 80% of depressed patients respond to at least one medication, although individual antidepressants are effective in only 50–60% of patients. Thus when one does not work, a switch should be made to another with a different profile (eg, if an SSRI, try buproprion or an SNRI), and so on.
- Factors to consider in selecting an antidepressant include prior response, family history of a response, anticipated side effects, efficacy, remission rates, dosing simplicity (promotes adherence), adherence,

TABLE 45–1 Medications for Depression

Tricyclics and Tetracyclics

Tertiary amine tricyclics
   amitripyline
   clomipramine*
   doxepine
   imipramine
   trimipramine
Secondary amine tricyclics
   desipramine
   nortriptyline
   protriptyline
Tetracyclics
   amoxapine
   maprotiline

Selective Serotonin Reuptake Inhibitors (SSRIs)

   citalopram
   escitalopram
   fluoxetine
   fluvoxamine*
   paroxetine
Dopamine–Norepinephrine Reuptake Inhibitors
   bupropion
Serotonin–Norepinephrine Reuptake Inhibitors (SNRIs)
   venlafaxine
   duloxetine†
Serotonin Modulators
   nefazodone
   trazadone
Norepinephrine–Serotonin Modulator
   mirtazapine
Monoamine Oxidase Inhibitors (MAOIs)
Irreversible, nonselective
   isocarboxazide
   phenelzine
   tranylcypromine
Reversible MAOI-A
   moclobemide*
Selective Noradrenaline
Reuptake Inhibitor
   reboxetine†

*Approved for treatment of obsessive–compulsive disorder (OCD) only.
†Not available in the United States.

and cost (if a patient cannot afford his or her expensive prescription antidepressant, the patient is likely to discontinue the drug).

- Anxiety and insomnia do not necessarily predict a better response to medications that have an enhanced sedative effect.
- The patient should be followed closely for a response to pharmaceuticals and the dose titrated upward if the patient does not respond in a couple of weeks.
- The patient's attitude toward antidepressants should be determined and that the patient is in fact taking the medication should be confirmed.
- Educating patients and their families (if possible) about the benefits of the drug and the risk of relapse helps promote adherence.

TRICYCLIC AND TETRACYCLIC ANTIDEPRESSANTS

- When prescribing tricyclic antidepressants (TCAs), *the potential for a lethal overdose* and *the possibility of inducing a manic episode* in patients with or without history of mania must always be considered.
- Data from 41 controlled trials indicate that TCAs are effective analgesics.[16]
- Amitriptyline is the most thoroughly studied, although desipramine, imipramine, clomipramine, nortriptyline, and doxepin have also been well studied.
- Controlled trials provide consistent evidence that TCAs are analgesic for diabetic neuropathy, postherpetic neuralgia, central pain syndromes, poststroke pain, and chronic headache.
- TCAs may also be efficacious as preemptive analgesia and for potentiating opioids for treatment of postoperative pain.
- Evidence of the pain-relieving efficacy of the tetracyclics maprotiline and amoxapine is limited. Maprotiline is more effective than paroxetine but is not superior to TCAs.
- Given that all TCAs and tetracyclic antidepressants are equally effective in treating depression and that most TCAs are efficacious in pain disorders, the choice of antidepressant is often influenced by the side effect profile:
  - Anticholinergic effects are common, though patients may develop tolerance, and include dry mouth, constipation, blurred vision, and urinary retention. Amitriptyline, imipramine, trimipramine, and doxepin are the most anticholinergic drugs; amoxapine, maprotiline, and nortriptyline are less anticholinergic; and desipramine is the least anticholinergic.
  - Sedation may be a welcome side effect in patients with sleep disturbances. Amitriptyline, doxepin, and trimipramine are most sedating; desipramine and protriptyline are the least sedating.
  - Autonomic effects due to α_1-adrenergic blockade result in orthostatic hypotension and are least to most likely to occur with amitriptyline, doxepine, clomipramine, amoxapine, and nortriptyline, in that order.
  - Cardiac effects, including tachycardia, prolonged QT intervals, and depressed ST segments on ECGs, contraindicate TCAs and tetracyclics in patients with prolonged conduction times. In patients with a history of cardiac disease, these drugs should be initiated at low doses, with gradual increase and monitoring of cardiac function.
  - The side effect burden and risk of untoward reaction with TCAs increases with patient age.
- Newer antidepressants are generally less toxic in cases of overdose but do not reduce the overall risk of suicide.

SELECTIVE SEROTONIN REUPTAKE INHIBITORS

- Since fluoxetine was introduced in 1988, the SSRIs fluoxetine, fluvoxamine, sertraline, paroxetine, and citalopram have captured more than 50% of the US prescription antidepressant market owing to their favorable side effect profile.
- Because of good efficacy rates and dosing simplicity, many patients with pain and depression receive SSRIs as initial treatment.
- Although SSRIs cost more than TCAs, the total cost of treatment is usually similar for patients who start with SSRIs and those who begin with TCAs but cannot tolerate them and must make additional office visits to switch to SSRIs.
- Although the antidepressant effects of SSRIs are not superior to those of TCAs and MAOIs, the more favorable side effect profile and overdose safety of SSRIs often make them the first-choice treatment of depression.
- The SSRIs differ primarily in their half-lives. At 2–3 days, fluoxetine has the longest, and its active metabolite has a half-life of 7–9 days. The half-lives of other SSRIs are approximately 20 hours.
- Because all SSRIs are metabolized in the liver by the cytochrome P450 isoenzyme, clinicians should be careful about drug interactions. Citalopram is least affected by cytochrome P isoenzymes.
- The most common side effects of SSRIs include agitation, anxiety, sleep disturbance, tremor, sexual dysfunction, and headache. Citalopram (Celexa) has been reported to have a lesser rate of sexual side effects than other SSRIs. Rarely, SSRIs have been associated with extrapyramidal-like symptoms, arthralgias, lymphadenopathy, inappropriate antidiuretic syndrome, agranulocytosis, and hypoglycemia.
- The interaction of SSRIs with MAOIs causes the central serotonin syndrome manifested by abdominal pain, diarrhea, sweating, fever, tachycardia, elevated mood, hypertension, altered mental state, delirium, myoclonus, increased motor activity, irritability, and hostility. Severe manifestation of this syndrome can include hyperemia, cardiovascular shock, and death.
- SSRIs have no α-adrenergic antagonistic effect and are essentially devoid of the Type 1A antiarrhythmic effect of tricyclics; therefore, SSRIs rarely are associated with orthostatic hypotension.

Analgesic Effects of SSRIs

- The analgesic effects of the SSRIs are not as pronounced as those of TCAs.
- Of 10 studies evaluating the efficacy of SSRIs in the treatment of chronic headache, 3 found SSRIs no better than placebo, 2 found SSRIs marginally better than placebo, and 5 found no improvement beyond the comparison drug.[16]

- Of three controlled trials examining SSRIs in the treatment of painful diabetic neuropathy, the larger study ($n = 46$) found no difference between fluoxetine and placebo, but the smaller studies found citalopram and paroxetine better than placebo.
- Studies comparing SSRIs with TCAs obtained consistently superior analgesia with TCAs.
- In 2000, Sindrup and Jensen identified all placebo-controlled drug trials involving treatment of pain in polyneuropathy and determined that the number of patients needed to treat to obtain one patient with more than 50% pain relief was 2.6 for tricyclics, 6.7 for SSRIs, 2.5 for anticonvulsant sodium channel blockers, 4.1 for gabapentin, and 3.4 for tramadol.[17]

DOPAMINE–NOREPINEPHRINE REUPTAKE INHIBITORS

- Bupropion (Wellbutrin) was synthesized in 1966 and emerged as an antidepressant without anticholinergic or cardiac effects. An increased incidence of drug-induced seizures in bulimic nondepressed subjects in one study, however, delayed its marketing. Subsequent studies of depressed patients did not replicate this finding, and the drug was reintroduced in 1989.
- Bupropion is as effective for depression as other antidepressants but is unique in that it is much less likely to cause psychosexual dysfunction.
- Because it blocks norepinephrine reuptake, bupropion has the potential for being an analgesic antidepressant, although this remains to be determined conclusively.
- In an open-label study, bupropion significantly reduced pain at 8 weeks, and a double-blind, placebo-controlled, crossover trial showed that 150–300 mg bupropion was effective and well tolerated for the treatment of neuropathic pain.
- In approximately 5% of the patients consuming 450–600 mg/d, bupropion causes the adverse effects of delusions, hallucinations, and the risk of seizures because of its potentiating effects on the dopaminergic system.

SEROTONIN–NOREPINEPHRINE REUPTAKE INHIBITORS

- The SNRI venlafaxine blocks reuptake as effectively as TCAs without causing the undesirable side effects associated with those agents.
- Venlafaxine has a faster-than-usual onset of action and demonstrated efficacy in seriously depressed patients.
- The norepinephrine reuptake-inhibiting properties of venlafaxine, particularly at higher doses, along with its structural similarity to tramadol, an analgesic with both opioid agonist and monoaminergic activity,

makes it a promising antidepressant for patients with chronic pain. In fact, norepinephrine reuptake inhibition may be crucial for relief of diabetic and postherpetic neuralgia pain.

- In healthy volunteers, venlafaxine increased the thresholds of pain tolerance to electrical sural nerve stimulation and of pain increase, indicating a potential analgesic effect for clinical neuropathic pain.[16]
- A number of case reports validate venlafaxine's efficacy in pain disorders, but controlled studies are lacking.
- Venlafaxine is generally well tolerated, and its side effects include nausea (37%), somnolence (23%), dry mouth (22%), and dizziness (22%).
- The most worrisome adverse effect is increased blood pressure, particularly in patients receiving more than 300 mg/d.

SEROTONIN MODULATORS
- The structurally related antidepressants trazodone and nefazodone are unrelated to the TCAs, MAOIs, or SSRIs.
- Trazodone has distinctive sedating properties and is used to treat insomnia in both pain and depression. Nefazodone is relatively free of this side effect and is generally well tolerated.
- No studies in humans have examined the analgesic effects of nefazodone.
- Four placebo-controlled trails support the analgesic effect of trazodone.
- Nefazodone is an effective antidepressant. Its half-life of 2–4 hours calls for twice-daily doses.
- The notable adverse reactions of nefazodone include liver failure, a drop in blood pressure, and drug interactions with triazolam (Halcion), alprazolam (Xanax), terfenadine/pseudoephedrine (Seldane), astemizole (Hismanal), and cisapride (Propulsid) due to its inhibition of cytochrome P450.

NOREPINEPHRINE–SEROTONIN MODULATOR
- The antidepressant mirtazapine (Remeron) antagonizes the central presynaptic α_2-adrenergic receptors, resulting in a potentiation of central noradrenergic and serotonergic transmission.
- Mirtazapine is an effective antidepressant, yet it lacks the anticholinergic effects of the TCAs and the anxiogenic effects of some SSRIs.
- Because of its broad neurotransmitter profile, mirtazapine has the potential to be an analgesic antidepressant, but this requires study.
- The adverse effects associated with mirtazapine include somnolence, which may be welcome in patients with sleep disturbances; increased appetite with weight gain, which may be welcome in cancer; increased serum cholesterol; and (among 0.3% of patients) agranulocytosis and neutropenia.

MONOAMINE OXIDASE INHIBITORS
- The MAOIs phenelzine (Nardil) and tranylcypromine (Parnate)inhibit the degeneration of biogenic amine levels.
- MAOIs may be effective for panic disorder with agoraphobia, posttraumatic stress disorder, eating disorders, social phobia, and atypical depression characterized by hypersomnia, hyperphagia, anxiety, and the absence of vegetative symptoms; however, these medications are generally not used because of their toxic potential (see below).
- Animal studies supporting the analgesic effects of MAOIs have not been replicated in pain patients.[16]
- The side effects of MAOIs and the potential for precipitating a toxic central serotonin syndrome when combined with other medications and certain foods limit their use to treatment-resistant depression.
- A tyramine-induced hypertensive crisis in patients taking MAOIs can be life-threatening. Other side effects include orthostatic hypertension, weight gain, edema, sexual dysfunction, and insomnia.

ANTICONVULSANTS
- Anticonvulsants have been used in pain management since the 1960s, very soon after they revolutionized the medical management of epilepsy.
- Anticonvulsants have an established role in the treatment of chronic neuropathic pain, especially when patients complain of shooting sensations or when the pain is lancinating or burning.
- The precise mechanism of action of anticonvulsants remains uncertain, but they may enhance γ-aminobutyric acid inhibition, thus producing a stabilizing effect on neuronal cell membranes, or they may act on *N*-methyl-D-aspartate receptor sites.
- Gabapentin, topiramate, and lamotrigine all have efficacy in one or more neuropathic pain conditions.
- Older anticonvulsants, such as phenytoin, clonazepam, and valproic acid, have not shown efficacy for pain in clinical studies and, because of their problematic toxicity, are generally not used, with the exception of carbamazepine, which is effective in trigeminal neuralgia.
- Many anticonvulsants have mood-stabilizing properties, but no controlled study supports the utility of mood-stabilizing agents as therapy in depression.
- The anticonvulsants lamotrigine and gabapentin may have antimanic and antidepressant activity.

- Gabapentin seems to be safe and well tolerated and has a favorable side effect profile, possible anxiolytic effects, and virtual absence of drug interactions.
- Lamotrigine requires careful dosing and close monitoring because it can cause a potentially severe skin rash. Lamotrigine is under investigation for treatment of various phases of refractory bipolar disorder, and many clinicians appear to be adding lamotrigine to the treatment regimens of bipolar patients with complex, treatment-resistant forms of illness.
- A double-blind study found lamotrigine (50 or 200 mg/d) effective in treating depression in patients with bipolar disorder, and a placebo-controlled study found it effective and safe in relieving pain associated with diabetic neuropathy.[17]

PSYCHOTHERAPEUTIC TECHNIQUES

- Although helpful, psychopharmacologic treatment of the psychiatric comorbidities associated with chronic pain is almost never successful alone because pain itself and the psychosocial contextual experience of pain both condition the neurophysiologic system.
- The successful treatment of chronic pain must be multidimensional, and psychotherapeutic interventions are helpful and often necessary for managing both pain and its psychiatric comorbidities.
- The psychotherapeutic techniques used in treating chronic pain patients include:
  ◦ Pain education.
  ◦ Supportive psychotherapy to strengthen patients' coping strategies.
  ◦ Cognitive behavioral therapy, which focuses on patients' maladaptive cognitions along with behavioral techniques, such as relaxation therapy and assertiveness training.
  ◦ Behavior therapy, based on behavior theory and social learning theory.
  ◦ Interpersonal therapy, which focuses on losses, role disputes and transitions, social deficits, and other interpersonal factors that may impact the development of depression.
  ◦ Dynamic psychotherapy, where the relationship with the therapist provides the context for the corrective emotional experience.
  ◦ Family therapy and couples therapy, which address the fact that chronic pain is a disruptive problem prone to affect the entire family.
  ◦ Group therapy, which can be educational and/or psychotherapeutic.
- Categorization of these strategies as distinct entities is useful for heuristic purposes only. In clinical practice,

psychiatrists individualize a combination of approaches to match their patients' needs.

COGNITIVE BEHAVIORAL THERAPY

- Cognitive behavioral therapy (CBT) is based on the theory that irrational beliefs and distorted attitudes toward the self, the environment, and the future perpetuate depression.
- Clinical studies show that CBT is effective in treating mild to moderate depression and in reducing pain-related impairments in pain disorder.
- The goal of CBT is to reduce depression by challenging these beliefs and attitudes.
- CBT can help patients recognize that emotional responses to pain are greatly influenced by their thoughts and that they can exercise control over the disruption produced by an unavoidable life event or chronic illness.
- Several investigators recommend providing CBT early in the course of illness to increase patients' confidence in managing symptoms and in their ability to reduce their health care utilization.

BEHAVIOR THERAPY

- Behavior therapy uses contingency management or operant conditioning to help patients modify pain-related behavior.
- These methods can also help rehabilitate pain patients by increasing their functional performance.

INTERPERSONAL PSYCHOTHERAPY

- Interpersonal psychotherapy (IPT), developed for treatment of depression, operates on the assumption that, because symptoms occur in a social context, addressing a problem or problems in the patient's interpersonal life may help alleviate symptoms.
- IPT for depression focuses on:
  ◦ Grief (a reaction to the death of a loved one)
  ◦ Role transition (giving up an old social role and adjusting to and embracing a new one)
  ◦ Role dispute (difficulty in a relationship arising from incompatible expectations)
  ◦ Role deficits (a paucity of interpersonal relationships)
- These principles can be applied to chronic pain patients whose symptoms and disability place them in a constant state of role transition exacerbated by depression or anxiety.

PSYCHODYNAMIC PSYCHOTHERAPY

- Psychodynamic psychotherapy includes all psychotherapeutic interventions that share a basis in psychodynamic theories about the cause of psychological vulnerabilities.

- This form of psychotherapy is most often long-term and has goals beyond immediate symptom relief.

PAIN AND ANXIETY DISORDERS

- Anxiety disorders are the most common form of mental illness in the United States (25% of the population have a history of an anxiety disorder vs 20% with a history of a mood disorder).
- Severe, acute pain activates stress-related noradrenergic systems in the brain and is often accompanied by cognitive–emotional reactions, such as fear and anxiety, which to some degree are contextually determined. For example, pain in childbirth usually does not evoke fear or anxiety, whereas pain associated with traumatic injury, with uncertain outcome, often does.
- The association of pain, anxiety, and depression may have a common neurochemical substrate in the serotonergic systems. Anxiety disorders, along with depression and substance abuse, are the most common comorbid conditions in patients with chronic pain.
- Patients commonly experience anxiety because of the stress of living with pain.
- The stress of severe trauma, for example, incurred in battle or a motor vehicle accident, may lead to posttraumatic stress disorder (PTSD) or a driving phobia, which can be comorbid with injury-related pain. The presence of comorbid obsessive–compulsive disorder with chronic pain can make both conditions worse if the patient has to undertake compulsive motoric acts (like cleaning rituals) to control the anxiety associated with the obsession.
- DSM-IV lists the following anxiety disorders:
  ◦ Panic disorder with or without agoraphobia
  ◦ Agoraphobia without panic disorder
  ◦ Specific and social phobias
  ◦ Obsessive–compulsive disorders
  ◦ Posttraumatic stress disorder
  ◦ Acute stress disorder
  ◦ Generalized anxiety disorder
  ◦ Anxiety disorders due to general medical condition
  ◦ Substance-induced anxiety disorders
  ◦ Anxiety disorders not otherwise classified
- These disorders can complicate a pain disorder and vice versa because the neurotransmitters implicated in panic disorders and phobic disorders, norepinephrine, serotonin, and γ-aminobutyric acid, are implicated in pain modulation.
- Consider also the challenges posed by a chronic pain patient whose pain management and pacing of activities are thwarted by (1) the compulsive cleaning rituals seen in obsessive–compulsive disorder; (2) posttraumatic stress disorder from a combat, rape, or motor vehicle accident; or (3) generalized anxiety or panic attacks further complicating disability.
- The management of anxiety disorders begins with a thorough assessment, including a detailed history.
- Depression is a frequent cause of anxiety.
- Other medical conditions that can present with anxiety, such as neurologic disorders (cerebral neoplasm, cerebrovascular accident), systemic conditions (hypoxia, hypoglycemia, cardiac arrhythmias, anemia), endocrine disturbances (thyroid, pituitary, parathyroid), and deficiency states (B_{12}, pellagra), must be excluded by physical exam and appropriate laboratory tests, including imaging studies.
- It is also important to rule out anxiety secondary to drugs, toxins, and psychoactive substance abuse.

PANIC DISORDERS

- Panic attacks occur in a variety of psychiatric disorders and, when recurrent or associated with significant apprehension and behavioral change, are the central manifestations of panic disorder.
- Because panic attacks are abrupt and intense, with symptoms referable to several bodily systems, they often present in the emergency room.
- The pharmacologic treatment of panic disorder includes high-potency benzodiazepines, TCAs, SSRIs, and MAOIs, and experience has revealed the superiority of the SSRIs and clomipramine. A few reports have suggested a role for nefazodone, venlafaxine, and buspirone but not for β-adrenergic antagonists.
- One approach is to start off with an SSRI and, if rapid control of anxiety is needed, to use a short-acting benzodiazepine until the SSRI is effective (keeping in mind the abuse potential and other potential negative effects of prolonged use of benzodiazepines).

PHOBIC DISORDERS

- Social phobia is a persistent and disproportionate fear that occurs in a performance or social setting and may include intense anticipatory anxiety.
- Often, social phobia is associated with hypersensitivity to criticism and low self-esteem.
- It may be generalized to involve multiple, slightly similar situations or be specific to a particular event.
- Social phobia is often a lifelong problem usually handled by avoidance, which limits opportunities.

- The condition responds well to SSRIs and high-potency benzodiazepines and may benefit from specific behavioral treatments. MAOIs are effective but are used rarely because of their relative toxicity and food restrictions. TCAs and β blockers often are used in clinical practice despite the lack of supporting evidence. Gabapentin and, perhaps, divalproex sodium are reasonable options for patients who fail the conventional medications.
- Double-blind, placebo-controlled studies have found paroxetine, fluvoxamine, and sertraline effective in social phobia. Of these, only paroxetine has been approved by the FDA for this indication.[16]
- Citalopram has not been tested in social anxiety disorder.

OBSESSIVE–COMPULSIVE DISORDER

- An estimated 2% of humans suffer from obsessive–compulsive disorder (OCD).
- An obsession is a recurrent and intrusive thought, feeling, idea, or sensation, and a compulsion is a conscious, standardized, recurring pattern of behavior.
- People with this disorder recognize that their reactions to these thoughts and acts are irrational and disproportionate.
- Recognition of and initiation of appropriate treatment for OCD are often delayed.
- The generally accepted hypothesis is that OCD involves abnormal serotonergic function regulation (although both serotonergic and nonserotonergic antidepressants effectively treat depression, only serotonergic drugs effectively treat OCD).
- Fluoxetine, fluvoxamine, sertraline, and paroxetine are all approved for the treatment of OCD, and high doses may be necessary, such as 80 mg/d fluoxetine.
- Of the TCAs, clomipramine is the most selective for serotonin reuptake and was the first FDA-approved drug for OCD. It is limited by its typical TCA side effect profile.
- The best outcome in OCD occurs in patients provided with both pharmacotherapy and behavior therapy.

POSTTRAUMATIC STRESS DISORDER

- Posttraumatic stress disorder (PTSD) results when a traumatic experience or exposure to a traumatic event is reexperienced persistently, causing avoidance of stimuli associated with the event and persistent symptoms of increased arousal.
- The treatment of PTSD requires that physicians give patients adequate time to disclose their stories.

- Education involves explaining to survivors and their families the nature of PTSD and responses to stress, as well as encouraging (not pressuring) survivors to discuss their traumatic experience with family and/or friends.
- Antidepressants such as amitriptyline, imipramine, and phenelzine are beneficial in treating PTSD. Also, SSRIs such as fluoxetine and sertraline often act rapidly to modulate affect, memory, and impulses in PTSD, both protecting against their overwhelming intensity and loosening excessive inhibitions.
- Reports of uncontrolled studies with small samples suggest a benefit with paroxetine, citalopram hydrochloride, fluvoxamine, nefazodone hydrochloride, trazodone hydrochloride, bupropion hydrochloride, and mirtazapine.
- Non-SSRI drugs are considered second-line or augmentative treatment, and trazodone has been suggested for managing insomnia in PTSD.

GENERALIZED ANXIETY DISORDER

- Generalized anxiety disorder (GAD) is characterized by excessive worrying that is difficult to control and is associated with somatic symptoms, such as muscle tension, irritability, difficulty sleeping, and restlessness.
- FDA–approved agents for the treatment of GAD include the benzodiazepines and buspirone.
- Although well-controlled data are lacking, long-term benzodiazepine use may be associated with tolerance, abuse, and dependence.
- Buspirone is effective in the treatment of GAD and avoids the disadvantages associated with benzodiazepines, but it has a slower onset of action—typically 1 to 3 weeks.
- TCAs, SSRIs, trazodone, and nefazodone have been evaluated in GAD, but data are extremely limited and, in some studies, complicated by the inclusion of patients with major depression.
- Among the newer antidepressants, only venlafaxine extended-release (XR) possesses unequivocal efficacy in GAD. The anxiolytic efficacy of venlafaxine XR has been demonstrated in two clinical studies in a defined population of patients with GAD without associated major depression.

PSYCHOTHERAPY FOR ANXIETY DISORDERS

- The principles of psychotherapy for patients with anxiety disorders are similar to those for patients with depression but place a greater emphasis on behavioral methods.

- The principles of treatment for anxiety and pain are similar in that the practitioner focuses on helping the patient learn specific cognitive and behavioral coping skills to prevent, abort, or ameliorate symptoms.
- In panic disorder, cognitive therapy challenges the patient's false beliefs and information about panic attacks and is used in conjunction with respiratory training, applied relaxation, and in vivo exposure and response prevention.
- In OCD, behavior therapy may be as effective as pharmacotherapy and may provide longer-lasting beneficial effects. The principal behavioral approaches in OCD are exposure and response prevention. Desensitization, thought stopping, flooding, and aversive conditioning have also been used.
- Psychodynamic psychotherapy may be useful in patients with PTSD. In some cases the reconstruction of the traumatic event along with abreaction and catharsis may be therapeutic. Other interventions for PTSD include those used for GAD: cognitive therapy, behavior therapy, and hypnosis.

CONCLUSION

- Pain activates emotions, and, in certain situations, emotions activate pain; thus, emotions and pain are inextricably intertwined in the phenomenology of chronic pain diseases and disorders.
- Emotions and pain share common neuroanatomic and neurophysiologic substrates.
- Managing unhealthy emotional responses to pain and the consequences of pain is part and parcel of the pain physician's daily work. To treat pain without managing emotions or to treat emotions without treating pain is usually futile, dooming the patient to chronic suffering and the clinician to chronic frustration.
- Thus, to manage most patients with chronic pain effectively, clinicians must identify, diagnose, and treat common comorbidities, such as uncomplicated depression.
- Because of the prevalence of comorbid depression and anxiety, easy access to mental health professionals with experience in treating pain and comorbidities is critical to success in a chronic pain practice.
- The physician must assure the patient that such referrals are common and expected in pain treatment, and the patient must understand that this is critical to the success of pain treatment.
- In the case of comorbidities, the physician should communicate a willingness to follow up the patient's emotional symptoms and psychosocial functioning with an interest equal to that expressed in the outcome of treatment of the pain symptoms.
- The physician should educate the patient without a comorbidity about the frequency of comorbidity and tell that patient to report the onset of depression or anxiety immediately.
- Because many pharmaceutical and psychotherapeutic strategies exist with a strong foundation of research support, physicians should prescribe with confidence in achieving a response and with the realistic goal of achieving depression remission and effective control of many anxiety symptoms and disorders.

REFERENCES

1. **Staats PS.** Pain management and beyond: Evolving concepts and treatments involving cyclooxygenase inhibition. *J Pain Symptom Manage.* 2002;24(1, Suppl):S4–S9.
2. **Gallagher RM.** Integrating medical and behavioral treatment in chronic pain management. *Med Clin North Am.* 1999;83:823–849.
3. **Rome H, Rome J.** Limbically augmented pain syndrome (LAPS): Kindling, corticolimbic sensitization, and the convergence of affective and sensory symptoms in chronic pain disorders. *Pain Med.* 2000;1:7–23.
4. **Fishbain DA.** Current research on chronic pain and suicide. *Am J Public Health.* 1996;86:1320–1321.
5. **Dohrenwend B, Marbach J, Raphael K, Gallagher RM.** Why is depression co-morbid with chronic facial pain? A family study test of alternative hypotheses. *Pain.* 1999;83:183–192.
6. **Picus T, Burton AK, Vogel S, Field AP.** A systematic review of psychological factors as predictors of chronicity/disability in prospective cohorts of low back pain. *Spine.* 2002;27:E109–E120.
7. **Mossey J, Gallagher RM, Tirumalasetti F.** The effects of pain and depression on physical functioning in elderly residents of a continuing care retirement community. *Pain Med.* 2000;1:340–350.
8. **Mossey JM, Gallagher RM.** Longitudinal evaluation of the effects of pain and depression on the physical functioning of continuing care retirement community residents: Implications for the treatment of pain in older individuals. *Pain Med.* 2001;2:247.
9. **Gallagher RM, Mossey J.** Inadequate pain care for elders: The need for a primary care–pain medicine community collaboration. *Pain Med.* 2002;3:180.
10. **Kroenke K, Spitzer RL, Williams JB, et al.** Physical symptoms in primary care: Predictors of psychiatric disorders and functional impairment. *Arch Fam Med.* 1994;3:774–779.
11. **Gallagher RM, Moore P, Chernoff I.** The reliability of depression diagnosis in chronic low back pain: A pilot study. *Gen Hosp Psychiatry.* 1995;17:399–413.

12. **Cano A, Weisberg J, Gallagher RM.** Marital satisfaction and pain severity mediate the association between negative spouse responses to pain and depressive symptoms in a chronic pain patient sample. *Pain Med.* 2000;1:35–43.

13. **Bruns D, Disorbio M.** Hostility and violent ideation: Physical rehabilitation patient and community samples. *Pain Med.* 2000;1:131–139.

14. **Fishbain DA, Cutler R, Rosomoff HL, Rosomoff RS.** Risk for violent behavior in patients with chronic pain: Evaluation and management in the pain facility setting. *Pain Med.* 2000;1:140–155.

15. **Thase ME, Entsuah AR, Rudolph RL.** Remission rates during treatment with venlafaxine or selective serotonin reuptake inhibitors. *Br J Psychiatry.* 2001;178:234–241.

16. **Lynch ME.** Antidepressants as analgesics: A review of randomized controlled trials. *J Psychiatry Neurosci.* 2001; 26:30–36.

17. **Sindrup SH, Jensen TS.** Efficacy of pharmacological treatments of neuropathic pain: An update and effect related to mechanism of drug action. *Pain.* 1999;83: 389–400.

SPECIAL TECHNIQUES IN PAIN MANAGEMENT

46 GENERAL PRINCIPLES OF INTERVENTIONAL PAIN THERAPIES

Richard L. Rauck, MD
Christopher Nelson, MD

OVERALL CONSIDERATIONS

- Informed consent is essential before any procedure is undertaken. (See below for a detailed discussion of the legal aspects of informed consent.)
- Practitioners should understand the difference between procedures with respect to expectation of therapeutic benefit versus desired diagnostic information.
- Practitioners should have the requisite skill set to perform intended interventional procedures. This skill set may come from a fellowship training, previous experience with similar techniques, and/or attendance at seminars, conferences, and cadaveric workshops. It is important that interventional pain practitioners understand their abilities and limitations in performing these procedures.
- Practitioners of interventional procedures should understand the potential risks and complications of the procedures they perform and have the knowledge and equipment necessary to resuscitate patients in an emergency.

GENERAL INDICATIONS FOR INTERVENTIONAL PROCEDURES

- Interventional procedures may be diagnostic and/or therapeutic.
- Interventional procedures are indicated for a variety of acute, chronic, noncancer, and cancer pain patients. Understanding the indications for interventional procedures is essential. Patient selection is pivotal for achieving long-term efficacy and positive outcome measures.
- Although some patients respond to interventional procedures as unimodality therapy, most chronic pain patients respond best when interventions are part of a multidisciplinary approach. Addressing the physical therapy, vocational needs, and psychological issues of the patient along with the indicated procedures enhances the long-term outcome.[1,2]
- Some patients should have interventions deferred until other serious issues (eg, severe depression) are managed.

USE OF NEW INTERVENTIONAL PROCEDURES

- New interventional procedures are continuously being developed and promoted by specialists in the field and industry.
- Caution should be used in employing new procedures. Proper indications can take years to fully understand with some procedures. Potential risks and complications may not be intuitive for a new procedure.
- Formal training may be necessary for some new procedures, while others may require only modification of existing practice.
- Practitioners should understand the differences in benefits and risks between existing and proposed techniques when evaluating new interventional procedures.

GENERAL TECHNIQUES FOR INTERVENTIONAL PROCEDURES

STERILE TECHNIQUE

- Sterile technique should be used for all interventional procedures. The degree of sterility may vary from a simple swab with an alcohol-soaked gauze to full operating room sterile procedure. The sterility required depends on several factors, including the likelihood of infection, patient factors (eg, diabetes mellitus), and the severity or difficulty of treating a resultant infection (eg, diskitis from a diskogram).
- Most interventional procedures are elective. Patients with concomitant, systemic infections should generally be rescheduled to a later date for a specific intervention. A risk/benefit analysis is necessary in some cases, such as for a patient with chest wall trauma and developing atelectasis who may benefit greatly from a thoracic epidural.

SEDATION

- Most awake patients experience some discomfort during an interventional procedure. Liberal use of local anesthetics decreases this discomfort to a tolerable level for most patients.
- The type of intervention has a significant role in the amount of discomfort the practitioner may expect a patient to experience; for example, a trigger point injection usually has significantly less associated pain than does provocative diskography.
- Some patients tolerate the pain of interventional procedures poorly. The term *needle phobia* is used for patients who experience excessive pain with any type of intervention. A larger percentage of patients cannot tolerate the more invasive procedures. A skilled and experienced clinician can usually determine the amount of pain expected during any given procedure.
- For any specific procedure or patient, the practitioner may decide to employ the use of sedation to help the patient tolerate the associated pain. Use of sedation is appropriate during interventional procedures but is an art that should be practiced carefully.
- Sedation is important, at times, for patient safety. Patients who move or jump during a procedure place themselves at risk of injury from the needle or cannula. This patient movement can be involuntary or reflexive to the needle invasion. Sedation often prevents this movement.
- An awake or semiconscious patient is important in many procedures to inform practitioners if the needle, catheter, and/or cannula are positioned in an unex-

pected place. Patients under appropriate levels of sedation can still interact with the practitioner and provide valuable feedback. For example, most sedated patients can inform the practitioner when a needle brushes along or contacts a nerve. Avoiding needle penetration of a nerve is often desired. If the patient is too heavily sedated or unconscious, the practitioner loses this important feedback.
- Appropriate levels of sedation often leave the patient amnestic of the procedure. Patients who reliably and routinely provide accurate information during the procedure develop retrograde amnesia. Clinically, this amnesia is acceptable and often beneficial, as patients often need repeat procedures. Unfortunately, in medicolegal cases, this amnesia is often interpreted as unconsciousness; thus documentation of this scenario may be helpful.
- Patients who have undergone sedation for interventions should be discharged in the care of a driver. Exceptions are rare and require sufficient recovery time for the effects of sedation to dissipate.
- Use of sedation always requires a risk/benefit analysis. The standard of care, however, does not require documentation of this risk/benefit analysis. In many cases, the benefits of sedation outweigh the risks.

FLUOROSCOPIC GUIDANCE

- Controversy exists regarding the necessity of fluoroscopic guidance for interventional procedures in pain medicine. Fluoroscopic guidance, however, has improved the efficacy of some interventions, such as celiac plexus and lumbar sympathetic nerve block.
- Certain procedures should only rarely be performed without fluoroscopic guidance. Examples include cervical and lumbar median branch blocks, where precise needle location can be guaranteed only with visualization of appropriate bony landmarks.
- Fluoroscopic guidance provides useful information when nerves, joints, or other intended targets are in proximity to bony landmarks. Many peripheral nerves, such as ilioinguinal/hypogastric nerves, are commonly blocked at a distance from a bony landmark. Use of fluoroscopic guidance in these situations is not as helpful as in other procedures, such as a selective nerve block.
- The use of fluoroscopic guidance for all nerve blocks in or around the spine is a subject of debate. The standard of care for access to the cervical, thoracic, and lumbar epidural space in perioperative or obstetric anesthesia is without fluoroscopic guidance. As many anesthesiology-trained interventionalists learned these techniques safely without fluoroscopy and have

practiced them for years in pain clinics without fluoroscopy, it has been difficult for many to see the need for change. Also, any radiation exposure carries some risk, and a substantial cost is associated with the use of fluoroscopy. This debate will undoubtedly continue.

- Fluoroscopic guidance has been extremely useful for many interventions. With the injection of appropriate contrast material, information can be gleaned about the characteristic spread of diagnostic and/or therapeutic injectate material.

- Radiation exposure from fluoroscopy can be significant to the patient and/or the practitioner.[3] Judicious use and continuous monitoring of live fluoroscopic times help limit this exposure. Practitioners should protect themselves with leaded gowns, thyroid shields, lined gloves, and protective glasses, when appropriate.

MONITORING

- Patients should be monitored following interventions. They may require nothing more than observation by office personnel prior to discharge or may require a formal recovery room and continuous vital sign monitoring.

- The level of monitoring depends on the procedure, the sedation used, and the individual patient. When intravenous sedation is used, heart rate, blood pressure, respiratory rate, and oxygen saturation are commonly monitored noninvasively.

MEDICATIONS

COMMONLY USED MEDICATIONS

- Local anesthetics and corticosteroids are the most frequently used medications in most interventional practices. Other medications, such as hyaluronidase, hypertonic saline, opioids, bretylium, and clonidine, are sometimes used. Many, if not most, of these drugs are used in interventional pain medicine for non-FDA-approved indications. This does not imply that they are not efficacious or that unacceptable risks exist. For a variety of business/legal reasons, many companies choose not to allocate the resources necessary to win FDA approval for a specific indication. The FDA does not limit the use of a drug to approved indications (the agency limits the ability of pharmaceutical companies to market a drug for a nonapproved indication).

- It is essential that interventional practitioners understand which drugs are safe for which procedures. For example, hypertonic saline is an effective drug in the epidural space but is rarely indicated for subarachnoid injection, and care should be taken to avoid intrathecal injection in most cases.

- Occasionally the indications for certain medications may change over time. For example, we use methylprednisolone acetate for cervical selective nerve root injections, but it is unclear whether there is an intravascular injection risk with a particulate steroid injection in this area. The use of intrathecal corticosteroids is controversial. Although clinical experience and the literature support the use of these agents in select situations,[4,5] older reports link neurotoxicity with the intrathecal injection of methylprednisolone acetate.[6]

- Interventional practitioners should stay abreast of the literature and alter their practices as findings emerge.

- When controversy exists, practitioners may have to decide whether or not to use selected drugs based on the local medicolegal environment.

MANAGING ANTICOAGULANTS

- Patients are prescribed intravenous (heparin, streptokinase), subcutaneous (low-molecular-weight heparins [LMWHs]), or oral (warfarin) anticoagulants/thrombolytic drugs for a variety of medical conditions.

- Many anticoagulants pose some undefined but increased risk for patients undergoing interventional procedures.

- Anticoagulants can be classified broadly as drugs that interfere with platelet function and those that interfere with the coagulation cascade as measured by prothrombin time and/or partial thromboplastin time. Many of these drugs have the potential to increase bleeding time and/or produce coagulopathy.

- Some agents, such as the nonsteroidal anti-inflammatory drugs, do not significantly increase the risk of perioperative interventions or of epidural steroid injections and can be continued safely during interventional procedures.[7,8]

- Drugs such as streptokinase, however, should be avoided in most patients scheduled to undergo an interventional procedure.

- LMWHs pose a significant risk in some patients. Practitioners should understand the risks associated with LMWHs and planned interventional procedures.[9]

- Because many interventions are elective, it is desirable and may be possible to stop anticoagulants 3–5 days beforehand. This may require clearance from the primary or prescribing physician. A bleeding history and/or PT/PTT/INR levels should be obtained in patients with recent excessive bleeding. Alternatively, the practitioner can hospitalize the patient and initiate intravenous heparin while discontinuing other anticoagulants. Once the effect of oral or subcutaneous drugs has dissipated, the heparin can be reversed with protamine for a short time while the procedure is performed. Anticoagulant therapy can be reinstituted following the procedure.

RISKS AND COMPLICATIONS

- Risks and potential complications should be explained to patients prior to interventional procedures, and alternative treatments should be discussed. This is often done outside the context of informed consent when the physician and patient discuss the treatment plan.
- Certain risks, including infection, trauma to a nerve from the needle, medication reaction, and death, are inherent to any procedure. Although death is a highly unexpected outcome of most procedures, its inclusion in a risk discussion or document implies some level of understanding by the patient that potentially serious complications can occur.
- Lack of efficacy is not a risk, but it is helpful to remind patients that no procedure guarantees improvement, and their symptoms could even become worse following the procedure, often for unclear reasons.

EMERGENCIES

- Interventional practitioners must be prepared to handle any potential complication.
- Resuscitative drugs, oxygen, airway management equipment, and suction should be maintained and readily available whenever interventional procedures and sedation are employed.
- The standard of care does not mandate that resuscitative equipment be available in each procedure room; however, transport of such equipment should occur with expediency in case of an emergency.
- Large, busy practices should have adequately trained personnel nearby to help in emergencies. Solo practitioners should know what trained personnel are readily available and how to get their help in case of an emergency.

MEDICOLEGAL RISK MANAGEMENT

- In today's environment, it is impossible to guarantee that anyone can expect immunity or protect himself or herself in all situations. Geography (practice loca-

tion), type of interventional practice (some procedures carry an inherently greater risk), and luck all play a role in avoiding the unpleasant experience of a medical malpractice lawsuit.[10–13]
- The burden rests on the plaintiff to prove that a physician committed malpractice by breaching the standard of care. To do this, a causal relationship must exist between the alleged breach, the injury, and the alleged damages. A breach in the standard of care that cannot be linked to the injury or damages usually results in a favorable verdict or settlement for the physician.
- Practitioners unfamiliar with the legal environment should obtain the best legal counsel they can afford whenever the possibility of a malpractice suit arises. In rare situations, a practitioner may want to hire legal representation soon after an intervention. Generally, one waits until a plaintiff has filed a complaint.

INDICATIONS
- Legal cases always involve examination of the indications for any procedure the plaintiffs allege resulted in malpractice.
- If plaintiff's counsel can establish a lack of medical indications for the procedure, standard of care was breached.
- Although this is often not a clearly won point, documentation of indications generally refutes this argument.

INFORMED CONSENT
- To perform any procedure without the consent of the patient is considered assault.
- Although informed consent can ethically and legally be obtained orally (by explaining the risks, complications, and alternative treatments, and documenting this explanation in office or progress notes) or be implied (eg, when a patient is undergoing the "*n*th" injection in a series and willingly lies on the bed in preparation for the injection), a legal debate can ensue whenever written documentation is poor.
- If adequate explanation is given but no documentation exists, the standard has been met, but credibility and the ability to remember the facts years later will be questioned if an unexpected event occurs and legal restitution is sought.
- Documentation of informed consent in writing, therefore, is preferred by legal experts.
- To avoid legal confrontation, therefore, the best informed consent is obtained in writing, is witnessed, and is documented in the patient's chart.

PERFORMANCE OF THE PROCEDURE
- Regardless of proper indications or informed consent, if the intervention is carried out in substandard fashion, the practitioner has violated the standard of care.

- Procedures should be carried out in a manner consistent with current textbooks and/or teachings.
- From the legal perspective, the more information documented about the performance of the procedure, the better.
- Many practitioners use legally accepted templates to document their procedures. Practitioners should always have the opportunity to individualize a template, however, when unusual events occur during an intervention.

COMPLICATIONS

- Complications can be expected to occur in any busy interventional practice.
- How the patient is managed following an alleged complication is often critical to the patient's outcome and to avoiding a possible medical malpractice suit or receiving a favorable verdict should one be filed.
- The first step is to listen fully and completely to the patient's complaint. Many physicians become defensive because they fail to realize that the patient is not trying to place blame but, instead, is simply trying to understand the situation.
- The physician should never compromise his or her honesty and integrity. If a complication occurs, it is almost always in the physician's best interest to acknowledge all of the facts and be straightforward and truthful with the patient.
- Patients generally want to know the cause of the complication, and the physician should explain that this is being explored.
- Often the cause of the complication cannot be clearly ascertained, particularly in the immediate postprocedural period.
- Sometimes, there is a causal relationship between the procedure and the event. This does not imply that a breach in the standard of care occurred. If the physician is clear about the cause, he or she should explain it to the patient after careful reflection and assimilation of the facts. It is usually better to wait several days or weeks and deliver accurate information to the patient and/or patient's family than to retract erroneous information given in haste.
- Maintaining a dialogue with the patient and/or patient's family is important as is keeping the patient coming for follow-up, which allows the interventionalist to maintain continuity of care.
- Continuing the doctor/patient relationship can be strained, particularly in the initial months following an event or if there is a lack of agreement on the facts, but it is often the best way to reach reconciliation and maintain a workable relationship.
- The physician should be very careful in discussions with patients and/or family members after an alleged complication. The relationship of a procedure to a complication may seem intuitive, but a true cause-and-effect relationship may not exist. For example, if a patient dies during a nerve block, the patient's family (and possibly the physician) may assume the procedure caused the death; however, a myocardial infarction, stroke, or malignant ventricular dysrhythmia may have been the actual cause. The physician should avoid accepting blame for an event until all the facts have been accumulated.

REFERENCES

1. **Wipf JE, Deyo RA.** Low back pain. *Med Clin North Am.* 1995;79:231.
2. **Manchikanti L, et al.** Evidence-based practice guidelines for interventional techniques in the management of chronic spinal pain. *Pain Physician.* 2003;6:3.
3. **Fishman SM, Smith H, Meleger A, Seibert JA.** Radiation safety in pain medicine. *Reg Anesth Pain Med.* 2002;27:296.
4. **Kotani N, Kashikata T, Hashimoto H, et al.** Intrathecal methylprednisolone for intractable postherpetic neuralgia. *N Engl J Med.* 2000;343:1514.
5. **Benzon HT, Gisson AJ, Strichartz GR, et al.** The effect of polyethylene glycol on mammalian nerve impulses. *Anesth Analg.* 1987;66:553.
6. **Nelson D.** Arachnoiditis from intrathecally given corticosteroids in the treatment of multiple sclerosis. *Arch Neurol.* 1976;33:373.
7. **Horlocker TT, Wedel DJ, Schroeder DR, et al.** Preoperative antiplatelet therapy does not increase the risk of spinal hematoma associated with regional anesthesia. *Anesth Analg.* 1995;80:303.
8. **Horlocker TT, Bajwa ZH, Ashraf Z, et al.** Risk assessment of hemorrhagic complications associated with nonsteroidal anti-inflammatory medications in ambulatory pain clinic patients undergoing epidural steroid injection. *Anesth Analg.* 2002;95:1691.
9. **Horlocker TT, Wedel DJ.** Neuraxial block and low-molecular-weight heparin: Balancing perioperative analgesia and thromboprophylaxis. *Reg Anesth Pain Med.* 1998;23 (6, Suppl 2):164.
10. **Swerdlow M.** Medico-legal aspects of complications following pain relieving blocks. *Pain.* 1982;13:321.
11. **Johnson SH.** Providing relief to those in pain: A retrospective on the scholarship and impact of the Mayday project. *J Law Med Ethics.* 2003;31:15.
12. **Mendelson G, Mendelson D.** Legal aspects of the management of chronic pain. *Med J Aus.* 1991;155:640.
13. **Vincent C, Young M, Phillips A.** Why do people sue doctors? A study of patients and relatives taking legal action. *Lancet.* 1994;343:1609.

47 ACUPUNCTURE

Albert Y. Leung, MD

INTRODUCTION

- Acupuncture is an ancient treatment modality for a variety of illnesses.
- Currently, in the United States, there are more than 3000 physicians (MD or OD) using acupuncture as a means of alternative therapy for different illnesses including chronic pain and cancer-related symptom management.
- Although the empirical principles that govern the practice of acupuncture are based largely on metaphysical doctrines within traditional Chinese medicine (TCM), the latest evidence from basic science research and controlled clinical trials in both the Eastern and Western medicine literature has provided insightful information regarding the clinical indications for and neurophysiologic mechanisms of acupuncture. In addition, this readily available information further facilitates the integration of acupuncture as a therapeutic tool into mainstream medicine.

HISTORICAL BACKGROUND

TRADITIONAL CHINESE MEDICINE

- It is estimated that acupuncture was first used in China 4000 to 5000 years ago.
- This modality of treatment was considered an integral part of TCM.
- *Huangdi Neijiang* (*Yellow Emperor's Classic of Internal Medicine*), published in 200 BC, was the first textbook that systematically described the concept of TCM and the principles that govern the practice of acupuncture.

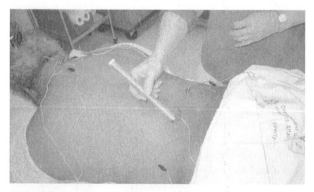

FIGURE 47–1 Electroacupuncture with moxibustion.

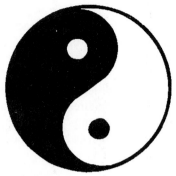

FIGURE 47–2 As perceived in traditional Chinese medicine, the symbol of Yin–Yang represents the duality that exists in nature, an imbalance of which leads to illness.

- With the advancement of medicinal tools throughout the history of civilization, different materials including stones, bronze, silver, and gold were used as tools in the practice of acupuncture. In addition, different methods of needle stimulation including manual manipulation, moxibustion (lighted sticks of an herb medicine, *artemis vulgaris*) (Figure 47–1), heat, and electroacupuncture (EA) have been applied to this ancient therapeutic technique.

MERIDIANS AND QI

- In TCM, the human body is considered a miniature model of the universe. Therefore, the laws and principles that govern the universe similarly regulate the human body.
- The main principles that form the foundation of TCM include Yin–Yang and the Five Elements.
  - The Yin–Yang principle is an expression of the duality that exists in nature; an imbalance in the duality was therefore thought to be the cause of illness (Figure 47–2).
  - The Five Elements principle, which embodies the elements of fire, earth, metal, water, and wood, is a system that complements the Yin–Yang principle. Within the Five Elements principle, each element exerts its unique regulatory effect on the other elements. The energy that exists or flows within these systems is called *Qi*. Furthermore, the channels that conduct the flow of Qi are called *meridians* (Figure 47–3).
- In TCM, the occurrence of illness is thought to be due to an imbalance in Qi, which can be either in excess or in a deficient state.
- By manipulating the acupuncture points along the meridians, one can correct the imbalance in Qi and thus reestablish the overall well-being of an individual.

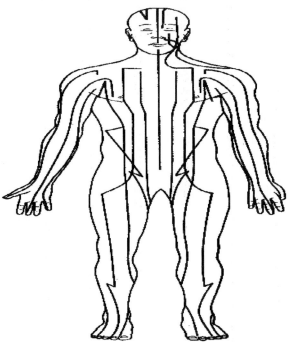

FIGURE 47–3 Distribution of classic acupuncture meridians, the channels in which Qi flows.

ACUPUNCTURE POINTS

- It has been estimated that there are approximately 360 classic acupuncture points in the human body.
- Although it is unclear how these points are selected, they appear to share some of the following characteristics:
  ○ Tenderness on palpation
  ○ High electrical conductance
  ○ Fibrillation and fasciculation potentials with electromyography
  ○ Erythema on insertion of a needle
  ○ Paresthesia in distant parts of the body
- A previous study also found a greater than 70% correlation between myofascial trigger points and acupuncture points.[1]
- In addition, a high correspondence also exists between motor points and acupuncture points.[2]
- Practitioners with various training backgrounds in acupuncture are also using other systems of acupuncture points including the ear (Figure 47–4), hand, and scalp.

ACUPUNCTURE IN THE UNITED STATES

- Despite the early acceptance of acupuncture as an alternative therapy in most Asian and European countries, acupuncture did not receive the same degree of attention in the United States until the early 1970s.

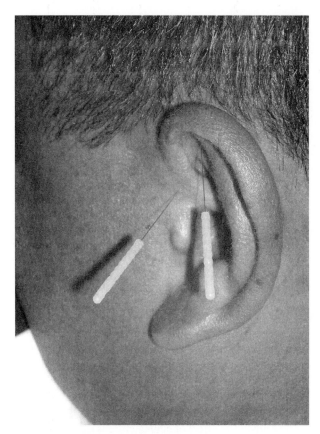

FIGURE 47–4 Auricular acupuncture.

- A report by James Reston of the *New York Times,* which described his own experience with pain and nausea relief with acupuncture after undergoing an appendectomy in China, prompted widespread interest in acupuncture in the United States.
- Since then, the National Institutes of Health (NIH) has funded several projects to study the mechanisms of acupuncture.
- In 1998, after reviewing current acupuncture-related literature, a panel of experts from NIH concluded that acupuncture is "effective" in two conditions: postoperative or postchemotherapy nausea and dental pain. In addition, the panel also concluded that acupuncture "may be effective" in a few other conditions as an adjunct treatment or an acceptable alternative therapy, which can be included in a comprehensive management program[3] (Table 47–1).

NEUROHUMORAL MECHANISM OF ACUPUNCTURE

PLACEBO OR NOT

- Because of the empirical nature of the principles that govern the use of acupuncture, the clinical effect of

TABLE 47–1 Summary of NIH Panel Consensus on the Efficacy of Acupuncture, 1998

Effective
   Adult postoperative and postchemotherapy nausea and vomiting
   Postoperative dental pain
May be effective
   Addiction
   Stroke rehabilitation
   Headache
   Menstrual cramps
   Tennis elbow
   Fibromyalgia
   Myofascial pain
   Osteoarthritis
   Low back pain
   Carpal tunnel syndrome
   Asthma

acupuncture has been doubted by some as a purely placebo response.

- Several lines of evidence provide strong arguments against this notion.
  - For example, acupuncture has been used in veterinary medicine in both surgical anesthesia and treatment of illness.
  - Numerous reports exist regarding the use of acupuncture in pediatric patients.
  - The analgesic effect of acupuncture is partially naloxone-reversible in both human and animal studies.
- All of this evidence argues against the notion that the clinical benefits of acupuncture observed for the past several thousand years represent a purely placebo effect.
- More recently, it has been postulated that the observed empirical clinical effect of acupuncture is mediated through a complex neurohumoral mechanism that involves both the peripheral and central nervous systems.
- There is evidence from both animal and human studies that supports a regulatory effect of acupuncture via the neuroenodocrinal system.

PERIPHERAL MECHANISM

- The modality specificity of different peripheral sensory fibers, namely, Aβ, Aδ, and C fibers, is well described in the literature.
  - Broadly speaking, high-frequency, low-threshold mechanostimulation is transmitted by the myelinated Aβ fibers.
  - Cool, well-localized pain is carried by the less myelinated Aδ fiber, whereas warm, hot, and cold pain sensations are carried by the unmyelinated C fiber.[4,5]

- Activation of myelinated primary afferent fibers (Aβ fibers) inhibits small unmyelinated primary afferent fibers (C fibers).
- It is known that acupuncture needles inserted into the skin, the subcutaneous tissue, and the deeper structures of fascia, muscle, tendon, and periosteum appear to stimulate primarily small myelinated Aδ afferent nerve fibers.
- High-frequency, low-intensity stimulation leads to a segmental inhibitory effect.
- Examples of such treatment modalities include high-frequency acupuncture and transcutaneous electrical nerve stimulation (TENS). However, unlike acupuncture, high-frequency TENS is usually not well tolerated in patients.
- Extrasegmental and suprasegmental inhibitory effects via the activation of descending inhibitory pathways of acupuncture can be achieved with high-intensity, low-frequency EA stimulation.

CENTRAL NEUROMODULATORY MECHANISM

- Although the exact central neuronal mechanism of acupuncture is still a matter of investigation, several central mechanisms have been proposed for the clinical benefits observed with acupuncture treatment.
- These mechanisms can be broadly classified as either endorphinergic or nonendorphinergic.

ENDORPHINERGIC SYSTEM

- Several lines of evidence strongly support β-endorphin involvement as the main mechanism of acupuncture analgesia.
- In a cross-perfusion experiment, an acupuncture-induced analgesic effect was transferred from the donor rabbit to the recipient rabbit when the cerebrospinal fluid (CSF) was transferred. In addition, the effect of acupuncture analgesia can be reversed with naloxone, and inhibition of the degradation of met-enkephalin by D-phenylalanine or D-leucine enhances the acupuncture analgesic effect, providing further evidence of endorphin system involvement.[6]
- Subsequent studies demonstrated that the release of different subtypes of endorphins appears to be frequency dependent. For example, antisera to met-enkephalin, dynorphin A, and dynorphin B reduce 2-, 15-, and 100-Hz acupuncture effects, respectively, suggesting frequency-dependent endorphin release in response to EA.[7]

- Evidence also suggests that EA analgesia is mediated through the periadqueductal gray (PAG) and shares some of the common descending inhibitory mechanisms of the exogenous opioids.
- The effect of acupuncture in managing withdrawal symptoms of narcotic addicts further implicates the endorphinergic mechanism of acupuncture.

NONENDORPHINERGIC MECHANISM
- The vasodilatory effect of acupuncture is blocked by the serotonin antagonist (cyproheptadine) but not by naloxone.
- On the other hand, inhibition of serotonin inactivation by clomipramine enhances acupuncture-induced analgesia.
- Acupuncture has also been shown to increase plasma cortisol levels in horses and induce the release of both endorphins and adrenocorticotropic hormones.[8]
- Such an effect appears to be bilateral and to have a nonsegmental craniocaudal gradient, and is non-naloxone-reversible.
- This result suggests the serotonin and sympathetic inhibitory mechanisms of acupuncture.

LATEST RESEARCH IN ACUPUNCTURE

- The neurophysical linkage of the neurohumoral mechanism of acupuncture at the supraspinal level is further supported by the latest research using functional MRI (fMRI) in which needle manipulation on either hand produces prominent decreases in fMRI signals in the nucleus accumbens, amygdala, hippocampus, parahippocampus, hypothalamus, ventral tegmental area, anterior cingulate gyrus, caudate, putamen, temporal pole, and insula. This preliminary evidence suggests that acupuncture may modulate the hypothalamus–limbic system and subcortical gray structures of the human brain.[9]
- In a more recent study investigating the neuronal specificity of acupuncture, both sham and real EA activated the reported distributed pain neuromatrix. However, real EA elicited significantly higher activation than sham EA over the hypothalamus and primary somatosensory–motor cortex and deactivation over the rostral segment of anterior cingulate cortex, suggesting the higher neuromodulatory effect of meridian points compared with the non-meridian points in the hypothalamus–limbic system.[10]
- Furthermore, the ability of EA to modulate expression of the c-*fos* gene in the central nervous system further substantiates the neurohumoral mechanism and the neuromodulatory effect of acupuncture analgesia.

CLINICAL APPLICATIONS

ACUTE INJURY PAIN

- According to the classic acupuncture literature, the anatomy of acupuncture is divided into different channels, so-called *meridians*, within which lie specific acupuncture points.
- The tendinomuscular meridian subsystem is located on the surface of the body.
- The tendinomuscular meridians can be used for treatment of pain, swelling, contraction, spasm, and other forms of acute trauma.
- The best results of this method of acupuncture are obtained when patients are treated within 12 to 24 hours of the injury.
- There are 12 tendinomuscular meridians, each starting at a toe tip or fingertip.
- The tendinomuscular meridians can be activated by:
  - Stimulating the point(s), that is Ting point(s), on the extremity with the tonification technique (turning a needle in clockwise rotations) to activate the meridian(s) transversing the lesion.
  - Stimulating the gathering point(s) appropriate for the meridian(s) using the neutral technique (turning a needle in alternating clockwise and counterclockwise rotations).
  - Surrounding the lesion with superficially placed needles.[11]

PERIOPERATIVE PERIOD

- Based on the NIH Consensus Conference in 1998, it is concluded that acupuncture can alleviate dental pain and postoperative nausea.
- In addition, it has been demonstrated that EA can decrease the postoperative opioid requirement and reduce analgesic-related side effects in low abdominal surgery.
- Anecdotal reports also indicate that acupuncture has been used in other types of surgical procedures such as craniotomy, tonsillectomy, thyroidectomy, and labor-related procedures either as a means of supplemental anesthesia or as a tool for managing postoperative associated side effects.

CHRONIC PAIN

- The use of acupuncture in chronic pain management is probably one of the most thoroughly studied areas in medicine.

- Acupuncture has been used to treat a variety of chronic pain conditions. Some of these chronic pain conditions have been studied more extensively than the others.
- For instance, in a randomized, single-blinded sham–controlled study, percutaneous electrical nerve stimulation (PENS) given with acupuncture needles was found to be significantly more effective in decreasing Visual Analog Scale (VAS) pain scores after each treatment than sham PENS, TENS, and exercise therapies with a decreased opioid requirement (Figure 47–5). Compared with the other three modalities, 91% of the patients reported that PENS was the most effective in decreasing their low back pain. PENS therapy was also significantly more effective in improving physical activity, quality of sleep, and sense of well-being. The SF-36 survey confirmed that PENS improved posttreatment function more than sham PENS, TENS, and exercise.

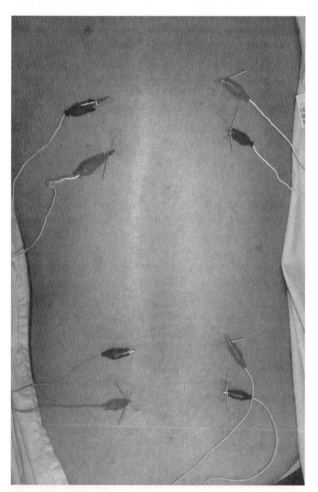

FIGURE 47–5 Percutaneous electrical nerve stimulation (PENS), a form of electroacupuncture for chronic low back pain.

The results of the same study suggested that PENS was more effective than TENS or exercise therapy in providing short-term pain relief and improved physical function in patients with long-term low back pain.[12]

- PENS is also a useful nonpharmacologic therapeutic modality for treating diabetic neuropathic pain. In addition to decreasing extremity pain, PENS therapy improves physical activity, sense of well-being, and quality of sleep while reducing the need for oral nonopioid analgesic medication.[13]
- Electrical stimulation at the specific dermatomal levels corresponding to the local pathology produces greater short-term improvements in pain control, physical activity, and quality of sleep in patients with chronic neck pain.[14]
- Although large-scale clinical trials have yet to be conducted, there is moderately strong evidence that acupuncture may be effective for treating both osteoarthritis and fibromyalgia.
- In the area of chronic headache management, a recent meta-analysis of 27 clinical trials that evaluated the efficacy of acupuncture in the treatment of primary headaches (migraine headaches, tension-type headaches, and mixed forms) concluded that acupuncture offers benefits in the treatment of headaches. However, additional clinical research is needed to further confirm the efficacy and indications for use of acupuncture in treating chronic headaches.

PALLIATIVE MEDICINE

- Aside from cancer-related pain management, acupuncture has also been used in cancer-related symptom management.
- One of the major benefits of acupuncture is the antinausea effect in cancer patients receiving chemotherapy.[3]
- Xerostomia is also a common and usually irreversible side effect in patients receiving radiation therapy for head and neck cancer. In one study of 38 patients with radiation-induced xerostomia, 20 in the experimental group were treated with classic acupuncture and 18 patients in the control group received superficial acupuncture as placebo. Within both groups the patients showed significantly increased salivary flow rates after the acupuncture treatment. In the experimental group 68% and in the control group 50% of the patients had increased salivary flow rates at the end of the observation period. Among those patients whose salivary glands had all been irradiated, 50% in both groups showed

increased salivary flow rates (>20%) by the end of the 1-year observation period. The improved salivary flow rates usually persisted after the acupuncture was discontinued. In an open pilot study conducted to investigate the safety and efficacy of acupuncture in 20 patients who suffered from dyspnea due to either primary or secondary malignancy, 70% (14/20) of patients reported marked symptomatic benefit from treatment. In addition, there were significant changes in VAS scores of breathlessness, relaxation, and anxiety more than 6 hours postacupuncture. There was also a significant reduction in respiratory rate, which was sustained for 90 minutes postacupuncture.[15]

- In another controlled study, 48 patients with mammary cancer after ablation and axillary lymphadenectomy were treated with acupuncture. The results showed a significantly higher range of arm movement immediately after acupuncture without pain. Acupuncture appears to be an effective treatment to relieve pain and improve arm movement after axillary lymphadenectomy.[16]

ADVERSE EVENTS RELATED TO ACUPUNCTURE

- Compared with pharmacologic interventions, side effects associated with acupuncture are quite minimal.
- Various adverse events associated with acupuncture have been reported in the literature. These adverse events, although rare, include pneumothorax, infection, and spinal lesions.
- A recent study, however, demonstrated that acupuncture, if conducted with caution and given by adequately trained practitioners, carries minimal risk for patients.[17]
- In another study, a total of 391 patients were treated in 1441 sessions, involving a total of 30,338 needle insertions. The incidence of recorded systemic reactions in individual patients was as follows: tiredness (8.2%); drowsiness (2.8%); aggravation of preexisting symptoms (2.8%); itching in the punctured regions (1.0%); dizziness or vertigo (0.8%); feeling of faintness or nausea during treatment (0.8%); headache (0.5%); and chest pain (0.3%). Recorded local reactions included: minor bleeding on withdrawal of the needle (2.6%); pain on insertion of the needle (0.7%); petechia or ecchymosis (0.3%); pain or ache in the punctured region after the treatment (0.1%); subcutaneous hematoma (0.1%); and pain or discomfort in the punctured region during needle retention (0.03%).[18]

REFERENCES

1. **Melzack R, Stillwell DM, Fox EJ.** Trigger points and acupuncture points for pain: Correlations and implications. *Pain.* 1977;3:3–23.
2. **Liu Y, Varela M, Oswald R.** The correspondence between some motor points and acupuncture loci. *Am J Chin Med.* 1975;3:347–358.
3. NIH Consensus Conference. Acupuncture. *JAMA* 1998; 280:1518–1524.
4. **Yarnitsky D, Ochoa JL.** Warm and cold specific somatosensory systems: Psychophysical thresholds, reaction times and peripheral conduction velocities. *Brain.* 1991; 114(pt 4):1819–1826.
5. **Verdugo R, Ochoa JL.** Quantitative somatosensory thermotest: A key method for functional evaluation of small calibre afferent channels. *Brain.* 1992;115(pt 3):893–913.
6. Medical Group of Acupuncture Anesthesia PMC. The role of some neurotransmitters of brain in finger-acupuncture analgesia. *Scientia Sin.* 1974;17:112–130.
7. **Fei H, Xie GX, Han JS.** Differential release of met-enkephalin and dynorphin in spinal cord by electroacupuncture of different frequencies. *Kexue Tongbo.* 1986;31: 1512–1515.
8. **Kaada B, Eielsen O.** In search of mediators of skin vasodilation induced by transcutaneous nerve stimulation: II. Serotonin implicated. *Gen Pharmacol.* 1983;14:635–641.
9. **Hui KK, Liu J, Makris N, et al.** Acupuncture modulates the limbic system and subcortical gray structures of the human brain: Evidence from fMRI studies in normal subjects. *Hum Brain Mapp.* 2000;9:13–25.
10. **Wu MT, Sheen JM, Chuang KH, et al.** Neuronal specificity of acupuncture response: A fMRI study with electroacupuncture. *NeuroImage.* 2002;16:1028–1037.
11. **Helms J.** The tendinomuscular meridian subsystem. In: Helms J, ed. *Acupuncture Energetics: A Clinical Approach for Physicians.* Berkeley: Medical Acupuncture Publishers; 1995:103–130.
12. **Ghoname ES, Craig WF, White PF, et al.** The effect of stimulus frequency on the analgesic response to percutaneous electrical nerve stimulation in patients with chronic low back pain. *Anesth Analg.* 1999;88:841–846.
13. **Hamza MA, White PF, Craig WF, et al.** Percutaneous electrical nerve stimulation: A novel analgesic therapy for diabetic neuropathic pain. *Diabetes Care.* 2000;23: 365–370.
14. **White PF, Craig WF, Vakharia AS, et al.** Percutaneous neuromodulation therapy: Does the location of electrical stimulation effect the acute analgesic response? *Anesth Analg.* 2000;91:949–954.
15. **Filshie J, Penn K, Ashley S, et al.** Acupuncture for the relief of cancer-related breathlessness. *Palliat Med.* 1996;10: 145–150.
16. **He JP, Friedrich M, Ertan AK, et al.** Pain-relief and movement improvement by acupuncture after ablation and axillary lymphadenectomy in patients with mammary cancer. *Clin Exp Obstet Gynecol.* 1999;26:81–84.

17. **Yamashita H, Tsukayama H, Tanno Y, et al.** Adverse events related to acupuncture. *JAMA.* 1998;280:1563–1564.

18. **Yamashita H, Tsukayama H, Hori N, et al.** Incidence of adverse reactions associated with acupuncture. *J Altern Complement Med.* 2000;6:345–350.

48 BOTULINUM TOXIN INJECTIONS

Charles E. Argoff, MD

INTRODUCTION

- The botulinum toxins are products of the anaerobic bacterium *Clostridium botulinum*.

- There are seven immunologically distinct serotypes of these extremely potent neurotoxins, types A, B, C1, D, E, F, and G. Only types A and B are available for routine clinical practice.

- Two type A preparations, Botox (Allergan, Inc., Irvine, Calif, USA) and Dysport (Ipsen Ltd., Berkshire, UK), have been developed for commercial use, but only Botox is available in the United States at this time. Type B is currently commercially available as Myobloc in the United States and as Neurobloc in Europe.

- These neurotoxins are proteins and vary with respect to molecular weight, mechanism of action, duration of effect, and adverse effects. The bacteria synthesize each toxin initially as a single chain polypeptide. Bacterial proteases then "nick" both type A and type B proteins, resulting in a dichain structure consisting of one heavy chain and one light chain. Type A is nicked more than type B and there is less than 50% homology between the two toxins.[1]

- Traditionally most of the known effects of these toxins have been attributed to their ability to inhibit the release of acetylcholine from cholinergic nerve terminals; however, this effect does not appear to explain the apparent analgesic activity of some of these toxins.[2] Inhibition of the release of glutamate, substance P, and calcitonin gene–related peptide reduced afferent input to the central nervous system through effects of the toxins on muscle spindles, and other possible effects on pain transmission independent of the effect on cholinergic transmission of these neurotoxins have been proposed based on the results of laboratory experiments.[3–5] In particular, Cui and colleagues recently reported in a placebo-controlled study that subcutaneous injections of botulinum toxin type A (BTX-A) into the paws of rats before exposure to the formalin model of inflammatory pain induced significant dose-dependent inhibition of both the acute and secondary pain responses. In addition to the demonstration that glutamate release in the periphery is reduced in treated as opposed to control animals, inhibition of the expression of c-*fos* was observed in the dorsal spinal cord in treated animals but not controls. These findings suggest indeed that one of the botulinum toxins (BTX-A) very likely operates by noncholinergic mechanisms, which helps to explain its analgesic effect.[4]

- The mechanism by which acetylcholine is released by these neurotoxins is a multistep process. It is much better understood at this point than the mechanism by which these neurotoxins may exert their analgesic effects. The toxin must be internalized into the synaptic terminal to exert its anticholinergic effect. The first step in this process is the binding of the toxin to a receptor on the axon terminals of the cholinergic terminals. Each specific botulinum toxin serotype binds specifically to its own receptor irreversibly, and neither binds nor inhibits the receptor for other serotypes.[5] After the toxin is bound, an endosome is formed that carries the toxin into the axon terminal. The final step involves cleavage of one of the known synaptic proteins that are required for acetylcholine to be released by the axon. Botulinum toxins A, E, and C cleave synaptosome-associated protein 25 (SNAP-25). Botulinum toxins B, D, F, and G cleave synaptobrevin, also known as vesicle-associated membrane protein (VAMP). Botulinum toxin type C also cleaves syntaxin.[1] The specific manner in which each toxin type may cleave the synaptic protein, as well the specific differences in effect on inhibiting acetylcholine release, is beyond the scope of this chapter. It has not yet been conclusively demonstrated how these differences translate into varied clinical responses including both beneficial and adverse effects.

- Once the toxin is injected into a muscle, weakness occurs within a few days to a week and peaks most often within 2 weeks, and then gradually muscle weakness resolves with a slow return to baseline. This recovery is associated with sprouting of the affected axon and return of synaptic activity to the original nerve terminals. Regeneration of the cleaved synaptic protein is also required for recovery to occur.

- The duration of the clinical effect of the currently available neurotoxins appears to be approximately 3 months but may clearly vary from individual to individual.[3,6] Additionally, the possible differences in duration of action of these toxins for different clinical conditions, for example, cervical dystonia versus migraine headache, have not been well studied to date.[7]

CURRENT FDA-APPROVED USES OF THE BOTULINUM TOXINS

- The first botulinum toxin to be approved by FDA for use in the United States was BTX-A (Botox) in 1989. Although originally FDA-approved for the treatment of strabismus, blepharospasm, and hemifacial spasm, FDA subsequently approved it for the treatment of cervical dystonia and, most recently, the treatment of glabellar wrinkles.
- The second botulinum toxin to be FDA-approved, botulinum toxin type B (BTX-B), is currently approved only for cervical dystonia.[8]
- Even among initial published studies on the use of either BTX-A or BTX-B for cervical dystonia, the analgesic effect of these agents, for example, the ability for these toxins to reduce the pain associated with cervical dystonia, was observed. In fact, the analgesic effect of the neurotoxins appeared to have a greater duration of action than other more direct neuromuscular effects.[8]
- The discussion that follows on the use of either BTX-A or BTX-B in the management of painful states other than those noted above concerns the off-label uses of these agents.

USE OF THE BOTULINUM TOXINS FOR TREATMENT OF CHRONIC HEADACHE

MIGRAINE HEADACHE

- The botulinum toxins have been used for a number of different headache types with varying responses according to the individual study.
- Initially, Dr. William Binder, a plastic surgeon, rather serendipitously made the observation that many of his patients who had undergone BTX-A injections for the treatment of glabellar lines reported notable improvement in their headache control. As a result of this observation, he and his colleagues coordinated a multicenter open-label trial of BTX-A in patients with migraine.[9] Thirty-six of seventy-seven (51%) patients with migraine as defined by the International Headache Society (IHS) noted complete relief of their headaches with a mean duration of effect of 4.1 months. Twenty-seven of seventy-seven (38%) reported a partial response. The site of injection varied from patient to patient but generally included the frontalis, temporalis, corrugator, and procerus muscles, and, in a few patients, suboccipital muscles. The dose of BTX-A also varied from patient to patient. Except for brow ptosis, no significant adverse effects were experienced.

- Silberstein et al reported the results of a multicenter, randomized, controlled study of BTX-A involving 123 patients with IHS-defined migraine who experienced between two and eight severe migraine headaches each month. Patients were randomized to one of three groups: placebo, 25 units of BTX-A, or 75 units of BTX-A. Eleven standard injection sites were used including the frontalis, temporalis, corrugator, and procerus muscles. Bilateral injections were performed. Compared with placebo, 25 units of botulinum toxin type A resulted in significantly fewer and less severe migraine headaches each month, a reduction in the amount of acute headache medication used, and a lower incidence of emesis. There was no difference between the group receiving 75 units of botulinum toxin type A and those receiving placebo. No adverse effects were noted except for 2 cases of diplopia and 13 cases of ptosis.[10]
- In a separate study, Brin and his colleagues presented the results of a randomized, placebo-controlled multicenter study of BTX-A in migraine prophylaxis. Patients received injections in either the frontal and temporal regions, frontal region only with placebo injections into the temporal region, temporal region only with placebo injections into the frontal region, or placebo injections into both regions. Only patients who received BTX-A injections into both temporal and frontal regions experienced significantly greater pain relief than the placebo group.[11]
- A variety of other studies have been reported more recently primarily, however, as abstracts only. Nevertheless, some interesting observations have been made. In a study of 30 patients with IHS-defined migraine headache experiencing between two and eight attacks each month, patients were randomized to receive either 50 units of BTX-A or placebo. Fifteen injection sites were used including the temporalis, frontalis, corrugator, procerus, trapezius, and splenius capitis muscles bilaterally. Patients were followed for up to 90 days. Compared with placebo-treated patients who did not experience any significant change in headache frequency or severity, those who received BTX-A injections had a significant reduction in headache frequency (at 90 days, 2.5 versus 5.8, $P<0.01$) as well as severity. No significant adverse effects were noted.[12]
- In an open-label study evaluating the effects of BTX-A on disability in episodic and chronic migraine, treatment with 25 units of BTX-A (frontalis, temporalis, and corrugator muscles) resulted in decreased migraine-associated disability in 58% of patients.[13]
- Two retrospective studies have emphasized the potential benefit of BTX-A as a "disease-modifying" treatment for patients with chronic migraine.[14,15] Each of

these reports suggests (based on nonrandomized data) that increasing benefit may be experienced with repeated treatments with BTX-A for patients with chronic migraine. These clinical observations, although not derived from randomized, controlled studies, are important to consider as many injectors do in fact believe that for maximal benefit to be realized from botulinum injections, a patient may indeed have to be treated at least several times.

- Only one open-label study involving the use of BTX-B for the treatment of chronic migraine headache has been reported. Forty-seven patients with at least four migraine headaches within a 4-week period were treated with a total of 5000 units of BTX-B into at least three injection sites. Injection sites were chosen on the basis of pain distribution, "trigger points," and glabellar lines. Thirty patients (64%) reported improvement in headache intensity and severity. One adverse effect experienced with BTX-B treatment in this study that was not experienced by BTX-A-treated patients was dry mouth.[16]

TENSION-TYPE HEADACHE

- Several studies involving the use of botulinum toxin for the treatment of IHS-defined tension-type headache have been reported.
- Smuts et al completed a randomized, controlled study of 37 patients with tension-type headache. Patients received either 100 units of BTX-A or placebo into six injection sites: two in the temporalis muscles and four in cervical sites. By the third month postinjection, the treated group experienced a statistically significant reduction in headache severity compared with the placebo-treated group.[17]
- A retrospective study of 21 patients with chronic tension-type headache with concurrent tenderness of the scalp or neck was conducted by Freund and Schwartz. Five injection sites were chosen and the patient received a total of 100 units of BTX-A. The injection sites were chosen based on the sites of maximal tenderness as reported by the patient. Eighteen of twenty-one patients experienced at least a 50% reduction in headache frequency and 20 of 21 experienced at least a 50% reduction in scalp/neck tenderness to palpation.[18]
- Although several other clinical reports have documented successful treatment of a small number of patients, another small study by Zwart et al reported on six patients with tension-type headache who were treated with BTX-A and failed to show any improvement in pain intensity following injection.[19] One reason for this outcome may have been that in this study,

patients received injections only into the temporalis muscle unilaterally.

- In a small randomized controlled study of 10 patients with tension-type headache, BTX-A was no more effective than placebo.[20]
- Porta evaluated the difference in response between BTX-A and methylprednisolone injections in patients with tension-type headaches. Although both groups improved, patients who had undergone the BTX-A injections experienced improvement for a greater duration (>60 days) compared with the methylprednisolone-treated patients.[21]

CLUSTER HEADACHE

- There have been three reports of treatment of cluster headache with botulinum toxin.
- In 1996, a single patient with cluster headache refractory to other treatment was reported by Ginies et al to respond to the injection of botulinum injection.[22]
- Two patients with intractable cluster headache were reported by Freund and Schwartz to respond to the unilateral injection of 50 units of BTX-A into five sites within the temporalis muscle on the affected side. Within 9 days of treatment, the headaches abated for both patients.[23]
- Robbins reported in a open-label study that for seven patients with chronic cluster headache who were treated with BTX-A or BTX-B, treatment was at least moderately effective in four of the seven and not effective in three. He also treated three patients with episodic cluster headache with botulinum toxin and two had at least moderate improvement.[24]

CHRONIC DAILY HEADACHE

- One open-label study, one randomized, controlled study, and one case series have been reported regarding the use of botulinum toxin for the management of chronic daily headache (CDH).
- Four of five treated patients in an open-label study by Klapper and Klapper benefited from injections.[25]
- In a randomized trial of 56 patients with CDH, patients were divided into four groups involving both forehead and suboccipital injections. Only patients who received botulinum toxin injections into each region experienced significant benefit.[26]
- Argoff reported on three patients with CDH who were successfully treated with a total of 5000 units of BTX-B injected into the frontalis, temporalis, corrugator, splenius capitis, splenius cervicis, levator scapular, and trapezius muscles.[27]

USE OF BOTULINUM TOXIN IN THE MANAGEMENT OF MUSCULOSKELETAL PAIN

- Painful musculoskeletal conditions that have been treated with botulinum toxin include chronic temporomandibular joint dysfunction, chronic myofascial pain, chronic cervicothoracic pain, and chronic low back pain.

TEMPOROMANDIBULAR DISORDERS

- Botulinum toxin type A has been used for a number of the temporomandibular disorders including myofascial dysfunction affecting this joint, bruxism, oromandibular dystonia, and masseter/temporalis hypertrophy.[28]
- In an open-label study of 46 patients with chronic temporomandibular pain, Freund et al injected BTX-A into both masseter muscles (50 units each) and into the temporalis muscles (25 units each) under electromyographic guidance. Outcome measures that showed improvement included pain level as assessed by Visual Analog Scale (VAS) scores, interincisal oral opening, and tenderness to palpation. Approximately 60% of those treated experienced at least 50% improvement in these areas.[29]
- In contrast, Nixdorf et al completed a double-blind, placebo-controlled crossover trial evaluating the use of BTX-A in the management of chronic moderate to severe orofacial pain of myogenic origin. Similar to Freund and colleagues' open-label study, 25 units of toxin was injected into each temporalis muscle and 50 units was injected into each masseter muscle. Crossover occurred at 16 weeks. Pain intensity and unpleasantness were the primary outcome variables used. No significant difference was determined between placebo and active treatment in this study; however, only 15 patients entered the study and only 10 patients completed it, and these small numbers may have made it difficult to see a statistical difference between the two groups.[30]
- The dose of botulinum toxin used for treatment of the temporomandibular disorders depends on the size(s) of the muscle(s) involved, as well as the type of toxin used. For the temporalis and medial pterygoid muscles, the recommended doses of BTX-A are between 5 and 25 units in multiple injection sites. For the masseter muscle, the recommended dose of BTX-A is 25 to 50 units, also in multiple injection sites. For the lateral pterygoid muscle, the recommended dose of type A toxin is between 5 and 10 units.[28] For each of these muscles, the recommended doses of type B toxin are between 1000 and 3000 units, again with multiple injection sites within each muscle.[31]

CERVICOTHORACIC DISORDERS

- A number of studies have examined the role of botulinum toxin in the treatment of chronic cervical or thoracic pain most often associated with myofascial dysfunction.
- In their study of the use of BTX-A injections into cervical paraspinal, trapezius, and thoracic paraspinal muscles, Wheeler et al were not able to detect any significant differences in pain reduction between treated and placebo patients.[32]
- Freund and Schwartz, in their randomized controlled study of 26 patients with chronic neck pain following "whiplash" injuries, demonstrated a statistically significant reduction in pain for the patients treated with BTX-A compared with placebo. One hundred units of toxin was injected into five "tender" sites and these were compared with a similar number of saline injections. Improvement was noted after 4 weeks.[33]
- Cheshire et al injected myofascial trigger points in the cervical paraspinal or shoulder girdle area in six patients with either BTX-A (50 units spread out over two to three areas) or saline. In this randomized, controlled, crossover study, crossover occurred at 8 weeks. Four of the six patients experienced at least 30% pain reduction in response to toxin but not saline injections.[34]
- In a previous study by Wheeler et al, 33 patients with cervical myofascial pain were injected with either 50 or 100 units of BTX-A or placebo. No significant differences were observed between the two groups.[35]
- Using a novel injection technique, injecting the whole muscle in a gridlike pattern instead of the areas of tenderness only, and using doses of BTX-A ranging from 20 to 600 units, Lang, in an open-label study of the use of type A toxin in the treatment of myofascial pain, noted that 60% of patients experienced good to excellent results 22–60 days following injection.[36]
- In a 12-week randomized, double-blind, placebo-controlled study, 132 patients with cervicothoracic myofascial pain were treated with BTX-A or saline by Ferrante et al. No significant differences in outcome were seen between the groups. Patients receiving BTX-A were treated with 50–250 units of toxin total divided among five injection sites.[37]
- Porta, in a single-blinded study, evaluated the difference between lidocaine/methylprednisolone injections and BTX-A injections in affected myofascial trigger points within the psoas, piriformis, and scalenus anterior muscles. Doses of 80–150 units of

toxin were used. Each group received benefit, but the toxin-treated patients experienced a greater duration of relief.[38]

- Opida has presented 31 patients with posttraumatic neck pain who he has treated with BTX-B injections in an open-label study. Seventy-one percent of his patients noted significant reductions in pain and headache frequency and severity.[39]
- Taqi et al have shown in two separate open-label studies that either type of botulinum toxin may be effective in the treatment of myofascial pain.[40,41]
- Several case reports on the use of BTX-B injections in the management of chronic myofascial pain have suggested generally good results.[42–44]

CHRONIC LOW BACK PAIN

- Use of botulinum toxin in the management of chronic low back pain has also been explored.
- Foster et al, in a randomized controlled study involving 31 patients with chronic low back pain, studied the effect of 200 units of BTX-A (five sites at paravertebral levels L1 to L5 or L2 to S1, 40 units/site) compared with placebo injections. Pain and extent of disability were noted at baseline as well as at 3 and 8 weeks using the VAS scale as well as the Owestry Low Back Pain Questionnaire. At both 3 and 8 weeks, more patients who had received botulinum toxin injections (73.3%/60%) experienced 50% or greater pain relief than the placebo-treated group (25%/12.5%). At 8 weeks there was less disability in the botulinum toxin-treated group than in the placebo-treated group.[45]
- Knusel et al treated patients with low back pain associated with painful muscle spasm with different doses of type A toxin and noted that only those treated with the highest doses (240 units) experienced greater relief than placebo-treated patients.[46]

PIRIFORMIS SYNDROME

- There have been reports of the use of botulinum toxin for the treatment of piriformis muscle syndrome as well.
- Childers et al concluded, following completion of a randomized, controlled, crossover study of 9 patients with piriformis muscle syndrome who were treated with both BTX-A (100 units) and placebo, that there was a trend toward greater pain relief for patients receiving toxin as opposed to placebo. Electromyographic and fluoroscopic guidance were used for the injections.[47]

- Fannucci et al reported that 26 of 30 patients with piriformis syndrome who were injected with BTX-A under CT guidance obtained relief of their symptoms within 5–7 days.[48]
- Fishman performed a dose ranging study with type B toxin in the management of piriformis syndrome using electromyographic guidance and observed notable symptom improvement as well.[49]

USE OF BOTULINUM TOXIN IN THE MANAGEMENT OF NEUROPATHIC PAIN AND OTHER PAINFUL CONDITIONS

- The use of botulinum toxin for the treatment of neuropathic pain is quite novel and there are only a few reports describing initial results in the management of postherpetic neuralgia, complex regional pain syndrome, and spinal cord injury pain.[50]
- Although reduction of pain is not the usual primary outcome measurement used in studies of botulinum toxin and spasticity, a study of patients treated with BTX-A for spasticity by Wissel et al noted the analgesic benefit of this treatment for 54 of 60 patients treated.[51]

GENERAL CONSIDERATIONS FOR TREATMENT

- Currently, neither of the available botulinum toxins is FDA-approved for a specific painful state; therefore, use is in an off-label manner. Patients should be informed of such prior to treatment.
- Significant side effects are uncommon. Pain, muscle weakness, and a flulike syndrome have been reported. Spread of toxin has been noted, with weakness sometimes involving muscles that were not directly injected. Autonomic side effects appear to be more commonly seen with type B toxin.
- Contraindications to treatment with botulinum toxin include pregnancy (category C), concurrent use of aminoglycoside antibiotics, myasthenia gravis, Eaton–Lambert syndrome, or known sensitivity to the toxins.
- Treating more frequently than the recommended interval of 12 weeks may lead to the development of antibodies to the toxin, which may also be associated with the development of clinical resistance.
- There is no valid way to reliably and consistently convert doses of type A toxin to doses of type B toxin at present.
- The use of botulinum toxin for pain management is as part of a comprehensive treatment program that has been developed based on an accurate diagnosis.

- Current storage/handling recommendations for each of the toxins should be followed.
- Whenever possible, an injection technique including needle size that is the least likely to cause additional pain should be used.
- Guidance techniques such as electromyography, CT, or fluoroscopy should be used at the discretion of the injector.
- Prolonged observation following the injections is generally not warranted.
- Follow-up should be arranged for 4–6 weeks following injections.
- More than one series of injections may be required to achieve maximal analgesic response.

REFERENCES

1. **Settler PE.** Therapeutic use of botulinum toxins: Background and history. *Clin J Pain.* 2002;18:S19–S24.
2. **Simpson LL.** Identification of the characteristics that underlie botulinum toxin potency: Implications for designing novel drugs. *Biochemie.* 2000;82:943–953.
3. **Guyer BM.** Mechanism of botulinum toxin in the relief of chronic pain. *Curr Rev Pain.* 1999;3:427–431.
4. **Cui M, Li Z, You S, et al.** Mechanisms of the antinociceptive effect of subcutaneous Botox®: Inhibition of peripheral and central nociceptive processing. *Arch Pharmacol.* 2002;365:33.
5. **Simpson LL.** Kinetic studies on the interaction between botulinum toxin type A and the cholinergic neuromuscular junction. *J Pharmacol Exp Ther.* 1980;212:16–21.
6. **Meunier FA, Schiavo G, Molgo J.** Botulinum neurotoxins: From paralysis to recovery of functional neuromuscular transmission. *J Physiol (Paris).* 2002;96:105–113.
7. **Tsui JKC.** Botulinum toxin as a therapeutic agent. *Pharmacol Ther.* 1996;72:13–24.
8. **Lew MF.** Review of the FDA-approved uses of botulinum toxins, including data suggesting efficacy in pain reduction. *Clin J Pain.* 2002;18:S142–S146.
9. **Binder WJ, Brin MF, Blitzer A, et al.** Botulinum toxin type A (BOTOX®) for treatment of migraine headaches: An open-label study. *Otolgolaryngol Head Neck Surg.* 2000;123:669–676.
10. **Silberstein S, Mathew N, Saper J, et al.** Botulinum toxin type A as a migraine preventive treatment. *Headache.* 2000;40:445–450.
11. **Brin MF, Swope DM, O'Brien C, et al.** Botox® for migraine: Double blind, placebo-controlled, region-specific evaluation (abstract). *Cephalalgia.* 2000;20:421.
12. **Barrientos N, Chana P.** Efficacy and safety of botulinum toxin type A (Botox®) in the prophylactic treatment of migraine. Paper presented at: American Headache Society 44th Annual Scientific Meeting; 2002; Seattle, Wash.
13. **Eross EG, Dodick DW.** The effects of botulinum toxin type A on disability in episodic and chronic migraine. Paper presented at: American Headache Society 44th Annual Scientific Meeting; 2002; Seattle, Wash.
14. **Mathew NT, Kallasam J, Kaupp A, et al.** "Disease modification" in chronic migraine with botulinum toxin type A: long-term experience. Paper presented at: American Headache Society 44th Annual Scientific Meeting; 2002; Seattle, Wash.
15. **Mauskop A.** Long-term use of botulinum toxin type A (Botox®) in the treatment of episodic and chronic migraine headaches. Paper presented at: American Headache Society 44th Annual Scientific Meeting; 2002; Seattle, Wash.
16. **Opida C.** Open-label study of Myobloc (botulinum toxin type B) in the treatment of patients with transformed migraine headaches (abstract). *J Pain.* 2002;3(suppl 1):10.
17. **Smuts JA, Baker MK, Wieser T, et al.** Treatment of tension-type headache using botulinum toxin type A. *Eur J Neurol.* 1999;6(suppl 4):S99–S102.
18. **Freund BJ, Schwartz M.** A focal dystonia model for subsets of chronic tension headache (abstract). *Cephalalgia.* 2000; 20:433.
19. **Zwart JA, Bovim G, Sand T, et al.** Tension headache: Botulinum toxin paralysis of temporal muscles. *Headache.* 1994;34:458–462.
20. **Gobel H, Lindner V, Krack PK, et al.** Treatment of chronic tension-type headache with botulinum toxin (abstract). *Cephalagia.* 1999;19;455.
21. **Porta M.** A comparative trial of botulinum toxin A and methylprednisolone for the treatment of tension-type headache. *Curr Rev Pain.* 2000;4:31–35.
22. **Ginies PR, Fraimout JL, Kong A, et al.** Treatment of cluster headache with subcutaneous injection of botulinum toxin. Paper presented at: 8th World Congress on Pain; 1996; Vancouver.
23. **Freund BJ, Schwartz M.** The use of botulinum toxin A in the treatment of refractory cluster headache: Case reports. *Cephalalgia.* 2000;20:329–330.
24. **Robbins L.** Botulinum toxin for cluster headache. Presented at: 10th Congress of the International Headache Society; New York; 2001.
25. **Klapper JA, Klapper A.** Use of botulinum toxin in chronic daily headaches associated with migraine. *Headache Q.* 1999; 10:141–143.
26. **Klapper JA, Mathew NT, Klapper A, et al.** Botulinum toxin type A (BTX-A) for the prophylaxis of chronic daily headache (abstract). *Cephalalgia.* 2000;20:292–293.
27. **Argoff C.** Successful treatment of chronic daily headache with Myobloc (abstract). *J Pain.* 2002;3(suppl 1):10.
28. **Schwartz M, Freund B.** Treatment of temporomandibular disorders with botulinum toxin. *Clin J Pain.* 2002;18: S198–S203.
29. **Freund B, Schwartz M, Symington J.** Botulinum toxin: New treatment for temporomandibular disorders. *Br J Oral Maxillofac Surg.* 2000;38:466–471.
30. **Nixdorf DR, Heo G, Major PW.** Randomized controlled trial of botulinum toxin A for chronic myogenous orofacial pain. *Pain.* 2002;99:465–473.

31. **WE MOVE.** Practical considerations for the clinical use of botulinum toxin type B: A self-study continuing medical education activity. February 2002.

32. **Wheeler A, Goolkasian P, Gretz S.** Botulinum toxin A for the treatment of chronic neck pain. *Pain.* 2001;94: 255–260.

33. **Freund B, Schwartz M.** Treatment of whiplash-associated neck pain with botulinum toxin A: A pilot study. *Headache.* 2000;40:231–236.

34. **Cheshire WP, Abashian SW, Mann JD.** Botulinum toxin in the treatment of myofascial pain syndrome. *Pain.* 1994; 59:65–69.

35. **Wheeler AH, Goolkasian P, Gretz SS.** A randomized, double blind, prospective pilot study of botulinum toxin injection for refractory, unilateral, cervicothoracic, paraspinal, myofascial pain syndrome. *Spine.* 1998;23:1662–1666;discussion, 1667.

36. **Lang A.** A pilot study of botulinum toxin type A (BOTOX®), administered using a novel injection technique, for the treatment of myofascial pain. *Am J Pain Manage.* 2000;10:108–112.

37. **Ferrante M, Bearn L, Rothrock R, King L.** Botulinum toxin type A in the treatment of myofascial pain. Presented at: Annual meeting of the American Society of Anesthesiologists; 2002.

38. **Porta M.** A comparative trial of botulinum toxin type A and methylprednisolone for the treatment of myofascial pain syndrome and pain from chronic muscle spasm. *Pain.* 2000;85:101–105.

39. **Opida CL.** Evaluation of Myobloc™ (botulinum toxin type B) in patients with post-whiplash headaches. Paper presented at: American Academy of Pain Medicine's 18th annual meeting; 2002; San Francisco.

40. **Taqi D, Gunyea I, Bhakta B, et al.** Botulinum toxin type A (Botox®) in the treatment of refractory cervicothoracic myofascial pain (abstract). *Pain.* 2002;3(suppl 1):16.

41. **Taqi D, Royal M, Gunyea I, et al.** Botulinum toxin type B (Myobloc™) in the treatment of refractory myofascial pain (abstract). *Pain.* 2002;3(suppl 1):16.

42. **Nalamachu S.** Treatment with botulinum toxin type B (Myobloc™) injections in three patients with myofascial pain. Paper presented at: American Academy of Pain Medicine's Annual Scientific Meeting; 2002; San Francisco.

43. **Smith H, Audette J, Dey R, et al.** Botulinum toxin type B for a patient with myofascial pain. Paper presented at: American Academy of Pain Medicine's Annual Scientific Meeting; 2002; San Francisco.

44. **Dubin A, Smith H, Tang J.** Evaluation of botulinum toxin type B (Myobloc™) injections in a patient with painful muscle spasms (abstract). *Pain.* 2002;3(suppl a):11.

45. **Foster L, Clapp L, Erickson M, Jabbari B.** Botulinum toxin A and chronic low back pain: A randomized, double blind study. *Neurology.* 2001;56:1290–1293.

46. **Knusel B, DeGryse R, Grant M, et al.** Intramuscular injection of botulinum toxin type A (Botox®) in chronic low back pain associated with muscle spasm. Paper presented at: American Pain Society Annual Scientific Meeting; 1998; San Diego, Calif.

47. **Childers MK, Wilson DJ, Gnatz SM, et al.** Botulinum toxin type A use in piriformis muscle syndrome: A pilot study. *Am J Phys Med Rehabil.* 2002;81:751–759.

48. **Fannucci E, Masala S, Sodani G, et al.** CT-guided injection of botulinum toxin for percutaneous therapy of piriformis muscle syndrome with preliminary MRI results about denervation process. *Eur Radiol.* 2001;11:2543–2548.

49. **Fishman LM.** Myobloc™ in the treatment of piriformis syndrome: A dose finding study. Paper presented at: American Academy of Pain Medicine's Annual Scientific Meeting; 2002; San Francisco.

50. **Argoff CE.** A focused review on the use of botulinum toxins for neuropathic pain. *Clin J Pain.* 2002;18:S177–S181.

51. **Wissel J, Muller J, Dressnandt J, et al.** Management of spasticity associated pain with botulinum toxin A. *J Pain Symptom Manage.* 2000;20:44–49.

49 NEUROLYSIS

Richard B. Patt, MD

BACKGROUND

- Neurolysis (neuroablation) refers to the intentional injury of a nerve(s) by chemical, thermal, cryogenic, or surgical means with the intent of relieving pain or spasticity.
- Neurolysis is performed at various anatomic sites to relieve refractory cancer pain, but because of its associated risks, it has been used infrequently to treat pain of nonmalignant origin.
- In vogue until recently, neurolysis is less commonly invoked in today's practice due to:
  - The dissemination and acceptance of pharmacotherapeutic strategies and guidelines
  - The widespread availability of safe analgesics
  - Increasingly liberal prescribing practices
  - The development and improvement of reversible neuromodulatory approaches (spinal analgesics and electrical stimulation)
- Neurolysis is now considered to be best reserved for discrete situations characterized by refractory pain or unremitting medication-mediated side effects.
- Although the sophisticated use of analgesics and complementary approaches has reduced the applications for neurolysis, it remains essential in a small proportion of patients with refractory pain or side effects, especially in the context of cancer pain when quality of life is often more important than longitudinal functional status.
- Neurolytic techniques are not a panacea nor can optimal results be achieved when these techniques are instituted in isolation.

- Neurolytic techniques are optimally regarded as a single component of a therapeutic matrix that includes disease-modifying therapies, pharmacologic strategies, neurosurgical and neuroaugmentative procedures, and behavioral and psychiatric approaches.
- Although detailed algorithmic approaches to decision making have been proposed for neurolysis, their utility is limited by a lack of controlled trials and the multiplicity of highly individualized determinants that are a consequence of the complexity of pain and the invasive, and, thus, hazardous, nature of this treatment.
- Generally provided by anesthesiologists and neurosurgeons, these therapies are most commonly considered after a diagnosis of advanced, irreversible disease has been established.
  - In specific situations, neurolysis is occasionally considered relatively early in the course of a progressive painful disorder.

NEUROABLATIVE MODALITIES

- In actual practice, the modalities used to produce neurolysis are, in most to least common order, chemical, thermal, cryogenic, and surgical.
- Chemical neurolysis is generally performed with either 100% (absolute or dehydrated) ethyl alcohol or phenol compounded with contrast medium, water saline, or, for intrathecal use, glycerine.
- Chemical neurolysis is less commonly performed with:
  - Ammonium salt solutions (pitcher plant distillate) and chlorocresol
  - Glycerol (its use is confined almost exclusively to the treatment of trigeminal neuralgia of nonmalignant origin)
  - Butamben, which is not readily available clinically and was thought to be neurodestructive but now appears to produce its long-lasting action based on a slow-release depot mechanism of local anesthetic
- Radiofrequency thermocoagulation, initially almost exclusively the realm of neurosurgeons performing percutaneous cordotomy, is now considered whenever a long-lasting block of a discrete neural target is desired.
  - Although equipment is costly and the technique complex, thermoablation may lower the risk of undesired deficits encountered with chemical ablation by increasing control over the resulting lesion because electrical stimulation and other parameters increase accurate localization and untoward spread after injection is eliminated.
  - Chemical neurolysis is preferred for interventions that depend on disrupting a more diffuse neural network, such as celiac plexus block.

- Cryoanalgesia is less commonly employed because the probes are bulky and practitioners believe that durable analgesia is more difficult to achieve with this technique.
  - Cryolysis be preferred for patients with longer life expectancies because preservation of the underlying neural architecture may reduce the risk of postablative dysesthesias.
  - Freezing under direct vision rather than percutaneously may enhance accuracy and outcomes.

RISKS AND LIMITATIONS

- The risks and limitations of neuroablation include impermanence, neuritis, neurologic deficit, damage to nontargeted neural and nonneural tissue, and failure due to overlapping nerve supply.
- Careful judgment and scrupulous technique must be exercised to endeavor to relieve pain without producing unwanted effects.
- Neurolytic substances and modalities damage tissue relatively indiscriminately.
  - An overzealous application (volume, drug concentration, sites) may lead to excessive neurologic injury that may persist.
  - The potential for undesired deficits can be assessed in advance, although incompletely, with prognostic local anesthetic blockade.
  - Careful assessment helps identify patients in whom weakness will be well tolerated, including those confined to bed, those with preexisting motor deficit or bladder diversion, and those with pain sufficiently severe to render an involved limb useless.
- Damage to nonnervous tissue may occur, such as skin slough after peripheral neurolysis, aortic dissection during celiac block, or renal infarct during sympathectomy.
- Aberrant spread and indiscriminate tissue injury can usually be avoided by verifying needle placement with imaging technology, serial aspiration, observation for paresthesias, manual appreciation of tissue compliance, electrical stimulation, and/or test doses of local anesthetic.
- Due to plasticity and because cell bodies are usually spared, pain relief is rarely permanent and averages only 3–6 months in patients with stable disease.
  - This duration is often adequate or can be extended by repetition in the preterminal patient.
- Spotty or transient pain relief may occur due to sheltering of neural targets by tumor and scarring, failure to appreciate overlapping sensory fields, and inadequate neurolysis.
  - Durability is maximized by targeting alternate sites unencumbered by tumor burden, by extending

blockade one or two levels beyond the dermatomal distribution of pain, by maximizing lesions by increasing the concentration of the injectate, or by ensuring adequate exposure time.

POTENTIAL ADVANTAGES

- Treatment with a single intervention targeted to a painful lesion that does not require continued administration or maintenance therapy potentially reduces:
  - The need for multiple drugs to control symptoms
  - High-dose requirements
  - Collateral effects on unrelated organ systems
  - Drug-mediated side effects
  - Disruptions to quality of life
  - Cost
  - The need for frequent outpatient visits
  - The need for ongoing home health care
  - Disruption of patient and family routines
  - Unwanted reminders of illness and illness behaviors
- Neuroablative techniques are especially useful in rural areas, developing nations, and any setting where health care technology or delivery is limited.

NEUROABLATION VERSUS SYSTEMIC PHARMACOTHERAPY

- Many of the cardinal benefits of pharmacotherapy relate to the dynamic nature of cancer and its attendant pain ("moving targets") characterized by unpredictably variable patterns of progression, regression, and recurrence.
- In contrast to ablative techniques, pharmacotherapy that relies especially on opioid analgesics as its mainstay is:
  - Effective for pain arising from a variety of etiologies (eg, tumor invasion, radiation fibrosis, stomatitis)
  - Effective for pain maintained by a variety of mechanisms (eg, nociceptive, neuropathic, mixed)
  - Effective for pain that is anatomically and topographically diverse (ie, bilateral, midline, and multifocal or disseminated pain)
  - Effective in diverse populations with applicability of the same basic principles in patients who span a wide age range (very young though very old) and fitness/performance status (ambulatory versus debilitated)
  - Effective across disparate cultures
  - Not reliant on costly technology and equipment or extensive, specialized training that may not be readily available.

NEUROABLATION VERSUS REGIONAL (INTRASPINAL) OPIOID PHARMACOTHERAPY

- The attributes of spinal opioid therapy and systemic pharmacotherapy are much more similar to each other than to those of neuroablative approaches.
- The effects of spinal and systemic analgesics are reversible, titratable, applicable to a wide variety of pain in diverse populations, and do not involve tissue destruction with its potential for lasting effects.
- In contrast to neurolysis, intraspinal opioid therapy more often provides effective relief of generalized pain, widely disseminated or multifocal pain, and pain that is bilateral or midline and is much more often applicable to pain arising from the limbs that are mostly underserved by nerves of mixed sensorimotor function.
- Although both neuroablation and spinal opioid therapy are interventional and, thus, are associated with greater cost, technical expertise, and risk than noninterventional therapy, neuroablation requires little aftercare and few specialized resources. In contrast, the more demanding maintenance therapy required for ongoing spinal drug administration requires a commitment on the part of the clinical team, patient, family, and institutions, including the hospital, home care nursing, and compounding pharmacies.
- On this basis, neuroablation may be more practical than spinal administration in rural areas, developing nations, and hospices that emphasize "low-tech" care.
- Although the relative pharmacoeconomics are poorly characterized, neuroablation may reduce the cost of ongoing care.

NEUROABLATION VERSUS LOCAL ANESTHETIC BLOCKADE

- The indications for local anesthetic blockade are relatively narrow for pain in the presence of cancer and other irreversible medical conditions and include diagnostic, prognostic, and therapeutic nerve blocks for premorbid chronic pain, secondary muscle spasm, sympathetically maintained pain, urgent relief in pain emergencies, and chronic catheter-based infusion.
- Although the utility of local anesthetic blockade can be extended by relying on chronic infusion, such therapies are limited by many of the same factors that limit the utility of spinal administration.
- In general, when neural blockade is indicated in populations with established progressive disorders, neuroablation is most often considered when pain is due to ongoing tissue injury and is expected to persist.

INDICATIONS, PATIENT SELECTION, AND DECISION MAKING

- Even with expert use of noninterventional therapies, a critical 10–30% of patients with cancer pain benefit from invasive approaches, including neurolysis.
- Evidence-based decision making is difficult due to a lack of controlled trials.
- The literature suggests that failure of conservative therapy may be predicted by the presence of various clinical features:
  ○ Movement-related pain appears to be most important.
  ○ Other features may include neuropathic pain, cutaneous ulcerative pain, massive tissue distortion, recent tolerance to analgesics, a history of alcohol or drug abuse, and severe psychological distress.
- Applicability can sometimes be extended to patients with noncancer pain, especially in the presence of another advanced, irreversible, or progressive illness.
- Decision making must be carefully individualized and should not be undertaken urgently.
  ○ Despite indications, treatment is not always routinely available due to uneven training and concerns regarding liability.
  ○ Despite their hazards, most neuroablative approaches are adaptations of techniques used for local anesthetic blockade and, other than the need for careful preparation and exquisite attention to detail, are not excessively technically demanding.

LIFE EXPECTANCY

- Life expectancy cannot be reliably and accurately ascertained even by experts.
  ○ Disease stage (especially metastatic status), treatability and performance status, and clinician experience help predict probable survival.
- The effects of neuroablation endure an average of 3–6 months, with a wide range.
  ○ Duration of relief may be influenced by incomplete neurolysis, new pain due to disease progression, and/or iatrogenic postdenervation neuropathic pain (neuralgia).
- Although treatment can be repeated, the optimal time to intervene, especially with procedures that may produce new pain (peripheral neurolysis), is probably within 6–12 months of predicted death.
- Cryoanalgesia or radiofrequency thermoablation is probably more appropriate than chemical or surgical ablation in patients with extended life expectancies because injury is more discrete, and, with cryoanalgesia, underlying neural architecture may be preserved.

- Sympatholysis and, to a lesser degree, subarachnoid neurolysis are less frequently implicated as causing deafferentation pain and, as a result, may be considered more liberally in patients with longer life expectancies.

WHEN DEATH IS IMMINENT

- Consideration of neurolysis must be carefully individualized based on the nature and severity of pain, functional status, the likelihood of efficacy relative to more conservative measures, and the goals and expectations of the patient and his/her family.
- The provision of comfort is the guiding therapeutic principle.
- When possible, treatment associated with extensive preparation, discomfort, or recuperation or that places undue demands on limited resources should be avoided.
- Treatment with a significant degree of inherent risk may be more liberally considered when conservative measures have proven unsuccessful.
- For patients unable to walk, neurolysis (eg, subarachnoid neurolysis, epidural analgesia) may sometimes be undertaken at the bedside, often with gratifying results.
- In contrast, procedures that rely on radiographic guidance or other extensive preparations are avoided.

PAIN CHARACTERISTICS

- Neurolytic procedures are most appropriate and effective for discrete, well-localized pain in a single area that the patient can reliably identify, ideally with a single finger or hand.
  ○ When extended to provide coverage for pain that is distributed more extensively or that is present in multiple areas, treatment is more prone to fail and is associated with increased risk for undesired neurologic deficit.
  ○ The exception is visceral pain, which, although it is often vague and broadly based, is generally amenable to neurolysis.
  ○ Although diffuse, visceral pain is typically well circumscribed and elicits a reliable, consistent report.
  ○ Although performed on a limited basis, epidural neurolysis can be successfully employed to manage segmental pain covering a relatively broad topography (eg, hemithoracic pain associated with mesothelioma) with a relatively low risk of neurologic morbidity.
  ○ Although subject to even more restricted availability, transnasal alcohol pituitary neurolysis,

cordotomy, myelotomy, and other even more esoteric neurosurgical procedures are sometimes considered for refractory pain that is diffused but reproducible.

- Patients with vague pain ("I can't describe it; it just hurts" or "It feels bad all over") or whose complaints are inconsistent or change over time are poor candidates for neurolysis.
  - Such a presentation confounds selection of the optimal intervention.
  - Rather than nociception and pain, such complaints may reflect a global experience of suffering dominated by spiritual, psychological, and/or social components.
  - Other indications that expressions of pain may reflect global malaise include selection of all the descriptors offered by assessment tools like the McGill Pain Questionnaire or Brief Pain Inventory or selection of predominantly affective (emotionally laden) descriptors (eg, wretched, cruel, agonizing, miserable).
  - Nevertheless, psychological disturbances commonly accompany established painful disorders and are not specifically contraindications, but when these disturbances are prominent and pharmacologic control is feasible, it is preferred to neurolysis.
- Neurolysis is best reserved for pain that is limited to a single site.
- Cancer pain is, however, often multifocal, especially with progressive disease.
  - Even with multifocal pain, treatment can be considered if a single source of pain is dominant, anticipating that reducing the foremost pain complaint may facilitate control of secondary pain with conservative treatment.
  - Despite the presence of multiple lesions, many patients appreciate pain in only a single site, especially in the case of bone metastases.
  - The clinician should be aware, especially in this setting, that despite a single apparent site of pain, neurolytic procedures are associated with the risk that "new" pain will be unmasked once the primary complaint is eliminated, perhaps as a consequence of spinal gating mechanisms,
  - When feasible, a preliminary local anesthetic block may help exclude this possibility
- The customary biologic behavior of the underlying malignancy and the growth pattern of a tumor in a given patient are other factors to consider before proceeding with neurolysis:
  - With rapid progression, pain may exceed the topographic boundaries of what would otherwise have been a successful procedure, or, alternatively, with rapid systemic progression, organ failure and metabolic abnormalities (eg, hypercalcemia, anemia) may render the urgent need for an aggressive procedure moot.
- Despite an absence of controlled trials, clinicians agree that somatic or visceral pain appears to respond more favorably to neurolytic blockade than does neuropathic pain.
  - Although often relieved by local anesthetic blockade, neuropathic pain responds less frequently to the additional nerve injury that occurs with neurolysis.
- Absolute contraindications to neurolysis, other than inadequate informed consent, are few, and even relative contraindications are plastic in the context of imminent death.
  - In addition to those discussed above, relative contraindications include local infection; bleeding diathesis; spinal cord compression; and, due to the risk of bleeding, embolism, sheltering (when local tumor growth or scarring "shelters" or prevents access to the neural target, rendering treatment effects unpredictable), and the extensive spread of solid tumor at or along the site of the injection.

SPECIFIC NEUROABLATIVE PROCEDURES

PERIPHERAL NERVES

- With a few exceptions, blockade of peripheral nerves is generally avoided due to:
  - Risk of new pain secondary to higher incidence of neuritis (more common with alcohol than phenol)
  - Risk of weakness due to predominance of mixed (sensorimotor) nerves
  - Risk of failure due to overlapping sensory distribution
- With intercostal blockade:
  - The risk of pneumothorax exists, but incidence is low.
  - Neighboring nerves must be destroyed to account for overlapping innervation.
  - The risk of neuritis exists.
  - Subarachnoid neurolysis is an alternative in experienced hands and may produce a predominantly sensory block with reduced risk of neuralgia.
- For cranial nerves.
  - Alcohol, phenol, or radiofrequency ablation of the fifth cranial nerve or its branches and, occasionally, of the ninth and tenth cranial nerves is performed.
  - This technique is used for orofacial pain that is unresponsive to radiotherapy.

○ Although its availability is limited, gamma knife irradiation (which produces delayed relief) has been recommended.

SYMPATHETIC NERVES

• Blockade of sympathetic nerves is used to treat refractory visceral pain, sympathetically maintained pain, hyperhidrosis, and peripheral ischemia.
  ○ Successful treatment is associated with a very low incidence of new pain and no numbness or motor weakness.
• Celiac plexus or splanchnic nerve block is often considered early in the course of treatment for abdominal and back pain secondary to visceral or retroperitoneal disease and can be accomplished by a variety of approaches.
  ○ Although usually performed percutaneously by an anesthesiologist, injections can be performed at the time of surgery, and splanchnic nerves can be sectioned via thoracoscopy.
  ○ While partially controlled trials suggest that pancreatic cancer pain may not vary significantly with pharmacotherapy versus neural blockade, better performance status and fewer side effects, presumably as a consequence of reduced opioid burden, are common.
  ○ One double-blind, placebo-controlled trial of celiac block serendipitously suggested a significant survival benefit in treated patients.[1]
• The superior hypogastric plexus block targets the sympathetic system near the sacral promontory bilaterally and is effective for visceral pelvic pain with no reported complications.
• Surprisingly, reflex sympathetic dystrophy (complex regional pain syndrome) infrequently accompanies a diagnosis of cancer.
  ○ Thus, stellate ganglion ablation, which is associated with risks of brachial plexus injury, is rarely required.
  ○ Likewise, most lower-extremity oncologic pain is somatically mediated, creating little role for lumbar sympatholysis.

CENTRAL NERVOUS SYSTEM/AXIAL

• Intrathecal (subarachnoid) neurolysis is a time-tested intervention that, although infrequently performed in contemporary practice, is in many respects straightforward.
  ○ When coupled with scrupulous decision making and technique, treatment is associated with highly rewarding outcomes, especially for chest wall pain, since targeted fibers are so distant from the outflow to the extremities and sphincters.
• Serial epidural neurolysis has some proponents, but intrathecal injections of absolute alcohol or phenol and glycerine are usually preferred because their respective hypobaricity and hyperbaricity confer much more exquisite control over drug spread.

CONCLUSION

• Neurolysis has an essential role in the management of specific pain syndromes in well-selected patients, usually in the context of multimodal therapy including, especially, pharmacologic management.
  ○ The paucity of data from controlled studies on neurolysis is a major barrier to the development of scientifically supported algorithmic approaches to decision making that integrate a full range of treatment approaches.
• A critical need exists for studies that accurately characterize the role of neurolysis with respect to the role of the more thoroughly investigated pharmacologic approaches.
• To begin reconciling these issues, discrete controlled comparisons among different treatment techniques for a variety of clinical syndromes are indicated.

REFERENCE

1. **Smith TJ, Staats PS, Deer T, et al.** Randomized clinical trial of an implantable drug delivery system compared with comprehensive medical management for refractory cancer pain: Impact on pain, drug-related toxicity, and survival, *J Clin Oncol.* 2002;20:4040.

50 COMPLEMENTARY AND ALTERNATIVE MEDICINE

Maneesh Sharma, MD

INITIAL APPROACH

• Many therapies can be drawn from complementary and alternative medicine (CAM) to treat pain.
• These therapies are being increasingly used by the public, and many are now subject to the same rigorous trials as allopathic treatments.

- Evidence indicates that the number of patients visiting alternative medicine practitioners nearly doubled from 1990 to 1997.
- Educated patients and patients with severe pain conditions are most likely to use CAM.[1]
- This increased prevalence of CAM behooves us to learn about these therapies and, at the very least, "integrate" them into our clinical thought processes, if not into our practices.[2]
- *Integrative medicine* is the term used to describe combined allopathic and complementary modalities for treatment of pain and disease.
- CAM therapies can be safely integrated with ongoing treatments. Just like other treatments, use of CAM therapies requires attention to drug interactions, cross-reactivity, and side effects.
- Always ask patients about their use of CAM and stop all supplements before initiating invasive or surgical procedures.
- Encourage patients to avoid use of CAM during pregnancy.

DIETARY THERAPY

- Diet modulation can alter pain by mechanisms involving oxidant production and cytokine biology.

WEIGHT LOSS

- Evidence indicates that body weight increases with chronic pain and that early weight gain may increase incidence of chronic pain later in life.
- Unhealthy weight gain early in life may increase the incidence of chronic pain later in life.[3]
- Excess body weight is a multifactorial problem that has reached epidemic proportions in the Western world. Thus, weight control must be part of any pain treatment plan.[4]

RAW VEGETARIAN DIET

- Increases fiber and antioxidant intake.
- May help reduce symptoms of fibromyalgia.[5]

OMEGA-3 FATTY ACIDS

- *Source*: flax seeds, walnuts, and fish.
- *Active ingredient*: α-linoleic acid (ALA).
- *Mechanism of action*: decrease prostaglandin E2 (PGE2) and leukotriene B4 (LTB4) inflammation;

increase prostaglandin inhibitor (PGI2) and PGI3; cause vasodilation, platelet inhibition, and blunt inflammatory response.[6]
- *Indications*: studied extensively in rheumatoid arthritis, in which they reduce morning stiffness and number of tender joints.[7]
- *Risks*: increased bleeding time, decreased thrombus formation.

SOY

- *Source*: soybeans.
- *Active ingredient*: soy is the only dietary source of isoflavones (phytochemicals similar in structure to mammalian estrogen).
- *Mechanism of action*: metabolized to its biologically active forms (genistein and daidzein) by intestinal bacteria. Approximately 30–50% of the ingested isoflavone is absorbed, and serum levels increase in a dose-dependent manner.[8–10]
- *Indications*: can be used as a primary source of protein because it meets human protein requirements.[11] Soy enhances pain suppression by reducing inflammation and decreasing production of tumor necrosis factor α (TNFα) in macrophages.[5,12,13]
- Soy is an antimutagenic, antioxidant agent with anti-inflammatory and cardioprotective effects.[8–10,14,15]
- *Contraindications*: soy allergies or hypersensitivities, pregnancy, lactation, presence of estrogen receptor-positive tumors.

SOY OIL

- *Active ingredient*: polyunsaturated fatty acids.
- *Mechanism of action*: decreases pain by reducing pro-inflammatory eicosanoids and cytokines and reducing TNFα.
- *Indications*: Analgesia supported by findings of increased paw-lick latency in rats fed soy oil.

ANTHOCYANINS

- *Source*: bright pigments found in plants and fruits, such as tart cherries, blueberries, bilberries, cranberries, elderberries, and grapes.
- *Active ingredient*: anthocyanin.
- *Mechanism of action*: inhibits prostaglandin synthesis with anti-inflammatory and antioxidant properties.
- *Indications*: Growing evidence indicates that fruits and vegetables help reduce the incidence of chronic pain, cancer, and cardiovascular disease. Studies

show anthocyanin extracts to be better anti-inflammatory agents than aspirin, better antioxidants than vitamin E, and better inhibitors of cyclooxygenases 1 and 2 than ibuprofen. Anthocyanins may be effective for treatment of chronic pain, such as arthritis pain.

- *Contraindications*: none known.

SUCROSE

- *Source*: carbohydrates, principally from cane sugar and cane beet.
- *Active ingredients*: glucose and fructose.
- *Mechanism of action*: decreases nociceptive transmission in the central nervous system, enhances levels of opioid-induced antinociception, and reduces tolerance to morphine.
- *Indications*: analgesia. Sucrose use significantly reduced the crying induced during infant heel lancing for blood collection. Rat studies also show a decrease in paw withdrawal from a hot plate.
- *Risks*: dental caries, diabetes, coronary artery disease, obesity.

HERBAL THERAPY

ST JOHN'S WORT

- *Source*: a flower containing flavonoids, naphthodianthrones, and glucinols.
- *Active ingredient*: hypericin, available as 0.3% hypericin (ie, LI 160).
- *Mechanism of action*: inhibits reuptake of norepinephrine, serotonin, and dopamine.[16]
- *Indications*: superior to tricyclic antidepressants with fewer side effects for depression and dysphoria; minor wounds; AIDS.[17]
- *Risks*: decreases concentration of protease inhibitors in HIV patients; may potentiate monoamine oxidase inhibitors[18]; photosensitization.
- *Contraindications*: pregnancy, excessive exposure to sunlight.

GINSENG

- *Source*: *Panax quinquefolius*.
- *Active ingredients*: the saponin glycosides known as ginsenosides and panaxosides, steroidal compounds, and coumarin.
- *Mechanism of action*: Ginsenosides stimulate and inhibit the central nervous system and stimulate TNFα production by alveolar macrophages.

- *Indications*: cancer prevention and treatment, diabetes treatment, stimulation of immune system, to increase stamina.
- *Risks*: may cause adverse drug interactions with monoamine oxidase inhibitors; increase effect of insulin and sulfonylureas, causing hypoglycemia; inhibit analgesic action of opioids; antagonize effect of anticoagulants.

BLACK CURRANT, EVENING PRIMROSE, AND BORAGE SEED OIL

- *Active ingredient*: γ-linolenic acid (GLA).
- *Indications*: GLA (1–3 g/d) has some efficacy in patients with rheumatoid arthritis and breast pain.[19]
- *Mechanism of action*: astringent, sequestering, and anti-inflammation properties.
- *Risks*: may exacerbate temporal lobe epilepsy and manic–depressive disorder.

MYROBALAN

- *Source*: bark extract of the plant *Terminalia arjuna* native to India.
- *Active ingredients*: tannins, triterpenoid saponins (including arjunic and terminic acid).
- *Mechanism of action*: reduces triglycerides and cholesterol; may enhance elimination of cholesterol.
- *Indications*: beneficial to patients with ischemic heart disease and chest pain; some evidence to support its use as a treatment of heart failure. A randomized, controlled, clinical trial indicated it is better than placebo and similar to isosorbide mononitrate in preventing provocable ischemia on the treadmill test.[20,21]
- *Dose*: 500 mg tid.
- *Risks*: no contraindications or interactions. Related *Terminalia oblongata*, at high doses, is linked to dyspnea. Hepatic necrosis may occur at high doses.
- *Contraindications*: none recorded.

KAVA KAVA

- *Source*: plant (*Piper methysticum*) cultivated in the Pacific islands.
- *Active ingredient*: kava lactones (pyrones 5–12%), chalcones. The extract used in studies, WS 1490, contains 70% kava pyrones.
- *Mechanism of action*: acts in the limbic system; binds to GABA receptors and increases GABA binding sites; also inhibits norepinephrine uptake, antagonizes

dopamine, inhibits monoamine oxidase B, and decreases glutamate release. Kava kava has anticonvulsant, anti-inflammatory, and antiplatelet properties.[16]

- *Indications*: treatment of anxiety (70 mg tid), sleeplessness (210 mg qhs),[22] and menopausal symptoms.
- *Risks*: oculomotor disturbance; may potentiate alcohol and psychotherapeutic agents; and, rarely, liver damage.
- *Contraindications*: liver disease, pregnancy.

CAPSAICIN

- *Source*: pepper plant.
- *Active ingredient*: capsaicin.
- *Mechanism of action*: inhibits substance P.
- *Indications*: topical treatment of postherpetic neuralgia, inflammation, diabetic neuropathy.
- *Risks*: skin rash.

DEVIL'S CLAW

- *Source*: roots, stems, leaves of South African plants in the sesame family (*Harpagophytum radix, Harpagophytum procumbens, Harpagophytum zeyheri*).
- *Active ingredient*: harpagosidelts such as harpagoside are metabolized into harpagogenin, which may be responsible for decreasing inflammation.
- *Mechanism of action*: not clear.
- *Indications*: inflammation, rheumatism (50–100 mg harpagoside/d), pain, and appetite, bile, and gastric stimulation.
- *Risks*: may cause miscarriage.
- *Contraindications*: duodenal or gastric ulcers, gallstones, heart disease, pregnancy, use of warfarin.

WILLOW BARK EXTRACT

- *Source*: bark from branches of willow tree, *Salicis alba*.
- *Active ingredient*: phenolic glycosides (salicin, salicortin, piecin, fragilin, tremulacin, triandrin) and tannins.
- *Mechanism of action*: similar to aspirin but slower to take effect than aspirin.
- *Indications*: rheumatoid arthritis, inflammation, fever, headaches, influenza, myofascial pain.
- *Risks*: gastrointestinal irritation and bleeding; interaction with anticoagulants.

ASPEN OR GOLDENROD (PHYTODOLOR)

- *Source*: Phytodolor is 3:1:1 preparation of *Populus tremula, Fraxinus excelsior*, and *Solidago virgaurea* derived from common ash, aspen, and goldenrod.
- *Active ingredient*: salicylic acid derivatives, phenolic acid, flavonoids, and triterpene saponins.
- *Mechanism of action*: thought to suppress inflammation by inhibiting arachidonic acid metabolism via the cyclooxygenase and lipoxygenase pathways.
- *Indications*: musculoskeletal pain, inflammation, rheumatoid arthritis, optimization of muscle and joint function.
- *Contraindications*: Some people experience gastrointestinal upset, allergic reactions, and other less common adverse effects.

MARIJUANA

- *Source*: cannabis plant, *Cannabis sativa*.
- *Active ingredient*: Δ9-tetrahydrocannabinol (THC).
- *Mechanism of action*: agonist to CB1 receptors (ie, arachidonyl cyclopropylamide).
- *Indications*: used to manage allodynia and chronic hyperalgesia associated with cancer pain[23]; may improve pain, mood, and sleep.[24]
- *Risks*: hallucinations at high doses.
- Further research on THC and marijuana use is needed.

OTHER THERAPIES

GLUCOSAMINE

- *Source*: Glucosamine is an amino sugar produced from shells of shellfish and is a key component of cartilage.
- *Active ingredient*: glucosamine, a constituent of proteoglycans in cartilage.
- *Mechanism of action*: stimulates chondrocytes to produce cartilage.
- *Indications*: osteoarthritis, inflammation, progressive joint space loss.
- *Risks*: may increase insulin resistance.
- *Contraindications*: pregnancy, shellfish allergy.[25–27]

ACUPUNCTURE

- *Mechanism of action*: neurohumoral hypothesis suggests that pain relief is partly mediated by stimulating Aδ afferents and initiating a cascade of endorphins and monoamines activated by stimulating *de qi* (a sensation of numbness and fullness).[28] Only limited evidence supports acupuncture as better than no treatment or placebo.[29]

- Injection of bee venom into an acupoint may cause an anti-inflammatory and antinociceptive effect by stimulating a dormant immune reaction.[30,31]
- *Indications*: chronic pain.
- *Risks*: relatively safe. Serious adverse events are rare.[32]
- *Contraindications to bee venom*: allergy.

EXERCISE, YOGA

- Increases strength, flexibility, feelings of well-being, and vitality.[33]

MASSAGE

- *Mechanism of action*: relaxation and release of tense and taut muscle fibers; activates large afferent fibers, releasing endorphins.
- *Indications*: myofascial pain and muscle fatigue.
- One study found a significant difference between visual analog scale pain scores during rest and massage, but no difference was observed on electromyogram.[34]

TRANSCUTANEOUS ELECTRICAL NERVE STIMULATION (TENS)

- *Mechanism*: pulsed electrical activity over the skin on a painful area activates large afferent fibers stimulating inhibitory dorsal horn neurons and releasing endorphins.
- *Indications*: TENS is a useful adjunctive treatment modality that helps many with chronic pain. It reduces scores on scales measuring anxiety and improves sleep.[35,36]

REFERENCES

1. **Rao JK, Mihaliak K, et al.** Use of complementary therapies for arthritis among patients of rheumatologists. *Ann Intern Med.* 1999;131:409.
2. **Eisenberg DM, Davis RB, Ettner SL, et al.** Trends in alternative medicine use in the United States, 1990–1997: Results of a follow-up national survey. *JAMA.* 1998;280:1569.
3. **Lake JK, Power C, Cole TJ.** Back pain and obesity in the 1958 British birth cohort: Cause or effect? *J Clin Epidemiol.* 2000;53:245.
4. **Jamison RN, Stetson B, Sbrocco T.** Effects of significant weight gain on chronic pain patients. *Clin J Pain.* 1990;6:47.
5. **Yagasaki K, Kaneko M, Miura Y.** Effect of soy protein isolate on cytokine productivity and abnormal lipid metabolism in rats with carrageenan-induced inflammation. *Soy Protein Res (Japan).* 2001;4:65.
6. **Simopoulos AP.** Omega-3 fatty acids in health and disease and in growth and development. *Am J Nutr.* 1991;54:438.
7. **Kremer JM, Lawrence DL.** Dietary fish oil and olive oil supplementation in patients with rheumatoid arthritis: Clinical and immunological effects. *Arthritis Rheum.* 1990;33:810.
8. **Jha HC, von Recklinghausen G, Zilliken F.** Inhibition of *in vitro* microsomal lipid peroxidation by isoflavonoids. *Biochem Pharmacol.* 1985;34:1367.
9. **Wu ES, Loch JT 3rd, Toder BH, et al.** Flavones. 3. Synthesis, biological activities, and conformational analysis of isoflavone derivatives and related compounds. *J Med Chem.* 1992;18:3519.
10. **Anderson JW, Johnstone BM, Cook-Newell ME.** Meta-analysis of the effects of soy protein intake on serum lipids. *N Engl J Med.* 1995;333:276–282.
11. **FAO/WHO/UNU Expert Consultation.** *Energy and Protein Requirements.* Geneva: World Health Organization; 1985: series 724.
12. **Seltzer Z, Dubner R, Shir Y.** A novel behavioral model of neuropathic pain disorders produced in rats by partial sciatic nerve injury. *Pain.* 1990;43:245.
13. **Shir Y, Ratner A, Raja SN, et al.** Neuropathic pain following partial nerve injury in rats is suppressed by dietary soy. *Neurosci Lett.* 1998;240:73.
14. **Rossi AL, Blostein-Fujii A, DiSilvestro RA.** Soy beverage consumption by young men: Increased plasma total antioxidant status and decreased acute, exercise-induced muscle damage. *J Nutraceuticals Functional Med Foods.* 2000; 3:33.
15. **Schofield D, Braganza JM.** Shortcomings of an automated assay for total antioxidant status in biological fluids. *Clin Chem.* 1996;42:1712.
16. **Katzung BG, ed.** *Basic and Clinical Pharmacology.* 8th ed. New York: Lange; 2001.
17. **Linde K, Mulrow CD.** *St John's Wort for Depression.* Oxford: Cochrane Collaboration, Cochrane Library; 2000; Issue 2.
18. **Pisticelli SC, Burstein AH, Chaitt D.** Indinavir concentrations and St John's wort. *Lancet.* 2000;355:547.
19. **Little C, Parsons T.** Herbal therapy for treating rheumatoid arthritis. *Cochrane Database Syst Rev.* 2001;1:CD002948.
20. **Bharani A, Ganguli A, et al.** Efficacy of terminalia arjuna in chronic stable angina: A double-blind, placebo-controlled, crossover study comparing terminal arjuna with isosorbide mononitrate. *Indian Heart J.* 2002;54:1705.
21. **Dwivedi S, Jauhari R.** Beneficial effects of terminalia arjuna in coronary artery disease. *Indian Heart J.* 1997; 49:507.
22. **Pittler MH, Ernest E.** Efficacy of kava extract for treating anxiety: Systematic review and meta-analysis. *J Clin Pharmacol.* 2000;20:84.
23. **Iversen L, Chapman V.** Cannabinoids: A real prospect for pain relief? *Curr Opin Pharmacol.* 2002;2:50.

24. **Ware MA, Gamsa A, Persson J.** Cannabis for chronic pain: Case series and implications for clinicians. *Pain Res Manag.* 2002;7:95–99.

25. **Reginster JY, Deroisy R, Rovati LC.** Long-term effects of glucosamine sulphate on osteoarthritis progression: A randomized, placebo controlled clinical trial. *Lancet.* 2001; 357:251.

26. **Schenk RC.** New approaches to the treatment of osteoarthritis: Oral glucosamine and chondroitin sulfate. *AAOS Instruct Course Lect.* 2000;49:491.

27. **Deal CL.** Neutraceuticals as therapeutic agents in osteoarthritis. *Rheum Dis Clin North Am.* 1999;25:379–395.

28. **Sims J.** The mechanism of acupuncture analgesia: A review. *Complement Ther Med.* 1997;5:102.

29. **Ezzo J, Berman B.** Is acupuncture effective for the treatment of chronic pain? A systematic review. *Pain.* 2000; 86:217.

30. **Lee J, Kwon Y.** Bee venom pretreatment has both an antinociceptive and antiinflammatory effect on carrageenan-induced inflammation. *J Vet Med Sci.* 2001;63:251.

31. **Kwon Y, Lee J.** Bee venom injection into an acupuncture point reduces arthritis associated edema and nociceptive responses. *Pain.* 2001;90:271.

32. **Ernest E, White AR.** Prospective studies of the safety of acupuncture: A systematic review. *Am J Med.* 2001;110:481.

33. **Wood C.** Mood change and perceptions of vitality: A comparison of the effects of relaxation, visualization and yoga. *J R Soc Med.* 1993;86:254.

34. **Tanaka T, Leisman G.** The effect of massage on localized muscle fatigue. *BMC Complementary Alternative Med.* 2002;2:9.

35. **Richards KC.** Effect of back massage and relaxation intervention on sleep in critically ill patients. *J Adv Nurs.* 1998; 7:288.

36. **Fraser J.** Psychophysiological effects of back massage on elderly institutionalized patients. *J Adv Nurs.* 1993;18:238.

51 CRYONEUROLYSIS

Lloyd Saberski, MD

INTRODUCTION

- Cryoneurolysis temporarily destroys a nerve through the application of extreme cold.
- When a cryoprobe touches a nerve, the extreme cold degenerates the nerve axons without damaging surrounding connective tissue.

PHYSICS

- The cryoprobe consists of an outer tube and a smaller inner tube that terminates in a fine nozzle.
- The working principle of a cryoprobe is based on the expansion of compressed gas (nitrous oxide or carbon dioxide).
- High-pressure gas (650–800 psi) is passed between the tubes and released via a small orifice into a chamber at the tip of the probe. Expansion of the gas within the chamber causes a substantial reduction in pressure (80–100 psi) and a rapid decrease in temperature that cools the probe tip surface to approximately $-70°C$. This causes an ice ball to form around the exterior of the probe tip.
- The low-pressure gas flows back through the center of the inner tube to the console where it is vented.
- The sealed construction of the cryoprobe ensures that no gas escapes from the probe tip, handle, or hose.
- Larger myelinated fibers cease conduction at 10°C, which is before unmyelinated fibers cease conduction, but at 0°C, all nerve fibers entrapped in the ice ball stop conduction. The clinical difference is moot as long as the temperature is below –20°C for 1 minute.

HISTOLOGY

- Histologically, the axons and myelin sheaths of the neurons degenerate after cryoneurolysis (wallerian degeneration), but the epineurium and perineurium remain intact, thus allowing subsequent nerve regeneration.
- The duration of the block depends on the rate of axonal regeneration after cryolesion, which is reported to be between 1 and 3 mm/d.
- Since axonal regrowth is constant, the return of sensory and motor activity is a function of distance between the cryolesion and the end organ.[1]
- The absence of external damage to the nerve and the minimal inflammatory reaction following freezing ensure that regeneration is exact. Thus, the regenerating axons are unlikely to form painful neuromas.

INDICATIONS

- Cryoneurolysis is best suited for clinical situations in which analgesia is required for weeks to months.
- The median duration of pain relief ranges from 2 weeks to 5 months.
- Cryoanalgesia is suitable for painful conditions that originate from small, well-localized lesions of peripheral nerves, such as neuromas, entrapment neuropathies, and postoperative pain.
- The longer than expected periods of analgesia that have been reported may arise from the patient's

enhanced ability to participate in physical therapy or from effect of prolonged analgesia on the central processing of pain (preemptive analgesic effect).
- Sustained blockade of afferent impulses with cryoanalgesia may reduce plasticity (windup) in the central nervous system and decrease pain permanently.

TECHNIQUE

- Cryoablative procedures can be performed open or closed (percutaneous), depending on the clinical setting. For management of chronic pain, however, open cryoneurolysis should be avoided if the procedure can be performed percutaneously.

OPEN CRYONEUROLYSIS FOR POSTOPERATIVE CRYOANALGESIA

- Most frequently, open procedures are performed to contribute to postoperative analgesia.
- Under direct visualization, the operator identifies the neural structure of concern and applies the cryoprobe for 1–4 minutes. (The time required is determined by tissue heat, blood supply, and the distance of the probe from the nerve.)
- Care is taken not to freeze adjacent vascular structures.
- The cryoprobe is withdrawn only after thawing, as removal with an intact ice ball can tear tissue.

POSTTHORACOTOMY PAIN
- Intraoperative intercostal cryoneurolysis is an easily performed open procedure on intercostal nerves just lateral to the transverse process, before branching of the collateral intercostal nerve. (A closed intercostal cryoneurolysis is much more difficult to perform and carries the risk of pneumothorax.)
- Postthoracotomy cryoanalgesia is an effective means of treating incisional pain but is not effective for pain from visceral pleura supplied by autonomic fibers or for ligamentous pain of the chest secondary to intraoperative rib retraction.

POSTHERNIORRHAPHY PAIN
- Cryoablation of the ilioinguinal nerve will decrease analgesic requirements during the postoperative period.
- After repair of the internal ring, the posterior wall of the inguinal canal, and the internal oblique muscle, the ilioinguinal nerve on the surface of the muscle is identified and elevated above the muscle for cryoablation.

PERCUTANEOUS CRYONEUROLYSIS FOR CHRONIC PAIN

- Percutaneous (closed) cryoablation is the technique of choice for outpatient chronic pain management. It has the advantage of easy application with few complications.

TEST BLOCKS
- Cryoanalgesia for chronic pain syndromes should always be preceded by diagnostic/prognostic local anesthetic test blocks.
- A favorable result occurs when the local anesthetic injection decreases pain and the patient can tolerate the numbness that replaces the pain.
- Care must always be taken regarding correct anatomic placement of the needles. When necessary, fluoroscopic guidance should be used.
- The smallest amount of local anesthetic required to achieve blockade must be used.
- A tuberculin syringe injecting tenths of a millimeter at a time ensures that the local anesthetic does not contaminate other structures, which would obfuscate interpretation of the block.

PERCUTANEOUS CRYOABLATION
- To perform a successful percutaneous cryoablation, it is essential to achieve proper placement of the cryoprobe.
- The preferred introducers are large-bore (12-, 14-, and 16-gauge) intravenous catheters, with the size based on the size of the cryoprobe.
- The nerve stimulator located at the tip of the cryoprobe can be used to determine if the cryoprobe is near a motor nerve.
- The operator freezes the nerve for 2–3 minutes.
- Often, patients feel an initial discomfort as the cooling begins, but this should quickly dissipate.
- Prior to removal of the probe, the tip should be thawed to prevent tissue damage from an ice ball sticking to the tissues.
- In general, with closed procedures, two freeze cycles each 2 minutes in duration, followed by their respective thaw cycles, are sufficient.

INDICATIONS FOR CRYONEUROLYSIS IN CHRONIC PAIN

INTERCOSTAL NEURALGIA
- Percutaneous cryoneurolysis of the intercostal nerves can be used to treat a variety of pain syndromes, including postthoracotomy pain, traumatic intercostal neuralgia, rib fracture pain, and, occasionally, postherpetic neuropathy.

PAINFUL NEUROMA

- Painful neuromas are typically associated with lancinating, shooting pain and are exacerbated by movement or deformation of nearby soft tissues.
- A cryoneurolysis is considered after careful mapping has isolated a discrete pain generator (neuroma).
- In these cases, cryoneurolysis is most effective when the volume of local anesthetic necessary for analgesia during the test block was 1 mL or less.

PAIN ASSOCIATED WITH HARVEST OF ILIAC CREST BONE FOR FUSION

- This pain is often responsive to cryoablation in cases where more conservative therapies have failed.

CERVICAL AND LUMBAR FACET AND INTERSPINOUS LIGAMENT PAIN

- Because this pain is typically exacerbated with movement, physiotherapy programs frequently fail.
- Fluoroscopically guided cryoneurolysis can improve analgesia, range of motion, and rehabilitation.

COCCYDYNIA

- The test injection should be performed bilaterally and should provide short-term analgesia.
- To perform cryoneurolysis of the coccygeal nerve, the probe must be inserted into the canal and contact the nerve.
- Accurate placement of the ice ball is facilitated by using the 100-Hz stimulator and by gauging patient response.
- Care should be taken to prevent bending the relatively large cryoprobe when inserting it in the canal.

PERINEAL PAIN

- Pain over the dorsal surface of the scrotum, perineum, and anus that has not been responsive to conservative management can at times be effectively managed with cryoneurolysis from inside the sacral canal with bilateral S4 lesions.
- Insertion of the cryoprobe through the sacral hiatus up to the level of the fourth sacral foramen for placement of a series of cryolesions can provide good analgesia for 6–8 weeks.[2]
- Bladder dysfunction is usually not encountered.

ILIOINGUINAL, ILIOHYPOGASTRIC, AND GENITOFEMORAL NEUROPATHIES

- These conditions often complicate herniorrhaphy, general abdominal surgery, or cesarean sections.
- Patients present with a sharp/lancinating or dull pain radiating into the lower abdomen or groin. The pain is exacerbated by lifting and defecation.

- Significant care and time must be spent in localizing the nerve, and use of the sensory nerve stimulator is required.
- The difficulty with localization has led to frequent misdiagnoses of the pain generator. In an effort to improve the accuracy of diagnosis, Rosser et al developed a "conscious pain mapping technique."[3] In a lightly sedated patient, a general surgeon working with a pain management specialist performs a laparoscopic evaluation of the abdomen in an operating suite. This allows easy visualization of the genitofemoral nerve, lateral femoral cutaneous nerve, and other structures.

NEURALGIA DUE TO IRRITATION OF THE INFRAPATELLAR BRANCH OF THE SAPHENOUS NERVE

- This condition occurs weeks to years after blunt injury to the tibial plateau or following knee replacement.
- The nerve is vulnerable as it passes superficially to the tibial collateral ligament, piercing the sartorius tendon and fascia lata, inferior and medial to the tibial condyle.
- Neuralgia due to irritation of the deep and superficial peroneal and intermediate dorsal cutaneous nerves can occur weeks to years after injury to the foot and ankle.
- These superficial sensory nerves pass through strong ligamentous structures and are vulnerable to stretch injury with inversion of the ankle, compression injury due to edema, and sharp trauma from bone fragments.

SUPERIOR GLUTEAL NERVE NEURALGIA

- This condition arises from irritation of the superior gluteal branch of the sciatic nerve and is commonly seen following injury sustained while lifting.
- The superior gluteal nerve is vulnerable as it passes in the fascial plane between the gluteus medius and gluteus minimus musculature and can be injured by shearing between the gluteal musculature with forced external rotation of the leg and by extension of the hip under mechanical load.
- The clinical presentation consists of sharp pain in the lower back, dull pain in the buttock, and vague pain to the popliteal fossa.

CRANIAL NEURALGIA

- Facial nerves can be cryolesioned.
- As these areas are relatively vascular, it is wise to inject a few milliliters of saline containing 1:100,000 epinephrine prior to insertion of the cryoprobe introducer cannula and to apply a postprocedural ice pack for 30 minutes to reduce pain and swelling.

SUPRAORBITAL NERVE NEURALGIA

- This condition often occurs at the supraorbital notch.
- Vulnerable to blunt trauma, this nerve is often injured by deceleration against an automobile windshield.
- Commonly confused with migraine and frontal sinusitis, the pain of supraorbital neuralgia often manifests as a throbbing frontal headache.

INFRAORBITAL NEUROPATHY

- The infraorbital nerve is the termination of the second division of the trigeminal nerve.
- An irritative neuropathy can occur at the infraorbital foramen secondary to blunt trauma or fracture of the zygoma with entrapment of the nerve in the bony callus.
- Commonly confused with maxillary sinusitis, the pain of infraorbital neuralgia usually manifests as pain exacerbated with smiling and laughter.
- A referred pain to teeth is common, and a history of dental pain and dental procedures is typical.

MANDIBULAR NEUROPATHY

- The mandibular nerve can be irritated at many locations along its path.
- Commonly injured as the result of hypertrophy of the pterygoids after chronic bruxism, it can also be irritated by loss of oral cavity vertical dimension from tooth loss and altered dentition.
- It is often associated with a referred pain to the lower teeth.

INJURY TO THE MENTAL NERVE

- The mental nerve is the terminal portion of the mandibular nerve.
- Injury to this nerve frequently occurs in edentulous patients.
- This pain can be reproduced easily with palpation.

AURICULOTEMPORAL NEUROPATHY

- The auriculotemporal nerve can be irritated at a number of different sites, such as immediately proximal to the parietal ridge at the attachment of the temporalis muscle and, less commonly, at the ramus of the mandible.
- Patients often present with temporal pain associated with retroorbital pain.
- Pain is often referred to the teeth.
- Patients frequently awake at night with temporal headache.

FUTURE DIRECTIONS

- Cryotechnology offers promise for a wide variety of pain management needs.

- Its unparalleled track record for safety is remarkable.
- Its effective and safe use on sensory and mixed nerves contrasts with the radiofrequency technology that potentially produces deafferentation.
- The preemptive anesthetic effect may make this a technique of choice for "winddown" (calming the central nervous system during neuropathic pain states).
- Lack of controlled studies, lack of uniform training, and poor communication among providers have impeded widespread adoption of the technology.

REFERENCES

1. **Evans P.** Cryo-analgesia: The application of low temperatures to nerves to produce anesthesia or analgesia. *Anaesthesia.* 1981;36:1003.
2. **Raj P.** Cryoanalgesia. In: *Practical Management of Pain.* Chicago: Year Book Medical; 1986:779.
3. **Rosser J, Goodwin M, Gabriel N, Saberski L.** Patient-guided mini-laparoscopy. *Pain Clin.* 2001;3(6):11.

52 SPINAL CORD STIMULATION

Richard B. North, MD

INTRODUCTION

- The goal of spinal cord stimulation (SCS) is to relieve pain by applying sufficient electrical stimulation to cause paresthesias covering or overlapping the area(s) of pain without discomfort or motor effects.
- As a reversible "neuromodulation" or "neuroaugmentation" technique, SCS impairs vibratory sensation but does not affect acute pain or facilitate insensible injury.

MECHANISM OF ACTION

- The "gate control theory of pain," published in 1965, provided a scientific basis for the use of electrical stimulation to treat pain by proposing that a "gate" regulates transmission of pain sensations from the dorsal horn in the spinal cord to the brain. This gate opens when small fiber afferents are unusually active and closes when large fiber activity is dominant.[1]
- By selectively depolarizing large fiber afferents in the dorsal columns, SCS can close this gate without causing motor effects.

- The gate control theory, however, fails to explain the fact that large fibers can signal hyperalgesia.
- A frequency-related conduction block may interfere with signals at the point where dorsal column fibers split off from dorsal horn collaterals. This would explain why SCS patients prefer a minimum stimulation rate of 25 pulses per second.[2]
- Animal studies using clinical range parameters indicate that the sympathetic nervous system and GABAergic interneurons may play a role when stimulation relieves ischemic or neuropathic pain.[3]
- Validated computer-generated models that predict the distribution of SCS current flow and voltage gradients in the spinal canal and cord have revealed the potential involvement of the pathways adjacent to the dorsal columns and of the dorsal roots.[4]
- SCS changes the neurotransmitter and neurotransmitter metabolite concentrations in cerebrospinal fluid (CSF).
- Administration of the opioid antagonist naloxone has no effect on SCS efficacy.

PATIENT SELECTION

GENERAL INDICATIONS

- An established and specific diagnosis should exist for the pain.
- All acceptable, less invasive treatment options should be exhausted.
- Psychiatric comorbidities, significant drug habituation, and issues of secondary gain should be addressed.
- Test stimulation with temporary electrode placement should relieve the pain.

SPECIFIC INDICATIONS

- The most common indication for SCS in the United States is "failed back surgery syndrome." In patients with associated axial low back pain, use of complex electrode arrays and careful psychophysical tests may help achieve coverage. Nociceptive or mechanical axial low back pain may not respond as well as neuropathic or deafferentation pain.
- In Europe, SCS is often used to treat ischemic pain arising from peripheral vascular disease in the lower extremities. In these patients, SCS also improves red blood cell flow velocity, capillary density, and perfusion pressures and may enhance limb salvage.[5]
- SCS provides pain relief and anti-ischemic effects when used to treat intractable angina pectoris.[6]

Fortunately, SCS does not mask the pain of myocardial infarction.

- SCS may relieve segmental pain from spinal cord injury, postcordotomy dysesthesias, and other spinal cord lesions (such as multiple sclerosis).
- Pain from peripheral nerve injury or neuralgia, causalgia, and "reflex sympathetic dystrophy" (complex regional pain syndrome) responds to SCS.[7]
- SCS is efficacious in most cases of postamputation pain syndrome, including phantom limb and stump pain.
- Other applications of SCS include the management of intractable pain associated with lower extremity spasticity, evoked potential monitoring, cerebral blood flow, autonomic hyperreflexia, and motor disorders.

CONTRAINDICATIONS

- Coagulopathy
- Sepsis
- Untreated, major comorbidity (eg, depression)
- Serious drug behavior problems
- Inability to cooperate or to control the device
- Secondary gain
- Demand cardiac pacemaker (without ECG monitoring or changing the pacemaker mode to a fixed rate)
- MRI needs

SYSTEM DESIGN AND USE

- Modeling studies show that:
  - The longitudinal position of an electrode dictates whether it achieves paresthesia at any given segmental level.
  - Bipolar stimulation is most effective on longitudinal midline fibers.
  - The optimal contact separation is 1.4 times the thickness of the meninges and CSF (6–8 mm).[4]
- Anatomic factors determine the appropriate position and spacing of spinal cord electrodes for the treatment of low back and leg pain. Although advancing electrodes cephalad would seemingly broaden the paresthesias, the decreasing thickness of ascending fibers in the dorsal column and the varying thickness of CSF may elicit excessive local segmental effects.[8]
- Bipoles should be closely spaced with the cathode cephalad and an anode(s) may be added cephalad to create a longitudinal tripole.[8,9] Creating a transverse tripole by adding lateral anodes should mitigate recruitment of lateral structures.[10]
- In patients with failed back surgery syndrome who have low back and lower extremity pain, low thoracic electrode placement is most effective.[11]

IMPLANTABLE DEVICES

ELECTRODES

- SCS electrodes are available as multicontact catheters (arrays of electrodes on a single carrier) inserted through a Tuohy needle or as insulated "paddles" or "plates" that require laminectomy (Figure 52–1).
- The percutaneous method offers longitudinal access to the spinal canal and, with fluoroscopy, allows the clinician to position the electrode optimally in a conscious patient.
- Insulated electrodes (requiring a small laminectomy) compare favorably with percutaneous electrodes for low back and lower extremity pain[12] and require half the battery power. Clinical outcome is significantly better at 1–2 years but not at 3 years.[13]
- "Dual-electrode" percutaneous arrays are inferior to a single electrode placed in the midline for the treatment of axial low back pain.[14]
- Intractable low back pain has been effectively treated with an insulated array of 2 parallel columns of 8 contacts (16 total).[15]

PULSE GENERATORS

- Multicontact pulse generators can be programmed postoperatively with the patient in the appropriate position to determine which anodes and cathodes should be active.
- "Multichannel" systems (single-channel generators gated to multiple outputs) are technically and clinically more reliable than single-channel systems.[2, 9]
- The radiofrequency-coupled passive implants used to deliver energy are not hampered by components with a limited life, but the external antenna can be inconvenient, can irritate the skin, and can cause fluctuations in stimulation amplitude.
- In contrast, the convenience of battery-operated "implanted pulse generators" (IPGs) may improve patient compliance unless patients compromise usage to maximize battery life (dictated by the amount of power required for a given amplitude, width, repetition rate, and time in use).
- Patients control IPGs with an external magnet (on–off and some adjustment in amplitude) or remote transmitter (for more complicated adjustments).

COMPUTERIZED STIMULATOR ADJUSTMENT

- The number of possible cathode and anode combinations increases disproportionately with the number of contacts (eg, 50 for an array of four, 6050 for an array of eight).
- Further adjustments must be made to pulse parameters (width, rate, and amplitude).
- Each combination must be considered for amplitudes ranging from first perception to discomfort.
- Computer analysis of these data for several populations of patients has resulted in the ability to make technical comparisons and in the development of rules and expert systems.[16]
- A patient can make computerized adjustments directly using a graphic input device to control stimulus amplitude, draw areas of pain and stimulation paresthesias, and rate pain on a visual analog scale.[17]
- The benefits of computerized adjustment include improved efficacy, battery life, and cost-effectiveness.[16]

TRIAL PROTOCOLS

- A temporary epidural electrode may be placed percutaneously for a trial of SCS.
- Power requirements and patient performance during a trial demonstrate the feasibility of implanting a device.
- During the trial, longitudinal mapping of the epidural space indicates the optimal placement of a permanent implant as well as which electrode and generator to use.
- An SCS trial is a third-party-payer prerequisite for long-term SCS treatment in the United States. This requirement may be met by test stimulation immediately before implantation.
- A percutaneous electrode placement allows:
  - The efficacy to be assessed in a fluoroscopy room (less expensive than an operating room).

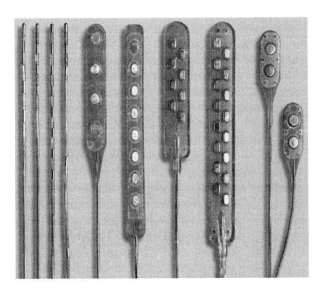

FIGURE 52–1 Some multicontact SCS electrode arrays are placed through a Tuohy needle; others require laminectomy.

○ The incremental withdrawal of the electrode at the bedside for assessment of a greater number of anode and cathode positions and pulse parameters.

○ Assessment under everyday conditions of activity and posture and with the patient's pain medications reduced.

○ The patient and the physician to gain information that will assist with implantation of the permanent device.

• Because a prolonged trial might increase the risk of infection and of epidural scarring that might compromise implantation, it is wise to limit a trial to 3 days, extending it on an individual basis.

• A percutaneous extension cable, intended for later removal, allows the temporary electrode to be adapted for a permanent system.

○ This option saves the expense of a second electrode but, unlike a simple percutaneous lead that can be removed at the bedside, requires one trip to the operating room for placement and another for internalization or removal.

○ Because percutaneous lead extensions increase the risk of infection, urgency to end the trial may lead to inappropriate implantation.

○ Increased incisional pain may confound trial results.

• Surgical electrode placement is sometimes required (eg, if prior spinal or peripheral nerve surgery precludes percutaneous access).

○ Surgical placement allows use of the insulated electrodes that prolong battery life and mitigate side effects, such as pain caused by unwanted recruitment of small fibers in the ligamentum flavum.[12]

• After a 2.5- or 3-day trial, clinicians should offer a permanent implant to patients who report at least 50% pain relief and have improved or stable analgesic requirements and activity levels.

• Other outcome measures are difficult to assess on the basis of a trial.

OUTCOMES

• Reported "success" rates (generally defined as a minimum of 50% pain relief) vary from 12 to 88% at follow-ups of 0.5–8 years.

• More than two decades of data address additional outcome measures of patient satisfaction with treatment, activities of daily living, work status, medication requirements, and changes in neurologic function.[2]

• Outcome results must be adjusted when the rate of permanent implantation is low (approximately 40%). This adjustment is less crucial when the implantation rate exceeds 75%.[2]

POTENTIAL COMPLICATIONS AND ADVERSE EFFECTS

• Generator failure
• Electrode fatigue fracture
• Electrode migration/malposition
• Exposure to electromagnetic fields (eg, diathermy, security systems)
• Spinal cord or nerve injury
• CSF leak
• Infection
• Bleeding

COST-EFFECTIVENESS

• According to the World Health Organization, "SCS appears to be cost-effective versus alternative therapies."[18]

• A similar conclusion can be reached by considering the cost associated with:

○ Initial screening and implantation
○ Battery replacement
○ Complications and hardware failure
○ Periodic adjustment of stimulation parameters
○ Medications

FUTURE DEVELOPMENTS

• Multicontact, multichannel stimulation devices that are functionally equivalent to multiple stimulators
• Automated, enhanced, patient-interactive adjustment methods
• Improved electrode designs
• Improved electronics
• Improved power source (eg, rechargeable)

REFERENCES

1. **Melzack R, Wall PD.** Pain mechanisms: A new theory. *Science.* 1965;150:971.

2. **North RB, Kidd DH, Zahurak M, et al.** Spinal cord stimulation for chronic, intractable pain: Two decades' experience. *Neurosurgery.* 1993;32:384.

3. **Linderoth B, Meyerson BA.** Spinal cord stimulation, I. Mechanisms of action. In: Burchiel K, ed. *Pain Surgery.* New York: Thieme; 1999.

4. **Holsheimer J, Struijk JJ.** How do geometric factors influence epidural spinal cord stimulation? A quantitative analysis by computer modeling. *Stereotact Funct Neurosurg.* 1991; 56:234.

5. **Jacobs MJ, Jorning PJ, Beckers RC, et al.** Foot salvage and improvement of microvascular blood flow as a result of epidural spinal cord electrical stimulation. *J Vasc Surg.* 1990; 12:354.

6. **Hautvast RWM, DeJongste MJL, Staal MJ, et al.** Spinal cord stimulation in chronic intractable angina pectoris: A randomized, controlled efficacy study. *Am Heart J.* 1998; 136:1114.

7. **Kemler MA, Barendse GAM, van Kleef M, et al.** Spinal cord stimulation in patients with chronic reflex sympathetic dystrophy. *N Engl J Med.* 2000;343:618.

8. **Holsheimer J.** Effectiveness of spinal cord stimulation in the management of chronic pain: Analysis of technical drawbacks and solutions. *Neurosurgery.* 1997;40:990.

9. **North RB, Ewend MG, Lawton MT, et al.** Spinal cord stimulation for chronic, intractable pain: Superiority of "multichannel" devices. *Pain.* 1991;44:119.

10. **Holsheimer J, Nuttin B, King GW.** Clinical evaluation of paresthesia steering with a new system for spinal cord stimulation. *Neurosurgery.* 1998;42:541.

11. **Barolat G, Massaro F, He J.** Mapping of sensory responses to epidural stimulation of the intraspinal neural structures in man. *J Neurosurg.* 1993;78:233.

12. **North RB, Kidd DH, Olin JC, et al.** Spinal cord stimulation electrode design: Prospective, randomized, controlled trial comparing percutaneous and laminectomy electrodes, Part I: Technical outcomes. *Neurosurgery.* 2002;51:381.

13. **North RB, Olin JC, Kidd DH.** Spinal cord stimulation electrode design: A prospective, randomized controlled trial comparing percutaneous and laminectomy electrodes. *Stereotactic Funct Neurosurg.* 1999;73:134.

14. **North RB.** Spinal cord stimulation for axial low back pain: Single versus dual percutaneous electrodes. In: *International Neuromodulation Society Abstracts.* Lucerne; 1998:212.

15. **Barolat G, Oakley JC, Law JD.** Epidural spinal cord stimulation with multiple electrode paddle leads is effective in treating intractable low back pain. *Neuromodulation.* 2001; 4:59.

16. **North RB, Calkins SK, Campbell DS, et al.** Automated, patient-interactive, spinal cord stimulator adjustment: A randomized controlled trial. *Neurosurgery.* 2003;52:572.

17. **North RB, Sieracki JM, Fowler KR, et al.** Patient-interactive, microprocessor-controlled neurological stimulation system. *Neuromodulation.* 1998;1:185.

18. **ECRI.** *Spinal Cord (Dorsal Column) Stimulation for Chronic Intractable Pain.* Health Technology Assessment Information Service, Plymouth Meeting, PA: ECRI; 1993.

53 EPIDURAL STEROID INJECTIONS

John C. Rowlingson, MD

INTRODUCTION

- Marked advances have been made in the management of chronic pain since the advent of pain management centers from which a practice model based on extensive workup of chronic pain sufferers has evolved, and private practice has made aggressive therapy available for a multitude of patients.

- Back pain is a common complaint for which patients are seen.[1]

- Most episodes of acute back pain resolve on their own in 4 to 6 weeks and extensive therapeutic intervention is not necessary.

- Assessment of "the pain" becomes more complex when the symptoms persist and attitudes, behaviors, and lifestyle changes as well as neuroplastic consequences in the nervous system perpetuate the pain.[1,2]

- The medical history must *then* encompass aspects of the consequences of activity interference, that is, disruption of activities of daily living, loss of independence, inability to perform one's job, and related psychosocial issues.

- The physical examination is more likely to reflect the components of pain-related deconditioning being endured by the patient.

- Deyo and Weinstein suggest that the workup must screen to answer three questions:
  - Is there systemic disease causing the pain?
  - Is there social or psychological distress that is amplifying or prolonging the pain?
  - Is there nerve compromise that might dictate surgical evaluation?[1]

- One bases the recommended therapy on the most likely of the differential diagnoses, which are vast for complaints of back pain.

- This process of *selecting* patients for specific therapies is particularly important in the potential application of interventional therapies such as nerve blocks.

- Not all patients referred or selected for epidural steroid injections (ESIs) manifest the classic symptoms of radiculopathy (see Table 53–1) or are considered appropriate candidates.

- The correlation of laboratory test findings, as to the efficacy of ESIs, is still not certain, so clinical judgment must be an additional and compelling component in the decision to suggest ESI.[1–3]

- The eternal hope is that treatment will eliminate the pain. However, when one is treating just the *symptoms*

TABLE 53–1   Classic Signs of Radiculopathy

Sharp, sudden, shooting pain
  Low back source: pain into the extremity below the knee
  Cervical spine source: pain into the upper extremity
Increased pain with coughing, sneezing, or straining
Onset often associated with lifting a heavy load while in an awkward position
Repetitive spinal motions can be causative in fatigued, anxious, poorly conditioned individuals

of pain, and not the cause, more appropriate, realistic expectations should prevail.

- In chronic pain, the reasonable goals of treatment include decreasing the frequency and/or the intensity of the pain, improving the patient's functional capacity, and enhancing the patient's ability to cope with residual pain.[2]

RATIONALE FOR EPIDURAL STEROID INJECTIONS

- It has long been held that radiculopathy may represent a toxic spill of inflammatory mediators from the disc more than a primary problem of mechanical compression of nerve roots by herniated discs.[2,4–7]
- Neuromuscular coordination defects are thought to cause inadequate distribution of physical forces that create pressures that exceed the viscoelastic characteristics of the annulus.[1]
- The posterior longitudinal ligament is thinner in the lumbosacral spine area, and a shift of weight bearing from the anterior elements of the spine to the more delicate posterior elements of the spinal arch, including the pedicles, lamina, and facet joints, leads to either frank herniation of the disc or a leak of nucleus pulposus contents.
- The disc contains phospholipase A-2 (PLA-2), interleukins, and proteoglycans.
- These are spilled into the epidural space, and are potent instigators of inflammation.
- It is also suggested that ingrowth of new nerves into the healing annulus may result in subsequent discogenic pain.
- Saal et al showed that PLA-2 from the disc was one of the offending agents in creating nerve root swelling after McCarron et al demonstrated that only small amounts of nucleus pulposus content were necessary to precipitate a marked inflammatory response.[5,8]
- The action of PLA-2 is to release arachidonic acid from cell membranes, so inhibiting this (which requires steroids) would help decrease the elaboration of inflammatory mediators.
- Chen et al demonstrated in an animal model that PLA-2 can "cause nerve root and corresponding behavioral and electrophysiologic changes consistent with sciatica."[9]
- The traditional concept impelling the injection of depo-steroids into the epidural space is that a localized placement of these most potent anti-inflammatory agents maximizes the anti-inflammatory effect and decreases the physical size of the nerve root, thereby decreasing the patient's symptoms.[6,7]

- Once this result is achieved, resumption of normal activity *and* participation in focused physical therapy and rehabilitation are expected.
- There have also been suggestions that the steroids provide a moderate block of nociceptive C fibers, stabilize membranes, decrease ectopic discharges from inflamed tissue, and perhaps decrease the CNS sensitization associated with acute and chronic pain.[4,6]
- Finally, the anti-inflammatory action of the local anesthetic frequently used has not been fully characterized.[10]

THE EVOLUTION OF DRUGS, NEEDLES, AND REFERRALS

- The two most common steroid preparations used are triamcinolone (Aristocort Intralesional) and methylprednisolone, yet there is no study comparing one with the other.[4]
- These are chemically altered such that their solubility is diminished, resulting in an estimated dwell time of 2–3 weeks.
- The drugs exert systemic effects so caution is advised with their use in patients with congestive heart failure, renal insufficiency, and diabetes secondary to the fluid retention and metabolic effects.[4]
- Cluff et al state "the ideal dose and type of steroid have yet to be determined."[11]
- Single-dose injections in animals failed to demonstrate evidence of tissue damage, and concerns about the toxicity of polyethylene glycol, at the concentrations used clinically, have been allayed.[2]
- Concern about the intrathecal placement of these compounds is prevalent based on historical and scientific data.[2–4,6,12]
- The potential for inducing adhesive arachnoiditis seems low and any such symptoms would be less common than the potential for procedure-related side effects such as backache, postdural puncture headache, paresthesias, bleeding, and infection, or even anxiety-related symptoms such as lightheadedness and nausea.[12]
- Abram advocates the use of a test dose of local anesthetic prior to the injection of depo-steroid in any patients in whom the determination of the accurate placement of the epidural needle is difficult, as in patients with previous back surgery.[4]
- Patients with back pain are often treating the musculoskeletal component of their pain with NSAIDs. A common question is, Can patients on such medications safely receive a needle-based therapy the magnitude of an epidural injection with a 17-gauge needle?

- Horlocker et al looked at the incidence of hemorrhagic complications related to NSAID use in patients receiving epidural steroid injections.[13]
- One thousand thirty-five patients underwent 1214 injections, the majority of them in the midline and at lumbosacral spine levels.
- Thirty-two percent had used NSAIDs within 1 week.
- Five and two-tenths percent of patients had a minor, hemorrhagic complication defined as blood appearing in the needle or catheter.
- No spinal hematomas were detected. Four percent of patients had worsening of the primary symptoms or a new neurologic deficit.
- Significant risk factors identified included increased patient age, needle gauge, the procedural approach used, needles tried at multiple levels, the number of needle passes, the volume of the injectate, and accidental dural puncture.
- The authors conclude that epidural steroid injections are safe in patients taking NSAIDs.
- One might worry about the potential increase in the intensity of symptoms if such drugs are withheld.
- This must be balanced against continuing their use *and* having some clinicians feeling obligated to obtain tests of coagulation that simply add expense.
- Liu et al reported on the benefit of using 20-gauge Tuohy needles.[14] Though effective in increasing patient comfort and lessening the risk of postdural puncture headache, their most successful use might also require confirmation of correct placement using fluoroscopy, adding at least expense if not scheduling issues and demanding greater expertise of the clinician. Parenthetically, the loss of resistance technique with these needles was most inaccurate in males and patients older than 70.
- A contemporary point of view holds that clinicians must establish a differential diagnosis for the patient's complaints through the distillation of data from history taking, physical examination, and laboratory tests.[1–4]
- Distinguishing internal disc disruption, with which patients complain of referred pain to the thigh and leg but with which there's no associated neurologic change, from obvious radiculopathy, with which there is positive straight leg raising, dermatomal pain, and peripheral sensory and/or motor changes, is important.[3,15]
- Epidural steroid injections are of minimal help in the former, as they would be in patients with neurogenic claudication, but of clearer benefit to patients with the latter diagnosis.[16]
- Fanciullo et al surveyed 25,479 patients referred to 23 specialty spine care centers with spinal and radicular pain as to the application of published guidelines that qualify patients for (mostly lumbar) epidural steroid injections.[17]
  - Whereas it is felt that younger patients with recent onset of radicular pain and no history of back surgery are best, these authors reported that epidural steroid injections were recommended for 7.9% of the studied patients.
  - These patients were characterized by complaints of radiating pain, a dermatomal distribution of pain, and neurologic signs on examination.
  - In addition, the patients had symptoms of greater than 1 year's duration *and* a higher incidence of comorbid conditions such as congestive heart failure, hypertension, peripheral vascular disease, and diabetes mellitus.
  - This is particularly significant since most of the reported cases of epidural abscess related to epidural steroid injections have been in diabetics.[4]
  - In his editorial preceding this study, Abram notes that the diagnosis of radiculopathy is the most consistent predictor of outcome with epidural steroid treatment, including patients with the provisional diagnosis of spinal stenosis.[3]
  - The application of guidelines, as documented by Fanciullo et al, resulted in a relatively small number of patients being referred and many of those having had protracted symptoms and/or previous surgical treatment—groups less likely to respond to epidural steroid injection.
  - A short-term response would generate frequent requests for repeated treatment, leading to risks of steroid-related and/or procedure-related complications in groups of patients perhaps already at risk.

TECHNIQUES FOR EPIDURAL STEROID INJECTION FOR SELECTED PATIENTS

- The original technique for the deposition of corticosteroids was a caudal approach with a large-volume injectate.
- There was clearly an intent to disrupt adhesions by fluid dissection.[2,4,6]
- Winnie refined the concept by showing that steroids placed at the level of pathology were more effective, and this became the prevalent technique.[2,4,6]
- Many, many studies have been published, but the lack of consistency of research design, type(s) of patients included, therapeutic protocol, and quality and duration of follow-up have been a significant problem in comparing the results and unifying the therapeutic approach based on randomized controlled trials.[2,3,6,7,11,18]

- The addition of fluoroscopy to the armamentarium theoretically limits the complications of this procedure by allowing confirmation of correct needle placement and demonstrating the clinically relevant spread of the injectate.
- The prolific availability of fluoroscopy has allowed the growth of a transforaminal/selective nerve root block (SNRB) technique.[11,19–22]
- This places depo-steroids at a site from which flow of the drug is more likely to include the anterior epidural space.
- Other stated (but unproven) advantages include a lower likelihood of dural puncture (5% for translaminar, not known for transforaminal) and use of less medication, thus decreasing the potential of drug-related side effects.
- Lutz et al advocated the (anatomically) "safe triangle" approach for transforaminal blocks, as enhancing the accuracy of drug deposition, providing a high steroid concentration at the chosen site, and doing so with a smaller dose of steroid.[20] Thus, there should be less need to add a diluent.
- Slipman et al studied 14 of 20 patients who were given cervical SNRBs at the pathologic level identified by clinical findings such as motor weakness and reflex change, MRI findings, and EMG, if necessary.[19] Overall, 60% of the patients had a good to excellent result as to pain reduction and functional improvement, after one to two injections over 2 weeks, as recorded during the average 21-month follow-up.
- Klein et al advocated the same technique for use in patients with cervical spine radiculopathy and published basically the same results.[21]
- Cluff et al recently completed a national survey on the technical aspects of ESI practice.[11]
  - The mix of 68 academic centers and 28 private practices lends the results applicability.
  - Their overriding summary was that after 50 years of clinical use, there still is no consensus as to the best technique for providing ESI.
  - The majority of practitioners use the loss of resistance technique to identify the epidural space, with patients in the prone more than the sitting position and with fluoroscopy used more in nonacademic venues.
  - The most frequent injectate was a combination of local anesthetics and corticosteroids.
  - Private practitioners were more likely to use a transforaminal approach in patients with failed back surgery syndrome in whom the chronicity of the pain and/or scar tissue may interfere with the patient's ability to get better.
  - Clinicians expressed concerns that too much injectate volume would dilute the corticosteroid whereas too little volume might not result in enough spread of the drug, giving the false impression that ESI was not effective.
  - In academic centers, the mean maximum number of ESIs in a patient in a year was 4.7, but the range was 0–20.
  - For private practice, the mean maximum number was 6.9 with a range of 3 to 40.
  - These data raise questions about how to most critically evaluate the effectiveness of ESI, so that only those patients truly benefitting from it continue to receive it, as well as the safety of repeated doses of depo-steroids.
- A cautionary tone is not unreasonable considering that closed claim data are beginning to indicate that ESIs are a major source of claims made, leading some insurance companies to apply up to a 25% surcharge for malpractice coverage for pain management physicians (personal communication).
- No study yet published can answer the question, Does an epidural steroid injection placed above or below a previous surgical site gain adequate access to the effective nerve roots?[11]
- A thorough, contemporary review comparing the transforaminal to the translaminar to caudal technique is provided in the evidence-based practice guidelines for interventional techniques for chronic spinal pain by Manchikanti et al.[22]
  - Based on their critical review, the transforaminal techniques have the best short- and long-term benefit, with caudal ESI techniques besting translaminar techniques thereafter.
- Straus provides insight about ESIs through the unique view of cost–benefit analysis.[23]
  - No review has been done that identifies the most economical practice setting (hospital, office, ambulatory surgery center) in which to provide ESI treatment.
  - The higher success rate for accurate placement of the epidural needle with fluoroscopy, alone, is *not* evidence of such benefit.
  - For economic success, there need to be data manifesting improved patient outcome, fewer complications, and actual cost reduction in care.
  - Straus's calculations don't justify the benefits of fluoroscopy, which impacts the decision about in which venue ESI therapy should be provided.
- Botwin et al published data from a retrospective study of complications in 207 patients who received 322 transforaminal lumbar ESIs.[24]
  - Nonpositional headache was the most common complaint, with short-term increase in back pain and increased leg pain the next most frequent.
  - The overall minor complication rate was 9.6% per injection (see Table 53–2).

TABLE 53–2   Incidence of Complications per Injection

COMPLICATION	LSS GROUP (259 INJECTIONS)	HNP GROUP (63 INJECTIONS)	COMBINED (322 INJECTIONS)
Transient nonpositional headaches that resolved within 24 h	7 (2.7)*	3 (4.8)	10 (3.1)
Increased postprocedure back pain at injection site	5 (1.9)	3 (4.8)	8 (2.4)
Facial flushing	3 (1.2)	1 (1.6)	4 (1.2)
Increased leg pain with radicular symptoms	1 (0.4)	1 (1.6)	2 (0.6)
Vasovagal reaction	1 (0.4)		1 (0.3)
Rash	1 (0.4)		1 (0.3)
Transient leg weakness	1 (0.4)		1 (0.3)
Dizziness	1 (0.4)		1 (0.3)
Increased blood serum (258 mg/dL) in an insulin-dependent diabetic	1 (0.4)		1 (0.3)
Intraoperative hypertensive episode	1 (0.4)		1 (0.3)
Episode of nausea	1 (0.4)		1 (0.3)

*n (%). LSS, lumbar spinal stenosis; HNP, herniated nucleus pulposus.

○ A more recent report by these authors on the complications of fluoroscopy-guided caudal ESIs showed a minor complication rate of 15.6% per injection, including insomnia on the night of the procedure, vasovagal reactions, infrequent nausea, and otherwise as in the study just mentioned.[25]

OUTCOMES

• Published success rates for ESI vary between 18 and 90%.[2,3,11,15,26]
• Koes et al reviewed 12 of 13 randomized controlled trials published on the use of caudal or lumbar ESIs.[26]
  ○ Eight of the 12 studies had methodologic flaws.
  ○ The 4 best studies were equally divided between showing a benefit and not.
  ○ Looking at all 12 studies, 6 were positive with respect to improved outcome and 6 manifested no benefit.
• Another contemporary review includes that by Buchner et al, who studied 36 patients less than 50 years of age with radicular pain, positive straight leg raising, MRI-proven prolapsed discs at L4–5 or L5–1, and no history of previous spinal surgery, spinal stenosis, cauda equina syndrome, or major motor deficits.[27]
  ○ Patients were randomized to conservative therapy (rest, NSAIDs, tramadol, physical therapy) or conservative therapy plus ESIs (100 mg methylprednisolone in 10 mL 0.25% bupivacaine, three injections in 14 days).
  ○ The ESI patients had a greater improvement in straight leg raising and a tendency to better pain relief and functional recovery, yet no statistically significant benefit was sustained at the 6-week or 6-month follow-up.

• Cannon and April have recently stated that lumbosacral ESIs "have a favorable role in the nonoperative treatment of true radicular pain," especially with the corticosteroid delivered to the pathologic site.
  ○ Of six qualified studies of ESIs, three are supportive of the treatment, three neutral as to the benefit, and two others are positive specifically for the caudal approach.
  ○ These authors state that there are fewer data as to the benefit of the transforaminal technique.
  ○ They advocate the caudal approach for L5–S1 pathology, the translaminar approach for patients with discs above L5–S1 (especially for patients with unilateral symptoms), placement of depo-steroid one level below in patients with central or posterolateral discs, and an at-the-level placement for anyone receiving a transforaminal approach.
• Based on these reviews, it is reasonable to suggest the following about ESI application:
  ○ Patients with a history of radiculopathy and a corresponding dermatomal sensory change, who have not responded to conservative therapy in 4 to 6 weeks, seem to be the most likely to benefit. As in all patients for interventional procedures, the absence of systemic infection or infection at the proposed needle insertion site and the absence of major coagulation defects must be documented.
  ○ Patients with a clinically significant herniated disc, diagnosed by both physical and laboratory findings, who have not improved with conservative therapy should be considered. The increased risk of infection in diabetics should be acknowledged.
  ○ Patients with a primary diagnosis of postural/musculoskeletal back pain who have intermittent radicular-like symptoms and who have not improved with conservative therapy measures over 8 to 10

weeks may benefit. Doses less than 80 mg methyl-prednisolone should be used.

○ Patients with established low back pain syndromes who develop a flare-up of symptoms that have radicular-like signs or symptoms should be evaluated carefully before ESIs are provided. The treatment may be of less benefit in those with longstanding pain, previous surgery, and preoccupation with vocational or legal issues and in patients who smoke heavily.

○ Patients with cancer-related pain who are thought to have tumor invasion of nerve roots (which causes an inflammatory pathology) may benefit from ESIs.

CONCLUSION

- Back pain is a common, pervasive, and expensive problem.
- The workup of any patient with acute, subacute, or chronic back pain must clarify whether the patient is seriously ill or not.
- It is essential to acknowledge that patients in pain want to know what is causing the pain, not so much what they do not have.
- Treating the *cause* of the pain is more likely to be successful than merely treating the *symptom* of pain.
- Patients should be actively selected for *all* procedures including ESIs, *each time* they present for treatment.
- The clinical decision at that time is based on assessment of their particular physical and nonphysical findings.
- ESIs are not to be viewed as generic treatment for all patients with back pain complaints.
- Rather, nerve blocks are but one component of a coordinated treatment program that balances the continuation of effective therapy with the cessation of any that is not working or that may be causing side effects.
- ESIs can help patients achieve the goals of acute and chronic pain management.

REFERENCES

1. **Deyo RA, Weinstein JN.** Primary care: Low back pain. *N Engl J Med.* 2001;344:363–370.
2. **Rowlingson JC.** Epidural steroids: Do they have a place in pain management? *Am Pain Soc J.* 1994;3:20–27.
3. **Abram SE.** Factors that influence the decision to treat pain of spinal origin with epidural steroid injections. *Reg Anesth Pain Med.* 2001;26:2–4.
4. **Abram SE.** Treatment of lumbosacral radiculopathy with epidural steroids. *Anesthesiology.* 1999;91:1937–1941.
5. **Saal JS, Franson R, Dobrow E, et al.** High levels of inflammatory phospholipase A2 activity in lumbar disc herniation. *Spine.* 1990;15:674–678.
6. **Cannon DT, Aprill CN.** Lumbosacral epidural steroid injections. *Arch Phys Med Rehabil.* 2000;81:S-87–S-98.
7. **Tonkovich-Quaranta LA, Winkler SR.** Use of epidural corticosteroids in low back pain. *Ann Pharmacother.* 2000; 34:1165–1172.
8. **McCarron RF, Wimpee MW, Hudkins PG, et al.** The inflammatory effect of nucleus pulposus: A possible element in the pathogenesis of low-back pain. *Spine.* 1987;12:760–764.
9. **Chen C, Cavanaugh JM, Ozaktay AC, et al.** Effects of phospholipase A2 on lumbar nerve root structure and function. *Spine.* 1997;22:1057–1064.
10. **Hollmann MW, Durieux ME.** Local anesthetics and the inflammatory response. *Anesthesiology.* 2000;93:858–875.
11. **Cluff R, Mehio A-K, Cohen SP, et al.** The technical aspects of epidural steroid injections: A national survey. *Anesth Analg.* 2002;95:403–408.
12. **Wilkinson H.** Intrathecal depomedrol: A literature review. *Clin J Pain.* 1992;8:49–56.
13. **Horlocker TT, Bajwa, ZH, Ashraf Z, et al.** Risk assessment of hemorrhagic complications associated with nonsteroidal antiinflammatory medications in ambulatory pain clinic patients undergoing epidural steroid injection. *Anesth Analg.* 2002;95:1691–1697.
14. **Liu SS, Melmed AP, Klos JW, Innis CA.** Prospective experience with a 20-gauge Tuohy needle for lumbar epidural steroid injections: Is confirmation with fluoroscopy necessary? *Reg Anesth Pain Med.* 2001;26:143–146.
15. **Mulligan KA, Rowlingson JC.** Epidural steroids. *Curr Pain Headache Rep.* 2001;5:495–502.
16. **Southern D, Lutz GE, Cooper G, Barre L.** Are fluoroscopic caudal epidural steroid injections effective for managing chronic low back pain? *Pain Physician.* 2003;6:167–172.
17. **Fanciullo GJ, Hanscom B, Seville J, Ball PA, Rose RJ.** An observational study of the frequency and pattern of use of epidural steroid injection in 25,479 patients with spinal and radicular pain. *Reg Anesth Pain Med.* 2001;26:5–11.
18. **Hopwood MB, Manning DC.** Lumbar epidural steroid injections: Is a clinical trial necessary or appropriate? *Reg Anesth Pain Med.* 1999;24:5–7.
19. **Slipman CW, Lipetz JS, Jackson HB, Rogers DP, Vresilovic EJ.** Therapeutic selective nerve root block in the nonsurgical treatment of atraumatic cervical spondylotic radicular pain: A retrospective analysis with independent clinical review. *Arch Phys Med Rehabil.* 2000;81:741–746.
20. **Lutz GE, Vad VB, Wisneski RJ.** Fluoroscopic transforaminal lumbar epidural steroids: An outcome study. *Arch Phys Med Rehabil.* 1998;79:1362–1366.
21. **Klein GR, Vaccaro AR, Cwik J, et al.** Efficacy of cervical epidural steroids in the treatment of cervical spine disorders. *Am J Anesthesiol.* 2000;9:547–550.
22. **Manchikanti L, Staats PS, Singh V, et al.** Evidence-based practice guidelines for interventional techniques in the management of chronic spinal pain. *Pain Physician.* 2003; 6:3–81.
23. **Straus BN.** Chronic pain of spinal origin: The cost of intervention. *Spine.* 2002;27:2614–2619.

24. **Botwin KP, Gruber RD, Bouchlas CG, et al.** Complications of fluoroscopically guided transforaminal lumbar epidural injections. *Arch Phys Med Rehabil.* 2000; 81:1045–1050.

25. **Botwin KP, Gruber RD, Bouchlas CG, et al.** Complications of fluoroscopically-guided caudal epidural injections. *Am J Phys Med Rehabil.* 2001;80:416–424.

26. **Koes BW, Scholten R, Mens JMA, Barter LM:** Epidural steroid injections for low back pain and sciatica: An updated systematic review of randomized clinical trials. *Pain Digest.* 1999;9:241–247.

27. **Buchner M, Zeifang F, Brocai DRC, Schiltenwolf M:** Epidural corticosteroid injection in the conservative management of sciatica. *Clin Orthop Relat Res.* 2000; 375: 149–156.

54 FACET JOINT BLOCKS

Somayaji Ramamurthy, MD

INTRODUCTION

- Back pain and neck pain are the most common causes of chronic pain and disability.
- Although radicular pain secondary to herniated disc is most commonly suspected, pain originating from facet joints is likely to be the etiology of 15 to 40% of nonradicular low back pain and 40 to 60% of nonradicular neck pain.
- These joints, also known as the zygapophyseal joints, are formed by the articulation of the articular processes of the adjacent vertebrae.
- These sinuarthrodial joints are subject to degenerative arthritis, thus becoming one of the factors contributing to nonradicular back and neck pain.
- Pain originating from facet joints can coexist with other causes of multifactorial back and neck pain including radicular, myofascial, sacroiliac, and intradiscal pathology.

DIAGNOSIS

- History and clinical examination findings have been shown unable to predict whether or not pain is originating from the facet joints.[1,2]
- Imaging studies including MRI have not been useful in pinpointing facet joints as the cause of pain, although SPECT scan findings have been reported to have a high correlation with the pain relief following joint injection with corticosteroids.[3]

- At present, state-of-the-art diagnosis can be established only by local anesthetic injections. Injection of local anesthetic and/or steroid either into the joint or blocking the nerve supply of the joint is used in establishing the diagnosis.

CONSERVATIVE THERAPY

- Nonradicular low back pain or neck pain is managed in our clinic using manual methods consisting of mobilization, physical therapy, and home exercises with significant success.
- In patients who have significant pain and restriction of motion it may be necessary to inject the facet joint or block the medial branches to provide analgesia for physical therapy and mobilization.

FACET JOINT INJECTION

- These injections are performed under fluoroscopic guidance using nonionic radiocontrast material.
- Greater than 50% pain relief with the injection of local anesthetic into the joint is considered diagnostic.[1]
- Steroids such as methylprednisolone acetate (Depo-Medrol), triamcinolone, and betamethasone are commonly mixed with the local anesthetic for therapeutic purposes.
- The role of the joint injections is controversial and the present trend is to use medial branch blocks for diagnostic and therapeutic purposes.

MEDIAL BRANCH BLOCKS

- Each lumbar facet joint is supplied by a branch of the posterior ramus from the nerve root at the corresponding level and the branches from the nerve root one level above (Figure 54–1).
- For example, the L4–5 facet joint receives a medial branch from the L5 posterior primary ramus and a branch from the medial branch of the L4 nerve root.
- The cervical facet joint receives innervation from the same level and one level above and below.
- To significantly denervate each joint, the medial branches of all the nerves supplying the joint have to be blocked.
- In the lumbar region the medial branches are blocked under fluoroscopic guidance at the junction of the transverse process and the superior articular process.
- In the cervical region the nerve is blocked at the waist of the articular process.

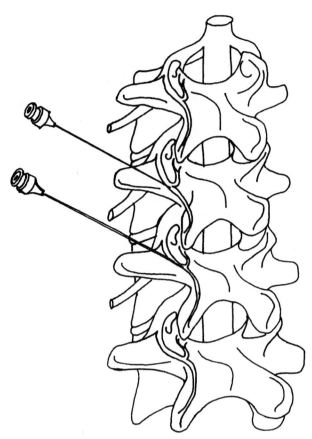

FIGURE 54–1 Medial branch blocks.

INTERPRETATION AND CONFIRMATION

- A single injection with the local anesthetic can produce false-positive results in 40% of patients.
- The most accurate technique consists of using double-blind, randomized injections of placebo, a short-acting local anesthetic such as lidocaine, and a longer-acting local anesthetic such as bupivacaine.
- In most clinical situations it is more practical to use short- and long-acting local anesthetic agents to assess whether the duration of pain relief corresponds to that of the local anesthetic agent.
- Some clinicians use corticosteroids such as methylprednisolone acetate (Depo-Medrol) and Sarapin (pitcher plant) to provide long-term pain relief.[2]
- Longer duration of pain relief has been achieved by using neurolytic techniques with 4% phenol, cryogenic nerve block, or most commonly radiofrequency lesions.
- Well-controlled studies indicate that radiofrequency lesion provides predictable long-term pain relief in patients with cervical facet joint pain secondary to trauma.[4]

- The role of radiofrequency lesions of the medial branches of the lumbar nerves in providing long-term relief of pain of lumbar facet origin is still being debated.

COMPLICATIONS

- The incidence of serious complications following injections into the facet joint is very low, although there are reports of infection and subarachnoid injection following facet joint injections.

REFERENCES

1. **Saal JS.** General principles of diagnostic testing as related to painful lumbar spine disorders: A critical appraisal of current diagnostic techniques. *Spine.* 2002;27:2538.
2. **Manchikanti L, Pampati V, Fellows B, et al.** The diagnostic validity and therapeutic value of lumbar facet joint nerve blocks with or without adjuvant agents. *Curr Rev Pain.* 2000;4:337.
3. **Dolan AL, Ryan PJ, Arden NK, et al.** The value of SPECT scans in identifying back pain likely to benefit from facet joint injection. *Br J Rheumatol.* 1996;35:1269.
4. **Lord S, Barnsley L, Walis B, et al.** Percutaneous radiofrequency neurotomy for chronic cervical zygapophyseal joint pain. *N Engl J Med.* 1996;335:1721.

55   INTRAVENOUS DRUG INFUSIONS

Theodore Grabow, MD

INTRODUCTION

- In the past decade, intravenous infusion therapy has been used to treat a variety of chronic pain conditions. The pharmacologic agents used for intravenous infusion therapy are diverse but reflect an ongoing accumulation of knowledge regarding the receptor pharmacology of nociceptive transmission.

LIDOCAINE

MECHANISM OF ACTION

- Following nerve injury and/or inflammation, abnormal expression of sodium channels alters sodium channel distribution.[1] This change in sodium channel expression leads to abnormal spontaneous firing of dorsal root ganglion neurons.

- Lidocaine, an amide local anesthetic, produces analgesia by blocking voltage-gated sodium channels to prevent the generation and conduction of nerve impulses. More than 20 types of sodium channels have been identified throughout the peripheral and central nervous system.
- Beyond its anesthetic use, lidocaine is indicated in the Advanced Cardiac Life Support protocol for resuscitation because of its antiarrhythmic activity.

TYPE OF PAIN TREATED

- Lidocaine can have significant analgesic effects against neuropathic pain.[2] Specifically, it seems to alleviate allodynia and hyperalgesia associated with complex regional pain syndrome (CRPS) types I and II as well as with postherpetic neuralgia.
- Lidocaine effectively treats spinal cord injury pain, chronic poststroke pain, adiposa dolorosa (Dercum's disease), phantom limb pain, proctalgia fugax, thalamic pain, trigeminal neuralgia, and diabetic neuropathy. Intravenous lidocaine can also be used to predict response to oral mexiletine.

DOSAGE

- No standard guideline exists for intravenous lidocaine infusion therapy for chronic pain. Dosage depends on clinical response and toxicity. Therapeutic plasma levels range from 0.62 to 5.0 μg/mL across diverse neuropathic pain states. The effective doses generally range from 1.5 to 5.0 mg/kg.
- Several paradigms for lidocaine infusion have been reported.[2] One method suggests a 3-mg/kg bolus over 3 minutes followed by a 4-mg/kg infusion over 60 minutes. Another describes a 500-mg total dose delivered over 60 minutes at the rate of 8.33 mg/min.

SIDE EFFECTS

- Lidocaine toxicity is generally accepted as 7 mg/kg.
- The side effects of lidocaine are directly related to the plasma levels (Table 55–1).
- Lidocaine can cause sedation, tinnitus, dry mouth, respiratory depression, and adverse central nervous system (CNS) (seizure, coma) and cardiovascular (increasing systolic blood pressure secondary to vasoconstriction and increase in heart rate) events.

TABLE 55–1   Side Effects of Systemic Lidocaine

SIDE EFFECT	PLASMA LEVEL (μg/mL)
Lightheadedness	~1.5
Perioral numbness	~2.0
Nausea	~2.3
Visual and auditory disturbances	~5.0
Muscular twitching	~8.0
Convulsions	~10
Coma	~15
Respiratory arrest	~20
Cardiovascular depression	~25

- The convulsant activity of lidocaine likely arises from selective depression of inhibitory neurons or networks within the CNS that allows excessive excitatory outflow.
- Low doses of lidocaine may prevent or treat dysrhythmias; however, higher doses may produce refractory dysrhythmias and cardiovascular collapse. True allergies to amide local anesthetics are rare.

KETAMINE

MECHANISM OF ACTION

- Ketamine is an noncompetitive, use-dependent antagonist of N-methyl-D-aspartate (NMDA) receptors[3] that blocks the NMDA channel in the open state by binding to the phencyclidine (PCP) site located within the lumen of the channel.
- Central NMDA receptors are located in the superficial dorsal horn on the terminals of primary sensory neurons and on the postsynaptic membranes of primary sensory neurons.
- Central NMDA receptor activation at the spinal cord level maintains a state of facilitated nociceptive processing after nerve injury or inflammation.
- Peripheral NMDA receptors, on cell bodies and nociceptive endings of primary sensory afferents, have been implicated in pain states caused by somatic inflammation and visceral distention.
- Antagonism of NMDA receptors produces antinociception in animal models of persistent or neuropathic pain and analgesia in certain pain states in humans.
- Other NMDA receptor antagonists include dextromethorphan, memantine, amantadine, methadone, dextropropoxyphen, and ketobemidone.
- Several other mechanisms might explain the analgesic effects of ketamine, which blocks voltage-sensitive calcium channels, depresses sodium channels and modulates cholinergic neurotransmission, has kappa

and mu opioid-like actions, and inhibits the uptake of both norepinephrine and serotonin.

TYPE OF PAIN TREATED

- Certain types of central and peripheral neuropathic pain (particularly allodynia and windup pain).
- Temporal summation of pain and hyperalgesia related to postherpetic neuralgia.
- Various clinical pain states, such as postoperative incisional pain, cancer-related pain, fibromyalgia, and experimentally induced pain.

DOSAGE

- No guidelines cover the starting bolus dose or infusion rate of intravenous ketamine therapy for chronic pain.
- Therapeutic serum concentrations of 0.31–0.55 μM can be achieved by an intravenous bolus of 60 μg/kg plus an intravenous infusion of 6 μg/kg/min.[4] Some clinicians start with a bolus of 0.1–0.2 mg/kg and the rate of 5–7 μg/kg/min.

SIDE EFFECTS

- Psychomotor agitation, motor incoordination, lacrimation, salivation, emergence reactions, bronchodilation, sympathoneuronal release of norepinephrine, myocardial depression, analgesia, CNS excitatory effects including sensory illusions, dizziness, sedation, dry mouth, blurred vision, and altered hearing.

PHENTOLAMINE

MECHANISM OF ACTION

- Phentolamine is a competitive nonselective α_1- and α_2-adrenergic receptor antagonist that antagonizes the effect of norepinephrine released from postganglionic sympathetic neurons and of circulating epinephrine released from the adrenal glands.
- Modulation of adrenergic neurotransmission produces analgesia in humans and antinociception in animal behavioral models of pain.
- Phentolamine promotes histamine release from mast cells, antagonizes serotonergic receptors, and blocks potassium channels. Other intravenous drugs used for sympathetic blockade include guanethidine, reserpine, and bretylium.

USE OF PHENTOLAMINE INFUSION

- Phentolamine infusion has diagnostic or therapeutic use in a wide variety of presumed neuropathic and inflammatory pain conditions.
- The phentolamine infusion test was developed to evaluate the presence of sympathetically mediated pain in patients with neuropathic pain. The rationale for the test is based on the presence of functional coupling between sympathetic efferent and nociceptive sensory afferent neurotransmission.[5]
- The phentolamine test is considered positive if the patient receives pain relief during the infusion trial. This suggests involvement of the sympathetic nervous system and adrenoceptor function in the generation or maintenance of the pain. If the infusion test is positive, an oral α_1-adrenergic receptor antagonist, such as doxazosin, may be prescribed.
- A series of treatments or prolonged continuous infusions may be therapeutic in certain sympathetically mediated pain states.

DOSAGE

- The standard dose is 1 mg/kg administered over 10 minutes (Table 55–2).[6]

TABLE 55–2   Phentolamine Infusion Test*

Preinfusion preparation	History and physical exam
	NPO; informed consent
	Resuscitative drugs and equipment
	Peripheral IV line (LR or normal saline)
	Supine or sitting position
	BP, ECG, SpO$_2$, peripheral temperature
	Baseline VAS for pain (repeat VAS every 5 min)
Saline infusion	LR 5-10 mL/kg (~500 mL) over 30 min
	Reassess VAS
	Continue LR if VAS decreases (possible placebo response)
	Initiate phentolamine infusion if VAS unchanged by LR
Phentolamine infusion	Propranolol 1-2 mg IV 15 min prior to phentolamine
	Phentolamine 1mg/kg IV in 100 mL normal saline over 10 min
	Patient "blinded" to start time of phentolamine infusion
	VAS every 5 min
Postinfusion care	LR infusion for 20 min (continue noninvasive monitoring)
	VAS every 5 min
	Monitor side effects and temperature change

*See Raja et al[6] for details.
NPO, nil per os (nothing by mouth); LR, lactated Ringer's; SpO$_2$, pulse oximetry; VAS, Visual Analog Scale.

- The analgesic effect of phentolamine may last several days.

SIDE EFFECTS

- Hypotension caused by a direct vasodilatory effect on vascular smooth muscle and subsequent baroreceptor-mediated reflex tachycardia.
- Phentolamine's direct inotropic and chronotropic effect on cardiac smooth muscle may exacerbate ischemia in patients with coronary artery disease.
- All adverse effects related to histamine release.

MAGNESIUM

MECHANISM OF ACTION

- Magnesium is a bivalent cation found throughout the body. Because magnesium is a pronounced voltage-dependent antagonist of the NMDA receptor channel at the resting membrane potential, it prevents subsequent influx of sodium and calcium ions.

TYPE OF PAIN TREATED

- Magnesium reduces nociceptive behaviors in animals and is analgesic in experimental pain, postoperative pain, headaches including migraines, and neuropathic pain in humans.

DOSAGE

- There are no protocols regarding bolus dose or infusion rates for magnesium therapy for pain.
- One study describes administration of a bolus dose of 30 mg/kg for neuropathic pain.[7] In another, a bolus dose of 0.16 mmol/kg followed by infusion of 0.16 mmol/kg/h failed to reduce pain significantly despite increasing serum magnesium concentration by a factor of 2.[8]

SIDE EFFECTS

- Heat or pain on injection and flushing.
- Lightheadedness and dizziness may occur.
- Hypermagnesemia results in muscle weakness, cardiac conduction delays, nausea, tocolysis, areflexia, respiratory paralysis, and coma.
- Magnesium depresses the CNS despite poor penetration of the blood–brain barrier and results in neuro-muscular blockade via interference with release of neurotransmitters in the peripheral nervous system.
- Magnesium also produces vasodilation, through a direct action on blood vessels and by a reduction in peripheral vascular tone by sympathetic inhibition.

ADENOSINE

MECHANISM OF ACTION

- Adenosine is an endogenous nucleoside used to terminate reentrant supraventricular arrhythmias.
- An intravenous bolus of adenosine slows sinus rate and atrioventricular nodal conductance velocities and increases the atrioventricular nodal refractory period.
- Adenosine can produce transient activation of the sympathetic nervous system by interacting with carotid baroreceptors.
- Adenosine receptors are expressed on the surface of many cells, including neurons, in the peripheral nervous system and CNS.[9] Peripheral administration of A1 receptor agonist produces antinociception in animals, whereas A2 and A3 receptor agonists are pronociceptive.
- With spinal administration, A1 receptor agonists produce antinociception in animal models of acute, persistent inflammatory and neuropathic pain. In humans, spinal delivery of adenosine analogs produces analgesia. Although the dorsal horn contains both A1 and A2 receptor subtypes, A1 receptors are located preferentially in the dorsal horn, particularly in the substantia gelatinosa. After spinal administration, adenosine produces inhibition of postsynaptic neurons by increasing inward potassium conductance.
- Adenosine produces presynaptic inhibition of primary sensory neurons and consequent reduction of release of pronociceptive transmitters, such as substance P and glutamate, through inhibition of inward calcium current.
- Because of the short half-life (~10 seconds in plasma) and considerable enzymatic degradation of adenosine at the blood–brain barrier, there is little entry of adenosine into the CNS. Thus, the systemic delivery of adenosine may produce analgesia in humans though action on peripheral A1 receptors rather than through a central mechanism.

TYPE OF PAIN TREATED

- Intravenous adenosine has been used to treat preoperative pain, experimental pain, and peripheral neuropathic pain.

DOSAGE

- For neuropathic pain, intravenous adenosine is infused at 50–70 µg/kg/min for 40–60 minutes.[10] The analgesic effects occasionally last several hours after termination of the infusion therapy.

SIDE EFFECTS

- Sinus bradycardia, sinus arrest, and sinus tachycardia. Noncardiac effects may include flushing, hyperpnea, headache, nausea/vomiting, and cough.

PAMIDRONATE

MECHANISM OF ACTION

- Bisphosphonates are potent inhibitors of bone resorption that inhibit osteoclast activity by a variety of mechanisms.
- The long-term analgesic effect likely is secondary to osteoclast inhibition.
- The short-term analgesic effect, which may be evident within days or weeks, likely is secondary to inhibition of various algogenic substances.

TYPE OF PAIN TREATED

- Pain caused by osteolytic bone metastasis and Paget's disease.
- A case report describes the treatment of pain secondary to CRPS with a monthly infusion of intravenous pamidronate.

DOSAGE

- The dosage is 15–30 mg/wk or 60 mg every 4 weeks.[11]
- The duration of infusion therapy generally is limited to 2-hour intervals, and the infusion therapy is repeated every 2–4 weeks over the course of several months.
- No protocols exist for the infusion of intravenous bisphosphonates in the outpatient setting for patients with chronic benign pain.

SIDE EFFECTS

- The transient side effects include myalgias, arthralgia, lymphopenia, neutropenia, injection site reaction, and febrile reaction.
- Rare side effects include hypocalcemia, uveitis, scleritis, and thrombophlebitis.

ALFENTANIL

MECHANISM OF ACTION

- Opioid receptors are located throughout the central and peripheral nervous system but are highly concentrated in the substantia gelatinosa of the spinal cord dorsal horn.
- Opioids decrease presynaptic voltage-sensitive calcium currents and subsequent release of pronociceptive transmitters, such as substance P and calcitonin gene-related polypeptide.
- Opioids increase postsynaptic potassium current and hyperpolarize dorsal horn neurons.

TYPE OF PAIN TREATED

- Opioids are the mainstay of postoperative pain management and have been administered by infusion therapy for several decades.
- Intravenous opioid infusion therapy has been used widely for the management of cancer-related pain.
- Opioids are effective analgesics in animal models of acute, postincisional, inflammatory, visceral, and neuropathic pain.
- Opioids are potent analgesics in a diverse array of pain conditions including acute, postincisional, chronic benign, cancer, and neuropathic pain.
- Alfentanil is a synthetic mu opioid receptor agonist that reduces experimental pain (ongoing pain, pinprick hyperalgesia, and mechanical allodynia) produced by intradermal injection of capsaicin.
- Although opioid infusion therapy has not gained widespread popularity as a diagnostic test to predict opioid responsiveness in patients who suffer from chronic pain, alfentanil administration may have prognostic utility in the decision to administer oral opioids for patients with neuropathic pain or other chronic pain conditions.

DOSAGE

- In one study, alfentanil was administered as a 500-µg bolus followed by infusion of 4000 µg/h for 85 minutes.[12]

SIDE EFFECTS

- Opioids can cause constipation, pruritus, nausea, urinary retention, somnolence, and respiratory depression.
- Higher doses of opioids can produce myoclonus and hyperalgesia.

TABLE 55–3 Intravenous Infusion Therapy

DRUG	RECOMMENDED DOSE*
Lidocaine	0.62–5.0 μg/mL plasma level
	1.5–5.0 mg/kg range
Ketamine	0.31–0.55 μM serum level
	60 μg/kg bolus followed by 6 μg/kg/min infusion
Phentolamine	1 mg/kg administered over 10 min
Magnesium	30 mg/kg bolus
Adenosine	50–70 μg/kg/min over 40–60 min
Pamidronate	15–30 mg/wk or 60 mg every 4 wk
Alfentanil	500-μg bolus followed by infusion of 4000 μg/h
	for 85 min

*There are no standard guidelines for dosing of intravenous infusion agents except for phentolamine. The recommendations listed above have been extracted from doses published in the literature.

CONCLUSION

- Most infusion therapies for chronic pain have not been studied systematically in randomized, controlled trials.
- We lack specific guidelines for the administration of these therapies, and only cautious recommendations can be provided (Table 55–3).
- Clinicians need to develop a thorough understanding of the rationale governing use of these therapies prior to instituting their routine use.

REFERENCES

1. **Waxman SG, Dib-Hajj S, Cummins TR, et al.** Sodium channels and pain. *Proc Natl Acad Sci USA*. 1999;96:7635.
2. **Mao J, Chen LL.** Systemic lidocaine for neuropathic pain relief. *Pain* 2000;87:7.
3. **Parsons CG.** NMDA receptor as targets for drug action in neuropathic pain. *Eur J Pharmacol*. 2001;429:71.
4. **Fisher K, Coderre TJ, Hagen NA.** Targeting the *N*-methyl-D-aspartate receptor for chronic pain management: Preclinical animal studies, recent clinical experience and future research directions. *J Pain Symptom Manage*. 2000; 20:358.
5. **Baron R, Levine JD, Fields HL.** Causalgia and reflex sympathetic dystrophy: Does the sympathetic nervous system contribute to the generation of pain? *Muscle Nerve*. 1999; 22:678.
6. **Raja SN, Turnquist JL, Meleka S, et al.** Monitoring adequacy of alpha-adrenoceptor blockade following systemic phentolamine administration. *Pain*. 1996;64:197.
7. **Brill S, Sedgwick PM, Hamann W, et al.** Efficacy of intravenous magnesium in neuropathic pain. *Br J Anaesth*. 2002; 89:711.
8. **Felsby S, Arendt-Nielsen L, Jensen TS.** NMDA receptor blockade in chronic neuropathic pain: A comparison of ketamine and magnesium chloride. *Pain*. 1996;64:283.
9. **Sawynok J.** Adenosine receptor activation and nociception. *Eur J Pharmacol*. 1998;347:1.
10. **Sjolund KF, Belfage M, Karlsten R, et al.** Systemic adenosine infusion reduces the area of tactile allodynia in neuropathic pain following peripheral nerve injury: A multicentre, placebo-controlled study. *Eur J Pain*. 2001;5:199.
11. **Strang P.** Analgesic effect of bisphosphonates on bone pain in breast cancer patients: A review article. *Acta Oncol*. 1996; 35:50.
12. **Park KM, Max MB, Robinovitz E, et al.** Effects of intravenous ketamine, alfentanil, or placebo on pain, pinprick hyperalgesia, and allodynia produced by intradermal capsaicin in human subjects. *Pain*. 1995;63:163.

56 NEUROSURGICAL TECHNIQUES

Kenneth A. Follett, MD, PhD

INTRODUCTION

- Neurosurgical techniques include "anatomic" (eg, spinal reconstruction, microvascular decompression), augmentative ("neuromodulation"), and ablative procedures.
- Neuroaugmentative therapies have largely replaced neuroablative therapies as treatments of choice for intractable pain, but ablative therapies may be appropriate for certain patients.
- Expertise overlaps among medical specialties involved in pain care. Thus, some techniques reviewed in this chapter (eg, spinal cord stimulation and intrathecal analgesic administration) are provided by pain physicians trained in specialties other than neurosurgery as well as by neurosurgeons.
- Pain medicine practitioners, however, should be familiar with the indications for common neurosurgical techniques and refer patients for such procedures when appropriate.

PATIENT SELECTION FOR SURGICAL PAIN THERAPIES

- A surgical procedure is not usually the first treatment option for intractable pain.
- Treatment of intractable pain should follow a rational process with the simplest, safest methods used first and interventional treatments reserved for later in the course. The approach to patients with pain should be flexible, however, and treatment should be tailored to meet individual needs. For some individuals, this

means that a surgical procedure may occur earlier rather than later in the course of treatment.

- In general, surgical treatment of intractable pain is appropriate for individuals in whom:
  - Conservative therapies have not provided adequate pain relief.
  - Other treatments are associated with unacceptable side effects (eg, medication side effects).
  - Further direct treatment of the underlying cause of pain is not possible, practical, or appropriate.
  - There are no contraindications to surgery (eg, infection, coagulopathy).
  - The pain has a definable organic cause.
- Surgical treatment is not appropriate in patients with significant or untreated psychological or psychiatric disorders or overt dysfunction, such as active psychosis, suicidal or homicidal behavior, major uncontrolled depression or anxiety, serious alcohol or drug abuse, and serious cognitive deficits. Thus, formal psychological evaluation is appropriate for many individuals being considered for surgical treatment of intractable pain. Other psychological "risk factors" include somatization disorders, personality disorders (eg, borderline or antisocial), history of serious abuse, major issues of secondary gain, nonorganic signs on physical examination, unusual pain ratings (eg, 12 on a 10-point scale), inadequate social support, unrealistic outcomes and expectations, and, in the case of implantable augmentative devices, an inability to understand the device or its use. Patients with psy-

chological risk factors are not necessarily precluded from surgical treatment, but the treatment program should address the psychological issues to facilitate good outcomes.[1]

NEUROSURGICAL TECHNIQUES FOR INTRACTABLE PAIN

- Indications for anatomic (eg, spinal reconstruction, microvascular decompression), augmentative (neuromodulation), and ablative procedures overlap in many instances (Table 56–1). Augmentative therapies are generally preferred as initial surgical treatments for pain management because of their relative safety and reversibility; however, ablative therapies have a role in the treatment of certain pain syndromes.
- Factors that must be considered when selecting a therapy include pain etiology (cancer-related vs nonmalignant); pain location; pain characteristics (nociceptive vs neuropathic); patient life expectancy; and psychological, social, and economic issues relevant to the pain complaint. The advantages and disadvantages of anatomic, augmentative, and ablative therapies should be weighed according to these factors before choosing a general approach. A specific intervention can then be selected from within one of these general approaches.
- Specific interventions vary in their appropriateness as treatments for pain in specific body regions (Table

TABLE 56–1   Neurosurgical Pain Therapies

PAIN THERAPY	HEAD/NECK	UPPER TRUNK, SHOULDER, ARM	LOWER TRUNK, LEG	DIFFUSE
Anatomic	X	X	X	X
Augmentative				
Peripheral nerve stimulation	X	X	X	
Spinal cord stimulation		X	X	X
Thalamus (PVG-PAG) stimulation	X	X	X	
Motor cortex/deep brain stimulation	X	X	X	
Intrathecal/epidural drug infusion		X	X	X
Intraventricular drug infusion	X	X	X	X
Ablative				
Neurectomy	X	X	X	
Sympathectomy	X	X	X	
Ganglionectomy	X	X	X	
Rhizotomy	X	X	X	
Spinal DREZ lesioning		X	X	
Cordotomy			X	
Myelotomy			X	
Nucleus caudalis DREZ lesioning	X			
Trigeminal tractotomy	X			
Mesencephalotomy	X	X		
Thalamotomy	X	X	X	X
Cingulotomy	X	X	X	X
Hypophysectomy		X	X	X

DREZ, dorsal root entry zone; PVG, periventricular gray matter; PAG, periaqueductal gray matter.

56–1). The specific treatment offered to a patient, whether correction of structural deformity, ablative, or augmentative, should be selected according to the needs of each individual patient and the skills of the treating physician.

ANATOMIC TECHNIQUES

- Anatomic techniques, such as spinal decompressive (eg, laminectomy, discectomy) and reconstructive procedures may be performed to treat pain, neurologic deficits, or orthopedic abnormalities.
- "Microvascular decompression" is an important treatment for trigeminal neuralgia, glossopharyngeal neuralgia, and nervus intermedius neuralgia and is a primary technique for classic neuralgia (paroxysmal, lancinating pain) that is refractory to pharmacologic treatment.
- Microvascular decompression is most appropriate for healthy patients, generally under the age of 65.
- The rationale of this surgery is to eliminate the compression of the cranial nerve by a blood vessel (usually a small artery) that generally occurs near the entry of the nerve into the brainstem.
- The advantage of microvascular decompression compared with percutaneous (eg, radiofrequency rhizotomy for trigeminal neuralgia) or open ablative procedures for cranial neuralgias is the absence of postoperative sensory deficit, which is an obligate outcome of most ablative procedures. Pain relief is achieved in more than 95% of patients.
- Pain may recur over months or years in some patients but relief is maintained in most patients.

AUGMENTATIVE TECHNIQUES

- Augmentative therapies involve either stimulation or neuraxial drug infusion.
- Compared with ablative therapies, augmentative therapies are:
  ○ Relatively safe, reversible, and "adjustable"
  ○ Cost more (initial device costs and upkeep)
  ○ Require maintenance (eg, refilling of infusion pumps, replacement of stimulation system battery packs)
  ○ Have the potential for device-related complications
- General indications for augmentative therapies are similar to those for other neurosurgical pain treatments.
- In addition, estimated patient life expectancy should be sufficient to warrant implantation of a neuroaugmentative device (eg, more than 3 months for a cancer patient).

STIMULATION THERAPIES

- FDA has approved spinal cord stimulation (SCS) and peripheral nerve stimulation (PNS) therapies.
- Other stimulation therapies in clinical use include deep brain stimulation and motor cortex stimulation.

SPINAL CORD STIMULATION
- SCS is appropriate for treatment of neuropathic pain that is relatively focal (eg, localized to one or two extremities or focal on the trunk) and static in nature.[2]
- Common applications include:
  ○ Radicular pain associated with failed back surgery syndrome.
  ○ Pain related to complex regional pain syndrome ("reflex sympathetic dystrophy").
  ○ Pain affecting the trunk (eg, postherpetic neuralgia, some types of postthoracotomy pain).
  ○ Extremity pain related to peripheral neuropathy, root injury, and phantom limb pain (postamputation stump pain does not improve consistently with SCS).
  ○ Ischemic extremity pain due to peripheral vascular disease may improve with SCS.
- In addition, SCS is gaining acceptance as a treatment for refractory angina pectoris and for interstitial cystitis, but it is not approved by FDA for these indications.
- Stimulation leads may be implanted percutaneously or surgically. Surgical ("laminotomy," "plate," or "paddle") leads offer the advantages of a lower incidence of dislodgement ("migration"), lower stimulation amplitude requirements, and longer pulse generator battery life.
- The success rate of SCS (more than 50% reduction in pain) in the failed back surgery syndrome population is approximately 60–65% at 5 years.
- Patients with complex regional pain syndromes have similar outcomes, although success rates as high as 70–100% have been reported.
- SCS is less consistently successful in the treatment of other pain syndromes, for example, phantom limb pain and postherpetic neuralgia, but warrants a trial because of its relative ease and safety.

PERIPHERAL NERVE STIMULATION
- The indications for PNS are similar to those for SCS except that the distribution of pain should be limited to the territory of a single peripheral nerve.
- Extremity pain that might be appropriately treated with PNS can sometimes be treated equally well with SCS, and many physicians find it easier to implant a percutaneous SCS lead than a PNS lead (which usually requires an open procedure).

- The outcomes of PNS are generally similar to those of SCS, and PNS can be very effective for the treatment of occipital neuralgia.

INTRACRANIAL STIMULATION

- Intracranial stimulation therapies include deep brain stimulation (DBS) of the somatosensory thalamus and periventricular–periaqueductal gray matter[3] and motor cortex stimulation.[4]
- These therapies are used primarily for treating pain of nonmalignant origin, such as pain associated with failed back surgery syndrome, neuropathic pain following central or peripheral nervous system injury, or trigeminal pain.
- Neither DBS nor motor cortex stimulation has the approval of FDA for the treatment of pain, although DBS has been used clinically for more than two decades.

Deep Brain Stimulation

- The targets for focal electrical stimulation of the brain include the ventrocaudal nucleus (ventroposterolateral and ventroposteromedial nucleus) and periventricular–periaqueductal gray matter (PVG–PAG).
- The DBS sites are chosen generally on the basis of the pain characteristics. Nociceptive pain and paroxysmal, lancinating, or evoked neuropathic pain (eg, allodynia, hyperpathia) tend to respond best to PVG–PAG stimulation, which may activate endogenous opioid systems. Continuous neuropathic pain responds most consistently to DBS of the sensory thalamus (ventrocaudal nucleus).
- Because many pain syndromes have mixed components of nociceptive and neuropathic pain, some physicians place electrodes in both regions, subject the patient to a trial of stimulation using externalized leads, and internalize the electrode that provides the best pain relief.
- Success rates of DBS for the treatment of intractable pain are difficult to determine from the literature because patient selection, techniques, and outcome assessments vary substantially among studies. Although 60–80% of patients undergoing a screening trial with DBS have sufficient pain relief to warrant implantation of a permanent stimulation system, 25–35% of patients undergoing a DBS trial have good long-term pain relief, and some investigators have reported 80% success rates.
- DBS results are better in patients with pain related to cancer, failed back surgery syndrome, peripheral neuropathy, or trigeminal neuropathy (not anesthesia dolorosa) than in patients with central pain syndromes (eg, thalamic pain, spinal cord injury pain, anesthesia dolorosa, postherpetic neuralgia, phantom limb pain).[3]

- The incidence of serious complications of DBS is generally low, but the combined incidence of morbidity, mortality, and technical complications can approach 25–30%.

Motor Cortex Stimulation

- Motor cortex stimulation (MCS) has received attention as an alternative to thalamic and PVG–PAG stimulation.[4] Overlap exists between indications for DBS and MCS, but MCS is thought to have a lower risk of serious complication because the electrode is placed epidurally rather than within the brain parenchyma.
- The primary indication for MCS is treatment of localized neuropathic pain. Because of technical issues related to electrode placement, the face is the easiest region of the body to treat, and MCS may be particularly effective for the treatment of trigeminal neuropathic pain. Treatment of focal pain affecting an arm may be possible, but treatment of pain affecting the trunk or, in particular, the legs is difficult because of technical difficulties in positioning the stimulation electrode over the appropriate region of motor cortex.
- Approximately 50–70% of patients undergoing MCS have good long-term pain relief. As with DBS, MCS seems to be most effective for patients with no anesthesia in the distribution of the pain being treated.
- MCS is a promising therapy, and its potential long-term efficacy is under active investigation at several centers.

NEURAXIAL DRUG INFUSION

- Neuraxial analgesic administration is indicated primarily for the treatment of pain syndromes with a significant nociceptive/somatic component (eg, cancer-related pain) because nociceptive/somatic pain typically responds to opioid therapy. However, neuropathic pain may improve with intrathecal analgesic administration as well.
- The most common application of intrathecal analgesic is management of pain related to failed back surgery syndrome, which typically includes both nociceptive (low back) and neuropathic (extremity) components.
- Although the use of intrathecal analgesics for the treatment of cancer-related pain is well-accepted, the use of this therapy for chronic nonmalignant pain remains controversial. In part, this reflects concern that neuropathic pain (common in chronic nonmalignant pain syndromes) does not respond adequately to opioids, and the efficacy and cost-effectiveness of the therapy have not been determined in controlled trials.

- The key advantage of neuraxial analgesic administration compared with other pain therapy is its versatility:
  - It has a wide range of indications, including nociceptive and mixed nociceptive/neuropathic pain syndromes.
  - It can be used to treat focal or diffuse pain as well as axial and/or extremity pain. It is used commonly to treat pain below cervical levels but can be effective for head and neck pain, especially if analgesic agents are delivered intraventricularly.[5]
  - It can be used in the setting of changing pain (eg, in a patient with progressive cancer).
- Significant disadvantages include device costs, medication costs, and need for maintenance (eg, pump refills and battery replacement).
- Most patients (60–80%) achieve good long-term relief of pain, and outcomes are similar (degree of pain relief, patient satisfaction, and dose requirements) for patients with cancer-related and noncancer pain.
- Serious complications of the therapy are uncommon.

ABLATIVE TECHNIQUES

- Ablative therapies are often considered the top and final rung on the pain treatment ladder (ie, the last resort), but in some instances they are procedures of choice. Thus, phantom-limb pain in the setting of spinal nerve root avulsion or "end zone" pain arising from spinal cord injury can be treated effectively by dorsal root entry zone (DREZ) lesioning.
- Lesioning and cordotomy might be more appropriate than intrathecal analgesia for the treatment of cancer-related pain in a patient with a short life expectancy
- Ablative therapies target almost every level of the peripheral and central nervous systems:
  - Peripheral techniques interrupt or alter nociception in the spinal cord (eg, neurectomy, ganglionectomy, rhizotomy).
  - Spinal interventions alter afferent input or rostral transmission of nociceptive information (eg, DREZ lesioning, cordotomy, myelotomy).
  - Supraspinal intracranial procedures may interrupt transmission of nociceptive information (eg, mesencephalotomy, thalamotomy) or influence perception of painful stimuli (eg, cingulotomy).
- Ablative therapies are most appropriate for the treatment of nociceptive pain rather than neuropathic pain. Neuropathic pain that is intermittent, paroxysmal, or evoked (eg, allodynia, hyperpathia) may improve after an ablative procedure, but continuous, dysesthetic neuropathic pain remains relatively unchanged in long-term follow-up.

PERIPHERAL TECHNIQUES

SYMPATHECTOMY

- Sympathectomy is indicated for the treatment of visceral pain associated with certain cancers.
- Although sympathectomy can be effective for noncancer pain associated with vasospastic disorders or sympathetically maintained pain (when sympathetic blocks reliably relieve the pain), the procedure has fallen into disfavor as a treatment for intractable nonmalignant pain because of inconsistent results.
- Because some data indicate that SCS provides a better long-term outcome with lower morbidity than does sympathectomy, SCS may become the treatment of choice for sympathetically maintained noncancer pain.

NEURECTOMY

- Neurectomy may be useful in individuals who develop pain following peripheral nerve injury, including that associated with limb amputation, or in cases where an identifiable neuroma is the cause of pain.
- Neurectomy is not useful for treatment of nonspecific stump pain after amputation or for other nonmalignant peripheral pain syndromes.
- The utility of neurectomy is limited because pain arising from a pure sensory nerve is not common, and mixed sensory–motor nerves cannot be sectioned without risk of functional impairment.
- As exceptions to this rule, however, sectioning the lateral femoral cutaneous nerve may provide good long-lasting relief of meralgia paresthetica, and sectioning the ilioinguinal and/or genitofemoral nerves may provide good relief of some inguinal pain syndromes (eg, postherniorrhaphy pain) in properly selected patients.

DORSAL RHIZOTOMY/GANGLIONECTOMY

- Dorsal rhizotomy and ganglionectomy serve similar purposes in denervating somatic and/or visceral tissues. Ganglionectomy, however, may produce more complete denervation than can be accomplished by dorsal rhizotomy because some afferent fibers enter the spinal cord through the ventral root and are not affected by dorsal rhizotomy. In contrast, ganglionectomy effectively eliminates input from dorsal and ventral root afferent fibers by removing their cell bodies, which are located within the dorsal root ganglion.
- Both rhizotomy and ganglionectomy can be used to treat pain in the trunk or abdomen, but neither procedure is useful for treatment of pain in the extremities unless function of the extremity is already lost, because denervation removes proprioceptive as

well as nociceptive input and produces a functionless limb.

- To be successful, denervation must extend over several adjacent levels. Limited denervation does not provide adequate pain relief, probably because of overlap of segmental innervation of dermatomes.
- In addition, these procedures are most appropriate for the treatment of cancer-related pain; noncancer pain does not improve consistently.
- When these procedures are used to treat neuropathic pain (eg, postherpetic neuralgia of the trunk), lancinating, paroxysmal, or evoked pain may improve, but continuous dysesthetic pain does not typically improve.
- In the setting of cancer, rhizotomy and ganglionectomy can be useful for thoracic or abdominal wall pain; for perineal pain in patients with impaired bladder, bowel, and sex function; and for pain in a functionless extremity. Multiple sacral rhizotomies can be performed (eg, to treat pelvic pain from cancer) by passing a ligature around the thecal sac below S1.

CRANIAL NERVE RHIZOTOMY

- Rhizotomy is especially useful in treating cranial neuralgias, especially trigeminal and glossopharyngeal neuralgia.[6] Classic trigeminal and glossopharyngeal neuralgia are unique among neuropathic pain syndromes in their uniformly good response to ablative procedures. In contrast, atypical facial pain syndromes (constant, burning pain) do not improve with ablative techniques and may intensify following rhizotomy.
- Percutaneous trigeminal rhizotomy can be accomplished with radiofrequency, glycerol injection, or balloon compression. These techniques are performed on an outpatient basis, are well tolerated, and have high success rates in relieving paroxysmal pain of cranial neuralgias.[6]
- Open rhizotomy (ie, via craniotomy or craniectomy) is usually performed for treatment of glossopharyngeal and nervus intermedius neuralgia and may be required for treatment of some trigeminal neuralgias.
- Stereotactic radiosurgery rhizotomy for the treatment of trigeminal neuralgia is an alternative to percutaneous or open rhizotomy or microvascular decompression.[7]
- Unlike other surgical treatments for trigeminal neuralgia, pain relief does not occur for several weeks following radiosurgical treatment. Radiosurgery is, therefore, not appropriate for patients with severe acute exacerbation of pain that cannot be controlled adequately with medications because it does not afford prompt pain relief.

- Early pain relief is achieved in more than 95% of patients undergoing percutaneous or open rhizotomy. Pain may recur after months or years in some patients, but relief is maintained in most patients.[6]

C2 GANGLIONECTOMY

- C2 ganglionectomy is indicated for the treatment of occipital neuralgia.
- It is especially effective for patients with posttraumatic occipital neuralgia who have no migraine component to their headache.[8]
- In most patients, long-term pain relief may be comparable to that achieved with occipital nerve stimulation without the need for implanted devices and long-term follow-up.

SPINAL TECHNIQUES

DORSAL ROOT ENTRY ZONE LESIONING

- DREZ lesioning of the spinal cord (for trunk or extremity pain)[9] or of the nucleus caudalis (for facial pain) can significantly relieve neuropathic pain in properly selected individuals.
- DREZ lesioning disrupts input and outflow in the superficial layers of the spinal cord dorsal horn where afferent nociceptive fibers terminate and some of the ascending nociceptive fibers originate. DREZ lesioning also disrupts the spontaneous abnormal activity and hyperactivity that develops in spinal cord dorsal horn neurons in the setting of neuropathic pain.
- DREZ lesioning is best reserved for localized pain with a neuropathic component. Certain types of cancer pain can be treated effectively with DREZ lesioning (eg, neuropathic arm pain associated with Pancoast tumor). The most successful applications, however, are related to treatment of neuropathic pain arising from spinal nerve root avulsion (cervical or lumbosacral) and "end zone" or "boundary" pain following spinal cord injury. These pain syndromes sometimes respond to SCS or intrathecal drug infusion, but DREZ lesioning can provide a similar result without the need for long-term device maintenance.
- DREZ lesioning has been used to treat other neuropathic pain syndromes (eg, postherpetic neuralgia), but good pain relief is not achieved consistently. DREZ lesioning of the nucleus caudalis can relieve deafferentation pain affecting the face (including postherpetic neuralgia), but outcomes are inconsistent. It is less helpful for facial pain of peripheral origin (eg, traumatic trigeminal neuropathy).
- As with other ablative procedures, DREZ lesioning is most effective for relieving paroxysmal or evoked neuropathic pain rather than continuous neuropathic pain.

CORDOTOMY

- Cordotomy can be an effective method of pain control, especially when pain is related to malignancy and for individuals with a short life expectancy for whom it is difficult to justify the costs of implanted drug infusion systems.
- Cordotomy disrupts nociceptive afferent fibers ascending in the spinothalamic tract in the anterolateral quadrant of the spinal cord.
- Cordotomy is a one-time procedure with no required long-term follow-up or maintenance. This is important for individuals who may find it difficult to return to a medical facility for refilling of an infusion system or for whom costs of ongoing medical care become burdensome.
- Cordotomy is used most commonly to treat cancer-related pain below the mid- to low cervical dermatomes. It is not generally used to treat noncancer pain, and cordotomy carries a significant risk of dysesthesias or neurologic complication.[10]
- Cordotomy can be performed as an open or percutaneous procedure.[10] Percutaneous techniques are less invasive, but some surgeons lack the required expertise and equipment.
- Pain relief following cordotomy varies with pain characteristics and location.
- Lancinating, paroxysmal, neuropathic pain and the evoked (allodynic or hyperpathic) pain that sometimes follows spinal cord injury or occurs as part of peripheral neuropathic pain syndromes can improve following cordotomy, but continuous neuropathic pain does not improve.[10] Laterally located pain responds better than midline or axial pain (eg, visceral pain). Midline and axial pain may require bilateral procedures to achieve pain relief.
- The risk of complications, including weakness; bladder, bowel, and sexual dysfunction; and respiratory depression (if the procedure is performed bilaterally at cervical levels), is significantly greater with bilateral procedures.[10] Bilateral percutaneous cervical cordotomies are usually staged at least 1 week apart to reduce the likelihood of a serious complication.
- The risk of respiratory depression subsequent to a unilateral high cervical procedure mandates that pulmonary function be acceptable on the contralateral side. For example, a patient who has undergone previous pneumonectomy for lung cancer should not undergo a cordotomy that would compromise pulmonary function of the remaining lung.[10]
- Cordotomy provides good pain relief in 60–80% of patients, but loss of pain relief may occur over time.[10] Approximately one-third of patients have recurrent pain in 3 months, half at 1 year, and two-thirds at longer follow-up intervals.

MYELOTOMY

- Myelotomy can provide significant pain relief in properly selected individuals, including some who fail treatment with intrathecal analgesics.[11]
- Commissural myelotomy was developed to provide the benefits of bilateral cordotomy without the inherent risk of lesioning both anterior quadrants of the spinal cord.[11] This is accomplished by sectioning spinothalamic tract fibers from both sides of the body with one lesion as they decussate in the anterior commissure. The advantage of myelotomy compared with cordotomy is that bilateral and midline pain can be treated with a single procedure with lower morbidity and mortality.
- Clinical observations revealed that a limited midline myelotomy (a lesion a few millimeters in length versus the several centimeters of a commissural myelotomy) or a high cervical myelotomy can be as effective as a commissural myelotomy in relieving abdominal, pelvic, and lower extremity pain.
- Identification of a dorsal column visceral pain pathway has led to the development of punctate midline myelotomy to treat abdominal and pelvic pain.
- These procedures are indicated primarily for cancer-related pain, generally in the abdomen, pelvis, perineum, and legs, and are most effective for nociceptive rather than neuropathic pain. Early, complete pain relief is achieved in most patients (more than 90%), but pain tends to recur, leaving only 50–60% of patients with good long-term pain relief.
- The risk of bladder or bowel complications or sexual dysfunction is less than that associated with bilateral cordotomy but remains sufficiently high that use of this procedure is restricted in most instances to patients with cancer-related pain who have preexisting dysfunction.

SUPRASPINAL CRANIAL TECHNIQUES

- Ablative neurosurgical procedures directed at the brainstem are not in widespread use, in part because relatively few patients require such interventions and because relatively few neurosurgeons have the expertise to perform them. They are reserved for patients who fail more conservative therapies or who are not candidates for less invasive procedures.

MESENCEPHALOTOMY

- Mesencephalotomy is indicated for intractable pain involving the head, neck, shoulder, and arm.[12] Most commonly, the procedure is used to treat cancer pain.
- Mesencephalotomy disrupts nociceptive fibers ascending in the brainstem and can be viewed as a supraspinal version of cordotomy.

- Pain relief is achieved in 85% of patients, but mesencephalotomy does not provide consistent long-term relief of central neuropathic pain.
- Side effects and complications, especially oculomotor dysfunction, are common.
- The utility of mesencephalotomy has diminished subsequent to the advent of neuraxial analgesic administration. Intraventricular morphine infusion can provide good relief of head, neck, shoulder, and arm pain with a lower incidence of complications.
- Mesencephalotomy may be preferable for some individuals, for example, those with a short life expectancy or for whom the costs or long-term follow-up required with neuraxial analgesic administration become burdensome.

THALAMOTOMY

- Thalamotomy has been used to treat both cancer and noncancer pain. In the setting of cancer, thalamotomy is most appropriate for patients who have widespread pain (eg, from diffuse metastatic disease) or who have midline, bilateral, or head/neck pain that other procedures are not likely to relieve.[13]
- The success rate of thalamotomy in relieving pain is slightly lower than that of mesencephalotomy, but the incidence of complications is lower with thalamotomy[13]; thus, thalamotomy may be preferable for the treatment of head, neck, shoulder, and arm pain in patients who are not candidates for neuraxial analgesia.
- Thalamotomy can also be useful for patients who are not candidates for cordotomy, for example, those with pain above the C5 dermatome or with pulmonary dysfunction.
- The procedure can be accomplished via stereotactic radiofrequency or radiosurgical techniques.
- Medial thalamotomy appears to be most effective for treating nociceptive pain (eg, cancer pain), with acceptable long-term pain relief obtained in 30–50% of patients.
- Overall, neuropathic pain syndromes respond less consistently to thalamotomy, with only approximately one-third of patients achieving long-term improvement.
- As with other ablative procedures, paroxysmal, lancinating neuropathic pain or neuropathic pain with elements of allodynia and hyperpathia (ie, evoked pain) may improve following thalamotomy, whereas continuous neuropathic pain tends not to improve.

CINGULOTOMY

- Cingulotomy is used less commonly to treat intractable pain than it is to manage psychiatric disorders. When used, it is most often to treat cancer pain, but it has been used for noncancer pain as well.[14]

- Approximately 50–75% of treated patients benefit from the procedure, at least short-term. In the cancer population, pain relief generally is maintained at least 3 months.
- The utility of cingulotomy for chronic noncancer pain is less certain; some studies indicate relatively good long-lasting pain relief and others only 20% long-term success.
- Because cingulotomy is performed to treat psychiatric disease and carries the stigma of "psychosurgery," formal review by an institutional ethics committee may be warranted before using this procedure to treat intractable pain.

HYPOPHYSECTOMY

- Hypophysectomy (surgical, chemical, or radiosurgical) can provide good relief of cancer-related pain.
- It is traditionally thought to be most effective for hormonally responsive cancers (eg, prostate, breast cancer) but may relieve pain associated with other tumors as well. It is indicated primarily for the treatment of diffuse pain associated with widespread disease.
- Hypophysectomy alleviates pain in 45–95% of treated patients. Pain relief occurs independent of tumor regression; the specific mechanism of pain relief is unknown.[15]

SUMMARY

- In general, augmentative neuromodulation techniques have supplanted ablative procedures as treatments of choice for intractable pain. The outcomes of augmentative therapies in properly selected patients are good, and the risk of serious or permanent complication is low, making neuromodulation therapies the first choice for many patients.
- Augmentative techniques, especially SCS and deep brain stimulation, are superior to ablative techniques for the treatment of neuropathic pain that has a continuous, dysesthetic component.
- Ablative therapies may be appropriate for some patients, for example, those with cancer-related pain who do not have a long life expectancy. Patients with a predominant nociceptive component of pain and those with neuropathic pain with paroxysmal or evoked components can also benefit from ablative techniques.
- Ablative techniques are very useful for certain pain syndromes:
  - Rhizotomy for trigeminal neuralgia
  - DREZ lesioning for "end zone" or "boundary" pain associated with spinal cord injury or phantom limb pain associated with avulsion of cervical or lumbar spinal nerve roots

○ Cordotomy or myelotomy for treatment of intractable cancer pain in patients with a short life expectancy or those who have failed treatment with neuraxial analgesics

- Pain management physicians should be familiar with the variety of neurosurgical techniques available to treat pain, their indications, and general outcomes and should incorporate these treatments into the care of their patients when appropriate. Otherwise, with the increasing amount of attention paid to augmentative therapies to treat intractable pain, ablative therapies that might be appropriate for some patients may be overlooked as treatment options.

REFERENCES

1. **Doleys DM, Olson K.** *Psychological Assessment and Intervention in Implantable Pain Therapies.* Minneapolis, Minn: Medtronic Inc; 1997.
2. **Deer TR.** The role of neuromodulation by spinal cord stimulation in chronic pain syndromes: Current concepts. *Tech Reg Anesth Pain Manage.* 1998;2:161.
3. **Kumar K, Toth C, Nath RK.** Deep brain stimulation for intractable pain: A 15-year experience. *Neurosurgery.* 1997; 40:736.
4. **Nguyen J-P, Lefaucheur J-P, Decq P, et al.** Chronic motor cortex stimulation in the treatment of central and neuropathic pain: Correlations between clinical, electrophysiological and anatomical data. *Pain.* 1999;82:245.
5. **Karavelis A, Foroglou G, Selviaridis P, et al.** Intraventricular administration of morphine for control of intractable cancer pain in 90 patients. *Neurosurgery.* 1996;39:57.
6. **Taha JM, Tew JM Jr.** Comparison of surgical treatments for trigeminal neuralgia: Reevaluation of radiofrequency rhizotomy. *Neurosurgery.* 1997;38:865.
7. **Maesawa S, Salame C, Flickinger JC, et al.** Clinical outcomes after stereotactic radiosurgery for idiopathic trigeminal neuralgia. *J Neurosurg.* 2001;94:14.
8. **Lozano AM, Vanderlinden G, Bachoo R, et al.** Microsurgical C-2 ganglionectomy for chronic intractable occipital pain. *J Neurosurg.* 1998;89:359.
9. **Rath SA, Seitz K, Soliman N, et al.** DREZ coagulations for deafferentation pain related to spinal and peripheral nerve lesions: Indication and results of 79 consecutive procedures. *Stereotact Funct Neurosurg.* 1997;68(1–4, Pt 1):161.
10. **Tasker RR.** Percutaneous cordotomy. In: Schmidek HH, Sweet WH, eds. *Operative Neurosurgical Techniques: Indications, Methods, and Results.* 3rd ed. Philadelphia: WB Saunders; 1995:1595.
11. **Watling CJ, Payne R, Allen RR, et al.** Commissural myelotomy for intractable cancer pain: Report of two cases. *Clin J Pain.* 1996;12:151.
12. **Bullard DE, Nashold BS Jr.** Mesencephalatomy and other brain stem procedures for pain. In: Youmans JR, ed. *Neurological Surgery.* Philadelphia: WB Saunders; 1996: 3477.
13. **Tasker RR.** Thalamotomy. *Neurosurg Clin North Am.* 1990;1:841.
14. **Hassenbusch SJ, Pillay PK, Barnett GH.** Radiofrequency cingulotomy for intractable cancer pain using stereotaxis guided by magnetic resonance imaging. *Neurosurgery.* 1990;27:220.
15. **Ramirez LF, Levin AB.** Pain relief after hypophysectomy. *Neurosurgery.* 1984;14:499.

57 RADIOFREQUENCY ABLATION

Sunil J. Panchal, MD
Anu Perni, MD

HISTORY

- Radiofrequency (RF) lesioning or ablation was first used in the treatment of pain to improve the predictability of the size of lesions created during percutaneous lateral cordotomy for unilateral malignant pain.
- RF lesioning is now used to treat a variety of pain disorders, including disk-related pain.
- The rationale for the use of RF in pain is straightforward: the destruction of the nerves that signal pain should relieve pain.
- This oversimplistic view of neural activity has led to less than satisfactory results with neuroablation and restriction of its use to certain conditions.

PRINCIPLES

- RF lesioning involves inserting a small insulated electrode with an uninsulated (active) tip through the tissue surrounding the target nerve.
- The tissue impedes the flow of current through the needle, causing the current to be dissipated as heat (Joule heating).
- Heat is not generated in the electrode tip because the electrode offers minimal resistance to flow. The tip absorbs heat from the surrounding tissue, however, eventually achieving thermal equilibrium with the entire system.
- The greatest density of current occurs adjacent to the tip of the electrode; as a result, the adjacent tissue becomes the hottest part of the lesion.
- The amount of heat generated controls the quality of the lesion; temperature control determines the size of the lesion.

- The lesion is spherical around the active tip and progresses only a very small distance beyond the cannula tip.
- Unlike direct current techniques, RF uses continuous high-frequency waves of about 1 MHz.[1]
  - Whereas direct current generates lesions by dielectric mechanisms similar to electrolysis, RF generates lesions by ionic means. Thus, compared with direct current lesions, RF lesions are more uniform in size, more predictable, and not complicated by the gas formation of electrolysis.
  - RF generators have automatic temperature controls that allow precise control over tissue temperature and the extent of the lesion.
  - Electrical stimulation can be used to locate the nerve and prevent unwanted nerve damage.
  - Tissue resistance (impedance) can be measured: high impedance (>2000 ohms) suggests electrical disconnection, and low impedance (<200 ohms) implies a short circuit.
- The most common reason for failure to generate a lesion is a poor electrical connection, usually related to cable damage.

CIRCUIT PRINCIPLES

- The circuit consists of a RF generator, which initiates the current; an active electrode, which delivers the current; a thermistor or thermocouple, which monitors the temperature; and a passive electrode with a large surface area, which returns the current.
- Current in the region of the active electrode generates heat, which in turn heats the electrode tip solely as a result of local tissue warming.
- The heat generated is a function of the amount of current that flows in the region of the electrode and the resistance of the surrounding tissue.
- Current flows from the active to the passive electrode, however, because, compared with the active electrode, the passive electrode has much greater surface area and less current density; thus, heating and tissue damage do not usually occur at the passive electrode.
- Tissue damage is related to the temperature generated; therefore, heating of the active electrode is an important safety feature that allows control of lesion size. Four factors affect the size of a lesion:
  - *Temperature*: At higher temperatures, the size of the lesion increases.
  - *Thermal equilibrium*: The more rapid the tissue equilibrium, the more uniform the lesion. Lesion size initially rises exponentially with time but becomes independent of time after approximately 30 seconds.
  - *Electrode size*: Larger electrodes generate larger lesions.
  - *Local tissue characteristics*: Lesions in tissues in contact with tissue of low electrical resistance, such as blood and cerebrospinal fluid, may be small or irregular in shape because the current was siphoned through paths with relatively little impedance. Similarly, lesions created next to heat-absorbing bone may suffer from irregular heating. Circulation of blood also provides a heat sink.
- Thus, choosing a proper electrode, achieving quick thermal equilibrium to a controlled temperature near nonconductive tissues, helps ensure optimal results.
- To ensure refinement of technique, it is essential, that the following parameters be recorded for every lesion: type of electrode, temperature, time, voltage, and current.
- The actual tip may not even be incorporated into the lesion, so nerves in contact with the tip may be only partially blocked; furthermore, electrodes placed tangential to the nerve often generate a more effective lesion.
- The effect of RF on tissue depends on the temperature generated: >45°C, irreversible tissue injury occurs; between 42 and 45°C, temporary neural blockade occurs.
- The larger the lesion, the larger the zone of irreversibility.[2] Early in its use, clinicians believed heat was selective for small-diameter neural fibers, but this was not borne out by histologic analysis.

EQUIPMENT

- Cannulas used for RF lesioning come in various lengths and diameters and may be straight or curved.
- Reusable and disposable needles are available.
- Selection depends on the depth of the intended target, the desired size of the lesion, and operator experience and comfort level with cannula placement.
- Cannula systems are available in 50-, 100-, and 150-mm lengths with both 5- and 2-mm active tips.
- When performing RF ablation, it is critical to have additional cannulas for backup, as well as backup connector cables to be prepared for possible defects/malfunctions.

ADVANTAGES

- With a typical temperature gradient of 10°C/mm, the lesion size can be effectively controlled and predicted by selecting the appropriate target temperature.

- Lesion temperature can be monitored with a thermocouple electrode, allowing for adjustment of energy output to maintain the target temperature.
- Appropriate placement of the electrode is facilitated with electrical stimulation and impedance monitoring.
- The stimulation feature allows the operator to determine if the active tip is too close to a neural target that is undesirable for lesioning, such as a nerve root.
- Conventional stimulation testing consists of sensory testing at 50 Hz up to 1.0 V and motor testing at 2 Hz up to 2.5 V. This range stimulates structures in a 1-cm radius of the active tip.
- Impedance monitoring provides additional information about the type of tissue in which the active tip is located (bone differs from muscle, etc) and assists in confirming appropriate location.
- The discomfort associated with this minimally invasive technique is of limited duration, and most RF lesions can be performed with mild sedation.
- It is very important to maintain the patient's ability to report his or her experience during sensory and motor testing to maintain safety.
- The incidence of morbidity and mortality is low when performed by a skilled operator.
- The procedure can be repeated if necessary.

GENERAL INDICATIONS, PROGNOSTIC TESTS, AND COMPLICATIONS

- RF ablation is a useful tool in the treatment of pain that occurs in a well-defined and fairly limited anatomic location where we have a clear understanding of the neuroanatomy involved for nociception.
- Appropriate patients are those in whom reasonable conservative treatment failed to provide adequate analgesia or was limited by side effects.
- Possible associated motor or sensory deficits must be discussed with the patient as part of the informed consent process prior to embarking on RF ablation.
- Psychological assessment helps eliminate patients who may not respond in a reliable manner to any intervention.
- A prognostic block is advised to assess possible magnitude of response to neuroablation.
- Some practitioners routinely perform a series of prognostic blocks using local anesthetics of different durations as well as a placebo injection to determine if the patient exhibits a consistent response.
- Complications associated with RF ablation include neurologic deficits from the intended target or nearby neural structures, deafferentation pain, neuritis, burn injury at breaks in the needle insulation, hematoma, and infection.

- All RF procedures are performed under sterile conditions with fluoroscopic guidance.

HEAD AND NECK PAIN

TRIGEMINAL NEURALGIA

- Idiopathic (typical) trigeminal neuralgia (ITN) is the most common form of cranial neuralgia, occurring with a mean annual incidence of 4 or 5 patients per 100,000 population.[3]
- Unilateral sharp, lancinating pain limited to the somatosensory territory of one or more divisions of the trigeminal nerve with short attacks and associated trigger points is characteristic of ITN. Other features include: absence of pain between attacks; frequent remissions, especially early in the course of the disease; normal neurologic examination; and high degree of pain relief in response to oral carbamazepine.
- The cause of ITN is unknown; however, in most patients, the trigeminal nerve root is compressed by adjacent vessels, most commonly the superior cerebellar and anterior inferior cerebellar arteries.
- Patients with ITN who no longer experience pain relief with medications or develop side effects can be treated effectively by percutaneous RF trigeminal rhizotomy, glycerol rhizotomy, or balloon compression. Each procedure has advantages and disadvantages; however, RF trigeminal rhizotomy has the highest selectivity.[4]

ANATOMY

- The trigeminal nerve originates in the brainstem and synapses in the gasserian ganglion before dividing into the ophthalmic, maxillary, and mandibular nerves, which pass through the foramen ovale.

TRIGEMINAL RHIZOTOMY TECHNIQUE

- Trigeminal rhizotomy,[5] used to treat ITN, can also effectively treat facial pain associated with tumors, multiple sclerosis,[6] and cluster headaches.[7]
- Oral intake is restricted 6 hours prior to the procedure, and atropine (0.4 mg intramuscularly) is administered 30 minutes before the procedure to reduce oral secretions and prevent bradycardia during sedation.
- Short-acting sedatives can be administered during the procedure.

- The patient lies supine with the head in neutral position.
- The patient's blood pressure, heart rate, and oxygen saturation are monitored continuously during the procedure.
- Three anatomic landmarks are marked on the face: 3 cm anterior to the external auditory meatus, beneath the medial aspect of the pupil, and 2.5 cm lateral to the oral commissure. The first two delineate the site of the foramen ovale, and the third delineates the site of needle entry.
- The needle is placed into the foramen ovale anteriorly. Positioning and adequate fluoroscopy are critical. The fluoroscope is positioned to obtain both submentovertex and lateral views.
- A standard 100-mm-long, 20-gauge cannula with a stylet penetrates the skin 2.5 cm lateral to the oral commissure.
- The surgeon's finger prevents the cannula from penetrating the oral mucosa and guides it into the medial portion of the foramen ovale.
- The needle is advanced toward the intersection of a coronal plane passing through a point 3 cm anterior to the tragus and a sagittal plane passing through the medial aspect of the pupil.
- Using lateral fluoroscopy, the cannula should be directed 5 to 10 mm below the sella floor along the clivus, toward the angle formed by the shadows of the petrous bone and the clivus.
- A needle depth of about 6 to 8 cm is enough to achieve entrance into the foramen ovale and is signaled by a wince and a brief contraction of the masseter muscle.
- Proper positioning of the cannula within the trigeminal cistern allows free flow of cerebrospinal fluid (CSF) once the stylet is removed; however, CSF may not be obtained in patients who have had a previous percutaneous ablative procedure.
- Paresthesia after stimulation at 50 Hz should be evident in the affected division at less than 1 V, and motor stimulation at 2 Hz should be minimal. Ideally, the threshold for motor stimulation should be at least twice the sensory stimulation threshold.
- Three sequential low-temperature burns are used, starting at 60°C for 1 minute, then increasing to 63° and 65°C.[1]
- The disappearance of the trigger zones and the development of the patient's inability to differentiate between sharp and dull stimulation are considered safe endpoints for the coagulation.
- Hypalgesia of 75% or more is a good endpoint.[4]
- After RF ablation, patients should receive half of the daily dose of anticonvulsant medications, which thereafter is slowly tapered and eventually discontinued.

- After RF ablation, mild facial numbness occurs in 98%, major dysesthesias in 10%, and anesthesia dolorosa (deafferentation pain) in up to 1.5%.
- Other complications include carotid artery puncture; injury to abducens, trochlear, or oculomotor nerves; epilepsy; infection; and alteration of salivation.

TRIGEMINAL RHIZOTOMY OUTCOMES

- Pain is immediately relieved in 99% of patients.
- The rate of pain recurrence is similar to that of microvascular decompression: approximately 15–20% in 10 to 15 years.[8]
- Kanpolat et al performed a 25-year follow-up in 1600 patients whose ITN was treated with RF and found that 97.6% had acute pain relief. Pain relief was reported in 92% of patients with single or multiple procedures at 5 years; 94.2% of the patients who underwent multiple procedures had pain relief; and at 20-year follow-up, 41% of single procedure and 100% of multiple procedure patients experienced pain relief.[9]

SPINE PAIN

OVERVIEW OF FACET ARTHROPATHY

- The pathophysiology of back pain is a complex issue, and the etiology of the pain is even more complex.
- The facet joint has a significant role in back pain, and the history and physical examination form the basis for the diagnosis of pain due to facet arthropathy. Unfortunately, neither is specific enough to make a decision leading to definitive therapy.
- Physical examination reveals tenderness over the facet joints and associated muscle spasm. The pain is exacerbated by extension or lateral bending, and the range of motion is limited in all directions.
- A sequence (usually two sets) of diagnostic injections of the medial branches is performed under fluoroscopy to help secure a more definitive diagnosis.
- The lack of a corresponding cutaneous innervation to the facet joint makes it impossible to determine when complete blockade has occurred; however, when the patient can extend the spine without reproducing the preblock pain, we can assume that the block has worked. The specificity of the test is also limited because the medial branch nerve innervates muscles, ligaments, and periosteum in addition to the facet joints.[10]

ANATOMY

- The facet joints are paired diarthrodial synovial joints formed by the inferior articular process of one vertebra and the superior articular process of the vertebra below.
- The facet joints are present from the C1–2 junction to the L5–S1 junction.
- Each facet joint has a dual innervation supply: the medial branch, from the posterior ramus of a spinal nerve root, divides into two branches that supply the facet joint at the same level and the joint at the level below. There is also some evidence of joint innervation from a third ascending branch, which originates directly from the mixed spinal nerve.[11]
- In the cervical facet region, the medial branch predominately supplies the facet joints, with minimal innervation of the posterior neck muscles.
- The C3 dorsal ramus is the only cervical dorsal ramus below C2 that regularly has a cutaneous distribution.
- The C3–4 to C7–T1 facet joints are supplied by the medial branches from the same level and the level above.
- The medial branches of the C3 ramus differ anatomically from those of lower cervical levels: the posterior rami nerve divides early in its course into deep and superficial (third occipital nerve) branches. The deep C3 medial branch descends to innervate the C3–4 facet joint, and the superficial medial branch traverses the C2–3 facet joint before entering the joint capsule.
- In the lumbar region, the medial branch is located in a groove at the base of the superior articular facet, and it sends a branch medially and to the inferior pole of the joint at the same level and a descending branch to the superior pole of the joint below.
- The thoracic facet joint innervation is similar to the lumbar region, except for the T5 to T8 levels, where the medial branches travel laterally from the foramen, cross the superior lateral border of the transverse process, and course medially to innervate the corresponding facet joint and the level below.

CERVICAL FACET DENERVATION

- Chronic cervical pain in one of the most difficult syndromes to treat.
- Percutaneous RF neurotomy has been increasingly used in the treatment of chronic cervical pain, especially pain originating from the cervical zygapophyseal joints. Few definitive data exist, however, on the efficacy of such procedures for several reasons: inadequate patient selection; inaccurate surgical anatomy; lack of controls; no controlled diagnostic blocks prior to RF ablation; and possible inaccurate placement of electrodes on the target nerve.
- In a controlled trial of the procedure, the outcomes were favorable for patients with chronic cervical zygapophyseal joint pain after percutaneous RF neurotomy with multiple lesions of target nerves. The median time that elapsed before the pain returned to at least 50% of the preoperative level was 263 days in the active treatment group compared with 8 days for the placebo group.[12]

TECHNIQUE

- In the traditional prone position, a 22-gauge, 5-cm needle with a 4-mm exposed tip is introduced 1–2 cm lateral to the waist of the articular pillar, guided by posterior–anterior and lateral views on fluoroscopy. This approach allows the practitioner to reach the desired target without encountering the vertebral artery.
- In the supine position, the head is rotated to the opposite side, and the fluoroscope is positioned approximately 10° obliquely. The needle is inserted into the posterior triangle and passed anteriorly under intermittent fluoroscopy until the transverse process is reached.[11] Compared with the prone position, the supine approach positions the needle more tangential to the nerve and should give better results.
- Stimulation should be performed at 50 and 2 Hz and should cause few radicular symptoms and no motor stimulation.
- Lesioning is at 80°C for 60 to 90 seconds.

THORACIC FACET DENERVATION

- The indication is thoracic facet joint syndrome; however, few data are available regarding the outcome measures of thoracic facet denervation. One report indicated that after a mean follow-up period of 31 months, 44% of patients were pain-free and another 39% of patients had greater than 50% pain relief.[13]

TECHNIQUE

- The patient is positioned prone with an abdominal cushion.
- The transverse process for each branch is identified using fluoroscopy, and the medial branch passes over the junction of the superior articular process and the transverse process.
- Stimulation should be at 50 Hz and less than 1 V, and motor stimulation should not be seen when 2 Hz is used at 2 V.
- Lesioning is at 80°C for 90 seconds.

LUMBAR FACET DENERVATION

- The indication for denervation is persistent facet-mediated low back pain with a good response to diagnostic blocks.[1]
- The lumbar facet is innervated by the medial branch of the posterior ramus of the corresponding nerve root and also the nerve root cephalad to it. The nerve loops over the junction of the transverse process and superior articular process.
- Reported long-term success rates include approximately 45% of patients achieving 50% relief at mean follow-ups of 2 years in one study and 3.2 years in another.[14,15]

TECHNIQUE
- The patient is positioned prone with an abdominal cushion to reduce lumbar lordosis.
- The patient's back is prepared in a sterile fashion, and the C-arm fluoroscopic device is used to identify the junction of the sacral ala with the superior articulating process of S1; the second and third targets are the superior and medial aspects of the transverse processes at L5 and L4.
- After the skin and subcutaneous tissues are anesthetized, the first cannula is placed so that it touches the groove between the sacral ala and superior articulating process of S1 (L5 dorsal ramus); the remaining cannulas are placed superomedial of the transverse processes of L5 and L4.
- At the level of the sacral ala and the transverse processes, the cannula is slipped over the leading edge of the periosteum.
- The RF cannulas should lie parallel to the nerve to be lesioned.
- The next step is checking the impedance and stimulation.
- Then lesioning is performed at 80°C for 90 seconds.

SACROILIAC JOINT DENERVATION

- The sacroiliac joint is a source of low back pain, with a referral pattern similar to that for pain originating in the lumbar facet joints.
- Interest is growing in using RF denervation to provide long-term analgesia for patients with this condition. Ferrante et al described a bipolar technique in which two needles are positioned approximately 1 cm apart, with multiple lesions performed along the length of the posterior surface of the joint. Over a 6-month follow-up period, 36.4% of patients achieved at least 50% pain relief.[16] In a pilot study, Cohen and Abdi

targeted the lateral branches as they exit the sacral neuroforamina to achieve more complete denervation of the joint.[10]
- Long-term outcome studies are not yet available.

NEUROPATHIC PAIN

- Fourouzanfar et al described the use of RF for ablation of the stellate ganglion, with 40% of patients achieving greater than 50% pain relief at a mean follow-up of 52 weeks.
- RF lesioning of the dorsal root ganglion has been reported to treat neuropathic pain, but prospective controlled trials are lacking.

PULSED RADIOFREQUENCY

- Observations of pain relief in patients who did not have evidence of complete nerve ablation led to theories that other mechanisms of pain relief may be associated with RF.
- Thus, investigators attempted to apply an RF field without increasing temperature (thereby avoiding tissue destruction).
- Pulsed RF achieves this goal by periodically interrupting the energy output, allowing time for heat to dissipate and avoiding a significant rise in temperature.
- Pulsed RF delivers two active cycles per second, with each cycle lasting 20 milliseconds.
- The optimal parameters for pulsed RF are unknown. Sluijter, who first described this technique, advocates using 45 V for 120 seconds, which is thought to be the highest setting that will not increase temperature.[17]
- Pulsed RF is used by clinicians in a variety of targets formerly treated with conventional RF with the hope of achieving analgesia while avoiding the complications associated with ablation.

FUTURE NEEDS

- Even though RF has been available for approximately 35 years, only a few controlled trials provide information on long-term outcomes for its use in a myriad of pain syndromes.
- Enough data exist to support the use of RF in trigeminal neuralgia and lumbar facet arthropathy, but there clearly is a need for further detailed investigation.
- Studies are also needed to determine the mechanism of action of RF and to compare pulsed RF with conventional RF.

REFERENCES

1. **Saberski L, Fitzgerald J, Ahmad M.** Cryoneurolysis and radiofrequency lesioning. In: Raj PP, ed. *Practical Management of Pain*. St. Louis: Mosby; 2000:759.
2. **Kline MT, Yin W.** Radiofrequency techniques in clinical practice. In: Waldman, ed. *Interventional Pain Management*. Philadelphia: WB Saunders; 2001:243.
3. **Maxwell RE.** Clinical diagnosis of trigeminal neuralgia and differential diagnosis of facial pain. In: Rovit RL, Murali R, Jannetta PJ, eds. *Trigeminal Neuralgia*. Baltimore: Williams & Wilkins; 1990:53.
4. **Slavin KV, Burchiel KJ.** Surgical options for facial pain. In: Burchiel KJ, ed. *Surgical Management of Pain*. New York: Thieme; 2002:855.
5. **Taha JM.** Percutaneous radiofrequency trigeminal gangliolysis. In: Burchiel KJ, ed. *Surgical Management of Pain*. New York: Thieme; 2002:841.
6. **Sweet WH.** The pathophysiology of trigeminal neuralgia. In: Gildenberg P, Tasker R, eds. *Textbook of Stereotactic and Functional Neurosurgery*. New York: McGraw–Hill; 1998: 1667.
7. **Taha JM, Tew JM Jr.** Surgical management of vagoglossopharyngeal neuralgia and other uncommon facial neuralgia. In: Tindall G, ed. *The Practice of Neurosurgery*. Baltimore: Williams & Wilkins; 1996:3065.
8. **Taha JM, Tew JM Jr.** A prospective 15-year follow up of 154 consecutive patients with trigeminal neuralgia treated by percutaneous stereotactic radiofrequency thermal rhizotomy. *J Neurosurg*. 1995;83:989.
9. **Kanpolat Y, Sauas A, Bekar A, Berk C.** Percutaneous controlled radiofrequency trigeminal rhizotomy for the treatment of idiopathic trigeminal neuralgia: 25-year experience with 1600 patients. *Neurosurgery*. 2001;48: 524–534.
10. **Cohen, Abdi S.** Lateral branch blocks as a treatment for sacroiliac joint pain: A pilot study. *Reg Anesth Pain Med*. 2003;28:113.
11. **Panchal SJ, Belzberg AJ.** Facet blocks and denervations. In: Burchiel KJ, ed. *Surgical Management of Pain*. New York: Thieme; 2002:666.
12. **Lord SM, Barnsley L, Wallis B, et al.** Percutaneous radiofrequency neurotomy for chronic cervical zygapophyseal-joint pain. *N Engl J Med*. 1996;335:1721.
13. **Stolker RJ, Vervest AC, Groen GJ.** Percutaneous facet denervation in chronic thoracic spinal pain. *Acta Neurochir (Wien)*. 1993;122:82.
14. **Goupille P, Cotty P, Fouquet B, et al.** Denervation of the posterior lumbar vertebral apophyses by thermocoagulation in chronic low back pain: Results of the treatment of 103 patients. *Rev Rhum Ed Fr*. 1993;60:791.
15. **North RB, Han M, Zahurak M, et al.** Radiofrequency lumbar facet denervation: Analysis of prognostic factors. *Pain*. 1994;57:77.
16. **Ferrante FM, King LF, Roche EA, et al.** Radiofrequency sacroiliac joint denervation for sacroiliac syndrome. *Reg Anesth Pain Med*. 2001;26:137.
17. **Sluijter M, Cosman E, Rittman W, et al.** The effect of pulsed radiofrequency fields applied to the dorsal root ganglion: A preliminary report. *Pain Clin*. 1998;11:109–117.

58 PERIPHERAL NERVE STIMULATION

Lew C. Schon, MD
Paul W. Davies, MD

INTRODUCTION

- Peripheral nerve stimulation (PNS) is used to treat chronic neurogenic pain that has failed to respond adequately to less invasive therapies.
- PNS can be an invaluable adjunct to conventional modalities, such as medications, injections, and creams, in the treatment of patients with chronic regional pain syndrome, type II.
- In 1967, Wall and Sweet reported the ability of electrical PNS to produce hypalgesia and abolish chronic pain.[1] After initial enthusiasm, the technique garnered little interest until the mid-1980s, when electrodes suitable for placement on peripheral nerves became commercially available.

THEORY

- The exact mechanism of action of PNS is not understood. Two possible mechanisms are outlined below.

CENTRAL MECHANISM

- Antidromic activation of large-diameter fibers in the spinal cord can block transmission of pain signals from small-diameter nociceptive afferent nerve fibers (gate-control theory).[2] PNS inhibits spinothalamic tract neurons within the spinal cord in animals.[3]

PERIPHERAL MECHANISM

- Spontaneous neuronal activity is seen in both A and C fibers in chronic pain conditions. PNS blocks nociceptive nerve fibers and, in neuroma models, stops neuronal discharge for a period beyond the duration of the stimulus.[4]

INDICATIONS

- PNS is indicated in the treatment of neuropathic pain involving one or two sensory or mixed nerves when more conservative nonoperative and operative therapies have failed.
- PNS can successfully treat pain in patients who have failed spinal cord stimulation (SCS) and other peripheral nerve procedures but should be used only after appropriate preoperative evaluation (see below), including a psychologic assessment.[5]

EVALUATION

- A preoperative evaluation is performed to ascertain which nerves are involved in pain transmission and to try to predict the response to PNS. The history and physical examination often reveal the affected nerves.
- Nerve involvement can be confirmed by an appropriate nerve block using local anesthetic. Although pain relief following a nerve block does not guarantee the success of PNS, failure to obtain pain relief is strongly suggestive that stimulation of the nerve is unlikely to be beneficial.[6]
- Transcutaneous electrical nerve stimulation (TENS) can be used to stimulate a nerve prior to implantation of the PNS components. It is generally believed that a positive response to this modality is predictive of a good response to PNS. If anatomical reasons, such as obesity and the depth of the nerve, impede a TENS trial, a temporary PNS lead may be placed.
- In PNS trials for occipital, cuneal, and lateral femoral neuralgia, temporary leads are often connected to an external reusable trial generator. Trials for upper and lower extremity neuralgias are usually performed in the operating room at the time of implantation. This is done by exposing the nerve and waking the patient up intraoperatively. The nerve is then stimulated and the patient's response monitored.[7] Depending on the degree of response to the stimulation, PNS is abandoned (no benefit), the lead is implanted permanently, or the lead is connected to an exterior reusable trial generator for a percutaneous trial.

PERIPHERAL NERVE STIMULATION VERSUS SPINAL CORD STIMULATION

ADVANTAGES OF PNS

- PNS limits paresthesias to the distribution of the nerve transmitting pain as opposed to a large portion of the extremity, as is frequently encountered in SCS.
- SCS lead placement can be complicated by delayed migration, which can cause inadequate coverage of the painful areas and bothersome paresthesias in other parts of the body.
- PNS is appealing to neurostimulation candidates who have undergone multiple failed surgeries and are reluctant to undergo spine surgery.

DISADVANTAGES OF PNS

- On very rare occasions, neuropraxia develops secondary to scarring induced from lead placement.
- Motor stimulation can occur when peripheral nerves are stimulated; however, this is very uncommon with correct lead placement and programming.
- PNS is more invasive than a percutaneously placed spinal cord stimulator. PNS is less invasive than SCS, however, when a laminectomy is used for lead placement.
- PNS generators and wires may be uncomfortable in certain patients, particularly those who are very thin. Wires may also be irritating near joints.

SURGICAL TECHNIQUE

ANESTHESIA

- Lead placement can be performed under general or local anesthesia. When general anesthesia is used, a wake-up test is necessary if an intraoperative trial is performed.
- Lead tunneling and generator placement may be performed under local anesthesia but are usually better tolerated with either supplemental deep sedation or general anesthesia.

LEAD PLACEMENT

- The affected nerve is carefully exposed without a tourniquet (to avoid damaging the nerve's blood supply). The exposed area of the nerve should correspond to the electrode length (Figure 58–1).
- If a plate electrode is used, some surgeons harvest a fascial flap and secure it with interrupted sutures over the exposed nerve prior to lead placement. This prevents the electrodes from directly contacting the nerve in a manner analogous with the dura mater in SCS. The plate electrode is then secured to soft tissues surrounding the nerve.

- Cuff/spiral electrodes usually circle the nerve without an intervening fascial flap.
- Some surgeons use interrupted sutures to connect the electrode to the nerve itself; others suture to the surrounding soft tissues.

WAKE-UP TEST

- When the electrode is in an appropriate position, the skin and soft tissues surrounding the incision are infiltrated with local anesthetic. The patient is then allowed to regain consciousness, and the lead is stimulated until the paresthesia covers the painful area. This is facilitated by preoperatively outlining the patient's area of pain with a skin marker and by using provocative testing.
- While the patient is awake, the joints of the limb should be put through a full range of motion to check that the stimulation is consistent (unchanged by movement). When optimal lead position has been achieved, it is secured to the epineurium.

LEAD TUNNELING AND GENERATOR PLACEMENT

- The generator pocket is fashioned in areas of fatty tissue along the anterior medial aspect of the thigh at a depth of approximately 1 to 2 cm from the skin surface in the subcutaneous fat (Figure 58–2). The correct depth ensures that the generator or radiofrequency device can communicate with the external remote control/energy source.

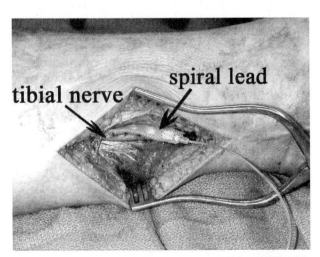

FIGURE 58–1 For appropriate lead placement, the length of the exposed nerve should match the length of the electrode.

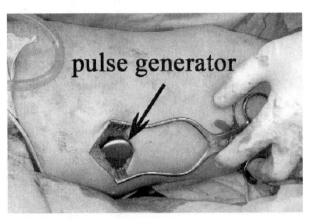

FIGURE 58–2 The pulse generator is inserted at a depth of 1 to 2 cm from the epidermis in a pocket of subcutaneous fatty tissue along the anterior medial aspect of the thigh.

- The pocket is usually created in an infraclavicular location for upper extremities and in the lower abdomen or medial thigh for lower extremities. It is important to ensure that the generator will not rub on bony protuberances, as this would cause pain.
- After the pocket is fashioned, a tunneling instrument is used to place an extension lead in the subcutaneous tissues to connect the generator to the electrodes. A third incision is often needed to aid with tunneling if the extension wire has to pass over the elbow or knee joint. The electrode lead is connected to the extension wire and attached to the generator.
- All joints in proximity to the PNS hardware should again be put through their full range of motion to ensure that there is no tension on the electrode plate that may encourage migration and/or device failure. The incision is closed and covered with a sterile dressing. If possible, a compression dressing is placed over the pulse generator to reduce the risk of a hematoma or seroma.

OUTCOME STUDIES

- A review of the literature from 1980 to 2002 reveals several papers on the outcome of PNS for neurogenic pain. Most of these studies are retrospective and defy comparison. With these limitations in mind, however, and defining "success" as greater than 50% pain relief, various authors report success rates of 32 to 89% (mean 61%) with complication rates of 5 to 27% (mean 17%).[6–13]
- In 1996, Hassenbusch et al[13] published results of a prospective trial of 32 patients with stage III reflex sympathetic dystrophy of whom 30 (90%) were considered appropriate candidates for PNS. Outcome was

measured in terms of pain relief, changes on physical examination, and activity levels. Patients were followed for 2.2±0.6 years. Nineteen (63%) patients gained fair to good pain relief, and six (20%) resumed part- or full-time employment.

CONCLUSION

- PNS is an invasive procedure that should be reserved for the treatment of neurogenic pain in patients who have failed to gain relief with medical and surgical therapies.
- Permanent implantation of a peripheral nerve stimulator should be performed only after appropriate preoperative evaluation and psychologic assessment.
- The technique of identifying and securing the optimal lead placement is meticulous.
- There is good evidence that appropriately selected patients can achieve substantial pain relief, enhanced functional ability, and improved work status with PNS.

REFERENCES

1. **Wall PD, Sweet WH.** Temporary abolition of pain in man. *Science.* 1967;155:108–109.
2. **Melzack R, Wall PD.** Pain mechanisms: A new theory. *Science.* 1965;150:971–979.
3. **Chung JM, Lee KH, Hori Y, et al.** Factors influencing peripheral nerve stimulation produced inhibition of primate spinothalamic tract cells. *Pain.* 1984;19:277–293.
4. **Wall PD, Gutnick M.** Properties of afferent nerve impulses originating from a neuroma. *Nature.* 1974;248:740–743.
5. **Levy RM.** Algorithms for treatment of neuropathic pain syndromes. In: North RB, Levy RM, eds. *Neurosurgical Management of Pain.* New York: Springer-Verlag; 1997: 337–339.
6. **Shetter AG, Racz GB, Lewis R, et al.** Peripheral nerve stimulation. In: North RB, Levy RM, eds. *Neurosurgical Management of Pain.* New York: Springer-Verlag; 1997; 261–270.
7. **Schon LC, Kleeman TJ, Chiodo CP, et al.** A prospective analysis of peripheral nerve stimulation for intractable lower extremity nerve pain. Paper presented at: 16th Annual Summer Meeting of the American Foot and Ankle Society; July 13–15, 2000; Vail (Colorado).
8. **Law JD, Swett J, Kirsch WM.** Retrospective analysis of 22 patients with chronic pain treated by peripheral nerve stimulation. *J Neurosurg.* 1980;52:482–485.
9. **Long DM, Erickson D, Campbell J, et al.** Electrical stimulation of the spinal cord and peripheral nerves for pain control: A 10-year experience. *Appl Neurophysiol.* 1981; 44:207–217.
10. **Nashold BS Jr, Goldner JL, Mullen JB, et al.** Long-term pain control by direct peripheral-nerve stimulation. *J Bone Joint Surg Am.* 1982;64:1–10.
11. **Waisbrod H, Panhans C, Hansen D, et al.** Direct nerve stimulation for painful peripheral neuropathies. *J Bone Joint Surg Br.* 1985;67:470–472.
12. **Gybels J, Kupers R.** Central and peripheral electrical stimulation of the nervous system in the treatment of chronic pain. *Acta Neurochir Suppl (Wien).* 1987;38:64–75.
13. **Hassenbusch SJ, Stanton-Hicks M, Schoppa D, et al.** Long-term results of peripheral nerve stimulation for reflex sympathetic dystrophy. *J Neurosurg.* 1996;84:415–423.

59 PROLOTHERAPY

Felix Linetsky, MD
Michael Stanton-Hicks, MB, BS
Conor O'Neill, MD

INTRODUCTION

- Regenerative injection therapy (RIT), also known as prolotherapy or sclerotherapy, is an interventional technique for the treatment of chronic musculoskeletal pain caused by connective tissue diathesis.[1–4]
- This technique originated in the United States in the mid-1840s for treatment of hernias.[5]
- RIT transitioned to musculoskeletal pathology in the 1930s.[1,3–5]
- Since then, the scope of applications has expanded gradually.[1–12]
- It has been proposed recently that pain reduction after RIT is due to chemomodulation or temporary neurolytic action of the injectate. The literature suggests that dextrose/lidocaine or dextrose/glycerine/phenol/lidocaine solutions have a more prolonged pain-relieving action compared with that of lidocaine alone.[2–4]

CLINICAL ANATOMY

- According to Willard, the connective tissue complex in the cervical, thoracic, and lumbar areas incorporates various ligaments and paravertebral fasciae to form a continuous connective tissue stocking surrounding, interconnecting, and supporting various soft tissue, vertebral, neurovascular, and osseous structures. This arrangement provides bracing and hydraulic amplification effect to the musculature, enhancing its strength by up to 30%.[13,14]

- The anterior compartment contains the paravertebral fascia muscles, vertebral bodies, intervertebral disc, and anterior and posterior longitudinal ligaments. The middle compartment includes the contents of the spinal canal. The posterior compartment begins medially at the ventral aspect of z-joint capsules and laterally at the posterolateral aspects of the transverse processes and converges at the apices of the spinous processes.[14]
- Movements of the cranium and spine are accomplished through various types of joints.[14] These include:
  ○ *Syndesmoses*, that is, anterior longitudinal ligament, posterior longitudinal ligament, anterior atlanto-occipital membrane, posterior atlanto-occipital membrane, ligamenta flava, interspinous ligaments, and supraspinous ligaments.[14]
  ○ *Synovial*, that is, atlanto-axial, atlanto-occipital, zygapophyseal, costotransverse, and costovertebral joints.[14]
  ○ *Symphysis*, for example, intervertebral discs.[14]
  ○ *Combined*, for example, sacroiliac joint, which is a synovial/syndesmotic articulation.[13,14]
- Connective tissues receive segmental innervation from the respective ventral and dorsal rami.[3,4,13,14]
  ○ Dorsal rami usually divide into medial and lateral branches (except the first cervical fifth lumbar that forms only a medial branch, fourth and fifth sacral and coccygeal).[14]
  ○ Medial branches of the dorsal rami (MBDR) innervate z-joints, multifidus muscles, intraspinous muscles and ligaments, and supraspinous ligaments.[13,14]
  ○ Free nerve endings and Pacini and Ruffini corpuscles have been identified in superficial layers of all ligaments, including supraspinous and interspinous, with a sharp increase in their quantity at the attachment to the spinous processes (enthesis), rendering them a source of nociception equal to that of z-joint capsules.[15]
  ○ Comparatively, the vascular supply is much less abundant. Such a relationship is essential for proper homeostasis.[16–18]
- Pain arising from affected connective tissue such as ligaments and tendons may mimic any referral pain patterns known.
  ○ Original patterns of referral pain from interspinous syndesmotic joints, that is, intraspinous ligaments, were published by Kellgren in 1939 and were subsequently confirmed in the 1950s by Feinstein and Hackett.[1]
  ○ Pain patterns from cervical synovial articulations were brought to light by Aprill, Dwyer, and Bogduk in 1990[19]; these were expanded to include upper cervical and thoracic articulations by Dreyfus in 1994.[20]

  ○ Also in 1994, Dussault described z-joint pain patterns in the cervical and lumbar areas, and Fortin described pain patterns from the sacroiliac joints.[21]
  ○ The size of this chapter precludes reproduction of the pain maps. There is a significant overlap between pain patterns from synovial and syndesmotic joints, as well as those from symphysial joints.

PATHOPHYSIOLOGY

- Connective tissues are bradytrophic; their regenerative capabilities are much slower than those of any other tissue.[16,17]
- The natural healing process consists of three overlapping phases: inflammation, granulation with fibroplasia, followed by contraction with remodeling.[1]
- Connective tissue response to trauma varies with the degree of injury[16–18]:
  ○ In the presence of cellular damage, regenerative response takes place.
  ○ In the presence of damage to the extracellular matrix, a combined regenerative, reparative response takes place.[3,4]
- Cell replication in combined regenerative, reparative processes is controlled by chemical and growth factors.[22]
- Natural healing, in the best circumstances, may restore connective tissue to its preinjury length but only to 50–75% preinjury tensile strength.[16,18]
- The most frequent degenerative changes in ligaments and tendons are hypoxic, followed by lipoid, mucoid, and calcific degeneration. A combination of all of these has been observed.[17]
- Modulation of regenerative and degenerative pathways remains a therapeutic challenge, and application of NSAIDs and steroids is of limited value.[18]
- Experimental studies have demonstrated that repeated injections of 5% sodium morrhuate at the fibro-osseous attachments (entheses) increased strength of the bone ligament junction by 28%, ligament mass by 44%, and thickness by 27% in comparison to saline controls.[10]

MECHANISM OF ACTION

- The RIT mechanism of action is complex and multifaceted. The three most important components are:
  ○ Chemomodulation of collagen through inflammatory proliferative, regenerative/reparative responses is induced by the chemical properties of the proliferants and mediated by cytokines and multiple growth factors.[2–4]

∘ Chemoneuromodulation of peripheral nociceptors provides stabilization of antidromic, orthodromic, sympathetic, and axon reflex transmissions. The literature suggests that a dextrose/lidocaine or dextrose/glycerine/phenol/lidocaine combination has a much more prolonged action than lidocaine alone.[2–4]

∘ Modulation of local hemodynamics with changes in intraosseous pressure leads to reduction of pain.[2–4]

INDICATIONS FOR RIT

- Discogenic low back pain.[7,8]
- Enthesopathy: a painful degenerative pathologic process that results in deposition of poorly organized tissue, degeneration and tendinosis at the fibro-osseous interface, and transition toward loss of function. (*Note*: Enthesis is the zone of insertion of ligament, tendon, or articular capsule to bone. The outer layers of the annulus represent a typical enthesis.)[2–4]
- Tendinosis/ligamentosis: a focal area of degenerative changes due to failure of the cell matrix adaptation to excessive load and tissue hypoxia with a strong tendency toward chronic pain and dysfunction.[2–4,12]
- Pathologic ligament softening and laxity: a posttraumatic or congenital condition leading to painful hypermobility of the axial and peripheral joints.[1–4,11,12]
- Chronic pain from ligaments or tendons secondary to repetitive or occupational sprains or strains, for example, "repetitive motion disorder."[1–4,11,12]
- Chronic postural cervical, thoracic, lumbar, and lumbosacral pain.[1–4,11,12]
- Lumbar and thoracic vertebral compression fractures with a wedge deformity that exert additional stress on the posterior ligamentotendinous complex.[1–4,11,12]
- Recurrent painful subluxations of the ribs at costotransverse, costovertebral, and/or costosternal articulations.[2–4,12]
- Osteoarthritis, spondylosis, spondylolysis, and spondylolisthesis.[2–4,12]
- Painful cervical, thoracic, lumbar, lumbosacral, and sacroiliac instability.[2–4,12]

SYNDROMES AND DIAGNOSTIC ENTITIES TREATED WITH RIT

- Cervicocranial syndrome: cervicogenic headaches, secondary to ligament sprain and laxity, atlantoaxial and atlanto-occipital joint sprains, and midcervical zygapophyseal sprains
- Temporomandibular pain and muscle dysfunction syndrome

- Barre–Lieou syndrome
- Torticollis
- Cervical disc syndrome without myelopathy
- Cervicobrachial syndrome (shoulder/neck pain)
- Hyperextension/hyperflexion injury syndromes
- Cervical, thoracic, and lumbar zygapophyseal syndromes
- Cervical, thoracic, and lumbar sprain/strain syndrome
- Costotransverse joint pain
- Costovertebral arthrosis/dysfunction
- Slipping rib syndrome
- Sternoclavicular arthrosis and repetitive sprain
- Tietze's syndrome/costochondritis/chondrosis
- Costosternal arthrosis
- Xiphoidalgia syndrome
- Acromioclavicular sprain/arthrosis
- Scapulothoracic crepitus
- Iliocostalis friction syndrome
- Iliac crest syndrome
- Iliolumbar syndrome
- Painful lumbar disc syndrome
- Interspinous pseudoarthrosis (Baastrup's disease)
- Lumbar instability
- Lumbar ligament sprain
- Spondylolysis
- Sacroiliac joint pain, subluxation, instability, and arthrosis
- Sacrococcygeal joint pain; coccygodynia
- Gluteal tendinosis with or without concomitant bursitis
- Myofascial pain syndromes
- Ehlers–Danlos syndrome
- Ankylosing spondylitis (Marie–Strümpell disease)
- Failed back syndrome
- Fibromyalgia syndrome
- Laxity of ligaments[1–4,6–8,11,23]

CONTRAINDICATIONS TO RIT

- Allergy to proliferant or anesthetic solutions or their components, for example, phenol, dextrose, or sodium morrhuate
- Acute nonreduced subluxations or dislocations, arthritis, bursitis, or tendinitis (septic, gouty, rheumatoid, or posttraumatic)
- Recent onset of a progressive neurologic deficit involving the segment to be injected, including but not limited to severe intractable cephalgia, unilaterally dilated pupil, bladder dysfunction, and bowel incontinence
- Request for a large quantity of narcotics before and after treatment
- Neoplastic and inflammatory lesions involving vertebral and paravertebral structures

- Lack of improvement after infiltration of the putative nociceptive structure with a local anesthetic or severe exacerbation of pain
- Febrile disorder or acute medical/surgical conditions that render a patient's status unstable[1–4,12]

COMMONLY USED SOLUTIONS

- The most common solution is commercially available 50% dextrose, which is diluted with a local anesthetic. For example, 1 mL of 50% dextrose mixed with 3 mL of 1% lidocaine produces a 12.5% solution. Gradual progressions to 25% dextrose solution have also been used.
- Five percent sodium morrhuate is a mixture of sodium salts of saturated and unsaturated fatty acids of cod liver oil and 2% benzyl alcohol. Note that the benzyl alcohol is chemically very similar to phenol and acts as a local anesthetic and preservative.
- Dextrose/phenol/glycerine (DPG or P2G) solution consists of 25% dextrose, 2.5% phenol, and 25% glycerine. In reference publications, DPG was diluted with a local anesthetic prior to injection. Dilution ratios are 1:1, 1:2, and 2:3. A 6% phenol in glycerine solution was used at donor harvest sites of the iliac crest for neurolytic and proliferative responses.
- Other solutions used include pumice suspension, tetracycline, and a mixture of chondroitin sulfate, glucosamine sulfate, and dextrose.[1–4,6–8,11,12]

TECHNICAL CONSIDERATIONS

- Any structure that receives innervation is a potential pain generator. To confirm that the structure is a pain generator, the structure proper or its nerve supply has to be injected with a local anesthetic, resulting in abolition of pain.[3,4]
- For RIT purposes, tissue pain generators are identified by reproducible local tenderness and are confirmed by needling and local anesthetic blocks of the tissue bed, taking its nerve supply into account.
- In experienced hands, using palpable landmarks for guidance, the following posterior column elements innervated by the dorsal rami may be safely injected without fluoroscopic guidance: spinous process, supraspinous and intraspinous ligaments, lamina, posterior zygapophyseal joint capsule, transverse process, and cervicodorsal fascia, as well as posterior sacroiliac, sacrotuberous, and sacrospinous ligaments and posterior sacrococcygeal ligaments.
- The dextrose/lidocaine solution is an effective diagnostic and therapeutic tool for pain arising from posterior column elements when used in increments of 0.2–1.0 mL injected at each bone contact in the following sequence:
  - In the presence of midline pain and tenderness, the interspinous ligaments are blocked initially in the midline.
  - If tenderness remains at the lateral aspects of the spinous processes, injections are carried out to the lateral aspects of the apices of the spinous processes, thus blocking off the terminal filaments of the MBDR of the dorsal rami.
  - Persistence of paramedial pain dictates blocks of the facet joint capsules, costotransverse joints, sacroiliac ligaments, and apices of transverse processes in the lumbar region and the posterior tubercle of the transverse processes in the cervical region with their respective tendon insertions.
  - Perseverance of lateral tenderness dictates investigation of the structures innervated by the lateral branches of the dorsal rami, that is, iliocostalis tendon insertions to the ribs.
- In this fashion, all potential nociceptors on the course of MBDR are investigated from the periphery to the center. Using the above-described sequence, the practitioner is able to make a differential diagnosis of pain arising from vertebral and paravertebral structures innervated by MBDR and lateral branches of the dorsal rami. (See Figures 59–1 and 59–2.)
- Pain from pathology of the upper cervical synovial joints presents a diagnostic and, more so, a therapeutic challenge. Because of the previously mentioned overlaps of pain patterns, it is usually a diagnosis of exclusion.
- Regarding therapeutic intervention, radiofrequency (RF) lesions and corticosteroid injections do not always produce the desired therapeutic value in upper cervical synovial joint pain.
  - It has recently been brought to light that intra-articular atlantoaxial and atlanto-occipital joint injections of 6% phenol have secured a long-lasting therapeutic effect in selected patients.[23]
  - Intra-articular injections of 25% dextrose into the above-mentioned joints, as well as into midcervical synovial joints, were reported to relieve persistent pain after RF and capsular injection failure.
- Painful lumbar disc syndrome also remains a therapeutic challenge.
  - Original studies in the 1950s advocated injection of irritating solutions into the lumbar intervertebral disc. Chemonucleoannuloplasty was revived in the last decade by the enthusiastic work of Klein, Eek, and Derby.
  - They reported significant pain improvement and return-to-work ratio after intradiscal injections of

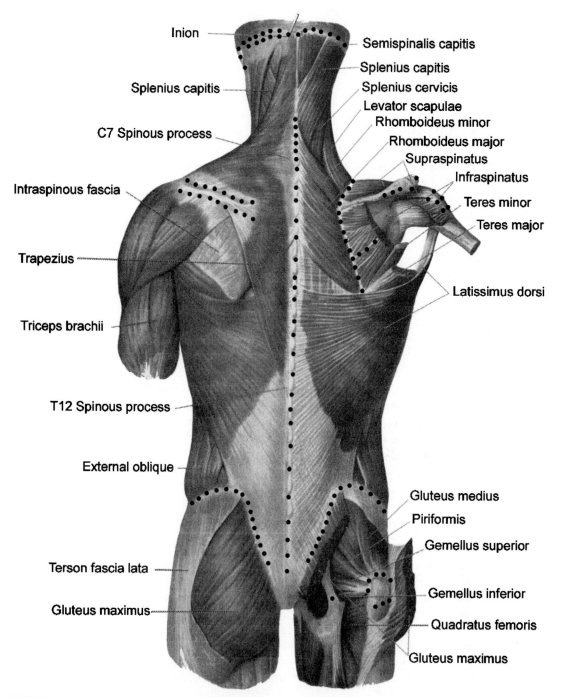

FIGURE 59–1 Dots represent some of the most common enthesopathy areas at the fibro-osseous insertions (enthesis) in the occiput, humerus, trochanter, iliac crest, and spinous processes. Dots also represent the most common location of needle insertions during RIT. (Please note: not all of the locations must be treated in each patient.) Dotted vertebral and paravertebral structures are innervated by their respective medial and lateral branches of the dorsal rami. From Sinelnicov. *Atlas of Anatomy.* Vol. 1. Meiditsina Moskow; 1972. Modified and prepared for publication by Tracey James.

25% dextrose mixed with chondroitin sulfate and glucosamine. The pilot group consisted of 30 patients with up to 2 years' follow-up. These patients have failed previous conservative care,

laminectomies, fusions at adjacent levels, or intradiscal electrothermal annuloplasty (IDET).[7,9]

○ Thirty patients were reported to have a significant pain improvement and return-to-work ratio after

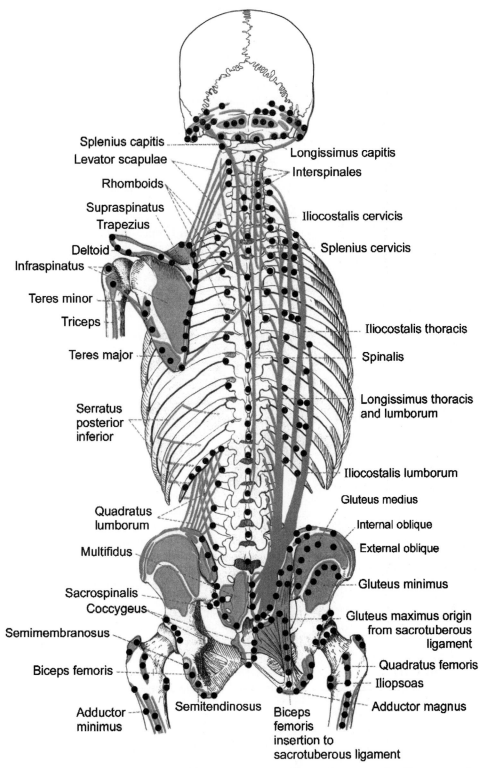

Splenius capitis
Levator scapulae
Rhomboids
Supraspinatus
Trapezius
Deltoid
Infraspinatus
Teres minor
Triceps
Teres major
Serratus
posterior
inferior
Quadratus
lumborum
Multifidus
Sacrospinalis
Coccygeus
Semimembranosus
Biceps femoris
Adductor
minimus
Semitendinosus
Biceps
femoris
insertion to
sacrotuberous ligament

Longissimus capitis
Interspinales
Iliocostalis cervicis
Splenius cervicis
Iliocostalis thoracis
Spinalis
Longissimus thoracis
and lumborum
Iliocostalis lumborum
Gluteus medius
Internal oblique
External oblique
Gluteus minimus
Gluteus maximus origin
from sacrotuberous
ligament
Quadratus femoris
Iliopsoas
Adductor magnus

FIGURE 59–2 Dots represent some of the most common enthesopathy areas at the fibro-osseous insertions of ligaments and tendons (enthesis) at the occiput, humerus, trochanter, iliac crest, and spine, ischial tuberosity, sacrum, and spinous processes. Dots also represent the most common location of needle insertions and infiltrations during RIT. (Please note: not all of the locations must be treated in each patient.) Dotted vertebral and paravertebral structures are innervated by their respective medial and lateral branches of the dorsal rami. From Sinelnicov. *Atlas of Anatomy*. Vol. 1, Meiditsina Moskow; 1972. Modified and prepared for publication by Tracey James.

lumbar intradiscal injection of a mixed solution containing dextrose, chondroitin sulfate, and glucosamine chloride. These patients had failed previous conservative care, laminectomies, fusions at adjacent levels, or IDET.[7,8]

- Pennsylvania researchers received and reported good results with lumbar intradiscal injections of 25% dextrose for treatment of painful mechanical and chemical discopathy, suggesting that 25% dextrose may provide an immediate and longlasting neurolytic action.

CONCLUSION

- RIT/prolotherapy is a valuable method of treatment for correctly diagnosed chronic painful conditions of the musculoskeletal systems.
- Thorough familiarity of the physician with clinical anatomy and pathophysiology, as well as anatomic variations, is necessary to use this technique affectively.
- Manipulation under local joint anesthesia and a series of local anesthetic blocks for diagnosis of somatic pain are other commonly used options in conjunction with RIT.
- RIT in an ambulatory setting is an acceptable standard of care in the community.
- Recent literature reports that NSAIDs and steroid preparations have limited usage in degenerative painful conditions of ligaments and tendons or chronic painful overuse injuries. Microinterventional regenerative techniques and proper rehabilitation up to 6 months or a year supported with acetaminophen and opioid analgesics may be more appropriate.

REFERENCES

1. **Hackett G, Hemwall GA, Montgomery GA.** *Ligament and Tendon Relaxation—Treated by Prolotherapy.* 5th ed. Springfield, Ill: Charles C Thomas; 1991.
2. **Linetsky FS, Botwin K, Gorfine L, et al.** Position Paper of the Florida Academy of Pain Medicine on regenerative injection therapy: Effectiveness and appropriate usage. *Pain Clin.* 2002;4(3):38–45.
3. **Linetsky F, Miguel R, Saberski L.** Pain management with regenerative injection therapy (RIT). In: Weiner R, ed. *Pain Management: A Practical Guide for Clinicians.* Boca Raton, Fla: CRC Press; 2002:381–402.
4. **Linetsky F, Eek B, Parris W.** Regenerative injection therapy. In: Manchikanti, ed. *Low Back Pain.* Paducah: ASIPP; 2002:420–519.
5. **Linetsky F, Mikulinsky A, Gorfine L.** Regenerative injection therapy: History of application in pain management. Part I. 1930s–1950s. *Pain Clin.* 2000;2(2):8–13.
6. **Klein R, Dorman TA, Johnson CE.** Proliferant injections for low back pain: Histologic changes of injected ligaments & objective measurements of lumbar spine mobility before and after treatment. *J Neurol Orthop Med Surg.* 1989;10:2.
7. **Klein R.** Intradiscal injection therapy for chronic discogenic pain, a prospective trial in progress. Paper presented at: American Association of Orthopedic Medicine Workshop. 2001; Daly City, CA.
8. **Klein RG, Eek B, O'Neill C, et al.** Biochemical injection treatment for discogenic low back pain: A pilot study. *Spine.* 2003;3:220–226.
9. **Linetsky F, Saberski L, Miguel R, Snyder A.** A history of the applications of regenerative injection therapy in pain management. Part II. 1960s–1980s. *Pain Clin.* 2001;3: 32–36.
10. **Liu Y, Tipton CM, Matthes RD, et al.** An in situ study of the influence of a sclerosing solution in rabbit medial collateral ligaments and its junction strength. *Connect Tissue Res.* 1983;11:95–102.
11. **Ongley MJ, Klein RG, Dorman TA, et al.** A new approach to the treatment of chronic low back pain. *Lancet.* 1987: 143–146.
12. **Reeves K.** Prolotherapy: Present and future applications in soft-tissue pain and disability. *Phys Med Rehabil Clin North Am.* 1995;6:917–926.
13. **Bogduk N.** *Clinical Anatomy of the Lumbar Spine and Sacrum.* 3rd ed. London/New York: Churchill Livingstone; 1997.
14. *Gray's Anatomy.* 38th British ed. Edinburgh/London: Churchill Livingstone, Pearson Professional Limited; 1995.
15. **Ashton I, Ashton A, Gibson S, et al.** Morphological basis for back pain: The demonstration of nerve fibers and neuropeptides in the lumbar facet joint capsule but not in ligamentum flavum. *J Orthop Res.* 1992;10:72–78.
16. **Best T.** Basic science of soft tissue. In: Delee J, Drez D, eds. *Orthopedic Sports Medicine Principles and Practice.* Vol 1. Philadelphia: WB Saunders; 1994:7–53.
17. **Jozsa L, Kannus P.** Human tendons, anatomy, physiology and pathology. In: *Human Kinetics.* Champaign, IL: 1997.
18. **Leadbetter WB.** Cell-matrix response in tendon injury. *Clin Sports Med.* 1992;11:533–578.
19. **Aprill C, Dwyer A, Bogduk N.** Cervical zygapophyseal joint pain patterns II: A clinical evaluation. *Spine.* 1990;15(6):458–461.
20. **Dreyfuss P, Tibiletti C, Dreyer SJ.** Thoracic zygapophyseal joint pain pattern. A study in normal volunteers. *Spine.* 1994;19:807–811.
21. **Dussault R, Kaplan PA.** Facet joint injection: Diagnosis and therapy. *Appl. Radiol.* 1994:35–39.
22. **Marui T, Niyibizi C, Georgescu H, et al.** Effect of growth factors on matrix synthesis by ligament fibroblasts. *J Orthop Res.* 1997;15:18–23.
23. **Stanton-Hicks M.** Cervicocranial syndrome: Treatment of atlanto-occipital and atlanto-axial joint pain with phenol/glycerine injections. Paper presented at: 20th AAOM Annual Conference and Scientific Seminar: A commonsense approach to "hidden" pain generators; 2003; Orlando, Fl.

60 REHABILITATION EVALUATION AND TREATMENT IN PATIENTS WITH LOW BACK PAIN

Michael Kaplan, MD

ASSESSMENT OF LOW BACK PAIN

SPINAL MOTION

- Accurate measurement is very important.
- Limitation of spinal motion correlates with the presence of lower back disability.
- Identification of palpable spasms and understanding nerve innervation are essential.[1]

PALPATION

- A positive Larson test, performed with the patient in the prone position, can indicate segmental instability common in degenerative disease of the lower lumbar discs.
- Active splinting of the segment reduces or eliminates the tenderness elicited with pressure over the spinous processes, which is suggestive of segmental instability.
- Tenderness from soft tissue injuries persists despite active splinting.
- Muscle spasm is defined by the presence of a persistent, palpable increase in muscle tone accompanied by localized tenderness.
- A digital rectal evaluation can detect pelvic floor myalgia or another pelvic pathology.
- Gentle and systematic palpation of the coccyx, sacrum, levator, ani, coccygeus, and piriformis muscles and their associated ligaments and attachments should be performed.

NEUROLOGIC ASSESSMENT

- Straight leg raising (SLR) tests should be performed to detect nerve root irritation. The classic positive SLR test is a reproduction of radicular pain at 30°–40°.
- Radicular pain reproduced at greater angles represents less significant nerve root irritation.
- Back and leg pain can be produced in the absence of nerve root irritation.
- Nonradicular pain may be caused by soft tissue tightness or spasms in the back, glutei, or hamstrings.
- Even with a soft tissue pain source, the SLR can still be used as an index of improvement during treatment.
- A positive crossed SLR test has the highest correlation with myelographic findings of a herniated disc.

- Significant inconsistency observed during sitting and supine SLR tests may provide insight into the psychogenic processes.
- Electromyography is a valuable adjunct in delineation and confirmation of neurologic findings.[2]

SPECIAL TESTS

- The Hoover test is of special interest and suggests the detection of malingering because it indicates the recognition of submaximal effort. The jolt test is a provocative method used to document pain enhancement or radiation due to sudden mechanical loading of the erect spine. While standing on tiptoes, the patient is asked to suddenly drop to a flat foot position. A positive jolt test is characterized by an exacerbation or radiation of pain.
- Leg length can be measured from the anterior superior iliac spine to the prominence of the medial malleoli (true leg length) or from the umbilicus to the medial malleoli (apparent leg length).

TRUNK STRENGTH

- Abdominal oblique muscles can be graded with the trunk rotated, as when a situp is performed.
- A similar method can be used to grade back extensors: lying prone with a pillow under the abdomen and hips, the patient extends the trunk and holds against resistance applied by the examiner.

RADIOLOGIC TESTS

- Plain radiography remains the cornerstone of radiologic tests.
- Plain radiography allows visualization of degenerative disc disease, spondylitis, compression fractures, metabolic bone disorders, bone tumors, congenital anomalies, and transitional vertebrae.
- Oblique views of the lumbosacral level can be added to visualize the facet and sacroiliac joints.
- Flexion–extension views are frequently added whenever spinal instability is suspected.[3]

COMMON BACK SYNDROMES

DEGENERATIVE DISC DISEASE WITH ASSOCIATED DEGENERATIVE JOINT DISEASE OF THE LUMBAR FACET JOINTS

- Degenerative disc disease is a consequence of the aging process and is, therefore, among the most common causes of mechanical back pain in middle-aged and older patients (Table 60–1).

EXAM

- Onset is insidious, and pain gradually increases with prolonged standing or sitting. Pain decreases when the patient is upright, moving about, or lying in the fetal position. Leg or foot radiating symptoms are minimal, and there are no cough/sneeze effects.
- The pain is located in the lumbosacral triangle and upper buttocks.
- The pain is symmetric and causes mild reduction in lumbar flexion as well as right and left trunk rotation and a moderate reduction in lumbar extension and lateral flexion bilaterally.
- Extension is the greatest arc of motion that increases pain.
- The Schober flexion test is 4.5 cm (normal is >5 cm).
- Lumbar lordosis is normal but fails to reverse on full voluntary flexion.
- Gait and heel-and-toe walking are normal.
- Radiographs reveal narrowed disc spaces at L4–5 and L5–S1, sclerosis of the facet joints, and hypertrophic changes.
- When disc material degenerates, the soft semiliquid, gel-like, hydrophilic nuclear pulposus is slowly replaced with a denser, less hydrophilic, less compressible, granular fibrous tissue.
- Degenerated discs also result in narrowing of the intervertebral spaces.
- Tolerance of vibration-related stress is particularly reduced.

PHYSIATRIC INTERVENTIONS

- Williams's exercises are the most popular lower back exercises (flexing the spine and reducing lumbar lordosis reduce axial loading on pain- and pressure-sensitive posterior spinal structures, such as the facet joints, which, in turn, reduce pain due to mechanical loading of these structures). Back flexion exercises, therefore, play a prominent role in the management of lower back pain secondary to degenerative disc disease.
- Trunk strengthening exercises improve the mechanical efficiency of the spinal muscular support system.
- Particular attention should be given to strengthening the abdominal oblique muscles, if strengthening is prescribed, as they are the major contributor to increased interabdominal pressure generated by trunk muscles during heavy lifting.
- Strengthening spinal extensors improves the efficiency of shock absorption by concentric and eccentric activity of the intersegmental spinal extensor muscles.
- Trunk strengthening should be predominantly isometric to reduce stress during active flexion in isotonic activities, such as situps.
- Lumbar supports can provide some reduction in mechanical stress on the lumbar spine by substituting for inactive or weak trunk musculature but should not be used routinely as they promote weakness in unused muscles.
- Lumbar rolls and pads are frequently used to increase sitting tolerance. Soft, shock-absorbing shoe inserts also reduce impact stress on the feet.
- Lumbar traction using a simple bar-hanging or pelvic gravity suspension device or any other gravity or low-friction controlled method may reduce lumbar facet loading and segmental muscle spasm but requires supervision.
- Essential interventions must include alterations in posture and improvements in body mechanics to minimize mechanical stress during daily activities.
- A rational exercise prescription for a patient with degenerative disc disease may, therefore, include:
  - Flexion exercises
  - Isometric strengthening of trunk muscles
  - Bar-hanging traction
  - Lumbar roll for sitting

TABLE 60–1 Signs That Aid in the Diagnosis of the Cause of Low Back Pain

DIAGNOSIS	PAIN INCREASED	PAIN DECREASED
Degenerative disc with incomplete lordosis	Positive Larson test (segmental instability) Extension	Knees and hips flexed (sitting)
Disc "protrusion" loss lordosis unilateral	Positive Schober <5 cm Flexion Sitting Crescendo/increasing pain	List to contralateral side Extension standing supine Knees and hips flexed
Spinal stenosis	Bilateral leg pain when walking Standing Extension	Sitting Squatting Flexion
Complete reversal lumbar lordosis	Spondylolysis positive reversal lordosis	Lumbar–sacral rigid bracing
Spondylolisthesis	Schober WNL Extension Positive step-off test Positive Larson	
Acute facet	Localized pain Sudden onset Lateral bend same side Extension	List with rotation to opposite side
Strain syndrome	Tenderness in multifidus muscle No segmental step-off (negative Larson)	List to ipsilateral side

- Lumbar support for repeated or heavier chores
- Shock-absorbing shoe inserts
- Heat
- Cryotherapy and analgesics for acute flares
- Patient education in posture and body mechanics[4]

LUMBOSACRAL STRAIN SYNDROME, MULTIFIDUS STRAIN (LORDOSIS)

EXAM

- Pulling in the back and left buttock immediately after transfer causes a constant pain of increasing intensity and stiffness.
- There are localized pain in the lumbosacral triangle, tenderness, and a slight list to one side; a slight antalgic gait; and a normal lordosis with incomplete reversal of lordosis on active trunk flexion.
- SLR tests are limited to >40°.
- The pain is probably due to muscle and ligament strains or facet joint sprains and usually resolves spontaneously without sequelae with curtailed activities and additional rest.

PHYSIATRIC INTERVENTIONS

- Bed rest is not always necessary. The traditional, full-week, bed rest trial for acute discogenic disorders may be inappropriate for acute muscle ligament or facet strains. Recent studies have shown no advantage with a prolonged period of bed rest.
- Activity is restricted, with a prescription for a soft lumbosacral support.
- Adherence to good posture is emphasized.
- Local heat cryotherapy, analgesics, and deep sedative massage may provide adjunctive temporary relief.
- Facet strains will likely heal if reinjury is avoided while healing is occurring. Some lumbosacral strain syndromes persist, and a few become chronic, possibly because of larger tears of muscles and ligaments.
- Prolonged or habitual muscle spasm may cause additional pain. An aggressive therapeutic program of deep heat, soft tissue mobilization, and muscle relaxation techniques, together with gentle, but progressive, lumbar stretching and isometric strengthening, may abort more ominous chronic back strain syndromes. General strengthening, with emphasis on knee extensor and leg strengthening, endurance training, and adoption of proper body mechanics are useful interventions.
- Physiatric treatment occurs in conjunction with maintenance of modified, appropriate work and activity levels.[5,6]

ACUTE LUMBAR DISC PROTRUSION (FREQUENTLY ACUTE LEFT L5 OR S1 RADICULOPATHY)

- Lumbar disc protrusions are due to degenerative or traumatic weakening and subsequent tearing of the anulus fibrosus.

EXAM

- This condition begins with deep, nagging pain in the lower back and posterior thigh. The next day, the patient is unable to straighten up and experiences pain in the lower back, buttock, posterior thigh, calf, and heel.
- Examination reveals localized pain to the lumbosacral triangle (one side more than the other), buttock, posterior thigh, and calf to the heel and lateral foot.
- The patient loses lumbar lordosis and develops an antalgic gait.
- Marked restriction occurs in trunk flexion and lateral flexion due to pain and moderate reduction occurs in all other arcs of motion.
- The jolt test is positive with radiating pain.
- Ankle jerk is diminished on the affected side.
- SLR causes lower back, left leg, and foot pain at 30°–40° or less.

MANAGEMENT

- Intradiscal pressure is reduced, allowing the nucleus material to retract and the associated edema of the nerve root to resolve.
- Strict bed rest is the most effective way to reduce disc pressures for an appropriate time.
- Oral analgesics are appropriate. Muscle relaxants, such as benzodiazepines, may be necessary, and their sedative side effects may improve psychological tolerance to enforced bed rest during the active phase.[7,8]
- Local heat may be effective in reducing associated muscle spasms.
- A bedside commode with armrests is preferable to bed pans for bowel and bladder care.
- Attention to proper body mechanics as well as a soft lumbar orthosis applied in bed before getting on the commode may provide support during toileting. Stool softeners and high-fiber foods or supplements reduce constipation.

PHYSIATRIC INTERVENTIONS

- Bed positioning should be arranged to avoid excessive lumbar flexion.
- Slight flexion may reduce small protrusions by tightening annulus fibers.
- Larger protrusions may not reduce with flexion, and some may instead protrude more if the annulus tear is large.

- Flexion of the hips and knees is allowed to reduce stretching of the nerve root over protruded disc material.
- The upper trunk should not be higher than the pelvis, except during meals, to avoid axial loading during the acute phase.
- Sitting is associated with high intradiscal pressure (more than double that of lying supine and 40% higher than when standing).
- The lowest intradiscal pressure occurs in a supine position with 90° hip and knee flexion.
- Attempts at reducing a disc protrusion with a progressive passive spinal extension program can be made in selected cases.
- A flexed position shifts vectors posteriorly, and extension may shift vectors anteriorly, reducing forces that are favorable to posterior or posterolateral protrusion.
- Appropriate lateral shifting may centralize lateral vectors.
- A small lumbar roll or pad may help maintain extension while supine.
- Lying prone may help reduce small disc protrusions.
- Lumbar traction is based on the premise of reduction of intradiscal pressure or the creation of a negative intradiscal pressure with the application of external distracting forces.
- External forces best exceed 50% of body weight to overcome body surface friction.
- Low-force traction (less than 20 kg) simply serves to keep the patient in bed.
- Heavy lumbar traction systems can reduce intradiscal pressures, but they cannot be tolerated for long periods.
- The prescription for an acute disc protrusion with severe symptoms could include 7 days of enforced bed rest; careful bed positioning; analgesics; muscle relaxants; stool softeners; a bedside commode; a progressive, passive extension program; and possible, periodic heavy lumbar traction.[9]
- Surgical intervention is reserved for patients who fail such a rest trial or those with progressive neurologic deficits, bowel or bladder involvement, or intractable pain.

EXERCISES

- The postrest management strategy includes gradual (not precipitous) and progressive mobilization (ambulation) of the patient from bed rest. Intradiscal pressure is higher during sitting than standing or walking, and when total bed rest is over, the patient should be helped to stand and walk. Ambulation with an assistant, walker, cane, or in parallel bars can transfer axial loading from the spine to the upper extremities. Soft lumbar support can further reduce intradiscal pressure while mobilizing the patient.

- Prolonged sitting should be delayed.
- Flexion and isometric exercises and bending, twisting, or lifting should be delayed until the annulus tear has had adequate opportunity to form a good scar, at least 6 weeks.
- At 6–8 weeks, if there is no sign of disc protrusion, root irritation, or muscle spasms, a very gentle isometric exercise program should commence.
- Patients are also instructed in ways to wean themselves from a corset or other assistive device.
- A protruded disc, even if managed successfully, will inevitably develop into a degenerative disk.

SPINAL STENOSIS (PSEUDO-CLAUDICATION)

EXAM

- Pain is worse with standing and especially worse with walking.
- Pain is often associated with a sensational weakness and numbness in both legs.
- The patient can walk 50–60 m before the pain prevents further walking.
- The patient gets prompt relief by sitting down and bending forward or squatting (relief by standing once ambulation is halted may suggest vascular etiology and lower-extremity symptoms).
- Lumbar lordosis decreases.
- Ankle jerks decrease or are absent on one or both sides.
- The condition is a consequence of advanced degenerative hypertrophic changes in a narrow spinal canal.
- The characteristic feature is claudication-like leg pain or weakness when walking relieved by rest and especially by spinal flexion.
- Surgical decompression is indicated if symptoms are sufficiently limiting, and the patient is medically able.

PHYSIATRIC INTERVENTIONS

- If surgery is ruled out, a program of flexion exercises and use of a lumbar corset, flexion jacket, or William brace and cane may reduce the neural element irritation.
- Shock-absorbing shoe inserts may help.
- Use of a transcutaneous electrical nerve stimulator during ambulation may further reduce pain but will not affect weakness or numbness.

BILATERAL SPONDYLOLYSIS WITH LOW-GRADE SPONDYLOLISTHESIS

- Spondylolysis does not usually cause symptoms; its consequence, spondylolisthesis, is frequently symptomatic, either from its associated mechanical instability or from traction on or compression of neural elements.

EXAM

- Pain is worse after jumping.
- Pain persists for days after exercise.
- Rest in bed for 2–3 hours usually relieves pain.
- During the past several months, pain has been constant.
- The pain has stopped exercise activity.
- Pain is bilateral in the midline, lower back.
- Pain extends to upper thighs.
- Pain is increased only on extension.
- There is no lateral list.
- There is complete reversal of lumbar lordosis on active spinal flexion.
- Deep tendon reflexes are normal.
- SLR test is negative.
- There is localized tenderness in the involved interspace, typically L4–5 or L5–6.
- Slight palpable step-off is detected at the same level.
- Jolt test is positive.
- Lumbar radiographs show (pars defect) spondylolysis and a spondylolisthesis at the level anterior or retrograde step-off. This is accentuated by flexion or extension on x-ray films.

MANAGEMENT

- Spondylolisthesis is graded according to Meyerding by the percentage of displacement of one vertebral body: grade 1 = 25%, grade 2 = 26–50%, grade 3 = 51–75%, and grade 4 = 76–100%.
- Surgical fusion is not always successful.

PHYSIATRIC INTERVENTIONS

- Effective nonsurgical treatment is available for low-grade spondylolisthesis. This involves a conservative program to reduce the lumbosacral angle and, thereby, reduce the anteriorly directed shear force on supporting soft tissues.
- A spine flexion program is appropriate and effective to maintain function.
- Therapy includes flexion exercises, posture training with emphasis on minimizing lumbar lordosis, isometric abdominal strengthening, and a lumbar support.
- Extension exercises are contraindicated.
- Bar-hanging and gravity traction systems in a flexed spine position may produce additional symptomatic relief but should be used with caution and may increase symptoms.
- Soft shock-absorbing shoe inserts are indicated.

- Activities that increase lordosis or are associated with sudden jolts should be avoided.
- Marked degenerative disc disease can cause spondylolisthesis without spondylolysis.
- Retrolisthesis, reverse spondylolisthesis, can also occur in the mid- and upper lumbar spine with significant degenerative disc disease.
- Management of degenerative spondylolisthesis is most similar to that of degenerative disc disease, with emphasis on isometric strengthening of trunk musculature and use of a lumbar orthosis. Surgical intervention is not frequently indicated. Spondylolisthesis may also result from multiple-level laminectomies.

ACUTE FACET SYNDROME

EXAM

- There are recurrent episodes of acute back pain.
- A sharp catch occurs when bending and twisting at the same time and then attempting to straighten up.
- A click is evident.
- Heavy lifting is not typically involved but bending backward and twisting are.
- Sudden-onset pain occurs when attempting to straighten from a flexed and twisted position (in contrast to disc protrusion pain, which involves a slow crescendo over several hours).
- Pain from acute muscle and ligamentous strain is not intense on onset but builds over minutes or hours.
- Acute disc herniations and acute facet syndromes cause the patient to list to the side opposite the pain.
- The painful arc pattern for a disc protrusion is pain on flexion.
- The painful arc pattern for muscle or ligamentous strain is pain with flexion, lateral flexion, and rotation to the opposite side (the motions that stretch the involved ligament or muscles) (Table 60–2).
- The painful arc pattern for acute facet strain is increased pain on extension, on lateral bending to the painful side, and on rotation to the opposite side (the motions that would increase loading on an ipsilateral facet joint).

TABLE 60–2 Painful Arcs in Acute Facet Syndrome

ORIGIN OF PAIN	MOVEMENTS THAT CAUSE PAIN
Disc protrusion	Flexion
Muscle or ligament strain	Flexion
	Lateral flexion
	Rotation to opposite side
Acute facet syndrome	Extension on lateral bending to same side
	Rotation to opposite side

- Acute facet syndrome is most common on the left side (probably because most people are right-handed).
- There is pain in the lumbosacral triangle.
- Pain extends into the left buttock and upper thigh.
- Gait is antalgic on the left with a list to the right side.
- Lordosis is reduced, and reversal is incomplete on attempted trunk flexion.
- Larson's test is normal.
- The SLR test is limited to 60° on the right by localized lower back pain and 80° on the left by tight hamstrings.
- There is localized tenderness at the spinous process and in the adjacent left paravertebral muscle belly.
- Increased pain restricts spinal extension, left lateral flexion, and right rotation.
- Resolution is prompt with simple readily available measures.
- Specific pathologic confirmation is not available.

PHYSIATRIC INTERVENTIONS
- Gentle lumbar manipulation, which relieves pain, except for mild residual soreness
- Lumbar mobilization without an end-arc thrust
- Flexion exercise home program, twice daily
- Lumbar rotation mobilization technique home program
- Body mechanic and lifting technique instruction[6]

TENSION MYALGIA (FIBROSITIS)

- "Lesion" is unidentifiable by laboratory tests, electromyography, radiography, direct biopsy, or electroencephalography.
- This is a diagnosis of exclusion.
- Other names include fibromyositis, fibromyalgia, tension myositis, and muscle attachment syndrome.
- The pain spasm cycle can be initiated by continuing muscle contraction.
- The cycle may begin when psychological stress or anxiety results in muscle tension.
- Persistently increased muscle tension may cause diffuse muscle pain in the involved muscles and their attachments. This explains the increased tenderness seen in many of the classic trigger points.
- Increased tenderness and pain in these sites might be a result of a lowered pain threshold associated with psychological tension.
- Tension myalgia can be derived from muscular or psychological tension.
- Posture is poor.
- Sleep disorder may contribute to a lowered pain threshold and increased pain.

EXAM
- Generalized morning stiffness
- Improvement in pain after getting up and moving.
- Worsening pain as day progresses.
- Continuous, but light, sleep at night; waking tired and unrefreshed
- Temporary relief provided by heat and rest
- No radicular features
- Mildly increased lumbar lordosis
- No list
- Manual muscle testing, deep tendon reflexes, negative jolt test, and normal Larson's test
- Spinal motions normal without painful arcs
- SLR test negative and limited to 70° bilaterally by tight hamstrings
- No true muscle spasms
- Multiple areas of increased tenderness in parascapular, paracervical, paralumbar, and gluteal trigger point sites
- Overreaction and regionalization in classic trigger point sites

PHYSIATRIC INTERVENTIONS
- The management strategy should break the pain–spasm cycle and reduce anxiety.
- Reassurance should be directed at answering questions to reduce anxiety.
- A thorough general and musculoskeletal exam should be conducted.
- Review normal and abnormal findings in detail.
- Tension myalgia should be discussed with the patient.
- Cryotherapy, local heat, and massage can be used for temporary pain relief and reduction of muscle tension.
- Trigger point massage, trigger point injections, and spray and stretch techniques also can be used.
- Temporary symptomatic relief is essential for achieving lasting results from learned relaxation techniques.

RELAXATION TECHNIQUES
- Relaxation techniques are designed to reduce resting muscle tension by conscious effort (general relaxation).
- Myoelectric biofeedback assists with this education process.
- Relaxation techniques improve the general level of fitness, body mechanics, and quality of sleep.

TRAUMATIC BACK STRAIN SYNDROME, SUPERIMPOSED GENERALIZED DECONDITIONING, AND SUPERIMPOSED PAIN AMPLIFICATION SYNDROME

EXAM
- Chronic post-traumatic soft tissue back injury
- Nonorganic regionalization in pain localization and on muscle testing.

- Nonorganic tenderness over the sacrum and on gentle superficial skin rolling.
- SLR sitting distraction test is positive.
- Overreaction on tandem walking evaluation.
- Passive trunk rotation simulation maneuver is negative.
- A Waddell score of 3 or more associated with significant nonorganic behavior is an indication for further psychological investigations; however, it is possible that the patient is not malingering or faking the pain.

PHYSIATRIC INTERVENTIONS

- The terms *pain amplification syndrome* and *symptom magnification syndrome* may be preferable to older terms like *function pain* and *chronic pain behavior*.
- A diagnosis of deconditioning is appropriate if it is documented by objective dynamometric testing or supported by a functional capacity or work capacity evaluation.
- This deconditioning may play as large a role in limiting rehabilitation as do nonorganic and psychological factors.
- Family and employer support, psychological and vocational counseling, relaxation, training in good body mechanics, physical reconditioning, a work-hardening program, and early settlement of litigation are all essential for return to a high-quality and productive life.

REFERENCES

1. **Johanning E.** Evaluation and management of occupational low back disorders. *Am J Ind Med.* 2000;81:258–264.
2. **Hoppenfeld S.** *Orthopedic Neurology: A Diagnostic Guide to Neurologic Levels.* Philadelphia: Lippincott;1977.
3. **Kendrick D, Fielding K, Bentley E, Miller P, Kerslake R, Pringle M.** The role of radiography in primary care patients with low back pain of at least 6 weeks duration: A randomized (unblended) controlled trial. *Health Technol Assess.* 2001; 5:1–69.
4. **Burton AK, Waddell G, Tillotson KM, Summerton N.** Information and advice to patients with back pain can have a positive effect. A randomized controlled trial of a novel educational booklet in primary care. *Spine.* 1999;24:2484–2491.
5. **Hsieh CY, Adams AH, Tobis J, et al.** Effectiveness of four conservative treatments for subacute low back pain: A randomized clinical trial. *Spine.* 2002;27:1142–1148.
6. **Zigenfus GO, Yin J, Giang GM, Bogarty WT.** Effectiveness of early physical therapy in the treatment of acute low back musculoskeletal disorders. *J Occup Environ Med.* 2000;42:35–39.
7. **Schnitzer TJ, Gray WL, Paster RZ, Karnin M.** Efficacy of tramadol in treatment of chronic low back pain. *J Rheumatol.* 2000;27:772–778.
8. **van Tulder MW, Scholten RJ, Koes BW, Deyo RA.** Nonsteroidal anti-inflammatory drugs for low back pain: A systematic review within the framework of the Cochrane Collaboration Back Review Group. *Spine.* 2000;25: 2501–2513.
9. **van Tulder MW, Blomberg SEI, de Vet HCW, van der Heijden G, Bronfort G, Bouter LM.** Traction for low back pain with or without radiating symptoms (Protocol for a Cochrane Review). *The Cochrane Library.* 2003;3.

61   PIRIFORMIS SYNDROME

Wesley Foreman, MD
Gagan Mahajan, MD
Scott M. Fishman, MD

INTRODUCTION

- Piriformis syndrome remains a controversial diagnosis of exclusion.
- Pain emanating from the other five short, external rotators adjacent to the piriformis muscle (superior and inferior gemelli, obturator internus and externus, and quadratus femoris) can make it challenging to decipher which muscle is involved.[1]
- To date, the diagnosis and definitive treatment options for piriformis syndrome remain ill-defined.
- In 1928, Yeoman was the first to publish that sciatica could be due to periarthritis involving the anterior sacroiliac ligament, the piriformis muscle, and the adjacent branches of the sciatic nerve.[2]
- Nine years later, Freiberg described two findings on physical examination believed to correlate with sciatic pain referable to the piriformis muscle:
  ○ Positive Lasègue's sign, as evidenced by pain and tenderness to palpation in the greater sciatic notch with the hip passively flexed to 90° and the knee passively extended to 180°
  ○ Positive Freiberg's sign, as evidenced by the reproduction of concordant gluteal and buttock pain with passive, forced internal rotation of the hip[3]
- In the same article, Freiburg also described how surgical release of the piriformis muscle relieved the symptoms.[3]
- In 1938, Beaton and Anson identified anomalies of the piriformis muscle and hypothesized that the cause of the pain could be the anomalous relationship between the piriformis muscle and the sciatic nerve.[4]

- However, it was not until 1947 that Robinson first introduced the term *piriformis syndrome*, which he assigned six signs and symptoms:
  - History of trauma to the gluteal and sacroiliac regions
  - Pain in the region of the sacroiliac joint, greater sciatic notch, and piriformis muscle that may travel down the limb causing gait difficulties
  - Acute exacerbation of the pain with stooping or lifting with some relief of pain by application of traction to the affected extremity
  - Palpable, tender, sausage-shaped mass over the affected piriformis muscle
  - Positive Lasègue's sign
  - Depending on the duration of symptoms, gluteal atrophy[5]
- Finally, in 1976, Pace and Nagle described a diagnostic maneuver now referred to as *Pace's sign*.[6] A positive test elicits pain and weakness of the affected side with resisted abduction and external rotation of the hip.
- It should be noted that the nerve entrapment pain associated with piriformis syndrome is distinct from the myofascial pain associated with a piriformis trigger point, though both entities often occur concurrently.[1]
- The pain referred from a piriformis trigger point may radiate to the sacroiliac region, laterally across the buttock and over the posterior aspect of the hip, and to the posterior two-thirds of the thigh.[1]

ANATOMY

- The name *piriformis* was created by the 16th and early 17th century anatomist Adriaan van der Spieghel, who based it on the Latin words *pirum* (pear) and *forma* (shape).[1]
- Co-localized with a series of five short, external rotator muscles (superior and inferior gemelli, obturator internus and externus, and quadratus femoris) below the posteroinferior edge of the gluteus medius muscle, the piriformis muscle has the uppermost position.[7]
- It originates medially from the anterior surface of the second, third, and fourth sacral foramina, exits the pelvis through the greater sciatic foramen, and inserts on the greater trochanter, filling most of the greater sciatic foramen as it passes from its point of origin to insertion.
- At rest, the piriformis muscle may have a snug fit in the foramen.
- When the muscle actively shortens, its diameter may significantly increase, compressing the muscle and the accompanying sciatic nerve.[1]

- Variability exists, however, in the course the sciatic nerve takes as it exits the greater sciatic foramen.
- Beaton and Anson found that among 1510 cadaveric extremities, the sciatic nerve exited below the piriformis muscle in 88%; in 11%, the piriformis muscle was divided into two parts such that the peroneal division of the sciatic nerve passed between both parts of the piriformis muscle and the tibial division passed below the bottommost part of the muscle; and in the remaining 1%, the peroneal and tibial divisions of the nerve either passed above and below the muscle, respectively, or the entire sciatic nerve pierced an undivided piriformis muscle (Figure 61–1).[8]
- Besides the sciatic nerve, other potentially vulnerable neurovascular structures pass through the greater sciatic foramen.
- These structures include the internal iliac artery, branches of the sacral plexus, superior and inferior gluteal nerves and blood vessels, pudendal nerve and blood vessels, posterior femoral cutaneous nerve, and nerves to the gemelli and obturator internus and quadratus femoris.
- Because all of the nerves (including the sciatic nerve) collectively supply the sensory and motor innervation to the gluteal, perineal, posterior thigh, and gastrocnemius regions, neural compression may produce buttock, inguinal, posterior thigh, and calf pain.[1]

INNERVATION

- The piriformis muscle is supplied by one or two small branches that come from the ventral rami of the first and/or second sacral nerves.

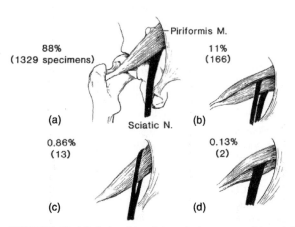

FIGURE 61–1 Relationship of the sciatic nerve and its subdivisions to the piriformis muscle in 1510 extremities studied. Reproduced, with permission, from Beaton and Anson.[4]

ACTION

- With the lower limb in a weight-bearing position, such as with ambulation, the piriformis muscle contracts to prevent rapid internal rotation of the hip.
- With the hip and knee extended, the piriformis muscle externally rotates the hip. However, when the hip is flexed to 90°, the piriformis muscle serves as a hip abductor.

DEMOGRAPHICS AND PATHOGENESIS

- Piriformis syndrome is reported to occur with a 6:1 female:male predominance.[6]
- It is commonly associated with direct trauma to the sciatic notch and the gluteal regions; prolonged sitting; prolonged combined hip flexion, adduction, and internal rotation; and certain sports activities.[1,9,10]
- The latter include cyclists, who ride for prolonged periods; tennis players, who constantly internally rotate their hip with an overhead serve; and ballet dancers, who constantly "turn out" (externally rotate their hip) while dancing.[1]
- While the mechanism of injury may be postulated, the etiology of the signs and symptoms remains less clear.
- One theory is that traumatic injury to the piriformis muscle generates inflammatory and edematous changes to the muscle and surrounding fascia, subsequently compressing the sciatic nerve against the wall of the pelvis and leading to a compression neuropathy.[10]
- The trauma itself may induce focal hyperirritability in the piriformis muscle, which can be further exacerbated by muscle spasm or hypertrophy.
- For those who do not sustain a direct injury to the muscle or those with anomalous piriformis anatomy, sciatic nerve irritation may occur by stretching of the piriformis muscle with passive internal or active external rotation of the hip.
- Entrapment of the superior gluteal nerve in the piriformis muscle may also produce similar pain.[11]

DIAGNOSIS

SYMPTOMS

- The most consistent symptom reported is that of a deep, aching pain in the buttock on the affected side.
- The pain may radiate to the hip, lower back, and posterior thigh, but rarely below the level of the knee.

- Squatting, climbing stairs, walking, and prolonged sitting (especially on hard surfaces) usually worsen the pain.
- The pain is typically unilateral, and is often associated with a limp on the affected side. In addition, the piriformis muscle's compression of the pudendal nerve and blood vessels may cause females to experience labial pain and dyspareunia, and males to experience scrotal pain and impotence.
- Painful bowel movements have also been reported, presumably due to the close proximity of the piriformis muscle to the rectum.

DIAGNOSTIC TESTS AND PHYSICAL EXAM FINDINGS

- *Freiberg's sign*: Buttock pain with passive, forced internal rotation of the hip.[3]
- *Pace's maneuver*: Buttock pain with resisted abduction of the affected leg while in the seated position.[6]
- *Lasègue's sign*: Pain and tenderness to palpation in the greater sciatic notch with the hip passively flexed to 90° and the knee passively extended 180°.[3]
- *Beatty maneuver*: With the patient lying in a lateral decubitus position on the unaffected side, buttock pain is elicited in the affected extremity when the patient actively abducts the affected hip and holds the knee several inches off the table.[12]
- *Rectal exam*: Tenderness to palpation along the posterolateral pelvic wall overlying the piriformis muscle.[13]
- *FA(d)IR*: An acronym for flexion, adduction, and internal rotation of the affected hip; the maneuver prolongs the H (Hoffman) reflex on a nerve conduction study.[14]
- *Gluteal atrophy*: When compression of the sciatic nerve has been long-standing, gluteal atrophy on the affected side may be observed.[9]
- *External rotation*: When the patient is lying supine, the affected hip is maintained in an externally rotated position, even in a relaxed state.[13]
- Unfortunately, there are no convincing studies assessing the sensitivity or specificity of any of these signs or tests in diagnosing piriformis syndrome.
- Benson and Schutzer noted the most common presenting symptoms were pain in the buttock area and intolerance to sitting on the involved side.[10]
- They also found that the two most consistent physical findings were tenderness to palpation at the greater sciatic notch and reproduction of pain with maximum flexion, adduction, and internal rotation of the hip.

- They went on to suggest that the most valuable pre-operative test was electromyographic evidence consistent with extrapelvic compression of the sciatic nerve at the level of the piriformis muscle.
- Jankiewicz et al showed that CT scans could have some diagnostic utility in suspected piriformis syndrome based on demonstrating asymmetric enlargement of the piriformis muscle on the affected side.[15]
- Benson and Schutzer, however, found that preoperative CT scans had no predictive value in the final outcome after surgery.[10]

TREATMENT

- Once properly diagnosed after other causes of low back, hip, and sciatic pain have been eliminated, treatment is undertaken in a stepwise approach.

TABLE 61–1 Rehabilitation Exercises for Piriformis Syndrome[24]

Piriformis stretch	Supine position with knees flexed and feet flat on the floor. Rest the ankle of the injured leg over the knee of the uninjured leg. Grasp the thigh of the uninjured leg and pull that knee toward the chest. The patient will feel stretching along the buttocks and possibly along the outside of the hip on the injured side. Hold for 30 s. Repeat three times.
Standing hamstring stretch	Place the heel of the patient's injured leg on a stool about 15 in high. Lean forward, bending at the hips, until a mild stretch in the back of the thigh is felt. Hold the stretch for 30 to 60 s. Repeat three times.
Pelvic tilt	Supine position with the knees bent and feet flat on the floor. Tighten the abdominal muscles and flatten the spine on the floor. Hold for 5 s, then relax. Repeat 10 times. Do three sets.
Partial curls	Supine position with the knees bent and feet flat on the floor. Clasp hands behind the head to support it. Keep the elbows out to the side and don't pull with the hands. Slowly raise the shoulders and head off the floor by tightening the abdominal muscles. Hold for 3 s. Return to the starting position. Repeat 10 times. Build up to three sets.
Prone hip extension	Prone position. Tighten the buttock muscles and lift the right leg off the floor about 8 in. Keep the knee straight. Hold for 5 s and return to the starting position. Repeat 10 times. Do three sets on each side.

- Initially, progressive stretching is employed, starting with 5 seconds of a sustained stretch and gradually building to 30 and 60 seconds (Table 61–1).
- This is repeated several times throughout the day and may be combined with physical therapy modalities, such as superficial and deep heat (ultrasound).
- It is important that any concomitant abnormal biomechanical problems, such as overpronation of the foot, also be addressed.
- Addition of nonsteroidal anti-inflammatory medications or acetaminophen should also be considered.
- If conservative management with physical therapy and medication fails to adequately relieve symptoms, intramuscular piriformis injections may be warranted.
- Various injection techniques performed under CT guidance, fluoroscopic guidance, or combined fluoroscopic and electromyographic guidance have been described (Table 61–2).[16]
- While traditional injections of a corticosteroid and a local anesthetic have proven to be effective, the duration of analgesia tends to be short-lived.[17]
- A promising addition to the treatment regimen, however, is botulinum toxin.

TABLE 61–2 Piriformis Injection Techniques

Approach 1:[10–25] Fluoroscopic Guidance Without EMG Localization

1. Place the patient in a prone position.
2. Prepare the skin and drape in a sterile manner.
3. Identify the expected position of the piriformis muscle under fluoroscopic guidance with the beam directed in an anteroposterior direction. As landmarks, use include the greater trochanter relative to the lateral border of the sacrum and sacroiliac joint on the affected side.
4. Visualize an imaginory line connecting the greater trochanter and the lower border of the sacrum.
5. Place a superficial skin wheal overlying the ischial bone, medial to the acetabulum and parallel to the target site of injection.
6. Advance a 22- or 25-gauge 3½-in (6-in if the patient is morbidly obese) spinal needle to a point along the imaginary line near the pelvic brim until the posterior ischium is contacted.
7. Inject contrast medium to visually confirm a classic sausage-shaped piriformis myogram (Figure 61–2).

Approach 2:[11] Fluoroscopic and EMG Guidance

1. Repeat steps 1–3 as described in approach 1.
2. Place superficial skin wheal overlying the 2 o'clock position (left side) or 10 o'clock position (right side) of the acetabulum of the affected extremity.
3. Advance an EMG needle until the 2 or 10 o'clock position of the acetabulum is contacted (Figure 61–3).
4. Ask the patient to contract the piriformis muscle by externally rotating and slightly abducting the affected hip.
5. Adjust placement of the EMG needle until maximum motor unit action potentials (MUAPs) are demonstrated while the patient is externally rotating and abducting the hip. Once the MUAPs are localized, ask the patient to stop contracting the piriformis muscle, and inject contrast medium to visually confirm a classic sausage-shaped piriformis myogram (Figure 61–2).

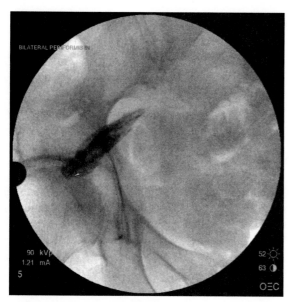

FIGURE 61–2 Piriformis myogram.

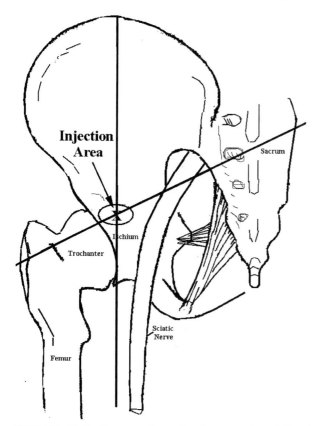

FIGURE 61–3 Diagram of needle placement for piriformis injection by approach 2.

• Botulinum toxin has been used in the treatment of spasticity in such conditions as cerebral palsy,[18] stroke,[19] and acquired brain injury.[20]

• Botulinum toxin is a potent neurotoxin that is produced by the gram-negative anaerobic bacterium *Clostridium botulinum.*[21]

• The two clinically available forms of botulinum toxin are type A (Botox) and type B (Myobloc), each inhibiting presynaptic release of acetylcholine, thereby leading to muscle relaxation.[21]

• A hypothetical direct analgesic effect of botulinum toxin is postulated to be due to inhibition of the release of substance P, which is co-released with acetylcholine into the nerve terminal, muscle, and its surrounding fascia.[22]

• Comparing intramuscular piriformis injection of 100 units of botulinum toxin A with injection of placebo (normal saline), Childers et al demonstrated significant analgesia in patients receiving the active agent.[23]

• Fishman and Zybert concluded that the combination of physical therapy and intramuscular piriformis injection of botulinum toxin A was more effective in reducing pain than physical therapy combined with either placebo or triamcinolone and lidocaine.[14]

• If conservative therapy or intramuscular piriformis injections fail to produce symptomatic relief, surgical consultation for evaluation of piriformis tendon release and sciatic neurolysis may be undertaken as a last resort.[10,11]

REFERENCES

1. **Travell JG, Simons DG.** *Myofascial Pain and Dysfunction: The Trigger Point Manual.* Vol 2. Baltimore: Williams & Wilkins; 1992:186–214.
2. **Yeoman W.** The relation of arthritis of the sacroiliac joint to sciatica. *Lancet.* 1928:1119–1122.
3. **Freiberg AH.** Sciatic pain and its relief by operations on muscle and fascia. *Arch Surg.* 1937;34:337–350.
4. **Beaton LE, Anson BJ.** The sciatic nerve and the piriformis muscle: Their interrelation and possible cause of coccygodynia. *J Bone Joint Surg.* 1938;20:686–688.
5. **Robinson DR.** Piriformis syndrome in relation to sciatic pain. *Am J Surg.* 1947:355–358.
6. **Pace JB, Nagle D.** Piriformis syndrome. *West J Med.* 1976;124:435–439.
7. **Jenkins DB.** *Hollingshead's Functional Anatomy of the Limbs and Back.* 7th ed. Philadelphia: WB Saunders; 1998:274–275.
8. **Beaton LE, Anson BJ.** The relation of the sciatic nerve and its subdivisions to the piriformis muscle. *Anat Rec.* 1938;70:1–5.
9. **Thiele GH.** Coccygodynia and pain in the superior gluteal region. *JAMA.* 1937;109:1271–1275.
10. **Benson ER, Schutzer SF.** Posttraumatic piriformis syndrome: Diagnosis and results of operative treatment. *J Bone Joint Surg Am.* 1999;81:941–949.

11. **Diop M, Parratte B, Tatu L, Vuillier F, Faure A, Monnier G.** Anatomical bases of superior gluteal nerve entrapment syndrome in the suprapiriformis foramen. *Surg Radiol Anat.* 2002;24:155–159.

12. **Beatty RA.** The piriformis muscle syndrome: A simple diagnostic maneuver. *Neurosurgery.* 1994; 34:512–514; discussion, 514.

13. **Kaul M, Herring SA.** Functional rehabilitation of sports and musculoskeletal injuries. In: Kibler WB, Herring SA, Press JM, eds. *The Rehabilitation Institute of Chicago Publication Series.* Gaithersburg, Md: Aspen; 1998: 209.

14. **Fishman LM, Zybert PA.** Electrophysiologic evidence of piriformis syndrome. *Arch Phys Med Rehabil.* 1992;73: 359–364.

15. **Jankiewicz JJ, Hennrikus WL, Houkom JA.** The appearance of the piriformis muscle syndrome in computed tomography and magnetic resonance imaging: A case report and review of the literature. *Clin Orthop.* 1991: 205–209.

16. **Fanucci E, Masala S, Sodani G, et al.** CT-guided injection of botulinic toxin for percutaneous therapy of piriformis muscle syndrome with preliminary MRI results about denervative process. *Eur Radiol.* 2001;11:2543–2548.

17. **Fishman LM, Anderson C, Rosner B.** BOTOX and physical therapy in the treatment of piriformis syndrome. *Am J Phys Med Rehabil.* 2002;81:936–942.

18. **Dursun N, Dursun E, Alican D.** The role of botulin toxin A in the management of lower limb spasticity in patients with cerebral palsy. *Int J Clin Pract.* 2002;56: 564–567.

19. **Brashear A, Gordon MF, Elovic E, et al.** Intramuscular injection of botulinum toxin for the treatment of wrist and finger spasticity after a stroke. *N Engl J Med.* 2002; 347:395–400.

20. **Francisco GE, Boake C, Vaughn A.** Botulinum toxin in upper limb spasticity after acquired brain injury: A randomized trial comparing dilution techniques. *Am J Phys Med Rehabil.* 2002;81:355–363.

21. **Davis LE.** Botulism. *Curr Treat Options Neurol.* 2003;5:23–31.

22. **Childers MK, Kornegay JN, Aoki R, Otaviani L, Bogan DJ, Petroski G.** Evaluating motor end-plate-targeted injections of botulinum toxin type A in a canine model. *Muscle Nerve.* 1998;21:653–655.

23. **Childers MK, Wilson DJ, Gnatz SM, Conway RR, Sherman AK.** Botulinum toxin type A use in piriformis muscle syndrome: A pilot study. *Am J Phys Med Rehabil.* 2002;81:751–759.

24. **White T.** *Piriformis Syndrome Rehabilitation Exercises: McKesson Clinical Reference Systems.* Ann Arbor: University of Michigan Health System; 2002.

25. **Saleemi S, Hernandez L, Rakesh V, Chandler E, Cork RC.** Medi-Dx 7000 V-sNCT a valuable aide in piriformis muscle syndrome diagnosis. In: *Piriformis Syndrome and Its Treatment by Botulinum Toxin-A, V-sNCT as an Aide to Diagnosis.* Shreveport: Louisiana State University; 2002.

62 SACROILIAC JOINT DYSFUNCTION

Norman Pang, MD
Gagan Mahajan, MD
Scott M. Fishman, MD

INTRODUCTION

- The sacroiliac joint (SIJ) has long been a controversial cause of low back pain, ever since Goldwaith and Osgood first reported it in 1905.[1]
- Whether or not SIJ dysfunction is a significant source of all cases of low back pain has not been clearly elucidated. Bernard and Kirkaldy-Willis concluded in their study of 1293 patients that the SIJ was the primary source of pain in 22.5%.[2]
- Others, however, believe the true sources of low back pain are hidden in the multitude of adjacent structures.

ANATOMY AND PHYSIOLOGY

- Five fused sacral vertebrae form the wedge-shaped sacrum.
- The sacrum articulates superiorly with the fifth lumbar vertebra and inferiorly with the triangle-shaped coccyx.
- In addition to supporting the lumbar spine, the sacrum transmits the forces from the lower limbs to the pelvis, and then to the vertebral column.[3]
- The SIJ itself is a C-shaped, diarthrodial structure located between the sacrum and the ilium and is a true synovial joint by virtue of the following features:
  - Presence of a joint cavity containing synovial fluid
  - Adjacent bones united by ligaments
  - A fibrous capsule surrounding the joint with an inner synovial lining
  - Surfaces that allow motion
- While SIJ mobility exhibits a few millimeters of glide and 2° to 3° of rotation, the SIJ is instead designed for stability.[4]
- Multiple major ligaments (iliolumbar, interosseous, anterior and superior sacroiliac, sacrospinous, and sacrotuberous) between the spine, sacrum, iliac bones, and pubic symphysis stabilize the SIJ.
- Muscles located in the same vicinity closely interact with these ligaments.
- There is no joint capsule posteriorly, and the interosseous ligament forms the posterior border of the joint space.

- The anterior SIJ surface is covered with a thin layer of hyaline cartilage on the sacral side and fibrocartilage on the iliac side.
- The ligaments, muscles, and joint capsules combine to enhance the SIJ's biomechanical function.

INNERVATION

- The SIJ and surrounding tissues are well innervated, posteriorly, by lateral branches of the posterior primary rami from L4 to S3 and, anteriorly, by lateral branches of the posterior primary rami from L2 to S2.[5]
- Innervation from multiple sources combined with wide individual variations in nerve supply accounts for the inconsistencies in pain referral patterns and thereby adds to the complexity of diagnosing SIJ pain.

CLINICAL PRESENTATION

- SIJ dysfunction may occur from an acute traumatic injury transmitted through the hamstring muscles, fall onto the buttocks, sudden heavy lifting, prolonged lifting and bending, rising from a stooping position, or repetitive shear and torsional forces on the SIJ during activities such as figure skating and golfing.[4]
- While pain of SIJ origin is often described as resulting from a combined rotation and axial loading injury to the lumbar spine,[6] studies have shown that history does not accurately correlate with the diagnosis of SIJ dysfunction.[7]
- The precise diagnosis of SIJ dysfunction is often difficult to make since it may also be associated with a herniated disc, spinal stenosis, facet arthropathy, or any other source of pain related to the spine, pelvis, hip, or lower extremity.
- Pain emanating from the SIJ is not exclusively limited to the lumbar and buttock region.
- It can be referred to the upper lumbar region, groin, thigh, and foot.[8]
- Depending on the portion of the SIJ injured, variable pain referral patterns may occur secondary to the inherent variability in innervation of the SIJ.
- SIJ pain may be worse in the morning and can be exacerbated by trunk flexion, prolonged sitting, weight bearing on the affected limb, and Valsalva's maneuver.[4]
- Symptoms may be relieved by flexing the affected leg and weight bearing on the contralateral leg.[4]

DIAGNOSIS

- While there is no definitive diagnostic test for SIJ dysfunction, numerous physical examination maneuvers have been described.[9]
- These tests include:
  - *Fortin's finger test:* The patient points to the area of pain with one finger. The result is positive if the site is within 1 cm of the posterior superior iliac spine.
  - *Patrick's test:* This maneuver is also known as the *fabere sign,* which is an acronym for the position in which the patient's hip is passively positioned for the test: *f*lexion, *ab*duction, *e*xternal *r*otation, and *e*xtension. With the patient lying supine, the ankle of the affected extremity is placed on the contralateral knee to create a figure-4 position. The examiner places his or her hand along the medial aspect of the knee of the tested extremity and applies downward pressure toward the examination table, while simultaneously providing counterpressure with his or her other hand on the contralateral anterior superior iliac spine (ASIS). The result is considered positive for SIJ pathology if pain is elicited along the ipsilateral SIJ. However, because this maneuver also stresses the hip joint, pain elicited in the ipsilateral groin suggests trochanteric pain.
  - *Gaenslen's test:* With the patient lying supine, the hip and knee of the unaffected extremity are maximally flexed toward the trunk, and the examiner passively extends the hip of the affected leg by allowing it to slowly drop off the edge of the examination table. This test maximally stresses the SIJ of the affected leg by allowing it to move through its full range of motion. The finding is considered positive if the patient experiences pain across the ipsilateral SIJ.
  - *Lateral compression test:* This test assesses for pathology localized at any of the major joints of the pelvic ring. The patient lies in a lateral decubitus position. The examiner applies downward pressure on the iliac crest, compressing it against the examination table. The finding is considered positive if the patient experiences pain across either the SIJ or the pubic symphysis.
  - *Anteroposterior pelvic compression test:* This test assesses for pathology localized at any of the major joints of the pelvic ring and is similar to the lateral compression test, but it is performed with the patient lying in a supine position. The examiner applies downward pressure on the pubic symphysis. The finding is considered positive if the patient experiences pain across either the SIJ or the pubic symphysis. Note that permission should be sought before applying pressure and having a witness in

the room may help avoid any misconception of inappropriate sexual contact.

◦ *SIJ compression test:* The patient lies prone. The examiner places his or her palm along the SIJ or on the sacrum and makes a vertical downward thrust. The finding is considered positive if the patient experiences pain along the ipsilateral SIJ line.

◦ *Distraction test:* The patient lies supine, and the examiner alternately presses on each ASIS in a posterolateral direction. The finding is considered positive if it produces pain or asymmetric movement.

◦ *Thigh thrust test:* Also known as the *fade test*, the patient is placed in a supine position with the hip on the affected side passively flexed and adducted to midline. The examiner applies downward pressure along the long axis of the femur to move the ilium posterior. The result is considered positive if it produces pain in the ipsilateral leg.

◦ *Passive straight leg raising:* The patient lies supine, and the examiner grasps the patient's heel and passively flexes the hip while keeping the knee in extension. The patient is asked to maintain the position and then to slowly lower his or her leg. The result is considered positive if it produces pain in the ipsilateral leg.

◦ *One-legged stork test:* Also known as *Gillet's test*. The patient is placed in a standing position with the examiner standing behind him or her. The examiner places one thumb slightly inferior to the posterior superior iliac spine (PSIS) of the affected extremity and the other thumb on the sacrum at S2 of the contralateral side. The examiner instructs the patient to actively flex the hip of the affected limb to 90°. If the thumb on the PSIS moves minimally or upward instead of inferolaterally as expected, it suggests hypomobility of the ipsilateral SIJ. Hypomobility can be a source of SIJ dysfunction.

◦ *Standing flexion test:* The patient is placed in a standing position with the examiner standing behind him or her. With the examiner's thumbs placed slightly inferior to each PSIS, the examiner instructs the patient to flex the trunk forward without bending the knees. The result is considered positive if asymmetric movement is detected at the PSIS.

◦ *Seated flexion test:* Also known as *Piedallu's test*, this maneuver is similar to the standing flexion test. The patient is placed in a seated position with the examiner standing behind him or her. With his or her thumbs placed slightly inferior to each PSIS, the examiner instructs the patient to flex the trunk forward. The result is considered positive if asymmetric movement is detected at the PSIS.

• Unfortunately, there is no consistent physical examination maneuver that has sufficient specificity to be used to diagnose SIJ dysfunction reliably in a clinical setting.[10]

• The reliability of these tests has been widely questioned based on poor inter- and intrarater reliability and demonstrating positive results in 20% of asymptomatic individuals.[4,11]

• The use of multiple tests, however, may improve the diagnostic reliability.

• When correlated to a positive diagnostic SIJ injection, Slipman et al found a positive predictive value of 60% if three exam maneuvers were positive.[12]

• Broadhurst and Bond demonstrated a sensitivity of 77 to 87% if three exam maneuvers were positive.[13]

• Although not specific for SIJ involvement, rectal examination may be necessary to search for referred pain from the prostate, uterus, or spasm in muscles of the pelvic floor.

• Piriformis muscle spasm can be localized at the end of the examiner's finger at the 2 or 10 o'clock position.

• Because of the piriformis muscle's close proximity to the SIJ, injury to the SIJ can trigger spasm of the piriformis muscle with subsequent irritation of the nearby sciatic nerve.

• Differential diagnosis for pain in the SIJ region includes pelvic fractures, infection, spondyloarthropathies, osteoarthritis, tumors, hip joint pathology, surrounding muscle dysfunction, and metabolic abnormalities (eg, gout/pseudogout) and referred pain from disc disease, spinal stenosis, or facet arthropathy.

• In the absence of the spondyloarthropathies, clinical lab work and diagnostic imaging of the SIJ are usually not helpful.

• Plain films and CT demonstrate abnormal degenerative SIJ changes in up to 24.5% of asymptomatic individuals over the age of 50, and bone scans have a variable sensitivity of 12.9 to 65%.[4]

• While bone scans have shown a low specificity for diagnosing sacroiliitis, single-photon emission computed tomography (SPECT) has shown high sensitivity in its early diagnosis.[14]

• Slipman et al, however, found the sensitivity dropped to 9.1% when SPECT was used for diagnosing SIJ dysfunction, which is not the same as sacroiliitis.[14]

• Finally, Battafarano et al and Hanly et al looked at MRI and sacroiliitis and reported sensitivities of 100 and 54%, respectively.[15]

• Many practitioners believe the only way to accurately diagnose SIJ dysfunction is by performing a diagnostic intraarticular injection with local anesthetic.

• Concordant pain occurring immediately on injection of the anesthetic is felt to be secondary to its distention of the joint capsule, whereas the subsequent analgesia is due to the local anesthetic effect.

- Sequential occurrence of these two symptoms is felt to further suggest the diagnosis.[16]
- Others, however, claim that pain relief following anesthetic injection does not necessarily indicate dysfunction of the SIJ since structures unrelated to the joint, but in the same region, also may be affected due to the infiltration and diffusion of anesthetic into the soft tissues surrounding the SIJ.[17]
- Finally, some practitioners may elect to concurrently mix a corticosteroid with the local anesthetic to offer a therapeutic, as well as a diagnostic, injection.

TREATMENT

- Conservative treatment may begin with nonsteroidal anti-inflammatory drugs (NSAIDs) and a course of physical therapy to assist with pelvic stabilization exercises, strengthening and stretching exercises for the lower extremities and spine, aerobic exercises, and correction of postural and gait abnormalities that may exacerbate SIJ pain.
- The use of a lumbar corset or SIJ belt may remind the patient to maintain proper posture. Unfortunately, no prospective studies have been done evaluating the efficacy of physical therapy and bracing in SIJ dysfunction.[4]
- Other conservative treatment options can include:
  - *Deep heat (ultrasound)*: Often better tolerated than ice and may be more likely to reach affected areas.
  - *Mobilization*: Many osteopathic, chiropractic, and physiotherapy techniques for restoring alignment and sacral position.
  - *Prolotherapy*: Involves injection of an irritant (often dextrose) along the joint line. The desired result is thickening of ligaments or muscle attachments to stabilize a "hypermobile joint." The operator must be familiar with technique and risks before attempting the procedure.
- When treatment with conservative therapies has plateaued or failed, injection therapies should be considered.
- While some SIJ injections are performed in office-based settings without the benefit of image guidance, this approach is not recommended because of the inability to confirm needle placement with access to the SIJ.
- Because of the thickness of the surrounding sacroiliac and interosseous ligaments and the convoluted joint surface, non-image-guided injections will most likely result in ligamentous or myofascial injections.[16]

- Although CT guidance has been used for this procedure, it can be safely performed at lower economic expense with fluoroscopic guidance.
- One of the many protocols for performing the injection is as follows[18]:
  - After informed consent is obtained, the patient is prepped and draped and placed in a prone position on the C-arm fluoroscopic table.
  - With the x-ray tube perpendicular to the table, the skin is marked over the distal 1 cm of the SIJ.
  - The fluoroscope tube is then angled about 20°–25° in the cephalic direction to displace the posteroinferior portion of the SIJ in a caudal direction. This allows the posteroinferior aspect of the joint to be clearly differentiated from the inaccessible anterior, which moves cephalad on the image.
  - Using sterile technique, a local anesthetic skin wheal is placed at the site previously marked. A 22-gauge 3.5-in (with a larger patient a 6-in needle should be used) straight or curved-tip spinal needle is advanced perpendicular to the fluoroscopic table.
  - With the tube in the cephalic position, the needle is directed toward the posterior aspect of the SIJ. As the needle contacts the firm tissues on the posterior aspect of the joint, it can be maneuvered through the ligaments and capsule into the joint by advancing it about 5–10 mm, usually by angling the needle tip slightly laterally to follow the natural curve of the joint.
  - Intraarticular placement is confirmed after injection of 0.2–0.5 mL of contrast (Figure 62–1). On demonstrating an arthrogram, a mixture of local anesthetic and corticosteroid is injected.
- While intraarticular injection of local anesthetic and corticosteroids can be effective, the duration of analgesia is often short-lived.
- Because repeated injections are not recommended as a long-term treatment plan, this has resulted in the application of novel techniques for treating SIJ pain.
- A case report of implanting a neuroprosthesis to stimulate the nerve supply (third sacral nerve roots) to the SIJ documented clinical success for two patients who were determined to have SIJ dysfunction by diagnostic SIJ block.[19]
- Intraarticular viscosupplementation with hyaluronic acid (Hylan) has also been reported to provide prolonged pain relief in some patients diagnosed with SIJ dysfunction.[20]
- Although hyaluronic acid did not resolve the pain permanently in those patients tested, the effect was significant and longer-lasting than the steroid response.
- Viscosupplementation may work by many putative mechanisms including:

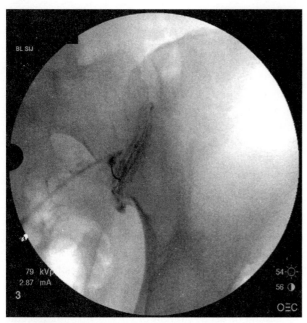

FIGURE 62–1 Intra articular spread of contrast in the sacroiliac joint.

○ Restoring or augmenting rheologic properties of the synovial fluid
○ Replacing pathologic synovial fluid
○ Supplementing elasticity and viscosity of synovial fluid
○ Independent analgesia (mechanism is yet unknown)
○ Slowing progression of osteoarthritis by inhibiting the diffusion of chondrocyte enzymes into the cartilage.[5,21]

• A recent pilot study by Cohen and Abdi described treatment of SIJ pain with continuous radiofrequency (RF) lesioning of the nerves innervating the SIJ.[22] In their study, 18 patients with SIJ pain, confirmed by a positive response to SIJ injection with steroid and a local anesthetic, first underwent diagnostic L4 and L5 dorsal rami and S1, S2 and S3 lateral branch block (LBB) with local anesthetic. Fifty percent or greater pain relief was needed prior to proceeding with continuous RF lesioning of the affected nerves at 80°C for 90 seconds. Thirteen of eighteen patients obtained significant pain relief with the diagnostic block, and two patients reported prolonged benefit. Nine patients who experienced greater than 50% pain relief with the diagnostic block underwent continuous RF lesioning of the nerves. Eight of the nine (89%) obtained 50% or more pain relief from continuous RF lesioning that persisted up to 9 months. While still a small pilot study, the results are encouraging. However, randomized, controlled trials are needed to further evaluate the efficacy of this procedure.
• Surgery should be considered only when pain is intractable and disabling, and the patient has failed to

respond to conservative treatments. Screw fixation of the ilium to the sacrum has been described.

CONCLUSION

• It has been said that the "SIJ has been a source of pain to both sufferers of low back pain and those who refuse to recognize its contribution to this common problem."[22]
• SIJ pain may present as a complex diagnostic problem that leads to elusive and controversial treatment options.

REFERENCES

1. **Goldwaith JAO, Osgood RB.** A consideration of the pelvic articulations from an anatomical, pathological, and clinical standpoint. *Boston Med Surg J.* 1905;152:593–601.
2. **Bernard TN Jr, Kirkaldy-Willis WH.** Recognizing specific characteristics of nonspecific low back pain. *Clin Orthop.* 1987:266–280.
3. **Bogduk N, Twomey LT.** *Clinical Anatomy of the Lumbar Spine and Sacrum.* New York: Churchill Livingstone; 1997: x, 261.
4. **Slipman C, Patel R, Shin C, Braverman D, Lenrow D.** Pain management: Studies probe complexities of sacroiliac joint syndrome. *BioMechanics.* April 2000.
5. **Calvillo O, Skaribas I, Turnipseed J.** Anatomy and pathophysiology of the sacroiliac joint. *Curr Rev Pain.* 2000; 4:356-361.
6. **Dreyfuss P, Cole A, Pauza K.** Sacroiliac joint injection techniques. *Phys Med Rehabil Clin North Am.* 1995;6:785–813.
7. **Schwarzer AC, Aprill CN, Bogduk N.** The sacroiliac joint in chronic low back pain. *Spine.* 1995;20:31–37.
8. **Slipman CW, Jackson HB, Lipetz JS, Chan KT, Lenrow D, Vresilovic EJ.** Sacroiliac joint pain referral zones. *Arch Phys Med Rehabil.* 2000;81:334–338.
9. **Reider B.** *The Orthopaedic Physical Examination.* Philadelphia: WB Saunders; 2001:195–197.
10. **Saal JS.** General principles of diagnostic testing as related to painful lumbar spine disorders: A critical appraisal of current diagnostic techniques. *Spine.* 2002;27:2538–2545; discussion, 2546.
11. **Dreyfuss P, Dryer S, Griffin J, Hoffman J, Walsh N.** Positive sacroiliac screening tests in asymptomatic adults. *Spine.* 1994;19:1138–1143.
12. **Slipman CW, Sterenfeld EB, Chou LH, Herzog R, Vresilovic E.** The predictive value of provocative sacroiliac joint stress maneuvers in the diagnosis of sacroiliac joint syndrome. *Arch Phys Med Rehabil.* 1998;79:288–292.
13. **Broadhurst NA, Bond MJ.** Pain provocation tests for the assessment of sacroiliac joint dysfunction. *J Spinal Disord.* 1998;11:341–345.

14. **Slipman CW, Sterenfield EB, Pauza K, Herzon R, Vresilovic EJ.** Sacroiliac joint syndrome: The diagnostic value of single photon emission computed tomography. *Int Spinal Inject Soc* 1994;2:2–20.

15. **Battafarano DF, West SG, Rak KM, Fortenbery EJ, Chantelois AE.** Comparison of bone scan, computed tomography, and magnetic resonance imaging in the diagnosis of active sacroiliitis. *Semin Arthritis Rheum.* 1993; 23:161–176.

16. **Lennard T.** *Pain Procedures in Clinical Practice.* Philadelphia: Hanley & Belfus; 2000:265–275.

17. **Freburger JK, Riddle DL.** Using published evidence to guide the examination of the sacroiliac joint region. *Phys Ther.* 2001; 81:1135–1143.

18. **Dussault R, Kaplan P, Anderson M.** Fluoroscopy-guided sacroiliac joint injections. *Radiology.* 2000; 214:273–277.

19. **Calvillo O, Esses SI, Ponder C, D'Agostino C, Tanhui E.** Neuroaugmentation in the management of sacroiliac joint pain: Report of two cases. *Spine.* 1998;23:1069–1072.

20. **Srejic U, Calvillo O, Kabakibou K.** Viscosupplementation: A new concept in the treatment of sacroiliac joint syndrome: A preliminary report of four cases. *Reg Anesth Pain Med.* 1999; 24:84–88.

21. **Fortin JD, Aprill CN, Ponthieux B, Pier J.** Sacroiliac joint: Pain referral maps upon applying a new injection/arthrography technique. Part II: Clinical evaluation. *Spine.* 1994; 19:1483–1489.

22. **Cohen S, Abdi S.** Lateral branch blocks as a treatment for sacroiliac joint pain: A pilot study. *Reg Anesth Pain Med.* 2003; 28:113–119.

63 SPINAL DRUG DELIVERY

Stuart Du Pen, MD

INDICATIONS

- The decision to use a spinal drug delivery system should build on the previous aggressive and optimized use of more conservative modalities.[1,2]
- The patient's pain-related diagnosis, other medical diagnoses or general health, previous treatment, and future potential treatment options are all considered in the process of evaluating the patient for spinal drug delivery.
- Patients who are often considered for spinal drug delivery:
  - Have neuropathic pain unrelieved by optimized oral medication management
  - Are opioid tolerant and require long-term opioid therapy
  - Have intractable side effects from oral analgesics and adjuvant medications
  - Are unable to comply with a conservative oral or transcutaneous treatment plan
  - Have intractable spasticity[3]

ADVANTAGES

- The advantages of spinal drug delivery must be examined in the context of patient-specific indications.
- In each case the advantages and risks must be balanced before considering the procedure.
- General advantages of the technique include:
  - Intrathecal opioid dose of morphine up to 300 times as potent as oral morphine
  - Choice of programmable or cost-efficient, nonprogrammable pumps
  - Completely implantable system
  - Programmable array from simple infusion to a complex infusion pattern
  - Ability to add adjuvant drugs, resulting in decreased opioid requirements
  - Precise delivery of intrathecal baclofen
  - Future ability to deliver PCA doses through the IT space

RISKS

- The risks of intraspinal catheterization and pump implantation should not be ignored. In experienced hands the risks are not only manageable, but can be limited.
- Externalized devices are associated with a higher rate of catheter-related infections.[4]
- Catheter-related intrathecal granulomas may be identified by MRI when abnormal and unexpected neurologic symptoms are detected.[5]
- Removal of the catheter from the granuloma usually results in complete relief of symptoms and resolution of the granuloma, whereas untreated granulomas may grow and result in cord compression.[6]
- As with all complications, diagnosis and treatment are paramount.
- General risks of the technique include:
  - Postoperative infections
  - Low-pressure spinal headaches
  - Catheter-related epidural space infections
  - Catheter-related granuloma formation
  - Dose escalation and tolerance
  - Possibly serious acute withdrawal symptoms due to pump or catheter failure (clonidine and baclofen)[3]

Table 63–1 Octanol Water Coefficient: Standard for Grading and Comparing Lipophilicity

Morphine	1.4
Hydromorphone	1.2
Meperidine	39
Fentanyl	813
Sufentanil	1788

From Carr and Cousins 1998.[1]

PATIENT SELECTION

- This is the most important part of the preimplant process. Careful selection of patients improves outcome results and builds trust in the patient–clinician relationship.[7]
- Patient selection begins with the process of examining indications in an individual patient and continues through the screening process and up to implantation.
- Patients are selected for implantation based on the following criteria:
  - Ineffective oral analgesia with multiple oral or transcutaneous trials including dose titration
  - Intolerable side effects despite opioid rotation
  - Functional analgesia during temporary trial infusion
  - Psychologic stability and realistic goals[8]
  - Access to care
  - Patient acceptance
  - Intractable spasticity unrelieved by oral antispasmodics with improved Ashworth scores at baclofen test dose[9]

DEVICE SELECTION

- Selection of the device depends on the duration of expected use, risk of infection, need for dose titration, and patient's access to health services and home support.
- The decision between epidural and intrathecal should be based on the patient's prognosis and expected therapeutic requirements. Here, a trial infusion gives the practitioner an estimate of the expected outcome.[7]
- Some options for device selection include:
  - Catheters, externalized for trial and therapeutic use: epidural, intrathecal
  - Catheters, internalized for intrathecal pumps or ports
  - Programmable and nonprogrammable intrathecal pumps
  - Ports: subcutaneous port connected to intrathecal and epidural catheters; trial or therapeutic infusion

PREIMPLANTATION ALGORITHM

- Experience indicates that a structured approach to the preimplant phase facilitates the best possible experience for patient and practitioner.
- Each clinic should establish a checklist algorithm to ensure that each patient has experienced a complete preimplantation evaluation.[7]

- Important components of that checklist include:
  - Does the patient meet appropriate patient selection criteria?
  - Has the patient been cleared by a knowledgeable psychologist?
  - Did the patient experience 50% pain reduction during the spinal infusion trial?
  - Did the patient get occupational therapy and physical therapy evaluations during the trial that showed acceptable functional gains?
  - Did nursing accomplish the preoperative teaching?
  - Was the preoperative infection risk assessment completed?

IMPLANTATION ISSUES

- The patient must be physically able to have the pump and catheter implanted.
- In some cases the patient may have had very extensive spinal or abdominal surgery which can increase the level of surgical complexity.
- The patient must be evaluated for the following:
  - Access to the intrathecal or epidural space
  - Access to a site for pump or device implantation
  - Patient positioning issues
  - Preoperative assessment of infection risk

DRUG SELECTION

- Generally morphine is the first drug used. Ideally, the choice of opioid should be based on the trial results.
- Health insurers may have limitations on drugs that are reimbursable.
- The trial opioid selection should be based on history of opioid tolerance, side-effect history, and the pain afferent spinal cord level compared with catheter tip location.
- Lipophilic opioids have limited spread, but a rapid onset of action. The duration of action depends on receptor affinity for the opioid, cord level lipid content, and lipid solubility.[1,7]
- The analgesic effect, onset of action, and relative equianalgesic doses of highly lipophilic drugs are dependent on the amount of spinal cord lipid and the accessibility of that lipid to the cerebrospinal fluid and blood supply.
- If the patient fails an opioid and there is a strong component of neuropathic pain, nonopioid agents may be added. These incude:
  - *Local anesthetics*: Bupivacaine is most commonly used. Limiting side effects may be sensory and motor impairment

- *Baclofen*: This GABA-B receptor agonist is FDA-approved for the treatment of spasticity. Case reports support analgesic effect in neuropathic pain.
- *Clonidine*: This α_2-adrenergic receptor agonist is FDA-approved for epidural delivery in cancer pain.
- *Ziconotide*: This N-type calcium channel blocker is currently in phase III trials.

DRUG COMPOUNDING ISSUES

- A mixing pharmacist with a special interest in pain management is an excellent resource for the pain specialist.
- Drug availability and compounding parameters are critical to fully use the scope of agents that may be required to manage intractable pain.
- Some issues are:
  - Knowledge of the commercially available concentrations of opioids, local anesthetics, clonidine, and baclofen is necessary.
  - A knowledge of how to combine commercially available concentrations of drugs safely is necessary.
  - Compounding of drugs should be done by well-trained personnel who understand the standards of intrathecal drug preparation.
  - Extreme drug concentrations, which may affect the spinal cord or have not been tested in the animal model, should be avoided.[10]
  - Only drugs and concentrations that have support in the clinical literature with published studies should be used.
  - Drug concentrations should allow reasonable time between pump refills.

COMPLICATIONS

- Managing complications begins with an understanding of the troubleshooting algorithms used to test catheter and pump function when faced with a failed infusion or unexpected withdrawal symptoms. A summary of troubleshooting steps is provided here for review.

CATHETER-RELATED COMPLICATIONS

- Aspirate the side port to check intrathecal catheter position.
- Obtain a lumbar spine film to check catheter position.
- Examine the catheter track by fluoroscopy during epidurogram or myelogram to check for catheter kinking or breaks.

- Obtain a pump myelogram or epidurogram.
- When epidural infection is suspected, aspirate the catheter for culture before it is removed.
- Aspirate the side port for culture when intrathecal infection is suspected.[11]

PUMP-RELATED COMPLICATIONS

- Make a computer inquiry of pump programming and battery status.
- Measure pump residual volume and compare with calculated residual volume.
- Do a rotor study to ensure pump motor function.
- Aspirate the pump pocket when infection is suspected.[12]

PORT-RELATED COMPLICATIONS

- Order a port myelogram to ensure continuity.
- Culture for infection.

CONTRAINDICATIONS

- Contraindications to intrathecal or epidural infusion are all relative, except for an allergy to the drugs.
- Infection risk is greatest with a history of frequent septicemia, but all patients are at risk.
- Anticoagulation issues with risk of compressive hematoma formation depend on the state of anticoagulation at the time of the catheter placement or removal.
- The risk of low platelet counts during chemotherapy has been shown not to increase the risk of hematoma formation if the catheter is not moved.[13]

REFERENCES

1. **Carr D, Cousins MJ.** Spinal route of analgesia, opioids and future options. In: Cousins MJ, Bridenbaugh PO, eds. *Neural Blockade*. 3rd ed. Philadelphia: Lippencott–Raven; 1998: 915–984.
2. **Bennet G, Serafini M, Burchiel K, et al.** Clinical guidelines for intraspinal infusion: Report of an expert panel. *J Pain Symptom Manage*. 2000;20:S37–S43.
3. **Becker WJ.** Long-term intrathecal baclofen therapy in patients with intractable spasticity. *Can J Neurol Sci*. 1995:22:208–217.
4. **Du Pen SL.** Implantable spinal catheter and drug delivery system: Complications. *Tech Reg Anesth Pain Manage*. 1998;2:152–160.

5. **Krames ES, Chapple I,** the 8703 W Catheter Study Group. Reliability and clinical utility of an implanted intraspinal catheter used in the treatment of spasticity and pain. *Neuromodulation.* 2000;3:7–14.

6. **Coffey RJ, Burchiel K.** Inflammatory mass lesions associated with intrathecal drug infusion: Catheters: Report and observations on 41 cases. *Neurosurgery.* 2002;50:78–87.

7. **Deer T, Winkelmuller W, Erdine S, Bedder M, Burchiel K.** Intrathecal therapy for cancer and nonmalignant pain: Patient selection and patient management. *Neuromodulation.* 1999;2:55–66.

8. **Doleys DM, Murray JB, Klapow JC, Coleton MI.** Psychological assessment. In: Ashburn MA, Rice LJ, eds. *Management of Pain.* New York: Churchill Livingstone; 1997:27–49.

9. **Gianino J, York M, Paice J.** *Intrathecal Drug Therapy for Spasticity and Pain.* New York: Springer-Verlag;1995.

10. **Naumann C, Erdine S, Koulousakis A, Van Buyten J-P, Schuchard M.** Drug adverse events and system complications of intrathecal opioid delivery for pain: Origins, detection, manifestations, and management. *Neuromodulation.* 1999;2:92–107.

11. **Follett KA, Naumann CP.** A prospective study of catheter-related complications of intrathecal drug delivery systems. *J Pain Symptom Manage.* 2000;19:209–215.

12. **Kulkarni AV, Drake JM, Lamberti-Pasculli M.** Cerebrospinal fluid shunt infection: A prospective study of risk factors. *J Neurosurg.* 2001;94:195–201.

13. **Enneking KF, Benzon HT.** Oral anticoagulants and regional anesthesia: A perspective. *Reg Anesth Pain Med.* 1998;23(suppl).

64 SYMPATHETIC BLOCKADE

Mazin Elias, MD, FRCA, DABA

INTRODUCTION

- The sympathetic nervous system is implicated in numerous pain syndromes.[1,2]
- Interruption of sympathetic flow has been proven to relieve certain pain syndromes.
- To optimize the outcome following sympathetic blockade, an accurate diagnosis of sympathetically maintained pain (SMP) should be made.
- SMP can be diagnosed clinically as any neuropathic pain, that is, burning in nature with allodynia.
- Laboratory tests can also confirm some degree of neuropathic pain component that is probably SMP (triple-phase bone scan).
- There is no gold standard criterion to determine if pain is SMP, although some have suggested a triple or quadruple test.

- The four tests include:
  - Good pain relief following sympathetic blockade that is directly related to the duration of the local anesthetic agent used (preferably a local anesthetic agent should be used versus a placebo)
  - Response to phentolamine infusion that produces system sympathetic blockade
  - Aggravation of the pain following infusion of norepinephrine
  - Relief of the pain with infusion of clonidine or application of a clonidine patch
- The classic targets of sympathetic blockade are[3]:
  - Sphenopalatine ganglia
  - Stellate (cervicothoracic) sympathetic ganglia
  - Celiac/splanchnic plexus (abdominal SMP and visceral pain)
  - Lumbar sympathetic ganglia (lower-extremity SMP and related pain syndromes
  - Superior hypogastric plexus (pelvic pain)
  - Ganglion impar (perianal and rectal pain)
- During sympathetic blockade, it is recommended that intravenous access be maintained should complications occur, and temperature of the extremities should also be monitored to indicate successful sympathetic blockade of an extremity.

SPHENOPALATINE GANGLION BLOCK

ANATOMY

- The sphenopalatine ganglion (SPG) is located in the pterygopalatine fossa (the sphenopalatine fossa), which is located posterior to the middle nasal conchae and anterior to the pterygoid canal.
- It lies close to the maxillary nerve.
- The sympathetic nerve passes through this ganglion to supply the sensory, vasomotor, and secretory fibers to the sphenopalatine, lacrimal, and nasal glands, and also to some of the sympathetic fibers along the cranial blood vessels.

TECHNIQUE

- The simplest technique is to advance two soft, cotton-tip applicators soaked with cocaine or viscous lidocaine through the nares, along the middle turbinate posteriorly.
- A second applicator is then applied superior and posterior to the first one, and both are left in position for 30 minutes.

- Fluoroscopic guidance can be used for both temporary and permanent block of the SPG, that is, neurolytic lesion and radiofrequency ablation (RFA).
- The needle is inserted between the mandibular rami, under fluoroscopy, and under the zygoma, aiming at the sphenopalatine fossa.
- Paresthesia to the maxillary nerve may occur and local anesthetic agent may reduce the pain.
- On AP view, the needle tip should lie just adjacent to the lateral nasal cavity wall. Application of 0.5 to 1 mL of contrast dye or 2 or 10 Hz of electrical stimulation through the radiofrequency needle can confirm the correct position of the needle tip.
- Stimulation should produce a tingling sensation in the nasal area and nasal cavity.
- Following that, 1 mL of local anesthetic agent or neurolytic agent can be applied. Alternatively, RFA can be performed.

COMPLICATIONS

- Mechanical
  - Traumatic injury to the maxillary nerve
  - Intravascular injection
  - Epistaxis
  - Pain at the site of injection
- Pharmacologic
  - Intravascular injection
  - Damage to the maxillary nerve by the neurolytic agent
  - Seizure from the local anesthetic agent

CERVICOTHORACIC/STELLATE GANGLION BLOCK

ANATOMY

- Sympathetic flow to the head and neck and to the upper extremities is derived from the upper five to seven thoracic spinal segments.
- Cell bodies are located in the gray matter of the dorsolateral spinal cord material.
- They exit with the anterior primary rami as white rami communicante.
- The fiber ascends along the anterior lateral surface of the spinal column, to the three cervical sympathetic ganglia (superior, middle, and inferior cervical sympathetic ganglia).
- In 80% of patients the inferior cervical and the first thoracic sympathetic ganglia fuse together to form the stellate ganglia.

- This is why the term *cervicothoracic sympathetic blockade* is more appropriate rather than *sympathetic stellate ganglion block*.
- The stellate ganglia lie in front of the neck of the first rib by the dome of the pleura.
- The cervicothoracic sympathetic ganglion supply the head and neck and most of the upper limb sympathetic flow, with the exception the nerve of Kuntz, which arises from T2 spinal segment and may bypass the cervicothoracic/stellate ganglia and pass to the upper extremity.
- This explains why stellate ganglion or upper cervical thoracic ganglion blockade sometimes may not provide total sympathectomy to the upper extremity.

INDICATIONS

- Head and neck if SMP
- Complex regional pain syndrome types I and II and other SMP syndromes of the upper extremities and anterior chest wall
- Vascular insufficiency/vascular disorders, including Raynaud's disease, and conditions of the upper extremities, head, and neck, including some vascular types of headache (migraine, cluster headaches)

TECHNIQUE

- The two classic techniques use either the C6 or C7 vertebra as a landmark.
- After identification of the level, either under fluoroscopy or by palpation, the C6 transverse process (Chassaignac's process) can be used as a landmark.
- At the junction of the body and the transverse process of either C6 or C7, the periosteum can be contacted using a 27-gauge short, beveled needle.
- The carotid artery can be retracted laterally with the sternomastoid to avoid puncture.
- Once the periosteum is contacted, the needle is withdrawn a few millimeters.
- After negative aspiration for both blood and cerebrospinal fluid, 1 mL of dye can be injected. If there is no intravascular or intrathecal spread, and if there is good spread along the sympathetic ganglia, 0.5 mL of local anesthetic is injected and the operator waits 2 to 3 minutes to exclude any signs of central nervous system toxicity (intravascular injection) or spinal analgesia (intrathecal injection). Then 2–10 mL of local anesthetic is injected.
- Sympathetic blockade of the head and neck can be confirmed by the development of Horner's syndrome.

- Sympathetic blockade of the upper extremity can be confirmed by measuring skin temperature, which should increase by at least 2° to 3°C.
- A modified posterior and anterior approach to the upper thoracic sympathetic ganglion can also be used for SMP of the upper extremities to avoid Horner's syndrome.[2]

COMPLICATIONS

- Mechanical
  - Pain from the injection
  - Hematoma
  - Pneumothorax
  - Pneumomediastinum
  - Injury to the esophagus
  - Brachial plexus
  - Vasovagal attacks
- Pharmacologic
  - Horner's syndrome
  - Spinal analgesia
  - Brachial plexus and phrenic nerve block leading to difficulty in breathing
  - Recurrent laryngeal nerve block leading to hoarseness of voice (this is why bilateral stellate ganglion/cervicothoracic ganglion blockade should not be attempted bilaterally)
  - Seizure because of intravascular injection

CONTRAINDICATIONS

- Contralateral phrenic nerve palsy
- Blood dyscrasia/coagulopathy
- Local sepsis
- Patient refusal

CELIAC/SPLANCHNIC NERVE PLEXUS BLOCK

ANATOMY

- Sympathetic supply to the abdominal viscera arises in the anterior lateral horn of the spinal cord.
- Preganglionic fibers from the spinal segment T5 to T10 give rise to the lesser splanchnic (T11, T12), greater splanchnic (T5 through T10), and least splanchnic (T12) nerves.
- These nerves hug the thoracic vertebrae, and then pass to the celiac plexus.
- The celiac ganglion is a meshlike structure that lies in front of the great abdominal vessel.

- It measures about 1 to 4.5 cm in diameter at the level of the first lumbar vertebra.
- From there, postganglionic fibers supply the abdominal viscera.

TECHNIQUE

- Multiple approaches have been used to block the celiac plexus, including anterior and posterior approaches and open techniques.
- The classic technique described here is the posterior approach.
- The posterior approach can be retrocrural, transcrural, or transaortic, where the needle lies in front of the aorta (celiac ganglion block). The transcrural approach is the celiac plexus block, and the retrocrural approach is the splanchnic nerve block.
- Although all provide effective sympathetic blockade, the splanchnic block is reserved for those patients who have abdominal pathology such as widespread metastasis of tumor, which makes the transaortic approach difficult, or where there is a vascular anomaly, that is, aortic aneurysm, which prohibits the transaortic approach.
- The posterior approach is done with the patient in the prone position.
- Either fluoroscopy or CT scan is used.
- The difference between the retrocrural and transcrural posterior approaches is the final position of the needle tip.
- If the needle is at the level of the T12 vertebra in the lower third of the anterior lateral area, then the posterior approach is transcrural.
- If the needle is at the middle to upper third of the L1 vertebra, the posterior approach is retrocrural.
- The needle is usually inserted at the edge of a triangle formed by the T12 rib, L1 transverse process, and tip of the T12 spinous process.
- The needle is directed so that the final position is in front of either the T12 or the L1 vertebra, depending on whether the approach is transcrural or retrocrural.
- Bilateral needles should be inserted.
- The position is confirmed by both AP and lateral views and by injection of dye.
- Following confirmation of the spread of dye, either local anesthetic agent is injected (8–15 mL on each side) or alcohol or phenol is injected for more permanent blockade.
- Before lytic block, local anesthetic agent should be injected initially to ensure that there is no intravascular or intrathecal epidural spread, as confirmed by the development of spinal analgesia; then the alcohol or phenol should be injected.

INDICATIONS

- Acute/chronic pancreatitis and hepatobiliary disorder including biliary sphincteric disorder
- Abdominal visceral pain syndrome including abdominal malignancies
- Abdominal angina

COMPLICATIONS

- Mechanical
  - Injury to the blood, kidney and ureter, lung, and pleura (pneumothorax, hemopneumothorax, pleurisy).
  - Paraplegia because of intravascular/intrathecal injection or because of trauma to the blood supply to the spinal cord (artery of Adamkeiwicz).
- Pharmacologic
  - Hypotension and diarrhea because of sympathetic blockade.
  - Intravascular injection (seizure).
  - Alcohol neurolytic block can cause alcohol withdrawal in those taking disulfiram for alcohol abuse therapy.
- Phenol should be avoided in patients who have vascular prosthesis, as it can attack the prosthesis.
- Intravenous access should be maintained and preload of fluid is also advisable to reduce the severity of hypotension.

LUMBAR SYMPATHETIC BLOCK

ANATOMY

- Preganglionic flow to the lower extremities arises from the dorsolateral part of the spinal cord (lower thoracic and upper two lumbar segments).
- They synapse into the lumbar sympathetic ganglion, which is located in the anterior lateral surface of the L2 to L4 vertebrae, anterior to the psoas muscle.
- There is some individual variation in the position.[4]
- Most postganglionic sympathetic fibers accompany nerve roots to the lower extremity.

TECHNIQUE

- In the lateral approach, with the patient in the prone position, the operator, under fluoroscopy and avoiding the transverse process of L2 or L4, inserts a 5-in spinal needle so that the final position of the tip of the needle is in front of and just lateral to the L2 vertebra (in the midfacetal line) or at the superior third of the L3 vertebra where, in most individuals, the sympathetic ganglion is located.[4]
- Injection of dye should confirm spread in front of and lateral to the vertebral body, on both AP and lateral views.
- To confirm sympathetic blockade, again, the temperature of the lower extremity should increase by at least 3°C, with 3 to 5 mL of local anesthetic agent.
- A small amount of local anesthetic agent is preferable to avoid spread to the somatic nerve, thus confusing the outcome of the block (somatic vs SMP).

INDICATIONS

- Complex regional pain syndrome types I and II (SMP)
- Vascular insufficiency/disorder of the lower extremity
- Neuropathic pain, that is, postherpetic neuralgia

COMPLICATIONS

- Mechanical
  - Infection
  - Trauma to the lumbar nerve and disc
  - Intravascular, intrathecal, and epidural injection
  - Kidney trauma (hematuria)
- Pharmacologic
  - Intravascular or intrathecal injection of local anesthetic agent or neurolytic agent
  - Hypotension
  - Paraplegia
  - In the case of neurolytic block, genitofemoral neuralgia
- Lumbar sympatholysis can be performed either by thermal lesion (RFA), lytic (phenol or alcohol) injection, or a combination of both to use less neurolytic solution and avoid spill on somatic nerves.[4]

SUPERIOR HYPOGASTRIC PLEXUS BLOCK

ANATOMY

- The plexus is located retroperitoneally in the lower third of the fifth lumbar vertebral body and the upper third of the sacrum in close proximity to the bifurcation of the common iliac vessel.
- It is supplied by the lumbar aortic and celiac sympathetic plexus.

- There are also some parasympathetic fibers from the ventral root of S2 to S4.
- The superior hypogastric plexus supplies the genital organs and the sigmoid colon and rectum.
- It also communicates with the inferior hypogastric plexus, which is located parallel to the pelvic floor. It is not feasible to block the inferior hypogastric plexus.

INDICATIONS

- Treatment of pelvic pain including malignancy, endometriosis, and pelvic inflammatory diseases/adhesions

TECHNIQUE

- With the patient in the prone position, on a pillow to flatten the lumbar lordosis, the x-ray beam is turned to 45° posterolateral view at the level of the L5 vertebra.
- Then, the cephalocaudal view is used to avoid the iliac crest, in such way that the view of the anterior lateral part of the L5 vertebra can be identified.
- With the gun barrel technique, a needle is inserted in such way that the tip lies in front of the vertebral body of L5. Sometimes, bending the needle tip by 50° can be used to bypass the transverse process of L4 or L5, if it is encountered.
- The position is confirmed by AP and lateral views and by injection of dye.
- Then, 3–10 mL of local anesthetic or neurolytic solution is injected on each side.

GANGLION IMPAR (GANGLION OF WALTHER) BLOCK

ANATOMY

- This solitary retroperitoneal structure is located at the level of the sacrococcygeal junction and marks the termination of the paravertebral sympathetic chain.

INDICATIONS

- Perianal pain that is sympathetically maintained
- Visceral pain

TECHNIQUE

- Two techniques have been described.
- The easiest is the transsacrococcygeal ligament technique, in which a needle is inserted through the

ligament until it lies just a few millimeters in front of the curvature of the sacrum.
- This is confirmed by the injection of dye (should resemble an apostrophe), followed by the injection of 2 to 4 mL of local anesthetic agent or neurolytic agent.
- An alternative technique is to insert a needle between the coccygeal and anal regions, through the anococcygeal ligament, and then direct the curvature toward the coccyx until the needle lies anterior to the surface of the bone.

COMPLICATIONS

- Caudal/epidural
- Injury to the rectum or periosteum
- Infection

POSTSYMPATHECTOMY SYNDROME

- Following sympathetic blockade, especially following neurolytic agent (although possible after RFA or surgical sympathectomy), the original pain may recur.
- A new neurologic deficit and new pain syndrome may also occur.
- This can be explained by reorganization and resprouting of the sympathic nerves with plasticity of the central and the peripheral nervous system.
- An alternative explanation is that during injection of lytic agent, some of the nearby somatic nerves are injured, producing a new neuropathic syndrome.
- Postsympathectomy syndrome is more common following sympathectomy for neuropathic pain, rather than following hyperhidrosis, although even sympathectomy for hyperhidrosis can be followed by neuropathic pain and by increasing hyperhidrosis as well.
- The best way to avoid these complications is to use a smaller volume of neurolytic agent or more localized RFA or surgical lesion.[5]

REFERENCES

1. **Waldman W.** *Interventional Pain Management.* Dannimiller Memorial Education Foundation. Philadelphia: WB Saunders; 2000.
2. **Elias M.** The anterior approach for thoracic sympathetic ganglion block using a curved needle. *Pain Clin* 2000; 12:17–24.
3. **Hahn M, McQuollan P, Sheplock GJ.** *Regional Anesthesia: An Atlas of Anatomy and Techniques.* St. Louis: Mosby; 1996.
4. **Rocco A.** Radiofrequency: Lumbar sympathiolysis. *Reg Anesth.* 1995;20:3–12.

5. Raj SN, Campbell JN. Risk–benefit ratio for surgical sympathectomy: Dilemmas in clinical decision-making. *J Pain.* 2000;1:261–264.

65 TRANSCUTANEOUS ELECTRICAL NERVE STIMULATION

Gordon Irving, MD

WHAT IS IT?

- Transcutaneous electrical nerve stimulation (TENS) is current is applied through electrodes placed on the skin that activates large-diameter sensory fibers.
- There are two main stimulation patterns: a low-frequency (also called acupuncture-like) 1- to 4-Hz, high-intensity, long-pulse-width signal that causes visible muscle contractions, and a high-frequency 50- to 120-Hz, low-intensity signal that causes a tingling or buzzing sensation.
- A small, portable device with two or four leads is used to produce the low-voltage electrical current.
- An estimated 250,000 units are prescribed annually in the United States.

HOW DOES IT WORK?

- TENS works by changing the body's perception of pain.
- The high-frequency, low-intensity mode is thought to work by "closing the gate."
- The gate theory states that when large Aβ fibers are stimulated, Aδ and C fiber nociceptive input is inhibited at the interneuron level of the substantia gelatinosa of the dorsal horn.
- The low-frequency, high-intensity mode works by recruiting both large- and small-diameter fibers and depends on supraspinal descending inhibitor mechanisms for its actions.

DOES IT WORK?

- Despite more than 600 published articles the methodology of most studies is poor and recent meta-analyses have recommended that better studies are urgently needed.
- Specific pain states for which there has not been shown to be evidence-based benefit include:
  - Labor pain[1]

- Chronic low back pain (Although there was a trend to greater pain reduction, better functional status, and better patient satisfaction with active TENS versus placebo, it was not statistically significant.)[2]
- TENS was shown to be of benefit in:
  - Primary dysmenorrhea, where high-frequency but not low-frequency TENS worked[3]
  - Osteoarthritis pain of the knee, where both high-frequency TENS and low-frequency TENS were found to be significantly better than placebo[4]
- Indeterminate studies in which the efficacy of TENS could neither be refuted nor confirmed included chronic pain of more than 3 months' duration, excluding angina, headache, migraine, and dysmenorrhea.[5]
- There are many studies suggesting long-term efficacy of TENS although these are not placebo-controlled.
- A positive effect on almost 8000 patients over periods from 6 months to 4 years has been reported.
- Measures included improved sleep and socialization, decreased pain, as well as decreased medication and utilization, of physical and/or occupational therapy.[6]

HOW IS IT USED?

TRIALING

- Place the electrodes with the pads placed around the painful area.
- With the TENS connected and turned on, a sensation should be felt covering the painful area.
- Use the electrical stimulus pattern that by trial and error was found to be the most successful in decreasing pain. This is usually the high-frequency, low-intensity mode.
- With this mode the intensity is increased until a buzzing or tingling is felt.
- The intensity is then reduced until it is barely felt.
- Continue this for 20–30 minutes.
- If the pain is lessened, 30 minutes or more of stimulation can be given.
- If there is no decrease in pain, move the pads to cover nearby trigger points or acupuncture points and retry the stimulation for an additional 20–30 minutes.
- If pain is felt along a nerve distribution, try placing the electrodes on the skin directly over the nerve.

LONG-TERM USE

- There are minimal side effects from the skin pads or use of the current.
- Tolerance may occur in the first few months with loss of efficacy.[7]

HOW MUCH DOES IT COST?

- The medical insurance company usually covers the leasing and subsequent costs.
- Purchase costs are $350 to 400, with ongoing costs for renewing the pads and electrode wires.

REFERENCES

1. **Carroll D, Tramer M, McQuay HJ, Bye B, Moore A.** Transcutaneous electrical nerve stimulation in labour pain: A systematic review. *Br J Obst Gynaecol.* 1997;104: 169–175.
2. **Brosseau L, Milne S, Robinson V, et al.** Efficacy of the transcutaneaous electrical nerve stimulator for the treatment of chronic low back pain: A meta-analysis. *Spine.* 2002;27: 596–603.
3. **Proctor ML, Smith CA, Farquhar CM, Stones RW.** *Cochrane Database Syst Rev.* 2002;CD002123.
4. **Osiri M, Welch V, Brosseau L.** Transcutaneous electrical nerve stimulation for knee osteoarthritis. *Cochrane Database Syst Rev.* 2000;CD002823.
5. **Carroll D, Moore RA, McQuay HJ, Fairman F, Tramer M, Leijon G.** Transcutaneous electrical nerve stimulation for chronic pain. *Cochrane Database Syst Rev.* 2001;CD003222.
6. **Chabal C, Fishbain DA, Weaver M, Heine L, Wipperman L.** Long-term transcutaneaous electrical nerve stimulation use: Impact on medication utilization and physical therapy costs. *Clin J Pain.* 1998;14:66–73.
7. **Fishbain DA, Chabal C, Abbott A.** Transcutaneaous electrical nerve stimulation treatment outcome in long term users. *Clin J Pain.* 1996;12:201–214.

66 DISCOGRAPHY/INTRADISCAL ELECTROTHERMAL ANNULOPLASTY

Richard Derby, MD
Sang-Heon Lee, MD, PhD

DISCOGRAPHY

CONCEPTS

- Discography is a diagnostic procedure for evaluating discogenic pain segments of the spine via injection of radiopaque contrast medium into the intervertebral disc nucleus.
- Conceptually, this method is an extension of clinical examination, tantamount to palpating for tenderness.[1]
- The cardinal component is reproduction of symptomatic pain via contrast medium injection.
- Patient cooperation is crucial for recognizing and reporting accustomed pain and pain reproduction.
- Discs with an intact normal anulus fibrosus usually do not hurt and have a firm injection endpoint, whereas abnormal discs are severely painful.[2]
- Normal psychometrics without chronic pain afford a low rate of false positives.

TERMS

- Provocative discography is the test for identifying the reproduction of concordant pain on intradiscal injection.
- Analgesic discography is the relief of disc pain via use of intradiscal local anesthetic.
- CT discography demonstrates the internal disc morphology by scanning.

DISCOGENIC PAIN

- In chronic low back pain, internal disc disruption (IDD) is 39%.[1]
- IDD is characterized by a the following:
  - A condition in which a disc may become painful as a result of disruption of internal architecture.
  - No external features: the contour of the disc remains normal.
  - The disc appears normal on CT and myelography, but nonetheless is painful.
  - Only provocative discography establishes the diagnosis.
- Excessive compression force may result in a fracture of the vertebral end plate.
- Disc degradation may occur, gradually extending to involve the entire nucleus.
- Disc degradation may spread radially into the anulus fibrosus, causing a fissure.
- Nerve endings are limited to the outer third of the anulus fibrosus.
- Nerves in discs contain peptides such as calcitonin gene-related peptide (CGRP), vasoactive intestinal peptide, and substance P, which are characteristic of nociceptive nerve fibers.[3]
- Inflammatory chemicals can sensitize nerve endings in the anulus fibrosus, rendering them activated at lower than normal mechanical thresholds.
- If remaining fibers of anulus fibrosus are breached, nuclear herniation may follow IDD.
- If a radial fissure completely erodes the annulus, the stage may be set for disc prolapse.

INDICATIONS

- Confirm diagnosis of discogenic pain when considering invasive intradiscal treatment options.
- Confirm diagnosis of discogenic pain for medicolegal purposes.
- Analysis of disc morphology.
- Identification of normal discs.

CONTRAINDICATIONS

ABSOLUTE
- The patient is unable or unwilling to consent to the procedure.
- Inability to assess patient reponse to the procedure.
- Untreated systemic or localized infections.
- Spinal cord compression causing myelopathy.
- Pregnancy.

RELATIVE
- Allergy to contrast medium, local anesthetic, or anitibiotics.
- Known bleeding diathesis.

EVALUATION

- The patient must be asked if he or she perceives pain during dye infiltration and if that pain is similar to, identical to, or different from the accustomed pain.
- A convincing, positive response occurs when the patient reports exact or similar reproduction of pain on stimulation of a given disc.
- Without an asymptomatic control disc, there is no evidence that the patient can discriminate between a symptomatic and an asymptomatic disc.
- New positive criteria for discography: reproducible VAS pain $\geq 6/10$ with <50 psi intradiscal pressure above opening and <3.5 mL total volume.
- Four categories of discs described by Derby et al[4] using pressure-controlled manometric discography are:
  - Chemical discs affording pain at minimal pressure of 15 psi
  - Mechanical discs characterized by pain provocation occurring at 15 and 50 psi when the patient is lying and standing, respectively
  - Intermediate discs, with pain occurring at 51–90 psi
  - Normal discs without pain.[4]
- The Dallas discogram scale[5] is used for annular disruption grading as follows:
  - Grade 0, where disruption, if any, is confined to the nucleus pulposus

- Grade 1, with disruption extending into the inner third of the anulus fibrosus
- Grade 2, with disruption extending as far as the inner two-thirds of the annulus
- Grade 3, where disruption extends into the outer third of the anulus fibrosus and may spread circumferentially between laminae of collagen

LUMBAR DISCOGRAPHY

- Lumbar discography is usually approached posterolaterally, although lateral (extrapedicular), posterior, and midline approaches may be employed (Figure 66–1).
- For the lumbosacral level, disc puncture is challenging and requires a double-needle technique, using both guide procedure needles.
- Once the tip of needle has been properly placed in the center of the nucleus pulposus, contrast medium is slowly injected.
- A normal disc accepts a limited volume of fluid, ranging from 1.5 to 2.5 mL.
- A variety of patterns occur in abnormal discs, whereas the normal nucleus assumes a globular or bilobed ("hamburger") pattern. However, none of these patterns are indicative of discogenic pain.
- Positive diagnosis can be ascertained only by the patient's subjective response to disc injection.
- Precise, pressure-controlled manometric discography may predict outcomes from treatment, surgical or otherwise, thereby greatly facilitating therapeutic decision making.[4]

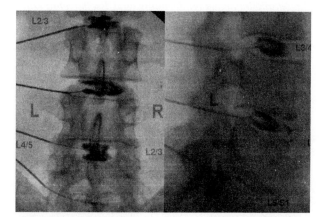

FIGURE 66–1 Posteroanterior and lateral views of a discogram of L3–4, L4–5, and L5–S1 discs. The L3–4 and 4–5 level discs manifest a normal nucleus with bilobed "hamburger" patterns. The L5–S1 disc shows narrow disc degradation, spreading to involve all of the nucleus pulposus with a relatively intact anulus fibrosus.

- Slow injection of contrast medium (~0.1 cc/s) is crucial to reduce false-positive findings in annular torn discs.

CERVICAL DISCOGRAPHY

- Cervical discs are embryologically and morphologically different from lumbar discs and the pathology of painful cervical discs remains elusive.
- During discography, the patient lies supine on the fluoroscopy table with gentle neck extension. As the esophagus lies to the left in the lower neck, the right-sided approach is used. The needle is advanced into the substance of the disc under direct fluoroscopic visualization. All needle movements should be slow and deliberate. Once the tip of the needle has been correctly placed in the center of the disc, pain response should be recorded at the time of distention and the volume of dye that the disc accepts should be noted. A normal cervical disc offers firm resistance and accepts less than 0.5 mL of solution.

COMPLICATIONS

- Complications may include:
  - Needle misplacement can result in penetration of the viscera and pneumothorax, arterial puncture, and damage of nerve roots.
  - Infection is usually inocculated from surface organisms or midadventure through bowel perforation, and may involve epidural abscess, retropharyngeal abscess, and discitis. The causative organisms of discitis are typically *Staphylococcus aureus, Staphylococcus epidermidis,* and *Escherichia coli.*[6]

PREVENTION OF DISCITIS

- To avoid infection, stringent attention to aseptic technique is critical.
- Prophylaxis with antibiotics before and after the procedure can be used. A sample regimen includes: 2 g cephalosporin IV 5 minutes preprocedure, 3–6 mg/mL cephalosporin included in the contrast medium, and 2 g cephalosporin IV postprocedure.

VALIDITY

- If strict criteria are applied, lumbar discography is very specific in subjects with normal psychometric profiles without chronic pain.[7]

- Cervical discography also accurately distinguishes painful, symptomatic, and anatomically deranged discs from asymptomatic discs.[8]

SCREENING

- MRI is a useful screening test prior to discography for revealing the nature of disc structure; however, CT does not reveal the internal architecture of the disc.
- Neither CT nor MRI establishes if the disc is painful.

UTILITY

- Pressure-controlled discography as a diagnostic test may identify patients who may benefit from surgical fusion. In the case of lumbar discography, the likelihood of success with anterior, lumbar, and interbody fusion for the treatment of internal disc disruption is higher in patients who exhibit a painful disc on provocation test.[9] Cervical discography can help the spine surgeon determine which disc requires cervical fusion.[10]

INTRADISCAL ELECTROTHERMAL ANNULOPLASTY

CONCEPTS

- Intradiscal electrothermal annuloplasty (IDET) is a minimally invasive procedure for the management of chronic low back pain of discogenic origin.[11] Potential candidates include patients failing conservative treatment regimens and those who may otherwise be candidates for spinal fusion.[11]
- Chemical and mechanical irritation to nociceptive nerves in the peripheral parts of the anulus fibrosus generates discogenic pain.[12] These nerve endings contain nociceptive neurotransmitters, substance P, calcitonin, and vasoactive intestinal peptide.[13] Thermal destruction of sensitized fibers may provide discogenic pain relief.

THEORY

- The proposed mechanisms of pain relief after IDET include[14]:
  - Thermal nociceptive fiber destruction.
  - Collagen modification with alteration of the biomechanics of the functional spinal segment.
  - Biochemical modification of the inflammatory process.

○ Cauterization of vascular ingrowth, or induction of healing of annular tears.
- Targeted thermal therapy can induce collagen fibril shrinkage at temperatures greater than 60°C and destruction of neural tissue at temperatures above 42 to 45°C.[15]
- The typical IDET procedure can generate only sufficient heat to produce nerve ablation. Collagen modification may not be a primary effect.[16]
- Current protocols might not cause either fissure closure or improved disc stability.
- The histologic findings are denaturation, shrinkage, and coalescence of annular collagen and stromal disorganization after IDET.[14]

PROCEDURE

- IDET uses a fluoroscopically guided intradiscal catheter placement technique to heat the intervertebral disc.[11] The flexible catheter traverses the inner annulus as a circular configuration.
- Proper catheter position is one of the key elements to obtaining a good result.
- The heating coil in the distal 5 cm of the catheter is heated to 90°C for 16 to 17 minutes.

INCLUSION CRITERIA

- Unremitting, low back pain of at least 6 months' duration
- No improvement with aggressive nonoperative care
- Negative straight leg raising (SLR) test; MRI without neural compressive lesion
- Discogram that reproduces concordant pain
- A < 30% decrease in disc height
- Absence of instability and stenosis[17]

EXCLUSION CRITERIA

- Inflammatory arthritis
- Nonspinal conditions that could mimic lumbar pain
- Medical or metabolic disorder that would preclude appropriate follow-up and participation
- Prior surgery at the symptomatic level(s)[17]

THERMAL CATHETER PROTOCOL

- With the patient under local anesthesia, a 17-gauge thin-wall needle is inserted under fluoroscopic guidance into the center of the disc. Catheter position is crucial (Figure 66–2).

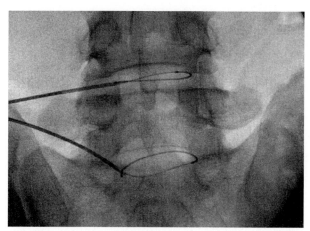

FIGURE 66–2 Fluoroscopy image of IDET procedure. The eletrothermal wires are placed within the L4–5 and L5–S1 discs.

- The coil in the distal 5 cm of the catheter is heated to 90°C for 16 to 17 minutes.
- About 40% of the time, bilateral deployment is required to cover the entire posterior annular wall.
- The patient must be alert enough to be observed for the development of radicular pain during the procedure.
- Most patients experience their typical back pain and referred leg pain during the procedure.
- After heating, intradiscal antibiotic injection (2–20 mg cefazolin) is recommended for prophylaxis against disc infection.[17]

POSTPROCEDURE CARE

- In the first month the patient may walk and perform low-intensity leg stretches, exercising the hamstrings and calf muscles.
- In the second month, low-intensity stabilization floor exercises may be gradually introduced.
- In the third month, the intensity of exercises may increase.
- In the fifth or sixth month, athletic activities such as skiing, running, and tennis may resume.
- Physical therapy typically less than 6 weeks in duration occurs during the second and third months.[17]

OUTCOMES

- An approximately 60% success rate is reported in selected patients.[18]
- Statistically significant improvements are observed in the pain Visual Analog Scale (VAS) and the 36-item Short-Form Health Survey (SF-36), particularly in physical function, bodily pain, and sitting tolerance scores.[19]

- Recently, using stringent criteria, about 50% of patients were significantly better, 40% the same, and ≤10% (6%) worsened.[20]
- Best outcomes are associated with excellent or good catheter position and low pressure-sensitive discs.[17]

COMPLICATIONS

- IDET is minimally invasive and the risk of major complications is low.
- Possible complications include:
  - Catheter breakage (0.05%)
  - Nerve root injury
  - Osteonecrosis of the vertebral body
  - Cauda equina syndrome

REFERENCES

1. **Schwarzer AC, Aprill CN, Derby R, et al.** The prevalence and clinical features of internal disc disruption in patients with chronic low back pain (see comments). *Spine.* 1995; 20:1878–1883.
2. **Carragee EJ, Tanner CM, Khurana S, et al.** The rates of false-positive lumbar discography in select patients without low back symptoms. *Spine.* 2000;25:1373–1380; discussion, 81.
3. **Weinstein J, Claverie W, Gibson S.** The pain of discography. *Spine.* 1988;13:1344–1348.
4. **Derby R, Howard MW, Grant JM, et al.** The ability of pressure-controlled discography to predict surgical and nonsurgical outcomes. *Spine.* 1999;24:364–371; discussion, 71–72.
5. **Sachs BL, Vanharanta H, Spivey MA, et al.** Dallas discogram description: A new classification of CT/discography in low-back disorders. *Spine.* 1987;12:287–294.
6. **Guyer RD, Collier R, Stith WJ, et al.** Discitis after discography. *Spine.* 1988;13:1352–1354.
7. **Walsh TR, Weinstein JN, Spratt KF, et al.** Lumbar discography in normal subjects: A controlled, prospective study. *J Bone Joint Surg Am.* 1990;72:1081–1088.
8. **Schellhas KP, Garvey TA, Johnson BA, et al.** Cervical diskography: Analysis of provoked responses at C2–C3, C3–C4, and C4–C5. *AJNR Am J Neuroradiol.* 2000; 21:269–275.
9. **Gill K, Blumenthal SL.** Functional results after anterior lumbar fusion at L5–S1 in patients with normal and abnormal MRI scans. *Spine.* 1992;17:940–942.
10. **Kikuchi S, Macnab I, Moreau P.** Localisation of the level of symptomatic cervical disc degeneration. *J Bone Joint Surg Br.* 1981;63:272–277.
11. **Djurasovic M, Glassman SD, Dimar JR 2nd, et al.** Vertebral osteonecrosis associated with the use of intradiscal electrothermal therapy: A case report. *Spine.* 2002;27: E325–E328.
12. **Konttinen YT, Gronblad M, Antti-Poika I, et al.** Neuroimmunohistochemical analysis of peridiscal nociceptive neural elements. *Spine.* 1990;15:383–386.
13. **Freemont AJ, Peacock TE, Goupille P, et al.** Nerve ingrowth into diseased intervertebral disc in chronic back pain. *Lancet.* 1997;350:178–181.
14. **Shah RV, Lutz GE, Lee J, et al.** Intradiskal electrothermal therapy: A preliminary histologic study. *Arch Phys Med Rehabil.* 2001;82:1230–1237.
15. **Troussier B, Lebas JF, Chirossel JP, et al.** Percutaneous intradiscal radio frequency thermocoagulation: A cadaveric study (see comments). *Spine.* 1995;20:1713–1718.
16. **Kleinstueck FS, Diederich CJ, Nau WH, et al.** Acute biomechanical and histological effects of intradiscal electrothermal therapy on human lumbar discs. *Spine.* 2001;26: 2198–2207.
17. **Derby R EB, Chen Y, O'Neill C, Ryan D.** Intradiscal electrothermal annuloplasty: A novel approach for treating chronic discogenic back pain. *Neuromodulation.* 2000; 3:82–88.
18. **Karasek M, Bogduk N.** Twelve-month follow-up of a controlled trial of intradiscal thermal anuloplasty for back pain due to internal disc disruption. *Spine.* 2000;25:2601–2607.
19. **Saal JA, Saal JS.** Intradiscal electrothermal treatment for chronic discogenic low back pain: Prospective outcome study with a minimum 2-year follow-up. *Spine.* 2002; 27:966–973; discussion, 73–74.
20. **Pauza K, Howell S, Dreyfuss P, et al.** A randomized, double-blind, placebo controlled trial evaluating the efficacy of intradiscal electrothermal anuloplasty for the treatment of chronic discogenic low back pain: 6-month outcomes. Paper presented at: International Spinal Injection Society, 10th annual scientific meeting; September 7, 2002; Austin, Tex; pp. 84–85.

67   NUCLEOPLASTY

Philip S. Kim, MD

INTRODUCTION

- Nucleoplasty is a novel technique of achieving percutaneous disc decompression that is gaining popularity among interventional pain physicians.
- Low back pain is one of the most common reasons patients visit a physician's office or emergency room or take time off from work.[1–4]
- Treating patients who have low back pain means addressing associated physiologic, psychological, and social issues. Successful medical and surgical interventions cannot restore function and relieve pain without the integration of specific therapeutic exercise

programs, education, and vocational rehabilitation. Thus, a multidisciplinary approach is needed to optimize therapeutic relief, allow patients to return to their preinjury state, and prevent further injury.

PHYSIOLOGIC ETIOLOGY OF LOW BACK PAIN

- The physiologic etiology of low back pain involves the vertebrae (posterior elements), muscles (quadratus lumborum, psoas), thoracolumbar fascia, dura mater, ligaments (interspinous, iliolumbar), sacroiliac joint, zygapophyseal joint, and discs.[5]
- The concept that lumbar intervertebral discs might be the source of pain was recognized in 1947 when a nerve supply was identified.[5] Unfortunately, multiple pain generators can present with similar clinical presentations, making it difficult to identify the true pain generator(s).
- A diagnostic dilemma occurs when an MRI or CT scan reveals degenerative discs (contained disc herniations, internal disruption, and bulging discs) because patients can have bulging discs without pain.[6]
- Combining clinical presentation with diagnostic imaging, one tries to devise an appropriate therapeutic medical and/or surgical intervention.
- A contained disc, bulging disc, or degenerative disc with persistent back/leg pain can call for a variety of interventions.
- Barring significant and progressive neurologic deficit and pain, it is appropriate to prescribe rest and physical therapy for a few weeks, and most patients recover within 1–3 months.[1,3]
- If pain persists and diagnostic images reveal disc disease with contained herniations and/or internal disc disruption, it is appropriate to consider surgical and minimally invasive interventions.

HISTORY OF PERCUTANEOUS DISC DECOMPRESSION

- During the past 20 years, clinicians have performed more than 500,000 percutaneous disc decompressions using various techniques.[7]

CHEMONUCLEOLYSIS

- By far the most widely used and studied is percutaneous disc decompression via chemonucleolysis,[7] which Lyman W. Smith introduced in 1963.[8]

- This procedure involves injection of chymopapain, a proteolytic enzyme derived from the papaya fruit, which cleaves proteogylcans into substituant mucoproteins and glycosaminoglycans.
- More than 400,000 chymopapain disc injections have been performed,[8] and the reported average success rate is 80%.[9–13]
- Unfortunately, inherent problems have reduced interest in this procedure in the United States. For example, a clinician cannot predict the amount of nucleus that chymopapain will digest, and overdigestion can lead to overdecompression, disc collapse, and instability. Chymopapain also fails to discriminate among the proteins it digests, and neural damage can result if the chymopapain contacts neural tissue.
- The rare, yet serious, complications associated with this procedure include episodes of transverse myelitis and paraplegia (in the first year, 55 were reported out of 100,000 procedures).[12] In addition, an estimated 0.5% of patients have an anaphylactic reaction to this enzyme.

AUTOMATED PERCUTANEOUS LUMBAR DISCECTOMY

- Automated percutaneous lumbar discectomy (APLD), which uses a fenestrated punch to manually decompress the nucleus pulposus, was first described by Hijikata.[14]
- More than 100,000 patients have undergone APLD, with pain relief obtained in 70–80%.[12,16–18]
- The primary effect of APLD is thought to be intradiscal pressure reduction.[15,19]
- APLD demonstrates that central disc decompression can, in turn, decompress a peripheral herniation.
- The popularity of this procedure has waned due to the cost and cumbersome nature of the equipment. Further studies are pending to validate the efficacy of APLD.

PERCUTANEOUS LASER DISCECTOMY

- Percutaneous laser discectomy, introduced by Choy in 1991, involves use of a YAG laser to vaporize the nucleus pulposus.[20,21]
- As with APLD, percutaneous laser discectomy centrally decompresses the disc to reduce a peripheral herniation.
- The overall success rate of percutaneous laser discectomy has been reported as more than 75%.[20,21]
- Studies using pressure transducers placed in the disc have reported a rapid drop in intradiscal pressure, which may be the reason for the relief of symptoms in many patients.[22]

- Concerns about the possible heat transfer throughout the disc and the adjacent bony endplate and nerve root (high temperatures have caused significant postoperative pain and spasm) plus the need for bulky, expensive equipment and specialized safety precautions have reduced the popularity of percutaneous laser discectomy.

INTRADISCAL ELECTROTHERMAL ANNULOPLASTY

- Intradiscal electrothermal annuloplasty (IDET) was developed in the 1990s by the Saul brothers.[23]
- IDET is performed by steering a curved resistive heating element around the posterolateral annulus under fluoroscopic guidance.
- By heating the posterolateral annulus to 70°C, annuloplasty attempts to denature collagen fibers and cause contraction of the annulus to seal annular tears.[23] By heating the posterolateral annulus above 45°C, annuloplasty also denervates posterior type C nerve fibers.[23]
- Several reasons exist for skepticism regarding IDET:
  - In vivo studies found that the temperature around the annulus during annuloplasty may not reach the 70°C thought to be necessary to shrink collagen and seal annular tears.[24]
  - Additionally, the sporadic annular temperature of 45°C noted in these studies is insufficient to destroy annular nerve endings.[24]

- A major drawback of annuloplasty is the technical difficulty and time involved in threading a curved 30-cm wire around the annulus.
- The amount of perioperative pain and back spasm are other drawbacks with IDET.
- Finally, there are also the concerns about the long-term outcomes and efficacy of IDET.

WHAT IS NUCLEOPLASTY?

- Nucleoplasty is a new, minimally invasive procedure that uses radiofrequency energy to ablate nucleus pulposus tissue in a controlled approach leading to a reduction of pressure on the nerve roots.

EQUIPMENT AND TECHNIQUE

- To perform nucleoplasty, a patented co-ablation technology is applied through a Perc-D wand, a l-mm-diameter bipolar instrument designed for ablation and coagulation of the nucleus using both energy and thermal technology (Figure 67–1).
- The wand is connected to the standard ArthroCare power generator available in most operating rooms.
- Using a posterior lateral approach, the disc is accessed with a 17-gauge Crawford needle.
- Through the wand, the clinician alternates power and voltage for two modes of action: ablation at 125 V and coagulation at 65 V.
- Following confirmed needle placement, the ablation mode is used while the wand is advanced to create a channel in the nucleus pulposus.

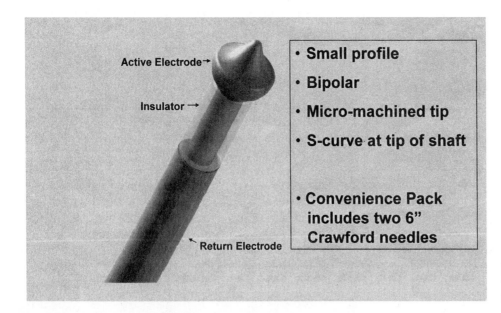

Active Electrode →
Insulator →
Return Electrode →

- **Small profile**
- **Bipolar**
- **Micro-machined tip**
- **S-curve at tip of shaft**
- **Convenience Pack includes two 6" Crawford needles**

FIGURE 67–1 Perc-D spine wand. Reprinted by permission from ArthroCare.

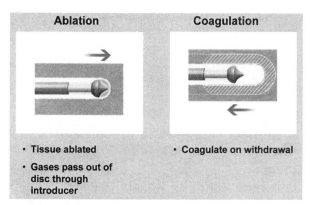

FIGURE 67–2 Nucleoplasty channeling. Reprinted by permission from ArthroCare.

- Ablation is a non-heat-driven process through which radiofrequency energy is applied to a conductive medium (saline) to generate a highly focused plasma field around the electrode at the tip of the Perc-D wand.[25]
- This plasma field contains sufficient energy to cleave molecular bonds at low temperatures (40–70°C) into various elementary molecules and low-molecular-weight gases, for example, oxygen, nitrogen, hydrogen, and carbon dioxide gases that escape through the introducer needle.
- The tip of the Perc-D wand has a small "C" curve that permits the clinician to create a series of six channels within the disc in various directions, removing a portion of the nucleus pulposus.
- The adjacent proteoglycans and collagen are denatured using bipolar radiofrequency energy in the coagulation mode during each withdrawal of the wand. This thermally seals the channels (Figure 67–2) and further decompresses the intervertebral disc.
- In all, approximately 1 cc of nuclear tissue or 10% of the nucleus pulposus is removed.
- The temperature measured from the tip of the Perc-D wand drops off steeply, which prevents inadvertent heating of the annulus (Figure 67–3). This, in turn, results in minimal or no intraoperative pain or spasm.

- The process takes approximately 3 minutes per disc, with an overall time of approximately 20 minutes.
- Usually, the procedure is performed under sedation or monitored anesthesia care.

PATIENT SELECTION

- Nucleoplasty is appropriate for patients who have the following characteristics and history[26]:
  ○ A positive MRI for contained disc herniation or disc bulge
  ○ A contained disc herniation, which measures less than 33% of the sagittal diameter of the spinal canal
  ○ Failure of conservative management of more than 6 weeks' duration
  ○ A positive discogram for recreation of concordant pain (pain that is identical in location and perception to that experienced in the patient's daily activities)
- In a study presented at the meeting of the International Society for the Study of Lumbar Spine (ISSLS) in Scotland in 2001, Carragee et al showed that nucleoplasty could complement microdiscectomy.[27] The success rate of microdiscectomy is 98% in patients with disc protrusion to an anterior posterior diameter greater than 9 mm and 24% in patients with disc protrusion to an anterior posterior diameter less than 6 mm. Thus, a patient who is unlikely to do well with microdiscectomy is the best candidate for nucleoplasty.

POSTOPERATIVE RECOVERY AND REHABILITATION

- Postoperatively, the patient goes home with the following instructions:
  ○ Rest for 1–3 days with limited sitting or walking 10–20 minutes at a time.

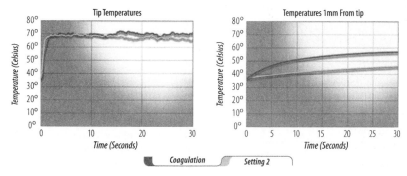

FIGURE 67–3 Temperature measures from tip of Perc-D wand. Reprinted by permission from ArthroCare.

○ Do not drive for the first 1–2 days.
○ Limit lifting to 5–10 pounds for the first 2 weeks.
○ Do not bend or twist the lower back.
○ Do not engage in chiropractic manipulation, massage, inversion traction, or traction for the first 12 weeks.
○ Practice gentle flexion and extension home exercises in 2–3 weeks.
○ Obtain formal physical therapy in 3–5 weeks.
○ After discharge from physical therapy, undertake an individual home exercise program to perform on an indefinite basis.

CONTRAINDICATIONS

• The contraindications for nucleoplasty include:
  ○ Disc space narrowing of more than 50%
  ○ Extruded or sequestered discs
  ○ Disc herniation greater than 33% of the sagittal diameter of the spinal canal
  ○ Obesity
  ○ Spinal stenosis
  ○ Spinal fracture or tumor
  ○ Coagulopathy[26]

BASIC AND CLINICAL STUDIES

BASIC STUDIES

• The basic science studies show that nucleoplasty is a safe, controlled, percutaneous method that achieves decompression of the disc.
• Disc histology postnucleoplasty reveals the volumetric removal of nucleus pulposus.[28]

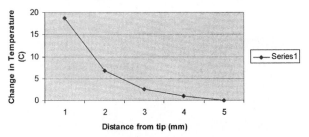

FIGURE 67–4 Nucleoplasty thermal profile in porcine model. Reprinted by permission from Chen et al.[28]

• The nucleoplasty channels show a clear coagulation border without necrosis of the nucleus.[28]
• Nucleoplasty does not disrupt or cause necrosis of the surrounding vital spinal structures of the nucleus, annulus, endplate, spinal cord, or nerve root.
• Photomicrographs show a normal disc endplate near the treated area.[28]
• A thermal mapping study of percutaneous disc decompression in a porcine model confirms the steep temperature drop-off from the tip of the Perc-D wand (Figure 67–4).[29] A similar finding was noted in human cadaver spine segments (Figure 67–5).[30]
• Intradiscal pressure studies in human cadaver spine segments revealed that nucleoplasty results in a significant drop in intradiscal pressure (Figure 67–6).[31]

CLINICAL STUDIES

• Emerging clinical studies show that nucleoplasty may play a role in the treatment of discogenic disease.[7,26,32–36]

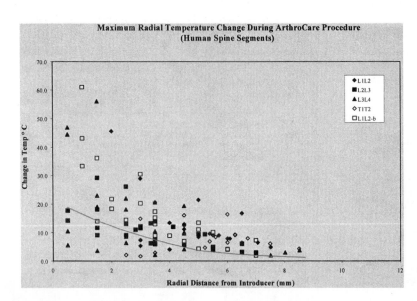

FIGURE 67–5 Nucleoplasty thermal profile in human model. Reprinted by permission from Diederich et al.[30]

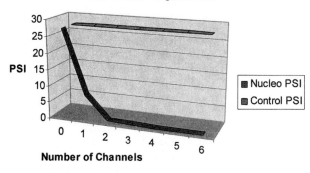

FIGURE 67–6 Nucleoplasty intradiscal pressure study in human cadavers. Reprinted by permission from Chen et al.[31]

• In one study of 45 patients who underwent percutaneous disc decompression using nucleoplasty, 9 had previously undergone fusion, percutaneous discectomies, or laminectomy.[26] The mean age of the patients was 39 years. All 45 patients were followed for 1 month, 33 for 3 months, 23 for 6 months, and 2 for a year. The author reported a 2-point reduction in the visual analog scale pain score, an increase in patient satisfaction, and a reduction in narcotic usage (Figure 67–7), for a success rate of 78%. The success rate was 81% for patients who had not undergone previous back surgery and 67% for those who had.

• In a study of 30 nucleoplasty patients (19 males, 11 females, mean age 37.6 years, age range 22–56 years) who were followed for 6 months,[32] the patients were divided into three groups: axial discogenic low back pain, axial discogenic low back pain with radicular symptoms, and pure radiculopathy without neurologic deficits. The clinicians treated 23 patients at one level, 4 at two levels, and 3 at three levels. Results included a 3.14 reduction in mean pain visual analog scale

score, total resolution of leg pain in 69% of the patients, no narcotic requirement in 86% after 6 months, and satisfaction with results in 89%. No complications were noted.

CONCLUSION

• Nucleoplasty is a safe, effective treatment for a select group of patients with lumbar discogenic pain.
• Additional clinical studies should determine the long-term outcome in patients who undergo nucleoplasty.
• Studies should compare nucleoplasty with conventional nonoperative and operative spine therapies.
• Nucleoplasty is being refined for thoracic and cervical disc disease.
• The US Food and Drug Administration has approved cervical disc decompression using co-ablation.

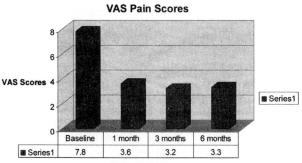

FIGURE 67–7 Results: VAS pain scores of patients undergoing nucleoplasty. Reprinted by permission from Sharps and Issac.[26]

REFERENCES

1. **Leroy N.** *The 50 Most Frequent Diagnosis-Related Groups (DREGS), Diagnoses, and Procedures: Statistics by Hospital Size and Location.* DHHS Publication No. (PHS) 90-3465, Hospital Studies Program Research Note 13. Rockville, Md: Agency for Health Care Policy and Research; 1990.
2. **Von Off M, Working S.** An epidemiological comparison of pain complaints. *Pain.* 1989;32:173.
3. **Nachemson AL.** Newest knowledge of low back pain: A critical look. *Clin Orthop.* 1992;279:8.
4. **Frymoyer J, Cats-Baril W.** An overview of the incidences and costs of low back pain. *Orthop Clin North Am.* 1991; 22:263.
5. **Bogduk N, Twomey L.** *Clinical Anatomy of the Lumbar Spine.* 3rd ed. New York: Churchill Livingstone; 1997.
6. **Wiesel S, Tsourmas N, et al.** A study of computer assisted tomography, I. The incidence of positive CAT scans in an asymptomatic group of patients. *Spine.* 1984;9:549.
7. **Sanders N.** *Percutaneous Disc Decompression: A Historical Perspective.* San Francisco: ArthroCare; 1999.
8. **Smith L.** Enzyme dissolution of nucleus pulposus in humans. *JAMA.* 1964;1:97.
9. **Fraser R.** Chymopapain for the treatment of intervertebral disc herniation: A preliminary report of a double blind study. *Spine.* 1982;7:608.
10. **Javid M.** Safety and efficacy of chymopapain (Chymodiactin) in herniated nucleus pulposus with sciatica: Results of a randomized, double-blind study. *JAMA.* 1983; 249:2489.
11. **Dabezies E, Langford K, Morris J, et al.** Safety and efficacy of chymopapain in the treatment of sciatica due to herniated nucleus pulposus: Results of a randomized double-blind study. *Spine.* 1988;13:561.

12. **Brown D.** Update on chemonucleolysis. *Spine.* 1996;21:625.
13. **Norby EJ, Manucher JJ, et al.** Continuing experiences with chemonucleolysis. *Mt Sinai J Med.* 2000;67:311.
14. **Hijikata S.** Percutaneous nucleotomy. A new concept technique and 12 year's experience. *Clin Orthop.* 1989;238:9–23.
15. **Onik G, Maroon JC, Vidovich DV.** Automated percutaneous discectomy. *Neurosurgery* 1990;26:228–232.
16. **Davis G, Onik G, Helms C.** Automated percutaneous lumbar diskectomy. *Spine.* 1991;16:359–363.
17. **Kaps H, Cotta H.** Early results of automated percutaneous lumbar diskectomy. In: Mayer HM, Brock M, eds. *Percutaneous Lumbar Discectomy.* Berlin/Heidelberg: Springer-Verlag; 1989:153–156.
18. **Hammons W.** Percutaneous lumbar nucleotomy. *West Neurol Soc.* April 1989:635.
19. **Onik G.** Percutaneous lumbar diskectomy using a new aspiration probe. *Am J Neuroradiol.* 1985;6:290.
20. **Choy DS.** Percutaneous laser disc decompression. *J Clin Laser Med Surg.* 1995;13:125.
21. **Choy D.** Percutaneous laser disc decompression. *Spine.* 1992; 17:949.
22. **Sherk HH.** Laser diskectomy. In: *Lasers in Orthopaedic Surgery. Orthopedics.* 1993;16:573–576.
23. **Saul JA, Saul JS.** Management of chronic discogenic low back pain with a thermal intradiscal catheter. *Spine.* 2000;25:382.
24. **Kleinstueck F, Diederich CJ, Nau WH, et al.** Acute biomechanical and histological effects of intradiscal electrothermal therapy on human lumbar discs. *Spine.* 2001;26:2198.
25. **Stadler K, Woloszko J, Brown IG, et al.** Repetitive plasma discharges in saline solutions. *Appl Phys Lett.* 2001;79:4503.
26. **Sharps L, Issac Z.** Percutaneous disc decompression using nucleoplasty. *Pain Physician.* 2002;5:121.
27. **Carragee EJ, Suen P, Han M, et al.** Can MR scanning in patients with sciatica predict failure of open limited discectomy? In: *Proceedings of the International Society for the Study of Lumbar Spine (ISSLS)*; Scotland; June 2001.
28. **Chen Y, Lee S, Chen D.** Histology of disc, endplate and neural elements post coblation of nucleus: An experimental nucleoplasty study. Paper presented at: *North American Spine Society/South American Spine Society Meeting of the Americas*; New York; 2002.
29. **Chen Y, Lee S, Chen D.** Experimental thermomapping study, in percutaneous disc decompression, nucleoplasty. Paper presented at: *North American Spine Society/South American Spine Society Meeting of the Americas*; New York; 2001.
30. **Diederich C, Nau W, Brandt L.** Disc temperature measurements during nucleoplasty and IDET procedures. *Eur Spine J.* 2002;11:418.
31. **Chen Y, Lee S, Chen D.** Intradiscal pressure study of disc decompression with nucleoplasty in human cadavers. Paper presented at: *North American Spine Society/South American Spine Society Meeting of the Americas*; New York; 2002.
32. **Chen Y, Lee S, Lau E.** Percutaneous disc decompression: Nucleoplasty for chronic discogenic back pain with or without sciatica: A preliminary 6-month follow-up study. Paper presented at: *North American Spine Society/South American Spine Society Meeting of the Americas*; New York; 2002.
33. **Chen Y, Lee S, Lau E.** Percutaneous disc decompression: Nucleoplasty for chronic discogenic back pain with or without sciatica: One year clinical follow-up study. Paper presented at: *International Spinal Injection Society*; Austin, TX; 2002.
34. **Slipman C, Sharps L, Isaac Z, et al.** Preliminary outcomes of percutaneous nucleoplasty for treatment of axial low back pain: A comparison of patients with versus without an associated central focal protrusion. *Eur Spine J.* 2002;11:416.
35. **Jones S, Fernau R, Buemi J.** Six month follow-up on lumbar disc nucleoplasty in 45 patients. Paper presented at: *North American Spine Society/South American Spine Society, NASS Meeting of the Americas*; New York; 2002.
36. **Singh V, Pioryani C, Liao L, et al.** Percutaneous disc decompression using coblation (nucleoplasty) in the treatment of chronic discogenic pain. *Pain Physician.* 2002; 5:250.

68 LYSIS OF ADHESIONS

Carlos O. Viesca, MD
Gabor B. Racz, MD
Miles R. Day, MD

INTRODUCTION

- Low back pain, with or without radicular symptoms, is a common medical condition that triggers mild to severe suffering, high health costs, and disability.
- The vast majority of low back pain sufferers recover in a relatively short period and are left without sequelae.[1,2]
- The less fortunate patients, in whom resolution of the condition does not occur despite aggressive therapy, find themselves without a definite (100%) effective treatment.
- Developing an understanding of the pathophysiology underlying the pain and designing target-specific treatment modalities may enhance the occurrence of successful outcomes.
- The past 15–20 years have seen tremendous progress in the understanding of neural pathways and the extent of tissue involvement in back pain. This understanding has triggered the development of new treatment techniques.

HISTORY

- Cathelin performed one of the first documented epidural injections for chronic pain in 1901.[3]
- Sicard and Forstier performed the first epidurography in 1921.[4]
- In 1950, when Payne and Rupp combined hyaluronidase with a local anesthetic in an attempt to alter the rapidity of onset, extent, intensity, and dura-

tion of caudal anesthesia,[5] they demonstrated maximal efficacy in a group receiving local anesthetic, hyaluronidase, and epinephrine. The hyaluronidase used in this study was relatively dilute at 6 U/mL, with an average volume of injection of 25 mL.

- In 1951, Moore added 150 U of hyaluronidase to enhance the spread of the local anesthetic he used in 1309 nerve blocks, including 20 caudal blocks.[6] His work confirmed that hyaluronidase is relatively nontoxic.
- Liévre and co-workers reported the first injection of a corticosteroid into the epidural space for the treatment of sciatica in 1957.[7] They injected a combination of hydrocortisone acetate (dose unknown) and radiopaque dye in 46 patients, with 31 positive results.
- In 1960, Goebert and colleagues reported good results after injecting 30 mL 1% procaine with 125 mg hydrocortisone acetate hydrocortisone into the caudal epidural space.[8]
- That same year, Brown injected 40–100 mL of normal saline followed by 80 mg methylprednisolone in an attempt to mechanically disrupt and prevent reformation of presumably fibrotic lesions in patients with sciatica.[9] He reported complete resolution of pain for 2 months in his four patients. This investigation laid the theoretical foundation for therapies in which specific catheter placement is crucial to the effective treatment of epidural adhesions.
- Administration of cold hypertonic saline intrathecally was first described by Hitchcock in 1967 for the treatment of chronic pain.[10] In 1969, he reported that the hypertonicity rather the temperature of the solution was the determining factor in its therapeutic effect.[11]
- Intrathecal hypertonic saline was subsequently employed by Ventafridda and Spreafico in 1974 for intractable cancer pain.[12] All 21 patients in this study had pain relief at 24 hours, although only 3 reported relief at 30 days.
- Racz and Holubec in 1989 reported the first use of epidural hypertonic saline to facilitate lysis of adhesions.[13]
- Stolker et al introduced hyaluronidase as an alternative agent in 1994.[14]

WHY ADHESIONS?

- Connective tissues, or any kind of tissue, naturally form fibrous layers (scar tissue) after disruption of the intact milieu.
- The tissues surrounding neural structures behave in the same fashion, trapping nerve roots and exposing them to continuous pressures as well as to stretching, which sensitizes the nerves.[15]

- In 1991, Kushlich et al published their observation that sciatica-like pain was generated by pressure on the anulus fibrosus and posterior longitudinal ligament, as well as by swollen, stretched, or compressed nerve roots.[16] All 193 of their patients who had undergone laminectomies under local anesthesia developed perineural fibrous tissue. While this scar tissue was never sensitive, the nerve root was frequently very tender. This led to the conclusion that pain to the nerve roots that are trapped by scar tissue might be associated with fixation of these affected nerve roots and susceptibility to tension and compression.

HOW TO DIAGNOSE THIS CONDITION?

- Radiologic studies, such as MRI and CT scan (including CT myelography), are of limited diagnostic value.
- Epidurography is more effective in diagnosing scar tissue because injected dye forms a filling defect. If this defect correlates with the neurologic abnormality, it helps formulate a diagnosis.[17]

WHAT TO DO?

- These tissue changes can trigger back pain and radicular symptoms, for which treatment might seem difficult. Thus, a great many patients are labeled with a diagnosis of "intractable chronic low back pain syndrome."
- Attempts to treat this pain range from increasing medical treatment by escalating drug dosages and submitting the patient to unsuccessful and frustrating physical therapy trials to conducting interventions, such as epidural steroid injections and selective nerve root blocks, both of which offer only very transient relief.
- If no attempt is made to release the neural structures from fibrous scar tissue, all of these treatment options are likely to be unsuccessful.
- This is why, in 1989, Dr. Gabor B. Racz developed the procedure known as "lysis of adhesions (epidural decompressive neuroplasty)" at Texas Tech University.[18]
- Lysis of adhesions can be performed in the cervical, thoracic, and lumbar epidural regions.

CAUDAL EPIDURAL DECOMPRESSIVE NEUROPLASTY (LYSIS OF ADHESIONS)

- At Texas Tech University, we have treated more than 5000 patients with this modality.

INDICATIONS

- Failed back surgery
- Disc disruption
- Traumatic vertebral body compression fracture
- Metastatic carcinoma of the spine leading to compression fracture
- Multilevel degenerative arthritis
- Facet pain
- Epidural scarring following the resolution of infection or meningitis
- Pain unresponsive to spinal cord stimulation
- Pain unresponsive to spinal opioids
- Pathologic vertebral compression fracture
- Osteoporotic vertebral compression fracture

CONTRAINDICATIONS

- Sepsis
- Coagulopathy
- Local infection at the site of the procedure

TECHNIQUE

- After informed consent is obtained, this elective operative procedure is performed under monitored anesthesia care. General anesthesia should be avoided to decrease the possibility of complications, as communication with the patient is crucial.
- Prophylactic antibiotics are administered intravenously with ceftriaxone sodium (Rocephin) 1 g within 30 minutes of the start of the procedure and continued every 24 hours while the patient is hospitalized. If the patient is allergic to penicillin, we prescribe oral quinolones 1 hour prior to the start of the procedure and both cephalexin (Keflex) 500 mg orally every 12 hours and quinolones orally for 5 days.
- The patient is placed in the prone position with a pillow under the abdominal area and ankles.
- C-arm fluoroscopy is available.
- The lumbosacral region is prepped and draped.
- The sacral hiatus is palpated, and a skin wheal is raised 1 cm lateral and 2 cm caudal to the sacral hiatus on the side opposite the suspected epidural scarring.
- The skin is pierced with an 18-gauge needle, and a 16-gauge RK epidural needle or a 16-gauge RX coudé needle is inserted through the sacral hiatus into the epidural canal.
- Correct needle positioning is confirmed with fluoroscopic views in the anteroposterior as well as the lateral planes. The tip of the needle should not be advanced beyond the S3 foramen.

- If, at this point, cerebral spinal fluid is aspirated or withdrawn from the needle, the needle should be removed and the procedure aborted and rescheduled.
- If venous runoff occurs, the needle should be repositioned, and additional iohexol should be injected for confirmation.
- After any negative aspiration of fluid (cerebral spinal fluid, blood, etc), we inject 10 mL of iohexol (Omnipaque 240 mg/mL).
- In a patient without pathology, the outline of the caudal epidural canal resembles a Christmas tree, with the branches being the nerve roots. In contrast, a patient with fibrosis of any origin will exhibit the filling defects (areas without contrast spread) that indicate adhesions created by scar tissue.
- A Tun-L-XL/24 or a stiffer Tun-L-XL (which will facilitate directional control) epidural catheter is inserted thorough the needle and guided ventrally to the area of the filling defect. (Before insertion, we have bent the catheter about 30° approximately 2.5 cm from the tip to aid with directional control.)
- A lateral view should be obtained to assist in placing the catheter in the ventral epidural space.
- When the position is confirmed, 10 mL of preservative-free normal saline with 1500 units of hyaluronidase is slowly injected.
- The final position of the tip of the catheter is confirmed by injecting 2–5 mL of iohexol, with fluoroscopic observation of the contrast spread into the previously nonvisualized area of the epidural space opened by removal of the scar tissue.[19]
- This is followed by injection of 3 mL of a solution of 9 mL 0.2% ropivacaine and 1 mL of 4 mg/mL dexamethasone. After 5 minutes, if there is no evidence of motor–sensory block, the remaining 7 mL of mixture is injected.
- The epidural needle is then removed under fluoroscopic guidance to ensure that the catheter remains at the site of adhesions, and the catheter is anchored to the skin with a nylon suture. Triple antibiotic ointment is applied at the catheter site, which is covered with a sterile dressing. A microfilter is connected to the end of the catheter hub, and the three pieces are taped together.
- In the postanesthesia care unit, after 20 minutes have passed, 10 mL 10% hypertonic saline is infused for a minimum of 30 minutes after administration of local anesthesia, and the catheter is flushed with 2–3 mL of normal saline and recapped sterile.
- If the patient complains of severe discomfort, the infusion is stopped, and 2–3 mL of 0.2% ropivacaine is administered. After 5 minutes, the infusion is restarted.
- In our institution, the patient is admitted for a 23-hour observation period, the second stage of the procedure

is performed the morning after the insertion prior to patient discharge, and the patient returns as an outpatient on the third day for the third stage.

- While the patient is hospitalized, a physical therapist assists in counseling and educating the patient on "neural flossing exercises" (manipulating the extremity to mobilize the nerve), which most patients are compliant with.
- Follow-up at our clinic is within 2 weeks postprocedure for general assessment and reinforcement to continue the physical therapy exercises.

TRANSFORAMINAL APPROACH

- A transforaminal approach is indicated when the suspected scar tissue cannot be reached through the caudal epidural approach or when severe scar tissue does not allow the caudal epidural catheter to open up the most cephalic areas (lumbar 3, lumbar 4 in most cases) that require this technique.
- When both caudal and transforaminal catheters are placed, the volume of injectate is 7 mL for each of the previously mentioned solutions, through each catheter.

EPIDUROSCOPY

- Epiduroscopy has utility as an adjuvant technique to assist in the specific placement of catheters at the caudal epidural level because it allows for direct visualization of the type of scar tissue and creates a bigger path of lysis of scar tissue.
- At present, epiduroscopy is considered an experimental technique by medical insurers and, thus, is not covered under any policy.

COMPLICATIONS

- Any reaction to the medications
- Unintended subdural or subarachnoid injection of local anesthetics or of any of the medications used for this procedure (this is avoidable when the practitioner has enough experience to recognize the fluoroscopic patterns that these injections cause)
- Bowel or bladder dysfunction from damage to neural structures
- Bleeding
- Infection
- Shearing of the catheter

REFERENCES

1. **Racz GB, Noe C, Heavner JE.** Selective spinal injections for lower back pain. *Curr Rev Pain.* 1999;3:333–341.
2. **Andersson GBJ.** Epidemiology of low back pain. *Acta Orthop Scand.* 1998;69:28.
3. **Burn JMB.** Treatment of chronic lumbosciatic pain. *Proc R Soc Med.* 1973;66:544.
4. **Sicard JA, Forestier J.** Méthode radiographique d'exploratione de la cavité épidurale par le lipiodol. *Rev Neurol.* 1921;28:1264.
5. **Payne JN, Rupp NH.** The use of hyaluronidase in caudal block anesthesia. *Anesthesiology.* 1951;2:164.
6. **Moore DC.** The use of hyaluronidase in local and nerve block analgesia other than spinal block: 1520 cases. *Anesthesiology.* 1951;12:611.
7. **Liévre JA, Block-Michel H, Attali P.** L'injection transsacrée, etude clinique et radiologique. *Bull Soc Med Paris.* 1957;73:110.
8. **Goebert HW, Jallo SJ, Gardner WJ, et al.** Sciatica: Treatment with epidural injections on procaine and hydrocortisone. *Cleve Clin Q.* 1960;27:191.
9. **Brown JH.** Pressure caudal anesthesia and back manipulation. *Northw Med.* 1960;59:905.
10. **Hitchcock E.** Hypothermic subarachnoid irrigation for intractable pain. *Lancet.* 1967;1:1133.
11. **Hitchcock E.** Osmolytic neurolysis for intractable facial pain. *Lancet.* 1969;1:434.
12. **Ventafridda V, Spreafico R.** Subarachnoid saline perfusion. *Adv Neurol.* 1974;4:477.
13. **Racz GB, Holubec JT.** Lysis of adhesions in the epidural space. In: Raj P, ed. *Techniques of Neurolysis.* Boston: Kluwer Academic; 1989:57.
14. **Stolker RJ, Vervest ACM, Gerbrand JG.** The management of chronic spinal pain by blockades: A review. *Pain.* 1994;58:1.
15. **Racz GB, Heavner JE, Raj P.** Nonsurgical management of spinal radiculopathy by the use of lysis of adhesions (neuroplasty). In: Aronoff GM, ed. *Evaluation and Treatment of Chronic Pain.* 3rd ed. 1999:533.
16. **Kushlich SD, Ulstrom CL, Michael CJ.** The tissue origin of low back pain and sciatica. *Orthop Clin North Am.* 1991;22:181.
17. **Racz GB, Heavner JE, Diede JH.** Lysis of epidural adhesions utilizing the epidural approach. In: Waldman SD, Winnie AP, eds. *Interventional Pain Management.* Philadelphia: WB Saunders; 1996.
18. **Lou L, Racz GB, Heavner JE.** Percutaneous epidural neuroplasty. In: Waldman SD, Lambert R, eds. *Interventional Pain Management.* 2nd ed. Philadelphia: WB Saunders; 2002.
19. **Lewandowski EM.** The efficacy of solutions used in caudal neuroplasty. *Pain Digest.* 1997;7:323.

Section IX
DISABILITY EVALUATION

69 DISABILITY/IMPAIRMENT

Gerald M. Aronoff, MD

PAIN IMPAIRMENT AND DISABILITY ISSUES

- Chronic pain is a major public health problem that inflicts tremendous personal suffering and, in the United States, has an annual cost exceeding $125 billion.[1]
- Between 1971 and 1981, the number of people with disabling back problems increased 168%, whereas the population increased only 12.5%.[2]
- In the United States and other countries where entitlement programs are viewed as appealing alternatives to gainful employment, individuals with chronic pain and disability frequently experience a complex and unrewarding journey through the health care system.[3]
- Often no direct correlation exists between objective impairment and an individual's request for disability status, and when economic conditions diminish job satisfaction and financial security, a "disability epidemic" can become a major public health problem.
- To reverse the "disability epidemic," our compensation and disability systems must offer incentives toward rehabilitation that encourage early intervention, prevention of chronicity, and timely return to work.[3–5]

PHYSICIAN-RELATED DISABILITY ISSUES

- Compounding this epidemic is the failure of some medical practitioners to distinguish between impairment and disability, as well as confusion about what constitutes maximal medical improvement.
- Clinically, physicians cannot prove the existence of a patient's pain. The "pain behavior" indicating an individual is in pain may be learned through conditioning and be goal-directed.
- Excessive pain behavior may lead to unnecessary diagnostic testing or invasive procedures and result in iatrogenic complications and prolonged disability.[3]
- Recipients of workers' compensation who have significant financial, psychosocial, and/or environmental reinforcement for their disability and little incentive to return to work may exhibit excessive pain behavior and be at increased risk of developing chronic pain syndromes unresponsive to conventional treatment.
- By overestimating impairment and imposing senseless limitations to activity, health care workers can reinforce a disability syndrome. In vulnerable individuals, this is a major factor leading to iatrogenic disability.
- Pain behavior may be modified or replaced by adaptive wellness behavior through behavioral intervention and psychotherapy. Therefore, patients with a chronic pain syndrome may need psychosocial treatment to achieve maximal medical improvement.

IMPAIRMENT AND DISABILITY ASSESSMENT

- Despite the need to adopt a biopsychosocial–economic perspective for evaluation and treatment of chronic pain,[6] disability evaluation systems continue to apply a biomedical perspective.[7]

KEY DEFINITIONS

- A "disability conviction" is the belief that chronic pain impedes the sufferer's ability to meet occupational demands, fulfill domestic and social responsibilities, or engage in avocational and recreational activities. A disability conviction is often based on cognitive distortions and abnormal behavior conditioned by being enmeshed in the health care system.[7]

- "Chronic pain syndrome" describes persistent pain accompanied by dysfunctional pain behavior, self-limitation in activities, and a degree of life disruption disproportional to the pathophysiology. A chronic pain syndrome occurs when pain is a focal point of a patient's life.
- Impairment is "A loss, loss of use, or derangement of any body part, organ system, or organ function."[8]
- Disability is "Alteration of an individual's capacity to meet personal, social, or occupational demands or statutory or regulatory requirements because of impairment. Disability is a relational outcome, contingent on the environmental conditions in which activities are performed."[8]
- Maximal medical improvement (MMI) is "A condition or state that is well stabilized and unlikely to change substantially in the next year, with or without medical treatment. Over time, there may be some change; however, further recovery or deterioration is not anticipated."[8]
- The "chronic disability syndrome," in which individuals who are capable of working choose to remain disabled,[9] often results from a fairly minor injury and actually represents an inability to cope with other problems.

CLINICAL IMPAIRMENT ASSESSMENT

- *The AMA Guides to Impairment and Disability Assessment* offers "a blend of evidence-based medicine and specialty consensus recommendations" for evaluating permanent impairment and is used throughout most of the United States and, increasingly, in other countries.[8]
- Physicians who evaluate patients in a clinical setting become the patients' advocates.
- Physicians evaluating individuals for impairment or disability are *not* patient advocates and should not rate impairment/disability in their own patients.
- Disability evaluators should avoid being overly influenced by subjective complaints, rate impairment on objective findings, and never refer to or consider the evaluee as a "patient."
- Evaluators should emphasize this situation to claimants prior to the assessment and should document this discussion in writing.
- Motivation should be evaluated as a very important link between impairment and disability.[8,10] Attitude, motivation, and support systems are often more

important prognosticators of disability and delayed recovery than are physical findings.

- There is no linear relationship between the degree of medical or psychiatric impairment and a disability rating.[9]
- It is essential to take a detailed medical, developmental, behavioral, and psychosocial history to assess an individual's current and premorbid level of functioning.
- Information about stressors, such as traumatic events, patterns of disability in the patient or other family members, patterns of self-defeating behavior, unmet dependency needs, childhood deprivation, and substance abuse, is important in understanding how the patient became the person being evaluated and prognosis, as well as in making statements about vocational matters and disability.[11]
- It should be determined if there appears to be significant suffering and demonstrable pain behavior.
- How the individual was functioning prior to the incident should be established.

MEASURING AND RATING PAIN

- Despite inherent limitations in self-report measures of pain, they are considered the most reliable tool.[12–14]
- Three useful questions are[15,16]:
  ○ What is the extent of the patient's disease or injury?
  ○ To what extent is the patient suffering, disabled, and unable to enjoy usual activities?
  ○ Is the illness behavior appropriate to the disease or injury or is there evidence of amplification of symptoms for psychologic or social reasons?

USING THE *AMA GUIDES* AND GENERAL ISSUES RELATED TO IMPAIRMENT FROM CHRONIC PAIN

- The *AMA Guides* and other rating systems (Social Security, private insurance companies, Veterans Administration) consider underlying medical (both organic and psychiatric) conditions rather than pain to be the cause of impairment.
- Despite the fact that this traditional biomedical model does not account for the subjective experience of the patient in pain, the *Guides* acknowledges that the reality of subjective experience challenges their system of impairment rating.
- The *Guides* chapter on pain presents an alternative conceptual model for painful conditions not based in mechanical failure and when the conventional rating system is inadequate for assessing the patient's

actual activities of daily living (ADLs) and assumes that:

- ◦ Pain is influenced significantly by psychosocial factors.
- ◦ There is often no direct correlation between pain and mechanical dysfunction.
- ◦ Pain may significantly impact patients' ability to perform ADLs.[7]
- The pain chapter guidelines are meant to evaluate pain-related impairment characterized by:
  - ◦ Excess pain in the context of verifiable conditions that cause pain
  - ◦ Well-established pain syndromes without significant, identifiable organ dysfunction to explain the pain
  - ◦ Associated pain syndromes (neuropathic pain states)[8]
- The pain chapter guidelines should not be applied to rate pain-related impairment in situations when:
  - ◦ Conditions are adequately rated in other chapters of the *Guides*.
  - ◦ Evaluees have low credibility.
  - ◦ The pain syndromes are ambiguous or controversial.[8]
- The guidelines may be used to rate ambiguous or controversial pain syndromes only if:
  - ◦ The symptoms and/or physical findings match a known medical condition.
  - ◦ The individual's presentation is typical of a widely accepted diagnosed condition with a well-defined pathophysiologic basis.
- The pain chapter provides detailed protocols for assessing mild, moderate, moderately severe, and severe pain-related impairments.[8]
- Although the pain chapter emphasizes that some pain may be real but not ratable, the chapter guidelines may frequently be used in a contrary attempt to rate such pain based on conditioned dysfunctional pain behavior, poor coping, and embellished self-reports.
- To make an impairment rating, the pain-related condition must have reached maximal medical improvement and the pain must result in significant diminished capacity to carry out ADLs (does not merely make daily activity painful).
- Individuals with chronic pain should not be considered to have reached maximum medical improvement unless they have:
  - ◦ Been evaluated by physicians knowledgeable about chronic pain
  - ◦ Had a multidisciplinary evaluation
  - ◦ Had an adequate trial of adjuvant analgesics in addition to primary analgesics
- The *AMA Guides* recognizes that emotional factors alter mental health, and rather than being the same as chronic pain, "psychogenic" pain is a psychiatric disorder that should be treated by specialists.

RETURN-TO-WORK ISSUES

- When a directive return-to-work approach is incorporated into the treatment of chronic pain patients receiving workers' compensation, most return to work and continue to work.[17]
- A less successful prognosis for successful return to work is a physician's recommendation for restricted or light duty.[18]
- Patients' physical, emotional, social, and spiritual well-being are more likely to be realized with the self-esteem that results from feeling useful because of gainful employment than with a disability award.[3]
- The probability of return to work is 50% after more than 6 months of disability, 25% after more than 1 year, and extremely unlikely after more than 2 years.[19]
- When chronic pain patients are treated in an interdisciplinary setting that combines treatment principles from physical, behavioral, and rehabilitation medicine using a biopsychosocial approach, return-to-work probability increases to the range of 68% despite prolonged absenteeism.[20]

TREATMENT ISSUES

- The initial noxious stimulus leading to nociception seems to be less important in the management of chronic pain syndromes than the patient's suffering, which reflects emotional distress, and pain behavior.[21] Thus, central factors may be more responsible than peripheral factors for delaying recovery and contributing to disability. Nociception, if present, may not be directly treatable by conventional techniques.
- If pain is intractable, both the health care professional and the patient become increasingly uncertain about the appropriate course of treatment and develop a sense of impotence and frustration that strains their interaction.[3]
- It is essential that treating physicians use established principles of behavioral and rehabilitation medicine to get to know their patients.
- Many who come to us with headaches, myalgias, or nonspecific pain syndromes are actually saying "my life hurts," and, instead of medicalizing their suffering, we should channel them into appropriate treatment.[22]
- Disability is more difficult to treat when it has continued for 6 months or longer. Thus, early recognition of features predicting poor prognosis and prompt intervention is important.

References

1. **Okifuji A, Turk DC, Kalauokalani D.** Clinical outcome and economic evaluation of multidisciplinary pain centers. In: Block A, Kremer E, Fernandez E, eds. *Handbook of Pain Syndromes.* Mahwah, NJ: Lawrence Erlbaum; 1999:77.
2. **Gatchel RJ, Polatin PB, Mayer TG, Garch PD.** Psychopathology and the rehabilitation of patients with chronic low back pain disability. *Arch Phys Med Rehabil.* 1994;75:666.
3. **Aronoff GM.** Chronic pain and the disability epidemic. *Clin J Pain.* 1991;7:330.
4. **Aronoff GM.** The role of the pain center in the treatment of intractable suffering and disability from chronic pain. *Semin Neurol.* 1983;3:377.
5. **Aronoff GM.** The disability epidemic (editorial). *Clin J Pain.* 1986;1:187.
6. **Aronoff GM, Feldman JB.** Preventing iatrogenic disability from chronic pain. *Curr Rev Pain.* 1999;3:67.
7. **Aronoff GM, Feldman JB, Campion T.** Chronic pain: Controlling disability. In: Randolph DC, ed. *Occupational Medicine.* 2000.
8. **Cocchiarella L, Anderson GBJ.** *American Medical Association Guides to the Evaluation of Permanent Impairment.* 5th ed. Chicago: AMA Press; 2000.
9. **Strang JP.** The chronic disability syndrome. In: Aronoff GM, ed. *The Evaluation and Treatment of Chronic Pain.* Baltimore: Urban & Schwarzenberg; 1985.
10. *American Medical Association Guides to the Evaluation of Permanent Impairment.* 4th ed. Chicago: AMA Press; 1993.
11. **Aronoff GM, Livengood J.** Pain: Psychiatric aspects of impairment and disability. *Curr Pain Headache Rep.* 2003;7:105.
12. **Hinnant DW.** Psychological evaluation and testing. In: Tollison CD, ed. *Handbook of Pain Management.* 2nd ed. Baltimore: Williams & Wilkins; 1994:18.
13. **Turk DC, Melzack R, eds.** *Handbook of Pain Assessment.* New York: Guilford Press; 1992:111.
14. **Hebben N.** Toward the assessment of clinical pain in adults. In: Aronoff GM, ed. *Evaluation and Treatment of Chronic Pain.* Baltimore: William & Wilkins; 1992:384.
15. **Turk DC, Rudy TE.** Persistent pain and the injured worker: Integrating biomechanical, psychosocial, and behavioral factors in assessment. *J Occup Rehabil.* 1991;1(2).
16. **Turk DC.** Evaluation of pain and disability. *J Disability.* 1991;2:24.
17. **Catchlove R, Cohen K.** Effects of a directive return to work approach in the treatment of workers' compensation patients with chronic pain. *Pain.* 1982;14:181.
18. **Hall H, McIntosh G, Melles T, et al.** Effect of discharge recommendations on outcome. *Spine.* 1994;19:2033–2037.
19. **Waddell G.** Biopsychosocial analysis of low back pain. *Baillieres Clin Rheumatol.* 1992;6:523.
20. **Flor H, Fydrich T, Turk DC.** Efficacy of multidisciplinary pain treatment centers: A meta-analytic review. *Pain.* 1992;49:221.
21. **Loeser J.** In: Stanton-Hicks M, Boas R, eds. *Chronic Low Back Pain.* New York: Raven Press; 1982:145.
22. **Aronoff GM, Tota-Foucette M, Phillips L, et al.** Are pain disorder and somatization disorder valid diagnostic entities? *Curr Rev Pain.* 2000;4:309.

70 MEDICAL/LEGAL EVALUATIONS

Richard L. Stieg, MD, MHS

INTRODUCTION

- It is impossible to practice pain medicine in 21st-century America and not be involved in medical/legal activity.
- To believe that we can practice in the isolated environment of an office/examination room or outpatient surgery center and avoid legal activity is to invite potential harm to ourselves and our patients.
- *Official* medical/legal evaluations are best conducted by experts, including pain medicine specialists who have developed expertise in this specialized area.
- Paying attention to the legal implications of our medical professional activity on a daily basis may help us avoid significant difficulties that can compromise a physician's time and a patient's care.

INFORMAL MEDICAL/LEGAL ACTIVITIES

MEDICAL RECORDS/REPORTS

- The medical record/report has far-reaching legal implications.
- The importance of careful, comprehensive, and timely recordkeeping of patient interactions cannot be overemphasized.
- The medical record should accurately reflect the time spent with the patient and the physician's thoughts about the evaluation and treatment plan.
- This record is a legal document that may well be scrutinized by fellow health care professionals, patients, payers, attorneys, or other third parties.
- A careful, comprehensive, and thoughtful report reflects positively on the physician and serves that professional well in ongoing treatment planning.
- On the contrary, a sloppy, poorly written report, particularly one that is generated days, weeks, or months after a patient encounter, serves no one well and may announce clearly to all who read it (assuming that it is

legible) that the doctor does not care or practices medicine inadequately.
- The obvious implications for doctor and patient may include:
  - Delayed payment of benefits to patients
  - Delayed payment of medical fees
  - An invitation for peer review of the doctor's practices
  - Increased risk of medical malpractice action
  - Loss of patient referral base
- When writing or dictating a medical report, it may be useful to imagine presenting it to a jury or peer review panel.

REQUESTS FOR MEDICAL RECORDS

- Now, business and regulatory demands on our time, coupled with legal requirements about how patient information may be shared, have changed the nature of cooperation among medical personnel.
- Confusion abounds over the federal HIPAA regulations that supersede many state laws.
- In addition to requests for patient care records, demands may arise for additional information and/or summarizing reports from the physician.
- This is especially true when patients' medical bills are being paid by workers' compensation or personal injury protection insurers.
- Such requests may come from third-party case managers (usually nurses) hired by these companies to help manage claims.
- These requests often appear to be onerous to physicians. Responding to them in a thoughtful and timely manner, however, is generally good business and may be helpful in securing appropriate medical benefits for your patients. Before responding it is wise to:
  - Understand your legal requirements
  - Arrange for appropriate payment of your services (these fees may be fixed by fee schedule)
  - Ascertain that your patient has signed a release to permit you to communicate this information
- My general advice to physicians is to establish a good working rapport with all your patients and have each one sign specific releases so that you can share your records with whomever you feel needs to help with patient care and medical claim management.
- Explain to the patient that you are trying to fulfill what may be competing business/regulatory/legal demands on you and that failure to do so could result in delayed payment to both of you or delayed or denied approval of recommended medical services.
- If the patient refuses, it would be wise to let other parties know why you are not sending records.

- A dilemma exists about what to do when such a scenario results in nonpayment or gross underpayment of fees for services that are not articulated in a contract or fee schedule. It is hoped that future regulatory relief and better business practices will solve such problems.

PRESENCE OF THIRD PARTIES DURING OFFICE VISITS

- Third parties, such as family members, friends, nurse case managers, insurance adjusters, "medical witnesses," and lawyers, may pay unannounced visits to your office during the course of a patient visit.
- You and your patient each have the right to refuse such interventions.
- Make it a point to:
  - Be sure you have the patient's permission for such individuals to be present.
  - Reserve the right to refuse admission to or excuse them from any portion of an interview or examination.
  - Disallow any electronic recording of the visit by patients or third parties.
- When the party present is viewed as an ally or may be important to patient care, you may wish to encourage such visits. Examples are family members who wish to be present or case managers who may be better able than you to secure medical benefits from the insurer for your patient.
- In the case of complex chronic pain patients, you may also try to facilitate case conferences at your office so that all parties playing a role in the patient's life can have a better understanding of the medical issues, including treatment plans.
- The medical/legal ramifications of this type of activity are self-evident.
- A carefully crafted document of such visits should include the names of the persons present and the purpose of their presence.
- Unfortunately, payment for this additional time and effort by pain medicine physicians varies considerably and must sometimes be viewed as a noncompensated, add-on service.

MEDICAL CREDENTIALS AND QUALIFICATIONS

- Many physicians have little or no interest in participating in medical/legal activities, such as being deposed and serving as a medical witness at a trial. They may even have an aversion to such activity. They may find themselves forced into such roles, however, by subpoena or feel morally obligated to participate on behalf of a patient or medical colleague.

- It is wise to document your credentials and qualifications for medical/legal activity to insulate yourself as much as possible from legal attack.

- Although you may be asked to produce new material, such as a clinical summary or an updated curriculum vitae (CV), *never* alter old records or documents. Copies may already be in the hands of legal parties, and altered documents can be personally damaging.

- Maintain an accurate CV that is absolutely factual, truthful, and contains no exaggerations or material omissions. You may be questioned about your CV by professionals who know much more about you than you might imagine (eg, calling yourself a "fellow" or "diplomate" of organizations that offer no such qualifications may be cannon fodder to an attorney seeking to discredit you).

FORMAL MEDICAL/LEGAL EVALUATIONS

- As in any other medical activity, training and/or credentialing for medical/legal evaluations is highly desirable and can be obtained from a number of different resources.[1–5]

- Engaging in medical/legal work, particularly when it involves peer review activity, carries a unique set of ethical standards and problems and is not for the fainthearted.

PEER REVIEW ACTIVITY

- All peer review activity has medical/legal implications. This activity includes participating in medical society ethics committees, credentialing or utilization review committees, and similar services for a variety of health-related institutions/organizations or conducting independent medical examinations or medical file reviews.

- These may require answers to questions about the reasonableness and appropriateness of colleagues' treatment.

- Such activity may be onerous but has long been recognized as acceptable and necessary to organized medicine.

- The American Medical Association advises that individuals engaging in such work "act ethically as long as principles of due process are observed," and that they "balance the physician's right to exercise medical judgment freely with the obligation to do so wisely and temperately."[6(p148)]

- With the advent of managed care, the number of such unclear situations seems to be increasing.

- A colleague issued an opinion (shared by two fellow physicians) during the course of a utilization review that a treating physician should be removed from a case because of unsound medical practice. Despite the fact that the panel members had been assured they were immune from legal attack because their activity was part of a state workers' compensation administrative process dictated by regulation, the treating physician sued the panel members. Although the case was dismissed, my colleague had to pay for her defense.

- There are few guarantees that peer review examiners whose opinions reflect unfavorably on their peers are immune from counterattack.

- Physicians engaging in a peer review, then, should understand the risks they face and determine whether such activity is worth their time.

- Before engaging in a peer review, it would be wise to contact your medical malpractice and professional liability insurance carriers as well as those representing the organizations requesting the review.

- All parties should be informed in writing about the scope of your expected activities and responsibilities.

- Any contracts should be reviewed, preferably by an expert who represents you.

- Do not assume that others have taken precautions for you.

- A little personal risk management could save a lot of time, effort, and even money should you find yourself under attack.

EXPERT TESTIMONY

- Answer questions simply, succinctly, and truthfully. The more unnecessary detail you add, the more likely you are to prolong your time and discomfort in the legal hot seat.

- Always stay within your area of expertise and do not try to overwhelm an examining lawyer or judge.

- Avoid jargon, editorial commentary, or illogical conclusions.

- Your examiner is usually much more informed about medical/legal matters than you are.

- It is better to say, "I don't know," or "that is beyond my area of expertise," than to have someone publicly demonstrate your weaknesses.

- *Come prepared*. Review the documents that are likely to be the foundation for your testimony (including that CV) and think through what you are going to talk about. The lawyer who has summoned you can help you prepare.

- Training as a professional witness is highly desirable and available via literature and training courses offered by professional societies.
- Remember the AMA believes that "as a citizen and as a professional with special training and experience, the physician has an ethical obligation to assist in the administration of justice," and that "medical witnesses should testify honestly and truthfully to the best of their medical knowledge." The medical witness must be nonpartisan and may not "accept compensation that is contingent upon the outcome of litigation."[6(p150)]
- Related ethical issues include: (1) promoting and advertising oneself as a professional medical witness; (2) obligations to speak up about perceived incompetence of fellow physicians; and (3) establishing reasonable fees for medical/legal services.

THE INDEPENDENT MEDICAL EXAMINATION

- The independent medical examination (IME) is a relatively recent phenomenon in the American health care system. Medical professional organizations, such as the American Academy of Disability Evaluating Physicians, offer such services as training, credentialing, and ongoing educational resources for IME physicians.
- Among the problems and challenges facing IME physicians and their clients articulated by a task force of 50 physicians in 1998 under the joint sponsorship of SEAK[1] and the American College of Occupational and Environmental Medicine are:
  - Objectively assessing and evaluating work capacity
  - Addressing malingering and symptom magnification
  - Obtaining needed medical reports in a timely manner
  - Preparing a cost-effective and time-efficient report
- As with any other professional medical activity, it is appropriate and desirable that physicians obtain comprehensive training in this highly specialized area to avoid:
  - Loss of respect from colleagues, clients (patients), and business associates
  - Loss of billable practice time while defending yourself against angry patients, lawyers, or colleagues
  - Increased legal scrutiny of the examiner's practice

CONCLUSION

- We live in a highly litigious society where medical activities are highly regulated. This makes medical/legal activity unavoidable to the practicing physician.
- Many have found medical/legal activities, such as peer review work, IME, and professional witnessing, to be challenging, interesting, and rewarding. Others dread it. The recognition that it is part of everyday practice will serve our patients and us well.
- Our patients also must cope with medical/legal issues, and, whether we are acting as their advocates or as independent reviewers of their care, we can better serve justice and the American health care system by being as familiar as possible with our medical/legal responsibilities.

REFERENCES

1. SEAK Incorporated Legal and Medical Information Systems, www.seak.com.
2. American Academy of Disability Evaluating Physicians, www.aadep.org.
3. American Academy of Pain Medicine, www.painmed.org.
4. American Medical Association, www.ama-assn.org.
5. **Babitsky S, Mangraviti JJ Jr, Todd CJ.** *The Comprehensive Forensic Services Manual: The Essential Resources for all Experts.* Falmouth, Mass: SEAK Incorporated Legal and Medical Information Systems; 2000.
6. American Medical Association. *Code of Medical Ethics: Current Opinions with Annotations 1996–1997.*

INDEX

Page numbers followed by italic *f* or *t* denote figures or tables, respectively.

A

Abdominal aortic aneurysm, 115
Abdominal epilepsy, 117
Abdominal migraine, 116
Abdominal pain
  acute, 113–115, 114*f*, 115*f*, 116*f*, 122
  AIDS-related, 177
  anatomy, 108–109, 109–111*f*
  chronic, 115–118, 117*t*, 118*t*, 122
  classification, 107–108
  differential diagnosis, 113
  from extraabdominal disease, 113,
    113*t*
  in geriatric patients, 115
  imaging, 122
  from intraabdominal disease, 113, 113*t*
  laboratory studies, 122
  patient evaluation, 111–113
  in pediatric patients, 115, 117*f*
  in pregnant women, 230, 230*f*, 231*f*
  treatment, 122–125, 123*f*, 124*f*
Abscess, vs. hematoma, 88*t*
Acetaminophen
  in geriatric patients, 201
  pharmacology, 46
  in pregnancy and lactation, 227
Action potential, 20
Acupuncture
  adverse events, 265
  bee venom, 280–281
  clinical applications, 263–265, 264*f*
  history, 260, 260*f*
  mechanisms, 261–263
  meridians, 260, 261*f*
  for myofascial pain, 206
  National Institutes of Health study, 261,
    262*t*
  points, 261, 261*f*
  Qi, 260, 261*f*
  research, 263
Acute facet syndrome, 329–330, 329*t*
Acute intermittent porphyria, 116
Adenosine, 299–300, 301*t*
Adhesions, in low back pain, 360–361
AIDS-related pain syndromes
  interventional therapies, 178
  multidisciplinary approach, 175
  musculoskeletal, 177
  neuropathic, 176
  treatment barriers, 177–178
  visceral, 177
Alfentanil, 300, 301*t*
Alpha agonists, 213*t*
Alternative medicine. *See* Complementary and
  alternative medicine (CAM)
American Board of Anesthesiology, 1–2, 2*t*

Amphetamines
  as analgesics, 75
  for pediatric patients, 213*t*
Analgesia
  epidural. *See* Epidural analgesia
  interpleural. *See* Interpleural analgesia
  intrathecal. *See* Intrathecal analgesia
  patient-controlled. *See* Patient-controlled
    analgesia (PCA)
Anorectal pain, 159
Antacids, 51*t*
Anthocyanins, 278–279
Antiarrhythmics, 193
Anticoagulants
  for interventional pain therapies, 257–258
  nonsteroidal anti-inflammatory drugs and, 51*t*
Anticonvulsants
  as analgesics, 56–59, 186*t*
  for central pain syndromes, 192–193
  for complex regional pain syndrome, 198
  for depression, 249–250
  for fibromyalgia syndrome, 208
  for headache, 135–136*t*, 138
  for myofascial pain, 206
  for pediatric patients, 213*t*
  in pregnancy and lactation, 229
  tramadol and, 66
Antidepressants
  as analgesics, 52–55
  for central pain syndromes, 193
  dosages, 53*t*
  for headache, 136*t*
  mechanisms of action, 53*t*
  numbers need to treat, 55*t*, 56
  pharmacology, 52–53
  in pregnancy and lactation, 229
  sexual function and, 154
Antidromic, 20
Antihistamines, 74
Antinarcoleptics, 213*t*
Antirheumatics, 51*t*
Anxiety
  assessment, 31
  chronic pain and, 251–253
  exam preparation and, 4
Arm pain. *See* Upper extremity pain
Arteriography, 30
Arthritis. *See also* Osteoarthritis; Rheumatoid
  arthritis
  common conditions, 179*t*
  evaluation, 17–180
  inflammatory vs. noninflammatory, 179*t*,
    180, 180*t*
Aspen, 280
Aspirin, 46–47
Axillary block, 103

B

Back pain. *See* Low back pain
Baclofen
  as analgesic, 75
  for headache, 136*t*
  for spasticity, 238*t*
Beatty maneuver, 333
Behavioral factors, 31–34
Behavioral therapy, 250
Benzodiazepines
  as analgesics, 74, 75
  for pediatric patients, 213*t*
  in pregnancy and lactation, 229
Beta-adrenergic blockers, 136*t*, 138
Bisphosphonates, 186*t*
Black currant, 279
Bone pain, AIDS-related, 177
Bone scintigraphy, 197
Borage seed oil, 279
Botulinum toxin injection
  FDA-approved uses, 267
  for headache, 137*t*, 138, 267–268
  pharmacology, 266
  treatment considerations, 270–271
Brain, ischemic injury of, 189–190, 190*f*
Breastfeeding
  acetaminophen use in, 227
  anticonvulsant use in, 229
  antidepressant use in, 229
  benzodiazepine use in, 229
  caffeine use in, 230
  ergot alkaloid use in, 230
  local anesthetics in, 228
  medication use in, 226, 226*t*
  nonsteroidal anti-inflammatory drug use in,
    227
  opioid use in, 228
Bupivacaine
  for interpleural analgesia, 100–101
  in peripheral nerve blocks, 102
Bupropion, 248
Butorphanol, 137*t*

C

Caffeine
  as analgesic, 75
  in pregnancy and lactation, 230
Calcium channel antagonists
  efficacy, 61–62
  for headache, 136*t*, 138
  intrathecal, 92
  mechanisms of action, 61
Calf pain, 130–131, 131*t*
Cancer pain
  adjuvant analgesics, 186*t*, 187–188
  assessment, 183

breakthrough, 187
  epidemiology, 183
  interventional management, 188–189
  intrathecal analgesia for. *See* Intrathecal
    analgesia
  neurolysis for, 275–276
  nonopioid analgesics for, 184, 186*t*
  opioids for, 184–187, 186*t*
  palliative care, 189
  treatment guidelines, 183–184, 184*f*, 185*f*
Capsaicin, topical, 280
  for arthritis, 41, 41*t*
  dosage and administration, 42
  evidence base, 41*t*
  formulation, 40
  mechanisms of action, 40
  for neuropathic pain, 40–41, 41*t*
  for periocular pain, 41
  for residual limb pain, 42
  side effects, 42
Carbamazepine
  as analgesic, 57, 58*t*
  for headache, 136*t*
  sexual function and, 154
Carpal tunnel syndrome, 24–25, 126
Catastrophizing, 31
Caudal epidural decompressive neuroplasty,
  361–363
Celiac/splanchnic nerve plexus block,
  346–347
Central pain syndromes
  in multiple sclerosis, 190–192, 191*f*
  poststroke, 189–190
  spinal cord, 192, 193*f*
  treatment approach, 191*t*, 192–194
Central poststroke pain (CPSP), 189–190,
  190*f*
Cervical disc herniation
  treatment, 149
Cervical discography, 352
Cervical spine
  imaging, 148
Cervical spondylosis
  treatment, 149
Cervicothoracic/stellate ganglion block,
  345–346
Chemonucleolysis, 355
CHEOPS scale, 211*t*
Children. *See* Pediatric patients
Chinese medicine, traditional, 47
Chronic disability syndrome, 366
Chronic pain syndrome
  acupuncture for, 263–264
  cryoneurolysis for, 283–285
  definition, 366
  epidural analgesia for, 85–86
  substance abuse and, 240–242*t*, 240–244, 242*f*
  treatment algorithm, 123–124, 124*f*
Chronic prostatitis, 156–157
Cingulotomy, 308
Clitoral pain, 158*t*, 164*t*
Clonidine
  epidural analgesia and, 85
  in peripheral nerve blocks, 102*t*
CMAP. *See* Compound muscle action potential
  (CMAP)
Coccydynia, 284
Cognitive behavioral therapy, 250

Complementary and alternative medicine
  (CAM), 277–278, 280–281
  dietary therapy, 278–279
  herbal therapy, 279–280
Complex regional pain syndrome (CRPS)
  clinical manifestations, 196
  diagnosis, 196–197
  electrodiagnostic tests, 25
  epidemiology, 195
  history, 195
  pathophysiology, 195–196
  spinal cord stimulation for, 286
  treatment, 197–199
  upper extremity, 127–128
Compound muscle action potential (CMAP), 20
Compressive neuropathy, 125–126
Computed tomography (CT)
  in acute abdominal pain, 122
  in pain evaluation, 29
Constant-flow-rate pump, 93, 95, 98
Continuous catheters, 105
Coping, 31–32
Cordotomy, 307
Corticosteroids. *See also* Epidural steroid
  injections
  as analgesic, 75
  for complex regional pain syndrome, 198
  intrathecal, 92
  for low back pain, 145
  nonsteroidal anti-inflammatory drugs and, 51*t*
  in pregnancy and lactation, 228–230
Costochondritis, 169–170
COX-2 inhibitors. *See* Cyclooxygenase-2
  (COX-2) inhibitors
CPSP. *See* Central poststroke pain (CPSP)
CPT. *See* Current perception threshold (CPT)
Cranial nerve rhizotomy, 306
Cryoneurolysis
  in chronic pain, 283–285
  histology, 282
  indications, 282–283
  physics, 282
  techniques, 283
Cubital tunnel syndrome, 126
Current perception threshold (CPT), 27–28
Cyclobenzaprine, 238*t*
Cyclooxygenase-2 (COX-2) inhibitors
  in geriatric patients, 201
  for osteoarthritis, 48
  for sickle-cell pain, 235*t*

D

Dantrolene
  as analgesic, 75
  for spasticity, 238*t*
Deafferentation syndrome, 153
Deep brain stimulation, 304
Degenerative disk disease, 325–327. *See also*
  Low back pain
Depression
  assessment, 31
  diagnosis, 245–246
  pain and, 244–245, 245*f*
  patient safety in, 246
  pharmacologic treatment, 246–250, 247*t*
  psychotherapeutic techniques, 250–251
  screening, 245
  therapeutic considerations, 246

Dermatomes, 19*f*
Devil's claw, 280
Diabetic neuropathy
  lidocaine patch 5% for, 38*t*
  topical capsaicin for, 41, 41*t*
Diazepam, 238*t*
Dietary therapy, 278–279
Disability
  assessment, 32, 366–367
  definitions, 365–366
  physician-related issues, 364
  treatment issues, 367
Discography, 30, 350–352, 351*f*
Diuretics, 51*t*
Dopamine-norepinephrine reuptake inhibitors,
  248
Dorsal column stimulation, 194
Dorsal rhizotomy, 305–306
Dorsal root entry zone lesioning, 194, 306
Durkan's test, 126
Dysmenorrhea, 157–158

E

Elastomeric reservoir pumps, 83
Elderly patients. *See* Geriatric patients
Electrodiagnostic tests, 20, 24, 25*t*. *See also*
  Needle electromyography (EMG); Nerve
  conduction studies
Electromyography. *See* Needle
  electromyography (EMG)
EMG. *See* Needle electromyography (EMG)
EMLA. *See* Eutectic mixture of local
  anesthetics (EMLA)
Epidural analgesia
  activation, 86–87
  additives, 85
  advantages, 341
  anatomy, 82, 82*f*, 83*t*
  for chronic pain patients, 85–86
  complications, 87–88, 88*t*, 343
  contraindications, 343
  delivery methods, 83, 341
  drug selection, 341*t*, 342
  equipment, 86
  history, 82
  indications, 341
  infusion rates, 84*t*
  labeling, 83
  local anesthetics, 84
  management, 88
  opioids, 84–85, 85*t*, 341*t*, 342
  patient selection, 342
  for pediatric patients, 215–216, 215*t*
  placement, 86, 87*f*
  risks, 341
  side effects, 84
  standarized orders, 89*f*
Epidural steroid injections
  complications, 293*t*
  drugs for, 290–291
  outcomes, 293–294
  patient selection, 289–290, 289–291, 289*t*
  rationale, 290
  techniques, 291–293
Epiduroscopy, 360, 363
Epinephrine
  epidural analgesia and, 85
  in peripheral nerve blocks, 102*t*

Ergotamine derivatives
  for headache, 136*t*, 138
  in pregnancy and lactation, 230
Esophagus pain, 167*t*, 169
Eutectic mixture of local anesthetics (EMLA)
  dosage and administration, 43
  evidence base, 43*t*
  formulation, 42
  mechanisms of action, 42
  for postherpetic neuralgia, 42, 43*t*
  for postoperative pain, 42–43, 43*t*
  side effects, 43
Evening primrose, 279
Examinations
  preparation, 2–3
  study technique, 3–5
Expert testimony, 370–371
Extraabdominal disease, 113, 113*t*

F
Fabere sign, 129, 337
FACES scale, 212*f*
Facet joint blocks, 295–296, 296*f*
Facial pain. *See* Orofacial pain
Fade test, 338
Familial Mediterranean fever, 117
Fear, assessment, 31
Fear-avoidance behavior, assessment, 32
Fentanyl
  for cancer pain, 186–187, 187*t*
  in geriatric patients, 202
Fibrillation potential, 20
Fibromyalgia syndrome
  clinical features and presentation, 207, 330
  diagnosis, 207–208, 208*t*
  electrodiagnostic tests, 25
  rehabilitation, 330
  tender point sites, 208*t*
  treatment, 208–209, 330
Fibrositis. *See* Fibromyalgia syndrome
Flecainide, 61
Fortin's finger test, 337
Fothergill's sign, 112
Freiberg's sign, 333
Functional dyspepsia, 118
Functional Pain Scale, 200*f*

G
Gabapentin
  as analgesic, 57, 58*t*
  for depression, 249–250
  for headache, 136*t*
Gaenslen's test, 337
Gamma knife radial surgery, 194
Ganglion impar blockade, 163–164, 348
Ganglionectomy, 305–306
Generalized anxiety disorder, 252
Geriatric patients
  abdominal pain in, 115
  adjuvant analgesics for, 203
  adverse drug reactions, 202–203
  nonopioids for, 201
  nonpharmacologic interventions, 200
  opioids for, 201–202
  pain assessment, 200–201, 200*f*
  pain vulnerability, 200
Gillet's test, 338
Ginseng, 279

Glossopharyngeal neuralgia, 152
Glucosamine, 280
Goldenrod, 280
Gout, 181*t*
Granuloma, 97
Growth hormone, 208

H
Headache
  AIDS-related, 176
  chronic daily, 133, 268
  cluster, 133–134, 133*t*, 138, 138*t*, 268
  diagnostic testing, 139, 139*t*
  epidemiology, 131
  hospitalization for, 139–140
  migraine. *See* Migraine headache
  opioids for, 140
  primary, 132
  rebound, 133
  secondary, 132
  tension-type, 132–133, 268
  treatment, 134–138, 135–137*t*
Health care providers, biases, 35
Heart pain, 167*t*, 168–169, 168*f*
Hematoma, vs. abscess, 88*t*
Herbal therapy, 279–280
Hip apprehension test, 129
Hip pain
  diagnosis, 129, 129*t*
  in pregnant women, 230–231
HIV-associated neuropathy, 38*t*, 39, 41, 41*t*
Hydromorphone, 186
Hypophysectomy, 308

I
Imaging, 28
Impairment, 366–367
Independent medical examination, 371
Infants. *See* Pediatric patients
Infraclavicular block, 103
Innervation
  gastrointestinal, 119*f*
  lower extremities, 19*t*
  upper extremities, 19*t*
Insertional activity, 20
Interpersonal psychotherapy, 250
Interpleural analgesia
  anatomy, 99–100, 100*f*
  complications, 101, 101*t*
  contraindications, 99
  indications, 99, 99*t*
  technique, 100–101
Interscalene block, 103
Interventional pain therapies. *See also* specific procedures
  complications, 258–259
  fluoroscopic guidance, 256–257
  indications, 255
  medications, 257–258
  monitoring, 257
  risk management, 258–259
  sedation for, 256
  sterile technique, 256
Intraabdominal disease, 113, 113*t*
Intracranial stimulation, 304
Intradiscal electrothermal annuloplasty, 352–353, 353*f*, 356

Intrathecal analgesia
  advantages, 341
  algorithm, 91*f*
  catheter placement, 95, 95*f*
  for central pain syndromes, 194
  for chronic pain, 304–305
  complications, 96–98, 343
  contraindications, 343
  delivery systems, 93, 341
  drug selection, 91–92, 341*t*, 342
  effects, 92–93
  implant procedure, 95–96
  indications, 341
  outcomes, 93
  patient selection, 94–95, 342
  risks, 341
  screening techniques, 94–95
  for spasticity, 238–239
Intravenous infusion therapy
  adenosine, 299–300, 301*t*
  alfentanil, 300, 301*t*
  ketamine, 297–298, 301*t*
  lidocaine, 296–297, 297*t*, 301*t*
  magnesium, 299, 301*t*
  pamidronate, 300, 301*t*
  phentolamine, 298–299, 298*t*, 301*t*

K
Kava kava, 279–280
Ketamine, 297–298, 301*t*
Knee pain, 129–130, 130*t*. *See also* Musculoskeletal pain; Osteoarthritis

L
Lamotrigine
  as analgesic, 57, 58*t*, 59
  for depression, 250
  efficacy, 61
Laparoscopic presacral neurectomy (LSPN), 158–159
Laparoscopic uterosacral nerve ablation (LUNA), 158
Laségue's sign, 333
Leg pain, 130–131, 131*t*. *See also* Musculoskeletal pain
Legal/medical evaluations, 368–371
Levator ani syndrome, 159
Levetiracetam, 58*t*
Levobupivacaine, 102
Lidocaine
  intravenous, 60*t*, 296–297, 297*t*, 301*t*
  in peripheral nerve blocks, 102
Lidocaine patch 5%
  dosage and administration, 40
  evidence base, 38*t*
  formulation, 37
  for low back pain, 39
  mechanism of action, 37–38
  for myofascial pain, 39
  for neuropathic pain, 38–39
  for osteoarthritis, 39
  side effects, 39–40
Lithium, 136*t*
Local anesthetics
  epidural, 84
  for pediatric patients, 214, 215*t*, 216*t*
  in pregnancy and lactation, 228

Low back pain
  acupuncture for, 264, 264f
  acute facet syndrome, 329–330, 329t
  assessment, 325
  botulinum toxin injection for, 270
  degenerative disk disease, 325–327
  differential diagnosis, 142t, 326t
  discography for, 350–352
  epidemiology, 141
  epidural steroid injections for, 290–291
  facet joint blocks for, 295–296
  imaging, 143–144, 144t
  intradiscal electrothermal annuloplasty for, 352–353, 353f
  lidocaine patch 5% for, 38t, 39
  lumbar disc protrusion, 327–328
  lumbosacral sprain, 327
  neuraxial drug infusion for, 304–305
  nucleoplasty for, 356–359
  pathophysiology, 141–142
  patient history, 142–143, 142t
  physical examination, 143, 143t
  physiology, 355
  in pregnant women, 231–233, 231f
  radiofrequency ablation for, 314
  rehabilitation, 325–330
  risk factors, 141
  spinal cord stimulation for, 286
  spinal stenosis, 328
  spondylolisthesis, 328–329
  tension myalgia, 330
  treatment, 144–146
Lower extremity pain
  hip, 129, 129t
  innervation, 19t
  knee, 129–130
  leg, 130–131, 131t
  peripheral nerve block, 104, 104t
  sacroiliac joint, 128–129
LSPN. See Laparoscopic presacral neurectomy (LSPN)
Lumbar disc protrusion, 327–328. See also Low back pain
Lumbar discography, 351, 351f
Lumbar plexus block, 104
Lumbar sympathetic block, 162, 347
Lumbosacral sprain, 327. See also Low back pain
LUNA. See Laparoscopic uterosacral nerve ablation (LUNA)
Lungs, visceral pain, 167–168, 167t
Lysis of adhesions, 360–363

M
Magnesium, 299, 301t
Magnetic resonance imaging (MRI)
  for low back pain, 144, 144t
  in pain evaluation, 29
MAOIs. See Monoamine oxidase inhibitors (MAOIs)
Marijuana, 280
Massage, 281
Maximal medical improvement, 366
Mechanical sensation testing, 26–27, 26t
Medial branch blocks, 295, 296f
Medical records/reports, 368–369
Medical/legal evaluations, 368–371
Melatonin, 137t
Mepivacaine, 102

Mesencephalotomy, 307–308
Methadone, 187
Methocarbamol, 238t
Mexiletine, 60–61
Migraine headache
  botulinum toxin injection for, 267–268
  pathophysiology, 132
  pharmacologic treatment, 134, 135–137t, 137–138
  in pregnant women, 233
  subtypes, 132
  symptoms, 132
  vs. cluster headache, 133t
Mirtazapine, 249
Modified Ashworth scale, 238t
Monoamine oxidase inhibitors (MAOIs)
  for depression, 249
  for headache, 138
Mood assessment, 31
Morphine. See also Opioids
  for cancer pain, 186
  for intrathecal analgesia, 91
Motor cortex stimulation, 304
Motor unit, 20
Motor unit action potential (MUAP), 20
Moxibustion, 260, 260f
MRI. See Magnetic resonance imaging (MRI)
MUAP. See Motor unit action potential (MUAP)
Multiple sclerosis pain, 190–192, 191f
Murphy's sign, 112
Muscle relaxants, 75–76
Muscle testing, 17
Musculoskeletal pain. See also specific anatomic regions
  AIDS-related, 177
  botulinum toxin injection for, 269–270
  in pregnant women, 230–233, 230f, 231f
Myelography, 29–30
Myelotomy, 307
Myofascial pain
  clinical features and presentation, 204–205
  diagnosis, 205
  electrodiagnostic tests, 25
  lidocaine patch 5% for, 38t, 39
  orofacial, 152
  pelvic, 159
  thoracic, 171–172
  treatment, 205–207, 205t
  trigger points, 172, 205–206, 205t
Myrobalan, 279

N
NCV. See Nerve conduction velocity (NCV)
Neck pain
  acceleration/deceleration injury, 150
  botulinum toxin injection for, 269–270
  diagnosis, 147–148
  facet joint blocks for, 295–296
  natural history, 147
  treatment, 148–150, 149t
Needle electromyography (EMG)
  analysis, 24, 25t
  contraindications, 23
  indications, 23
  principles, 23, 23f
  spontaneous activity, 23–24, 24f
Nefazodone, 249

Nerve conduction studies
  contraindications, 21
  F wave, 22
  H reflex, 22, 22f
  indications, 21
  limitations, 22
  motor, 21, 21f
  principles, 21
  repetitive nerve stimulation, 22–23
  sensory, 21, 22f
  types, 21–22
Nerve conduction velocity (NCV), 20
Nerve root impingement, 143t
Neuraxial drug infusion. See Intrathecal analgesia
Neurectomy, 305
Neuritis, 153
Neuroablation. See Neurolysis; Neurosurgical techniques
Neurogenic pain
  residual limb. See Postamputation pain syndrome
  thoracic, 172
Neurolysis, 272–273. See also Cryoneurolysis
  advantages, 274
  for cancer pain, 275–276
  indications, 275–276
  life expectancy factors, 275
  modalities, 273
  risks and limitations, 273–274
  specific procedures, 276–277
  vs. local anesthesia, 274
  vs. regional analgesia, 274
  vs. systemic pharmacotherapy, 274
Neuromas, 153, 284
Neuromodulation, 199
Neuropathic pain
  abdominal, 107
  adjuvant analgesics for, 187–188
  AIDS-related, 175
  anticonvulsants for, 56–59, 58t
  botulinum toxin injection for, 270
  electrodiagnostic tests, 25
  lidocaine patch 5% for, 38–39, 38t
  physiology, 9–12
  topical capsaicin for, 40–41, 41t
Neuropathy
  compressive. See Compressive neuropathy
  diabetic. See Diabetic neuropathy
  HIV-associated. See HIV-associated neuropathy
  peripheral. See Peripheral neuropathy
Neurosurgical techniques, 302–303, 302t
  ablative, 305–308
  anatomic, 303
  neuraxial drug infusion, 304–305
  patient selection, 301–302
  peripheral, 305–306
  stimulation, 303–304
  supraspinal cranial, 307–308
Nimodipine, 62
NMDA receptor antagonists
  as analgesics, 75–76
  for central pain syndromes, 194
  for visceral pain, 120
Nociceptive pain
  pharmacology, 8–9
  physiology, 7–9

Nonsteroidal anti-inflammatory drugs
(NSAIDs)
  adverse effects, 49–51
  dosage, 47*t*
  drug interactions, 51*t*
  in geriatric patients, 201
  half-lives, 47*t*
  for headache, 135*t*
  for low back pain, 145
  for myofascial pain, 206
  pediatric doses, 50*t*
  for pediatric patients, 212, 212*t*
  pharmacology, 47–48
  in pregnancy and lactation, 227
  structure, 48, 49*t*
  surgical stress response and, 51
  topical, 44
  toxicity scores, 49*t*
Norepinephrine-serotonin modulator, 249
NSAIDs. *See* Nonsteroidal anti-inflammatory
  drugs (NSAIDs)
Nucleoplasty, 356–359, 356–359*f*

O
Obsessive-compulsive disorder, 252
Odontalgia, atypical, 153
Omega-3 fatty acids, 278
One-legged stork test, 338
Opioids
  for cancer pain, 186
  for central pain syndromes, 193–194
  for complex regional pain syndrome, 198
  conversion table, 188*t*
  in epidural analgesia, 84–85
  for geriatric patients, 201–202
  for headache, 140
  intrathecal, 91–93
  for low back pain, 145
  mechanisms in humans, 73
  for myofascial pain, 206
  in patient-controlled analgesia, 78*t*
  for pediatric patients, 212–213, 217*t*
  peripheral action, 72, 72*f*
  in peripheral nerve blocks, 102*t*
  pharmacology, 67–69, 68*t*
  in pregnancy and lactation, 228
  receptors, 68–69, 68*t*
  rotation, 187
  sexual function and, 154
  for sickle cell pain, 236*t*
  side effects, 187
  sites of action, 69
  spinal action, 71, 71*f*
  supraspinal action, 70–71, 70*f*, 71*f*
Oral hypoglycemic agents, 51*t*
Orchialgia, 157*t*, 164*t*
Orofacial pain, 41, 151–153
  AIDS-related, 177
  cryoneurolysis for, 284–285
Orthodromic, 20
Osteoarthritis
  acetaminophen for, 48
  chronic inflammatory, 181, 181*t*
  evaluation, 180
  lidocaine patch 5% for, 38*t*, 39
  topical capsaicin for, 41, 41*t*
  treatment, 181
Oxcarbazepine, 58*t*

Oxycodone, 186. *See also* Opioids
Oxygen inhalation, 136*t*

P
Pace's maneuver, 333
Pain
  gate control theory, 285–286
  neuropathic. *See* Neuropathic pain
  nociceptive. *See* Nociceptive pain
  psychiatric comorbidities, 244
Pain fibers, afferent, 7–8
Pain medicine
  expert testimony, 370–371
  medical credentials, 369–370
  medical records/reports, 368–369
  peer review activity, 370
  subspecialty certification examination, 1–5,
  2*t*
  third parties during office visits, 369
Pain scales, 16–17, 17*f*
Palliative medicine, 265–265
Pamidronate, 300, 301*t*
Panic disorders, 251
Parietal pain, abdominal, 107
Paroxysmal neuralgia, 152
Patient history, 15–16, 31–34
Patient-controlled analgesia (PCA)
  advantages, 77
  contraindications, 78
  disadvantages, 77–78
  discontinuation, 80–81
  indications, 78
  intravenous opioid, 78–80, 78*t*
  patient education, 80*t*
  for pediatric patients, 214, 216*t*
  rationale, 77
  side effect management, 80*t*
  subcutaneous opioid, 81
Patient-provider interactions, 34–35
Patrick's test, 129, 337
PCA. *See* Patient-controlled analgesia (PCA)
Pediatric patients
  abdominal pain in, 115, 117*f*
  adjuvant agents for, 213, 213*t*
  local anesthetics for, 215*t*, 216*t*
  multidisciplinary approach, 210–211
  nonsteroid anti-inflammatory drugs for, 212,
  212*t*
  opioids for, 212–213, 217*t*
  pain assessment, 211–212, 211*t*, 212*f*
  pain factors, 211
  patient-controlled analgesia for, 214, 216*t*
  undertreatment of pain in, 210
Peer review, 370
Pelvic examination, 113
Pelvic joint dysfunctions, 160
Pelvic pain
  cryoneurolysis for, 284
  differential diagnosis, 161
  in females, 157–159, 158*t*, 159*t*
  interventional blocks, 161–165
  in males, 156–157, 157*t*, 159*t*
  malignant causes, 161
  neuroanatomy, 154–155
  nonmalignant causes, 155–156, 155*t*, 156*t*
  in pregnant women, 231
Penile pain, 157*t*, 164*t*
Percutaneous disc compression, 355–356

Percutaneous electrical nerve stimulation
  (PENS), 264, 264*f*
Perimedullar block, 164
Perineal pain, 164*t*, 284
Peripheral nerve blocks
  agents, 102*t*
  benefits and risks, 102
  continuous catheters, 105
  lower extremity, 104, 104*t*
  methods, 102–103
  by neurolysis, 276–277
  for pelvic pain, 165
  upper extremity, 103, 103*t*
Peripheral nerve stimulation
  indications, 316
  outcome studies, 317–318
  patient evaluation, 315–316
  technique, 316–317, 317*f*
  theory, 315
  vs. spinal cord stimulation, 316
Peripheral nerves, 19*f*
Peripheral neuropathy
  AIDS-related, 176
  clinical features, 219
  diagnosis, 219
  epidemiology, 218
  pathophysiology, 218–219
  treatment, 219–220
Peristaltic pumps, 83
Phalen's test, 126
Phase, 20
Phenoziathines, 74
Phentolamine, 298–299, 298*t*, 301*t*
Phenytoin, 51*t*
Phobic disorders, 251–252
Physical examination, 17–19, 18*t*, 19*f*, 19*t*,
  112–113
Physical therapy
  for complex regional pain syndrome, 197–198
  for fibromyalgia syndrome, 208
Phytodolor, 280
Piriformis syndrome
  anatomy, 332, 332*f*
  botulinum toxin injection for, 270, 335
  diagnosis, 333, 335*f*
  history, 331
  pathogenesis, 333
  rehabilitation exercises, 334*t*
  treatment, 334–335, 334*t*, 335*f*
Plain radiography
  in complex regional pain syndrome, 197
  in pain evaluation, 28–29
Polyradiculopathy, AIDS-related, 176
Positive sharp wave, 20
Postamputation pain syndrome
  characteristics, 221
  incidence, 221, 221*t*
  prevention, 222
  risk factors, 222
  spinal cord stimulation for, 286
  topical capsaicin for, 42
  treatment, 222
Post-breast surgery pain, 172
Postcholecystectomy chronic pain, 223–224
Postherpetic neuralgia
  eutectic mixture of local anesthetics for, 42, 43*t*
  lidocaine patch 5% for, 38–39, 38*t*
  topical capsaicin for, 40

Postinguinal hernia pain syndrome, 224, 283

Postmastectomy pain syndrome
characteristics, 223
incidence, 223
risk factors, 223
topical capsaicin for, 41, 41*t*, 223

Poststernotomy pain syndrome, 224

Postsurgical pain syndrome
criteria, 220
eutectic mixture of local anesthetics for, 42–43, 43*t*

Postsympathectomy pain syndrome, 224, 348

Postthoracotomy pain syndrome, 171
characteristics, 222
cryoneurolysis for, 283
incidence, 222, 222*t*
prevention, 223
risk factors, 223
treatment, 223

Posttraumatic stress disorder, 252

Postvasectomy pain syndrome, 225

Pregnancy
abdominal pain in, 230, 230*f*, 231*f*
acetaminophen use in, 227
anticonvulsant use in, 229
antidepressant use in, 229
benzodiazepine use in, 229
caffeine use in, 230
corticosteroid use in, 228–229
ergot alkaloid use in, 230
hip pain in, 230–231
local anesthetics in, 228
low back pain in, 231–233, 231*f*
medication use in, 226, 226*t*
migraine headache in, 233
musculoskeletal pain in, 230–231*f*, 230–233
neurodiagnostic imaging in, 232*t*
nonsteroidal anti-inflammatory drug use in, 227
opioid use in, 228
pelvic pain in, 231

Probenecid, 51*t*

Procaine, 61

Proctalgia fugax, 159

Programmable pump, 93, 95–96, 98

Prolotherapy. *See* Regenerative injection therapy (RIT)

Prostadynia, 157*t*, 164*t*

Prostatitis, 157*t*, 164*t*

Psoriatic arthritis, 181*t*

Psychodynamic psychotherapy, 250–251

Psychological evaluation, 31–34

Psychosocial history, 16, 33–34

Psychotherapeutic techniques
for anxiety disorders, 253
for depression, 250–251

Pudendal nerve block, 165

Pudendal nerve entrapment, 160–161

Pumps
for epidural analgesia, 83
for intrathecal analgesia, 93, 97–98

Q

Quinine sulfate, 75–76

R

Radiculopathy
electrodiagnostic tests, 25
epidural steroid injections for, 289–290
symptoms, 289*t*

Radiofrequency ablation
advantages, 310–311
complications, 311
equipment, 310
future developments, 314–315
for head and neck pain, 311–312
history, 309
indications, 311
for neuropathic pain, 314
principles, 309–310
pulsed, 314
for spine pain, 312–314

Radionuclide scanning, 30

Raw vegetarian diet, 278

Raynaud's phenomenon, 127

Recruitment, 20

Reflex sympathetic dystrophy. *See* Complex regional pain syndrome (CRPS)

Regenerative injection therapy (RIT)
anatomy, 318–319, 322*f*, 323*f*
contraindications, 320–321
indications, 320
mechanisms of action, 319–320
pathophysiology, 319
solutions used, 321
technical considerations, 321–324, 322*f*, 323*f*

Rehabilitation
in low back pain, 325–330
in piriformis syndrome, 334, 334*t*

Residual limb pain, neurogenic. *See* Postamputation pain syndrome

Rheumatoid arthritis, 182, 182*t*

Rheumatologic conditions, 179*t*

RIT. *See* Regenerative injection therapy (RIT)

Ropivacaine, 102

S

Sacroiliac joint pain, 160
anatomy, 336–337
clinical presentation, 337
diagnosis, 128–129, 337–339
treatment, 339–340, 340*f*

Sciatic nerve block, 104

Sclerotherapy. *See* Regenerative injection therapy (RIT)

Secondary gain, 34

Selective serotonin reuptake inhibitors (SSRIs)
as analgesics, 54, 186*t*, 248
for depression, 248
dosages, 53*t*
for headache, 138
mechanisms of action, 53*t*
side effects, 248
tramadol and, 66

Sensory nerve action potential (SNAP), 20

Sensory testing
current perception threshold (CPT), 27–28
mechanical, 26–27, 26*t*
quantitative, 26–28
thermal, 26*t*, 27

Serotonin modulators, 249

Serotonin-norepinephrine reuptake inhibitors, 248–249

Shoulder pain. *See* Upper extremity pain

Sickle cell anemia
causes of death, 235*t*
clinical manifestations, 234–235
pain management, 235–236, 235–236*t*
vaso-occlusive crises, 234–236, 234*t*

Sinemet, 238*t*

Sleep disturbance
assessment, 32–33
in fibromyalgia syndrome, 209

SNAP. *See* Sensory nerve action potential (SNAP)

Sodium bicarbonate, 102*t*

Sodium channel antagonists
efficacy, 60–61
mechanisms of action, 59–60
side effects, 60*t*

Soy, 278

Spasticity
differential diagnosis, 237
evaluation, 237
history, 237
muscle groups involved, 239*t*
quantification, 237, 238*t*
treatment, 238–239, 238*t*

Sphenopalatine ganglion block, 344

Spinal anatomy, 82*f*, 83*t*

Spinal cord
lesions, 192, 193*f*
sensory cells, 8–9
syringomyelia, 192
traumatic ischemic injury, 192

Spinal cord stimulation
implantable devices, 287, 287*f*
indications, 303
mechanism of action, 285–286
outcomes, 288, 303
patient selection, 286
system design, 286
trial protocols, 287–288
vs. peripheral nerve stimulation, 316

Spinal drug delivery. *See* Epidural analgesia; Intrathecal analgesia

Spinal stenosis, 328. *See also* Low back pain

Spondyloarthropathy, 181*t*

Spondylolisthesis, 328–329. *See also* Low back pain

Spontaneous activity, 20

SSRIs. *See* Selective serotonin reuptake inhibitors (SSRIs)

St. John's wort, 279

Stimulants, 186*t*

Stinchfield test, 129

Stress, exam preparation and, 4

Study techniques, 3–4

Substance abuse
assessment, 241–242, 242*t*
behaviors, 241*t*
in chronic pain patients, 240, 240*t*
optimizing drug therapy in, 242–243, 242*f*
psychiatric complications, 240–241

Sucrose, 279

Sudomotor testing, 197

Superior hypogastric plexus block, 162–163, 347–348

Supraclavicular block, 103

Surgical scars, 172

Sympathectomy, 305

Sympathetic dystrophy, 171
Sympathetic nerve blocks
    celiac/splanchnic nerve plexus, 346–347
    cervicothoracic/stellate, 345–346
    in complex regional pain syndrome, 197,
        198–199
    ganglion impar, 163–164, 348
    indications, 344
    lumbar sympathetic, 162, 347
    by neurolysis, 277
    sphenopalatine ganglion, 344
    superior hypogastric plexus, 162–163, 347–348
Symphysis pubis, 160
Syringe pumps, 83
Systemic lupus erythematosus, 181*t*

T
TCAs. *See* Tricyclic antidepressants (TCAs)
Temporomandibular disorders, 269
TENS. *See* Transcutaneous electrical nerve
    stimulation (TENS)
Tension myalgia. *See* Fibromyalgia syndrome
Tetracyclic antidepressants, 247
Thalamotomy, 308
Thermal sensation testing, 26*t*, 27
Thermography, 197
Thigh thrust test, 338
Thoracic pain
    musculoskeletal, 169–170, 170*f*
    myofascial, 171–172
    postoperative, 172
    visceral, 167–169, 167*t*, 168*f*
Thyroid supplementation, 208
Tiagabine, 58*t*
Tietze's syndrome, 169, 170*f*
Tinel's test, 126
Tissue injury, 7
Tizanidine
    as analgesic, 75–76
    for headache, 136*t*
    for myofascial pain, 206
    for spasticity, 238*t*
Topical analgesics. *See also* specific agents
    for complex regional pain syndrome, 198
    rationale, 37

Topical capsaicin. *See* Capsaicin, topical
Topiramate
    as analgesic, 58*t*
    for headache, 136*t*
Trachea, visceral pain, 167–168, 167*t*
Tramadol
    benefits, 66
    dosage and administration, 64
    drug-drug interactions, 66
    indications, 64–66
    mechanisms of action, 63
    pharmacology, 63–64
    side effects, 64–65
    titration schedule, 65–66, 65*t*
Transcutaneous electrical nerve stimulation
    (TENS)
    for central pain syndromes, 194
    definition, 349
    efficacy, 349
    mechanism and indications, 281, 349
    procedure, 349
Trazodone, 249
Tricyclic antidepressants (TCAs)
    as analgesics, 54, 186*t*
    for complex regional pain syndrome, 198
    for depression, 247
    dosages, 53*t*
    for fibromyalgia syndrome, 208
    in geriatric patients, 201
    for headache, 136*t*, 138
    mechanisms of action, 53*t*
    side effects, 247
Trigeminal neuralgia, 152, 311–312
Trigger point needling, 205–206, 205*t*
Triptans, 135*t*, 137*t*

U
Ultrasonography, 122
Upper extremity pain
    complex regional pain syndrome, 127–128
    compressive neuropathy, 125–126
    innervation, 19*t*
    peripheral nerve block for, 103, 103*t*
    posttrauma, 127
    vasculopathy, 127

Urethral syndrome, 159*t*, 164*t*
Urine toxicology screening, 243
Urogenital pain, 156–159, 157–159*t*,
    164*t*

V
Valproic acid
    as analgesic, 58*t*
    for headache, 136*t*
Vaso-occlusive crises, 234–236, 234*t*
Venlafaxine
    as analgesic, 54–55
    for depression, 248–249
Verapamil, 62
Visceral pain
    AIDS-related, 176
    biochemistry, 120
    central sensitization, 120–121
    characteristics, 107
    mediators, 121–122
    neurophysiology, 118–119, 119*f*, 120*f*
    peripheral sensitization, 121, 121*f*
    transmission, 119–120
Visual analog scale, 17*f*
Vocational history, 16
Von Frey hairs, 26–27
Vulvar hyperesthesia, 158*t*, 164*t*
Vulvodynia, 158*t*, 164*t*

W
Wartenberg's sign, 126
Weight loss, 278
Willow bark extract, 280
Work-related issues, 33
World Health Organization
    analgesic ladder for cancer pain, 184*f*
    pain management guidelines, 123, 123*f*

Y
Yin-Yang, 260, 260*f*
Yoga, 281

Z
Ziconotide, 61–62
Zonisamide, 58*t*